ATLAS OF CLINICAL GROSS ANATOMY

ATLAS OF CLINICAL GROSS ANATOMY

Kenneth P. Moses MD
Staff Physician
Southern Inyo Hospital
Southern Inyo Healthcare District
Lone Pine, California, USA
Assistant Professor of Anatomy
Department of Pathology and Human Anatomy
Loma Linda University School of Medicine
Loma Linda, California, USA

John C. Banks Jr. PhD
Professor of Anatomy and Physical Therapy
Department of Physical Therapy
Andrews University
Berrien Springs, Michigan, USA

Pedro B. Nava PhD
Professor of Anatomy and Co-Chair
Department of Pathology and Human Anatomy
Loma Linda University School of Medicine
Loma Linda, California, USA

Darrell Petersen
Instructor
Department of Pathology and Human Anatomy
Biomedical Photographer
Loma Linda University School of Medicine
Loma Linda, California, USA

**Prosections of the Head, Neck, and Trunk
prepared by Martein Moningka**
Division of Anatomy
Loma Linda University School of Medicine
Loma Linda, California, USA

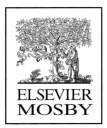

ELSEVIER
MOSBY

ELSEVIER
MOSBY

An imprint of Elsevier Ltd.

Publishers:	Inta Ozols, Richard Furn
Project Development Managers:	Duncan Fraser, Alison Whitehouse
Production Managers:	Colin Arthur, John Richardson
Design Management:	Jayne Jones, Andy Chapman
Illustration Manager:	Mick Ruddy
Illustrations:	Paul Banville and Mandy Miller
Dissection color overlays:	Gus Gomes, Bruce Hogarth
Cover Design:	Andy Chapman
Cover Illustration:	Paul Banville
Copyeditors:	Eleanor Flood, Lindy van den Berghe
Proofreaders:	Christian Simpson, Andrew Johnston
Index:	Jill Halliday, Liza Furnival

First published 2005

ISBN 0323037445

British Library Cataloguing in Publication Data
A catalogue record for this book is available from the British Library

Library of Congress Cataloging in Publication Data
A catalog record for this book is available from the Library of Congress

Printed in Spain

Notice
No responsibility is assumed by the Publishers, Editors or Contributors for any loss or injury and/or damage to persons or property arising out of or related to any use of the material contained in this book. It is the responsibility of the treating practitioner, relying upon independent expertise and knowledge of the patient, to determine the best treatment and method of application for the patient.

The Publisher

Last digit is the print number: 10 9 8 7 6 5 4 3 2 1

Working together to grow
libraries in developing countries

www.elsevier.com | www.bookaid.org | www.sabre.org

ELSEVIER   BOOK AID International   Sabre Foundation

The publisher's policy is to use **paper manufactured from sustainable forests**

ABOUT THIS BOOK

A solid foundation in anatomy is essential to everyone entering the health sciences. However, more and more health science programs are reducing the amount of time being devoted to the teaching of anatomy. As one-time students and teachers of anatomy, we have therefore long felt that there is a need for a new atlas of human anatomy.

Leading atlases today present the human body either through idealized colored drawings or by using a rich mixture of dissection photographs. Although these atlases have been well received and have many strengths, we believe that our new atlas built on the following key features is unique and will offer something particularly useful for students:

1 **Large, single-page macroscopic photographs** of cleanly dissected cadaveric material, presented from the surface and down through the superficial and deeper layers, to the skeleton. This is how readers encounter anatomy in the dissection laboratory and is, we feel, truer to life than reliance on the use of idealized drawings, particularly where access to cadaveric material is reduced.
2 **Deliberately concise text** to accompany each set of dissection photos and radiological images. This is not intended to be a textbook in disguise, and the aim of the text, illustrated with simple supporting diagrams, is to prepare readers for the detailed photographs to come. Brief clinical correlations also put the anatomy directly into the context of common clinical presentations.
3 **Consistent organization within each chapter:** orientation text, then surface anatomy, followed by superficial to deep dissections, and finally radiological imaging. This consistent format and order will improve readers' self-directed learning – increasingly important at a time when the time given over to the direct teaching of anatomy is under pressure.

We created our team – a clinician, two professors of anatomy, and a medical photographer – with these aims in mind. We also brought in the considerable dissection skills of Martein Moningka, a prosector in the Loma Linda Department of Pathology and Human Anatomy, to add to our own.

PHOTOGRAPHS
Within each chapter, the anatomy photographs are presented in the same consistent way:

- Surface topography photographs, with 'ghosting', show major palpable features and prominent bony landmarks.
- Full-page dissection photographs progress from the superficial layers through to the deeper layers. In selected dissections important vessels, nerves, and other structures have been digitally color enhanced to improve the clarity and understanding of complex or difficult areas. Each photographic image has been carefully crafted with respect to size, orientation and labeling to allow for immediate orientation by the reader and an easy understanding of the anatomy presented.
- Osteology photos taken from the same visual perspective as the dissections allow students to put the structures of the skeleton and soft tissues together easily and improve their visualization of each body region.

- Radiological images include several imaging modalities – plain film radiographs, computed tomography scans (CTs), and magnetic resonance images (MRIs), in recognition that, for the students, imaging is an early point of contact with, and has become essential to, the teaching of clinical anatomy.

All photographs and diagrams of one side of the body show the right side, unless stated otherwise in the captions.

TEXT AND TABLES
The text has been kept deliberately concise and clear:

- Orientation text, together with specially commissioned summary diagrams, concisely describes the major anatomical features of each body system: muscles, nerves, arteries, and veins and lymphatics. This allows readers to 'place' the information immediately without needing to flip back and forth between text and photographs.
- Selected clinical correlations, which put anatomical understanding in a clinical context, represent clinical presentations that a practitioner is likely to encounter.
- A review table of important structures is located around the midpoint of each chapter. In chapters containing many muscles, this table lists each muscle and cites its origin, insertion, innervation, action, and blood supply. In other chapters, where there are no large named muscles, the table describes other major structures: for example, in the chapter on the lungs, the table details the bronchopulmonary segments.
- Cross-references, which allow students to integrate knowledge from one area to another and gain a deeper understanding of anatomy, and commonly used mnemonics, have been included to facilitate learning.

We have made a deliberate omission of the brain and spinal cord because these areas are covered in great detail in neuroanatomy courses, and the focus of this text is the study of general gross human anatomy.

For uniformity we have chosen to use the terminology presented within *Terminologia Anatomica* (Thieme, Stuttgart/New York, 1998), a joint publication by the Federative Committee on Anatomical Terminology and the 56-member association of the International Federation of Association of Anatomists.

ORGANIZATION
The organization of *Atlas of Clinical Gross Anatomy* follows a logical and consistent plan:

- Overall, the book takes a regional approach to the human body. It is divided into four sections arranged in a logical (from head to toe) order – head and neck, upper limb, trunk, and lower limb. Chapters within each section also flow in a head-to-toe order.
- Each section begins with an introductory chapter that provides an overview of general regional principles and relationships. This foundation acts as a framework for the more detailed concepts that follow in the succeeding chapters.
- Specific chapters are given over to descriptions of the major joints of the extremities: shoulder, elbow, wrist, hip, knee, and

ankle. To the best of our knowledge this is the only current atlas to do so.

- Within each chapter, the anatomy photographs are presented in the same way – from surface anatomy to the superficial layers of a dissection through to the deeper layers.

This atlas has been peer reviewed by an international review panel of anatomy instructors and by general surgeons and specialists in otorhinolaryngology, urology, gynecology, and oromaxillofacial, orthopedic, plastic and reconstructive, and cardiothoracic surgery. In addition, we are grateful for comments from reviewers in the fields of dentistry, dental hygiene, nursing, physical therapy, occupational therapy, audiology and optometry, as well as many student reviewers.

The resulting *Atlas of Clinical Gross Anatomy* is, we hope, an attractive, student-oriented anatomy atlas with a consistent, well-organized layout. It has been prepared not only for students and instructors in professional programs, i.e. medical, dental, physical therapy, and chiropractic, but also other allied-health programs such as occupational therapy, audiology, optometry, and undergraduate anatomy. Additionally, we believe it should be useful as a source of review to resident surgeons, and resident and attending physicians in family practice, internal medicine, pediatrics, obstetrics and gynecology, and psychiatry.

This atlas has been, in total, eight years in the making and is, we think, an exciting new tool for the understanding and appreciation of the human body. It is our hope that our collective enjoyment of the subject has produced an anatomical work that will be appreciated and used by students of anatomy for many years to come.

K. P. Moses
J. C. Banks Jr.
P. B. Nava
D. K. Petersen
November 2004

CONTENTS

Section 1 *Head and neck*

Section 2 *Upper limb*

Section 3 *Trunk*

Section 4 *Lower limb*

EDITORIAL REVIEW BOARD

Liliana D. Macchi, PhD
Second Chair
Department of Normal Human Anatomy
Faculty of Medicine
University of Buenos Aires
Buenos Aires, Argentina

Bradford D. Martin, PhD
Associate Professor of Physical Therapy
Department of Physical Therapy
School of Allied Health
Loma Linda University
Loma Linda, California, USA

Martha D. McDaniel, MD
Professor of Anatomy, Surgery and Community and
Family Medicine
Chair, Department of Anatomy
Dartmouth Medical School
Hanover, New Hampshire, USA

Jan H. Meiring, MB, ChB, MpraxMed(Pret)
Professor and Head
Department of Anatomy
University of Pretoria
Pretoria, South Africa

John F. Morris, MB, ChB, MD
Professor
Department of Human Anatomy and Genetics
University of Oxford
Oxford, UK

Juanita P. Moses, MD FAAP
Assistant Professor Department of Pediatrics and
Human Development
Michigan State University College of Human
Medicine
Staff Physician, Department of Pediatrics
Devos Children's Hospital
Grand Rapids, Michigan, USA

Helen D. Nicholson, MB, ChB, BSc, MD
Professor and Chair
Department of Anatomy and Structural Biology
University of Otago
Dunedin, New Zealand

Mark Nielsen, MS
Biology Department
University of Utah
Salt Lake City, Utah, USA

Wei-Yi Ong, DDS, PhD
Associate Professor
Department of Anatomy
Faculty of Medicine
National University of Singapore
Singapore

Gustavo H. R. A. Otegui, MD
Department of Anatomy
University of Buenos Aires
Buenos Aires, Argentina

Ann Poznanski, PhD
Associate Professor
Department of Anatomy
Midwestern University
Glendale, Arizona, USA

Matthew A. Pravetz, OFM, PhD
Associate Professor
Department of Cell Biology and Anatomy
New York Medical College
Valhalla, New York, USA

Reinhard Putz, MD, PhD
Professor of Anatomy
Chairman Institute of Anatomy
Ludwig-Maximilians-Universitat
Munich, Germany

Ameed Raoof, MD, PhD
Lecturer
Division of Anatomy and Department of Medical
Education
The University of Michigan Medical School
Ann Arbor, Michigan, USA

James J. Rechtien, DO
Professor
Division of Anatomy and Structural Biology
Department of Radiology
Michigan State University
East Lansing, Michigan, USA

Walter H. Roberts, MD
Professor Emeritus
Department of Pathology and Human Anatomy
Loma Linda University School of Medicine
Loma Linda, California, USA

Rouel S. Roque, MD
Associate Professor
Department of Cell Biology and Genetics
University of North Texas Health Sciences Center
Forth Worth, Texas, USA

Lawrence M. Ross, MD, PhD
Adjunct Professor
Department of Neurobiology and Anatomy
The University of Texas Medical School at Houston
Houston, Texas, USA

Phillip Sambrook, MD, BS, LLB, FRACP
Professor of Rheumatology
University of Sidney
Sidney, Australia

Mark F. Seifert, PhD
Professor of Anatomy and Cell Biology
Indiana University School of Medicine
Indianapolis, Indiana, USA

Sudha Seshayyan, MS
Professor and Head
Department of Anatomy
Stanley Medical College
Chennai, India

Kohei Shiota, MD, PhD
Professor and Chairman
Department of Anatomy and Developmental
Anatomy
Director, Congenital Anomaly Research Center
Kyoto University Graduate School of Medicine
Kyoto, Japan

Allan R. Sinning, PhD
Associate Professor
Department of Anatomy
The University of Mississippi Medical Center
Jackson, Mississippi, USA

Bernard G. Slavin, PhD
Course Director, Human Gross Anatomy
Keck School of Medicine
University of Southern California
Los Angeles, California, USA

Terence K. Smith, PhD
Professor
Department of Physiology and Cell Biology
University of Nevada School of Medicine
Reno, Nevada, USA

Kwok-Fai So, PhD(MIT)
Pofessor and Head
Department of Anatomy
Faculty of Medicine, The University of Hong Kong
Hong Kong, China

Susan M. Standring, PhD, DSc
Professor of Experimental Neurobiology
Head, Division of Anatomy, Cell and Human Biology
Guy's, King's and St Thomas' School of Biomedical
Sciences
King's College
London, UK

Mark F. Teaford, PhD
Professor of Anatomy
Center for Functional Anatomy and Evolution
Johns Hopkins University School of Medicine
Baltimore, Maryland, USA

Nagaswami S. Vasan, DVM, PhD
Associate Professor
Department of Cell Biology and Molecular Medicine
New Jersey Medical School
Newark, New Jersey, USA

Ismo Virtanen, MD, PhD
Professor of Anatomy
Anatomy Department
Haartman Institute
University of Helsinki
Helsinki, Finland

Linda Walters, PhD
Professor, Preclinical Education
Midwestern University
Glendale, Arizona, USA

Joanne C. Wilton, PhD
Director of Anatomy
Department of Anatomy
The Medical School, University of Birmingham
Birmingham, UK

Susanne Wish-Baratz, PhD
Senior Teacher
Department of Anatomy and Anthropology
Sackler Faculty of Medicine
Tel Aviv University
Tel Aviv, Israel

Henry K. Yip, PhD
Associate Professor
Department of Anatomy
Faculty of Medicine
The University of Hong Kong
Hong Kong, China

David T. Yew, PhD, DSc, DrMed(Habil), CBiol, FIBiol
Professor and Chairman
Department of Anatomy
The Chinese University of Hong Kong
Hong Kong, China

SPECIALIST REVIEWERS

Anatomy
Brad Martin PhD
Ralph Perrin PhD

Audiology
Heather L. Knutson MA CCC-A FAAA

Cardiology
Mil Dhond MD FACC
Husam Noor MD

Cardiothoracic surgery
Leonard Bailey MD FACS
Anees Razzouk MD FACS

Dietetics
Arlene Campbell RD

Dentistry
Carlos Moretta DDS RDH

Dental hygiene
Jolene N. Bauer RDH

Emergency medicine
Michael Dillon MD FACEP
Greg Goldner MD FACEP
Eliot Nipomnick MD FACEP

Family practice
Tricia Scheuneman MD

General surgery
Nathaniel Matolo MD FACS
Clifton Reeves MD FACS
Mark Reeves MD FACS
Hamid Rassai MD FACS

Internal medicine
Sofia Bhoskerrou MD
Joseph Selvaraj MD MPH

Nursing
Robin Hoover RN ADN
Pam Ihrig RN BSN
Joanna Krupczynski RN BSN
Sandy Manning RN BSN

Obstetrics and gynecology
Tricia Fynewever MD
Wilbert A.Gonzalez MD FACOG
Jeffrey S. Hardesty MD FACOG
Kathleen M. Lau MD FACOG
Sam Siddighi MD

Occupational therapy
Kristina Brown OT

Ophthalmology
Julio Narvaez MD FAAO
Wendell Wong MD FAAO

Oromaxillofacial surgery
Allen Herford MD DDS FACS

Orthopedics
Raja Dhalla MD FACS
Christopher Jobe MD FACS
Richard Rouhe MD FACS

Otorhinolaryngology
George Petti MD FACS
Mark Rowe MD FACS

Pathology
Jeff Cao MD

Plastic and reconstructive surgery
Subhas Gupta MD FACS
Brett Lehocky MD FACS
Duncan Miles MD FACS
Michael Pickart MD FACS
Andrea Ray MD FACS
Frank Rogers MD FACS
Arvin Taneja MD FACS

Physical medicine and rehabilitation
Jien-sup Kim MD

Physical therapy
James Ko PT

Urology
H. Roger Hadley MD FACS AUA

STUDENT REVIEWERS

Bart Abriol
Rishi Agrawal
Idalia Alaniz
Emma Bellchambers
Fiona Blackburn
Holly Blake
Bryan D. Brewer
Naomi Bullen
Rianna Burrill
Doug Campbell
Sarah Clark
Joanna Coyne
Richard Crane
Paul H. Dahm
Oliver Dale
Silvia de Faria
Amy E. Ellis
James Ellison

Allen Eshmoili
Ann Figurski
David T. Foster
Kathryn Friday
Robert Michael Galbraith
Matthew Garget
Joseph Gerbrandt
Bryan Glick
Jenece Gungl
Antonia Hargadon-Lowe
Mark Higgins
Grove L. Higgins III
B.J. Ho
Lacy Huff
Crystal Kiefer
Alison Lawton
Arden Lay
Zsuzsanna H. McMahan

Karen Memmelaar
Edsel Montemayor
Joseph Muñoz
David P. Nieson
Elizabeth O'Connor
Edward Palafox
Adriane A. Ramirez
Sasha Rodriguez
Sarah Elizabeth Rood
Lynne Selmser
Heather Smith
Nicole Tribhuwan
Gina Voci
Linda Walden
Melanie Worth
Tom Zrilli

ACKNOWLEDGMENTS

The idea to write this book came to me while a first year medical student. Thank you to each person who encouraged me to write this book: John, who was my anatomy professor in college and one of my favorite teachers; Ben, my medical school gross anatomy professor who is an excellent lecturer and now a good friend; and Darrell, who is in my opinion the world's best medical photographer.

Thank you to the Elsevier Staff – Inta Ozols, Richard Furn, Duncan Fraser, Colin Arthur, Alison Whitehouse and others – for being such friendly co-workers on this large task and for being mindful of this author's words and opinions. I truly enjoyed the entire process.

Thank you to Kendra Fisher, MD for all of your assistance in helping us obtain and also review all of the radiographic anatomy in this book.

Thank you to my sister Juanita Moses, MD who has a great understanding of practical clinical medicine and an impeccable attention to detail; she edited the entire manuscript at each of the three proof stages.

And above all, a special thank you to my mother Dr Gnani Ruth Moses for raising a son to believe that 'all things are possible'.

K. P. Moses

Thanks must go to everyone who has assisted in the proofreading and checking of the manuscript.

Grateful thanks to Michigan State University for supplying the cadavers for the chapters on the upper and lower limbs. Special thanks go to the Department of Radiology in the Division of Anatomy and Structural Biology, its Chair, E. James Potchen MD, and Faculty Coordinator, Gerald Aben MD. Also, Kristin Liles, Director of Anatomical Resources and Bruce E. Croel, Anatomical Preparation Technician.

I would also like to thank Andrews University and the Department of Physical Therapy for the use of their anatomy lab space, and for the interest and encouragement of its Chairs, Daryl W. Stuart EdD, and Wayne L. Perry PhD.

J. C. Banks Jr.

I would like to express my appreciation to all of the individuals within the Division of Anatomy at Loma Linda University who supported this endeavor. A special thanks to Martein Moningka, Curator, for his many hours of hard work on numerous, detailed dissections for this atlas.

A grateful thanks to Linda Durham, Willed Body Administrator, and to Zina Trochanowski for her typing of the manuscript.

Dawn, thank you for your inspiration and support.

P. B. Nava

I would first like to thank Ken for asking me to be a part of such a great project. Thanks also to my fellow authors – it has been a pleasure working with you over the years and I look forward to many more.

Dave, for being a mentor/instructor in school and most importantly for being my friend, I owe you many thanks.

Additionally I would like to thank: Heather, Denise, Jim, Mesfen, Julie, Natalie, Kristina, Carlos, Jolene, Joanna, Cynthia, Todd, EJ, Linda, Zina, Tom, Samantha, Bob, Mary, Gary, Warren and everyone that helped, even in a small way, with this project.

D. K. Petersen

DEDICATIONS

This book is dedicated to the One
who has been there to assist and guide me
throughout the entire process.
K. P. Moses

To my wife Patricia and
daughters Erin and Kirsten,
for allowing me to spend so
many hours in my anatomy lab.
J. C. Banks Jr.

To the many teachers, professors and
mentors, who have had faith in me
during my academic career.
P. B. Nava

To my mother, for all of her love and support;
and to my grandparents, Lester and Carrie,
for giving me my first camera at age 6.
D. K. Petersen

1 Introduction to anatomy

Anatomy is the study of the structure of the body. Like any other discipline, it has its own language to enable clear and precise communication. Anatomists base all descriptions of the body and its structures on the 'anatomical position'. In this position the body is erect, arms at the sides, the palms of the hands facing forward and the feet together. The anatomical position is used by anatomists and clinicians as a frame of reference to place anatomy in a three-dimensional context and to standardize the terms for anatomical structures and their functions.

Anatomical planes pass through the body in the anatomical position and are used for reference. The three main descriptive planes (Fig. 1.1) are:

- **the median plane** – a vertical plane that divides the body into left and right halves (strictly speaking, this is called the **median sagittal plane**);
- **sagittal planes** – any vertical plane parallel to the median plane, for example midway between the median plane and the shoulder;
- **the frontal** (or **coronal**) **plane** – a vertical plane oriented at 90° to the median plane that divides the body into front (anterior) and back (posterior) sections;

- **the horizontal** (**transverse** or **axial**) **plane**, which divides the body into upper (superior) and lower (inferior) sections, and in some situations is referred to as a 'cross-section'.

Specific terms of description and comparison, based on the anatomical position, describe how one part of the body relates to another:

- **anterior** (ventral) – toward the front of the body;
- **posterior** (dorsal) – toward the back of the body;
- **superior** (cranial) – toward the head;
- **inferior** (caudal) – toward the feet;
- **medial** – toward the midline of the body;
- **lateral** – away from the midline of the body;
- **proximal** – toward the point of origin, root, or attachment of the structure;
- **distal** – away from the point of origin, root, or attachment of the structure;
- **superficial** (external) – toward the surface of the body;
- **deep** (internal) – away from the surface of the body;
- **dorsum** – superior surface of the foot and posterior surface of the hand;
- **plantar** – inferior aspect of the foot;
- **palmar** (volar) – anterior aspect of the hand.

There are also terms for movement. Movements take place at joints, where bone or cartilage articulate. Most movements occur in pairs, with the movements opposing each other:

- **flexion** decreases the angle between body parts, and **extension** increases the angle;
- **adduction** is movement toward the median plane of the body, while **abduction** is movement away from the median plane;
- **medial rotation** turns the anterior surface medially or inward;
- **lateral rotation** turns the anterior surface laterally or outward;
- **supination** is lateral rotation of the limb, for example such that the palm starts the movement facing down and ends the movement facing up, whereas **pronation** is medial rotation of the limb, for example such that the palm starts the movement facing up and ends the movement facing down;
- **inversion** is movement of the foot so that the sole faces medially, and **eversion** is movement of the foot so that the sole faces laterally;
- **opposition** is action whereby the thumb abducts, rotates medially, and flexes so that it can meet the tip of any other finger.
- **circumduction** is circular movement of the limbs that combines adduction, abduction, extension, and flexion (e.g. 'swinging the arm around in a circle');
- **elevation** lifts or moves a part superiorly, whereas **depression** lowers or moves a part inferiorly;
- **protrusion** (protraction) is to move the jaw anteriorly, while **retrusion** (retraction) is to move the jaw posteriorly.

Structures may be unilateral or bilateral. The heart is an example of a **unilateral structure**: it exists on only one side of the body. **Bilateral structures**, for example the vessels of the arm, are present on both (*bi*-) sides of the body. Two similar adjectives **ipsilateral**, meaning

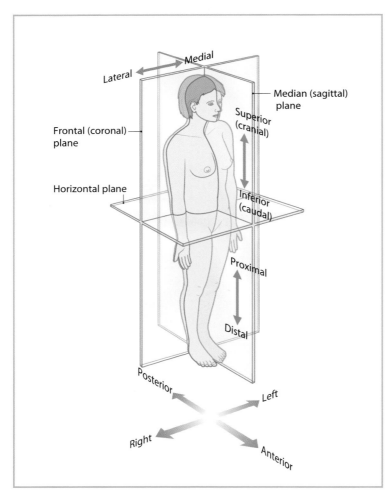

Figure 1.1 Anatomical planes and orientation

on the same side of a structure, and **contralateral**, meaning on the opposite side, are often used in anatomical descriptions.

BODY SYSTEMS

A body system is a combination of organs with a similar or related function that work together as a unit. Body systems work together to maintain the functional integrity of the body as a whole.

Musculoskeletal system

Skeleton

The human skeleton of 206 bones comprises:

- the **axial skeleton** – the skull, vertebrae, ribs, sternum, and hyoid bones; and
- the **appendicular skeleton** – the pectoral and pelvic girdles, and the upper and lower limbs.

Muscles

Muscle cells contract. Movement is produced when the contraction occurs in a muscle that is attached to a rigid structure, for example a bone.

There are three types of muscle, which differ in location, histological appearance, and how they are controlled (voluntary vs involuntary control).

- **Skeletal muscles** are mainly under voluntary – conscious – control, and are the muscles of most interest in gross anatomy. They are attached at each end – either to bone or connective tissue – via tendons and aponeuroses. They usually span a single joint so that contraction causes the joint to move in a specific direction.
- **Smooth muscle** occurs in the digestive, respiratory, and cardiovascular systems, and is under involuntary control. It helps maintain and change the lumen of the gut, bronchi, and blood vessels. In the gut, rhythmic contractions of smooth muscles generate the peristaltic waves that push food through the gastrointestinal tract.
- **Cardiac muscle** occurs only in the heart and is under involuntary control. Contractions of cardiac muscle are the driving force behind the circulation of blood.

Muscle names

Muscles generally have descriptive names that give an indication of their shape, number of origins, location, number of bellies, function, origin, or insertion. Muscles are classified according to the arrangement of their bundles of muscle fibers (fasciculi), which affects the degree and type of movement of an individual muscle. The fiber arrangements may be:

- **straplike** (parallel)
- **fusiform** (spindle-like)
- **fan-shaped**
- **pennate** (feather-like)
- **bipennate**
- **multipennate**
- **sphincter** (circular).

The attachment of a muscle that moves least is the **origin**; the more mobile attachment is the **insertion**. In some instances these roles are reversed.

Connective tissue

Individual muscle cells are covered by specialized connective tissue (**endomysium**). Because each cell is extremely long, the term fiber is used more often than cell. A bundle of several fibers (a **fascicle**) is surrounded by a sheet of connective tissue (**perimysium**). The entire muscle is surrounded by a sheath of connective tissue (**epimysium**). These three levels of connective tissue (also known as **investments**) are interconnected and provide a route for nerves and blood vessels to supply the individual muscle cells. They also transmit the collective pull of individual muscle cells, fascicles, and entire muscles to the points of muscle attachment.

Muscle groups

Muscles combine in groups to perform complex or powerful movements. Groups of muscles that initiate a movement are **prime movers**; those that oppose the movement are **antagonists**. Muscles that contract to support a primary movement are **synergists**. **Paradox muscles** are muscles that relax against the pull of gravity.

Nervous system

The nervous system consists of the brain, spinal cord, and all peripheral nerves (Fig. 1.2). It is the main control center for the body's numerous functions, processing all external and internal stimuli and responding appropriately. Its main structural and functional subdivisions are:

- the **central nervous system** (**CNS**), comprising the brain and spinal cord;
- the **peripheral nervous system** (**PNS**), composed of 12 pairs of cranial nerves arising from the brain and 31 pairs of spinal nerves arising from the spinal cord;
- the **autonomic division** (see below), composed of elements from both the CNS and PNS.

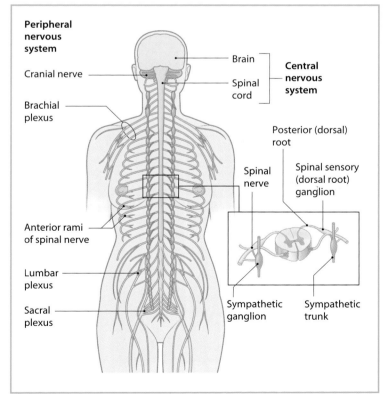

Figure 1.2 Nervous system

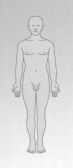
A **neuron** (nerve cell) comprises a cell body, an axon, and dendrites. The **axon** is the long fiber-like part of the nerve between the cell body and the target organ. In special circumstances, for example in the autonomic division (autonomic part of the PNS, see below) when two neurons meet, the axon of one neuron meets the **dendrites** of another at a junction called the **synapse**.

Motor nerves (efferent nerves) carry impulses from the CNS to the PNS and innervate muscles. **Sensory nerves** (afferent nerves) receive information from sense receptors throughout the body and relay it back to the CNS for processing and interpretation.

Autonomic division

The **autonomic division** is subdivided into two parts – the **sympathetic** and **parasympathetic nervous systems** – and allows the body to respond appropriately to any given set of circumstances with very little conscious control.

Axons from neurons in the CNS (**preganglionic fibers**) run to autonomic ganglia outside the CNS. The preganglionic fiber from a central neuron synapses with a second neuron within the ganglion. Nerve fibers (**postganglionic fibers**) then travel from this second neuron to the target organ or cell. A **ganglion** is therefore a collection of neuron bodies outside of the CNS that acts as a point of transfer for neuron stimulation. Both the sympathetic and parasympathetic subdivisions of the autonomic division contain ganglia. Most organs receive input from both subdivisions of the autonomic division, however the body wall does not receive parasympathetic nerve fibers.

Sensory (e.g. pain) fibers from the viscera reach the CNS via either or both of the autonomic pathways, but there is no peripheral synapse for visceral sensory nerves. Their cell bodies are located in either the **spinal ganglion** (dorsal root ganglion) or the sensory ganglion of certain cranial nerves.

The sympathetic nervous system sends signals from the CNS to prepare the body for action – dilating the pupils, increasing the heart and respiratory rates, and causing sweating, vasoconstriction, cessation of gastrointestinal movements, and constriction of urinary and anal sphincter muscles.

Parasympathetic nerve fibers do the opposite – they relax the body, constricting the pupils, slowing the heart rate, promoting salivary secretion, increasing peristalsis (gastrointestinal tract stimulation), and relaxing the urinary and anal sphincters.

Cardiovascular system

The **heart** is in the middle mediastinum between the lungs. It has four chambers that pump blood throughout the body. The right side of the heart receives deoxygenated blood from the body and pumps it to the lungs: **pulmonary circulation**. The left side receives oxygenated blood from the lungs and sends it to the body: **systemic circulation**, in which **arteries** carry blood from the heart to the tissues and organs, and **veins** return blood to the heart.

Arteries

The **aorta** is the largest artery in the body. It carries oxygenated blood from the left ventricle of the heart to the rest of the body. Ascending from the heart, the aorta forms an arch that curves toward the left side of the body and then descends in the chest toward the abdomen. The first arteries that branch from the aorta are the relatively small **coronary arteries**, which supply blood to the heart itself. The first large branch from the aorta is the **brachiocephalic trunk**, which gives rise to the **right common**

carotid and **right subclavian arteries**. These supply blood to the head, neck, and right upper limb, respectively (Fig. 1.3). The **left common carotid** and **left subclavian arteries** are the next arterial branches and supply blood to the left side of the head and neck and to the left upper limb, respectively. After these branches, the aorta turns inferiorly toward the abdomen. Branches of the descending thoracic aorta supply the viscera within the thorax and the chest wall, mediastinum, and diaphragm.

The thoracic aorta pierces the diaphragm at the level of thoracic vertebra TXII to become the abdominal aorta. The abdominal aorta gives rise to three main unpaired arteries:

- the **celiac trunk** (at vertebral level TXII);
- the **superior mesenteric artery** (at vertebral level TXII/LI); and
- the **inferior mesenteric artery** (at vertebral level LIII).

These three arteries supply blood to the abdominal viscera and are derivatives of the embryonic foregut, midgut, and hindgut, respectively. The abdominal aorta also supplies blood to the body wall via paired lumbar segmental arteries. The **renal arteries** (at LI level), **suprarenal arteries**, and gonadal arteries (at LII/LIII vertebral level) are paired arteries that supply the viscera of the posterior abdominal wall. Inferiorly, the abdominal aorta divides into the **left and right common iliac arteries** at the level of LIV vertebra. As the

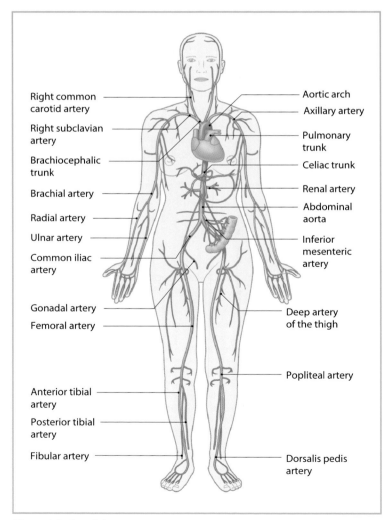

Figure 1.3 Arterial system

common iliac arteries descend into the pelvis they subdivide into vessels that supply the pelvis and both lower limbs.

Veins

Veins transport deoxygenated blood from the tissues and organs back to the heart (Fig. 1.4). Systemic veins direct blood from the body to the superior and inferior venae cavae, which drain to the right atrium of the heart. The pulmonary vein, unlike the rest of the veins, transports oxygenated blood from the lungs to the left atrium of the heart.

The **superior vena cava** receives blood from the head and neck, chest wall, and upper limbs via the **internal jugular**, **azygos**, **subclavian**, and **veins brachiocephalic**. The **inferior vena cava** receives blood from the pelvis, abdomen, and lower limbs.

The **portal system** is a special set of veins that drains blood from the intestines and supporting organs. Its venous blood is rich in absorbed nutrients from the digestive tract. The **hepatic portal vein** is formed by the union of the **splenic** and **superior mesenteric veins**. Blood flows from the hepatic portal vein to the liver. From the liver, hepatic veins drain into the inferior vena cava.

Lymphatic system

The lymphatic system is composed of a series of **lymphatic vessels** and **lymph nodes** (filters), which transport excess tissue fluid (**lymph**) from the tissue spaces to the venous system (Fig. 1.5). Lymphatic vessels also transport nutrient-rich lymph from the intestines to the blood and play a role in immunity.

Lymph flow through the body is slow. In many areas it is unidirectional because of the presence of one-way valves in the vessels. Flow is promoted by the massaging of lymph vessels by adjacent arteries and – in the limbs – skeletal muscle, and by vessels, and pressure differences between the abdominal and thoracic cavities.

Lymphatic vessels begin as blind-ended capillaries within the tissue spaces. Excess tissue fluid enters them to become a colorless, clear fluid – lymph. This then passes through a series of lymph nodes as they convey lymph toward the venous system:

- the **jugular trunks** lie beside the internal jugular vein and receive lymph from each side of the head and neck;
- the **subclavian trunks** drain the upper limbs and chest;
- the **bronchomediastinal trunks** drain the organs of the thorax.

In the abdomen, the **thoracic duct** drains lymph from the lower limbs, pelvis, and abdomen. Lymph from the thoracic duct drains to the junction of the left subclavian and left internal jugular veins. The thoracic duct receives the left jugular lymph trunk, left subclavian lymph trunk, and left bronchomediastinal lymph trunks. Essentially it drains the lower part of the body, the left upper limb, and the left side of the head and neck. Lymph from the right upper limb and right side of the head and neck drains to the right jugular lymph trunk via reciprocal vessels, which enter the venous system at the union of the right internal jugular and right subclavian veins.

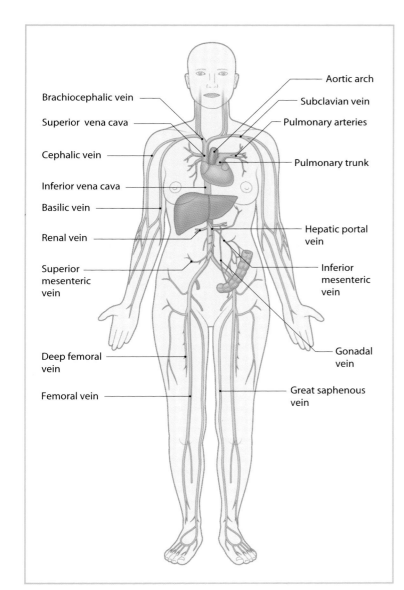

Figure 1.4 Venous system

Labels: Brachiocephalic vein; Superior vena cava; Cephalic vein; Inferior vena cava; Basilic vein; Renal vein; Superior mesenteric vein; Deep femoral vein; Femoral vein; Aortic arch; Subclavian vein; Pulmonary arteries; Pulmonary trunk; Hepatic portal vein; Inferior mesenteric vein; Gonadal vein; Great saphenous vein

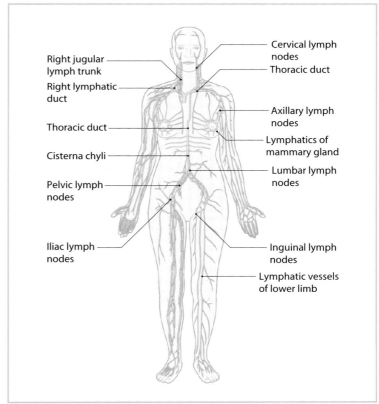

Figure 1.5 Lymphatic system

Labels: Right jugular lymph trunk; Right lymphatic duct; Thoracic duct; Cisterna chyli; Pelvic lymph nodes; Iliac lymph nodes; Cervical lymph nodes; Thoracic duct; Axillary lymph nodes; Lymphatics of mammary gland; Lumbar lymph nodes; Inguinal lymph nodes; Lymphatic vessels of lower limb

Introduction to the head and neck

The head and neck are two distinct anatomical regions of the body, but they have related nerve and blood supply.

HEAD

The head is a highly modified structure with several important functions. It houses and protects the special sense organs – the eyes, ears, nose, tongue, and related structures. The **skull** is specially adapted to enclose, support, and protect the brain (Fig. 2.1). It has numerous foramina for cranial nerves and vascular structures to pass into and out of the cranium, contains cavities that carry out some of the functions of the upper gastrointestinal tract and respiratory tracts (e.g. oral and nasal cavities), and provides a foundation for the face. Anatomically, the skull is divided into two main parts:

- the **neurocranium** houses the brain, forms the base of the skull and cranial vault, and is formed from eight bones – the occipital, sphenoid, frontal, and ethmoid bones, a pair of parietal bones, and a pair of temporal bones;
- the **viscerocranium** (facial skeleton) contributes to the structure of the orbits and the nasal and oral cavities, providing a foundation for the face; it comprises the mandible and vomer, and a pair each of maxilla, palatine, nasal, zygomatic, lacrimal, and inferior nasal concha bones.

The **paranasal sinuses** are cavities within the maxillary, ethmoid, frontal, and sphenoid bones that communicate with the nasal cavity through small ostia (openings).

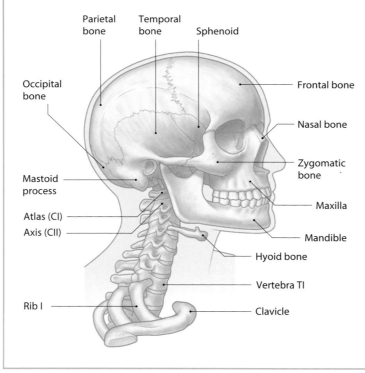

Figure 2.1 Bones of the head and neck

NECK

The head is mobile because the skull is balanced on the flexible bony spine. The neck extends from the base of the skull (a circular line joining the superior nuchal line, mastoid process, and lower border of the mandible) to the chest (sternum, clavicles, spine of scapula, and spinous process of vertebra CVII). It is a flexible conduit for blood vessels, the spinal cord, and cranial and spinal nerves passing between the head, thorax, and upper limb.

The neck is supported by muscles, ligaments, and the cervical vertebrae, which provide a strong, flexible skeletal framework without sacrificing stability. The seven cervical vertebrae have **vertebral foramina** (for the vertebral arteries to pass through) within their transverse processes (see Chapter 26). The cervical segment of the vertebral column is strongly supported by numerous ligaments and muscles (both extrinsic and intrinsic). Intermediate parts of the respiratory tract (larynx and trachea), digestive tract (pharynx and esophagus), and endocrine glands (thyroid and parathyroid glands) are located within the neck.

For descriptive purposes, the neck is subdivided into **anterior** and **posterior triangles**. These two large triangles are further subdivided into minor triangles: **submandibular, submental, carotid, muscular, occipital,** and **omoclavicular (subclavian) triangles** (see Chapter 12).

The fascia of the neck is multilayered and encloses the muscles, glands, and neurovascular structures. The relationships between the different fascial layers determine how infection and cancer spread in the neck. The **deep cervical fascia** subdivides the neck into **vascular, vertebral,** and **visceral compartments.** This arrangement allows movement between adjacent structures and compartments, and facilitates the surgical approach to specific areas. The **investing layer** of cervical fascia encircles all structures of the neck by investing the sternocleidomastoid and trapezius muscles, the fascial roofs of the anterior and posterior cervical triangles, and the parotid and submandibular salivary glands. Deep to the investing fascia and surrounding the visceral compartment is the **pretracheal layer** of cervical fascia, which invests the trachea, thyroid and parathyroid glands, and the **buccopharyngeal fascia**, which extends from the base of the skull and envelopes the buccinator muscle and pharyngeal constrictors.

The cervical part of the vertebral column and its contents form the vertebral compartment of the neck, and are surrounded by the **prevertebral layer** of fascia. The **brachial plexus** passes between the anterior and middle scalene muscles and is enclosed in a prolongation of the prevertebral fascia – the **axillary sheath**. The **suprapleural membrane**, which covers the apex of the lungs, is continuous with the prevertebral fascia and continues into the thorax as the **endothoracic fascia**.

Two special fascial units – the **carotid sheaths** – extend from the base of the skull to the superior mediastinum. These sheaths enclose the common and internal carotid arteries, the internal jugular vein, and the vagus nerve [X], and are surrounded by the deep cervical lymph nodes (see p. 9).

MUSCLES

The major muscles of the head and neck are derived embryologically from two major sources:

- pharyngeal arches;
- somites.

Mesoderm from the first, second, third, fourth, and sixth pharyngeal arches gives rise to muscles of mastication and facial expression, stylopharyngeus, and muscles of the larynx and pharynx, respectively. These muscle groups are innervated by the trigeminal [V], facial [VII], and glossopharyngeal [IX] nerves, and the cranial root of the accessory nerve, respectively.

The extraocular muscles are derived from pre-otic somites and are innervated by the oculomotor [III], trochlear [IV], and abducent [VI] cranial nerves.

The intrinsic and extrinsic muscles of the tongue are derived from post-otic somites, and are innervated by the hypoglossal nerve [XII].

NERVES

The head is innervated by the cranial and spinal nerves, which contain sensory, motor, and autonomic components. The 12 pairs of cranial nerves [I to XII] emerge from the brain and brainstem to innervate the head and neck (Table 2.1).

Spinal nerves originate from the spinal cord and enter the neck through intervertebral foramina between the cervical vertebrae. They provide general sensation to the occipital region (see Chapter 27), posterior and anterior neck, and part of the lateral face.

Autonomic nerves to the head (both sympathetic and parasympathetic) regulate the size of the pupil and lens of the eye, secretion by the salivary and lacrimal glands, glands in the upper respiratory and gastrointestinal tracts, and the diameter of extracranial vessels in the head.

- Preganglionic parasympathetic nerve fibers in the brainstem follow the same pathway as the oculomotor [III], facial [VII], glossopharyngeal [IX] and vagus [X] nerves, and synapse with postganglionic neurons in the autonomic ganglia. These ganglia provide postganglionic nerve fibers for the target organs (see Chapter 1).
- Preganglionic sympathetic nerve fibers to the head and neck arise from the upper part of the thoracic spinal cord and synapse in the superior cervical ganglia (see Chapter 13).

Postganglionic fibers emerging from the **superior cervical ganglion** form periarterial plexi, which run with blood vessels to the target organs in the head and neck, providing their autonomic supply.

Nerve control of the neck overlaps with that of the head because cranial nerves also innervate this area. In addition, spinal nerves supply the neck segmentally. Several cranial nerves – the glossopharyngeal [IX], vagus [X], accessory [XI], and hypoglossal [XII] nerves – pass through foramina in the base of the skull and into the neck and beyond.

Sensory innervation of the head and neck is shown in Figure 2.2.

ARTERIES

Blood supply to the head and neck (Fig. 2.3) is from:

- the common carotid artery, which arises from the aorta;
- the vertebral arteries, which arise from the subclavian arteries.

Number	Name	Function
TABLE 2.1 CRANIAL NERVES AND THEIR FUNCTIONS		
I	Olfactory	Sense of smell
II	Optic	Vision
III	Oculomotor	Eye movements
IV	Trochlear	Eye movements
V	Trigeminal	Motor to muscles of mastication and sensation from the head and neck
VI	Abducent	Eye movements
VII	Facial	Motor to muscles of facial expression and taste
VIII	Vestibulocochlear (auditory)	Sense of hearing and sense of balance
IX	Glossopharyngeal	Motor to muscles of swallowing and sensory from pharynx and lateral face
X	Vagus	Motor to vocal muscles: sensory from pharynx, larynx, and lateral face; parasympathetic innervation to the gastrointestinal tract
XI	Accessory	Motor to some muscles of pharynx, larynx, and palatal musculature and some muscles of the neck
XII	Hypoglossal	Motor to most tongue muscles

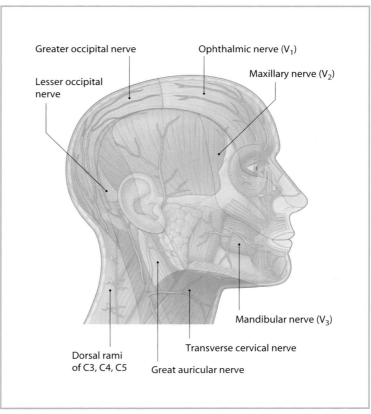

Figure 2.2 Sensory innervation of the head and neck

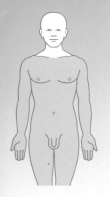

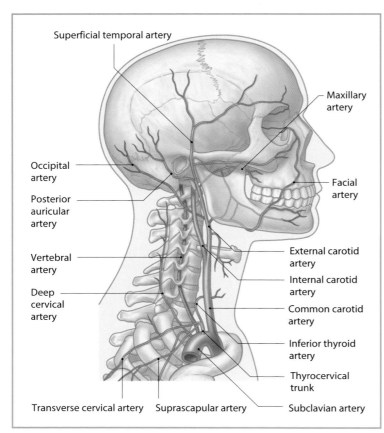

Figure 2.3 Arteries of the head and neck

The **common carotid arteries** ascend from the arch of the aorta on the left and the brachiocephalic artery on the right and divide into the internal and external carotid arteries. The **internal carotid artery** ascends to the skull, where it branches to supply intracranial structures. Branches of the **external carotid artery** are the **superior thyroid artery** (supplying the thyroid gland), **lingual artery** (supplying the tongue), **facial artery** (supplying the face), **ascending pharyngeal artery** (supplying the pharyngeal muscles), **occipital artery** (supplying the upper posterior neck), and **posterior auricular artery** (supplying the ear and surrounding area). The two terminal branches of the external carotid artery are the **maxillary artery** (supplying the temporal, infratemporal, and pterygopalatine fossae, see Chapter 5) and the **superficial temporal artery** (supplying the scalp and lateral face, see Chapter 3).

Multiple anastomoses between branches of the internal and external carotid arteries ensure that the head and its structures have a rich blood supply.

The **vertebral artery** is a branch of the subclavian artery. It ascends in the neck and segmentally supplies the cervical spinal cord, adjacent neck structures, and the brain. Other branches of the subclavian artery – the **thyrocervical trunk**, **costocervical trunk**, and **dorsal scapular arteries** – also provide blood to the neck.

- The branches of the thyrocervical trunk supply blood to the region after which they are named: the **suprascapular artery** supplies the base of the neck and the scapula, the **transverse cervical artery** supplies the scalene and deep neck muscles, the **inferior thyroid artery** supplies the inferior part of thyroid gland.

- The costocervical trunk branches to form the **supreme intercostal artery** (which supplies the first intercostal space) and the **deep cervical artery** (which supplies muscles of the deep posterior neck).
- The dorsal scapular artery primarily supplies the muscles of the scapula.

VEINS

Venous blood from within the cranial cavity drains into venous dural sinuses, which are formed by a splitting of the dura mater. Subsequently, the venous blood drains into the large **internal jugular vein**, which commences at the jugular foramen of the skull and into which drain vessels from the neck that correspond to the branches of the carotid arterial system.

The veins of the head are numerous and are named after the associated arteries. They contain very few valves; this permits venous flow in either direction (Fig. 2.4) and allows extracranial drainage to the intracranial vessels.

LYMPHATICS

The exterior surfaces of the head and neck are richly supplied with lymphatic vessels, lymph nodes, and tissue (Fig. 2.5). In contrast, the central nervous system lacks a lymphatic drainage system; instead **cerebrospinal fluid** (**CSF**) serves this function.

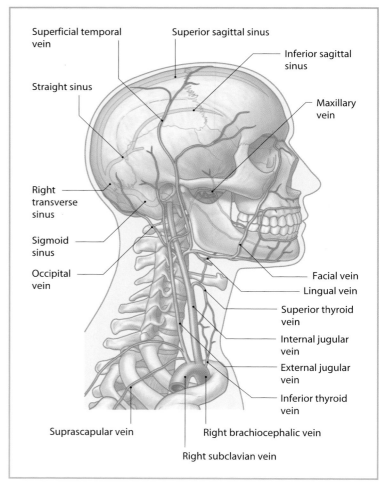

Figure 2.4 Veins of the head and neck

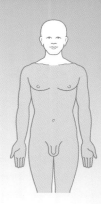

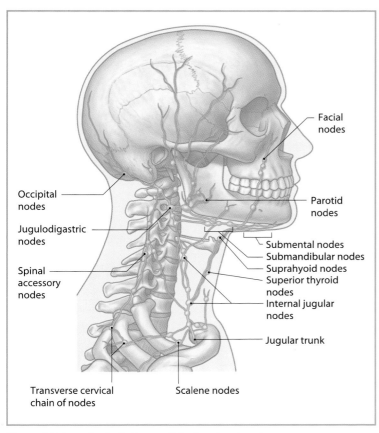

Facial
nodes

Occipital
nodes

Parotid
nodes

Jugulodigastric
nodes

Submental nodes
Submandibular nodes
Suprahyoid nodes

Spinal
accessory
nodes

Superior thyroid
nodes

Internal jugular
nodes

Jugular trunk

Transverse cervical
chain of nodes

Scalene nodes

Figure 2.5 Lymphatic drainage of the head and neck

The face and scalp drain along unnamed lymphatic vessels to a superficial horizontal ring of nodes at the junction of the head and neck. The corresponding deep horizontal ring of nodes is located deep to the superficial tissues in the visceral compartment of the neck. These nodes drain the oral cavity, pharynx, and larynx. From here, lymph flows to the deep cervical lymph nodes on the carotid sheath (see Chapter 12).

On each side of the neck vessels from the deep cervical nodes join to form a **jugular trunk**, which enters the venous system at the junction of the internal jugular and subclavian veins. The jugular trunks also receive lymphatic flow from the chest, limbs, abdomen, and pelvis.

MNEMONIC	
Cranial nerves:	**On Old Olympus Towering Tops A Few Virile Germans View A lot of Hops** (**O**lfactory, **O**ptic, **O**culomotor, **T**rochlear, **T**rigeminal, **A**bducent, **F**acial, **V**estibulocochlear, **G**lossopharyngeal, **V**agus, **A**ccessory, **H**ypoglossal)

3 Skull

The skull (Figs 3.1 and 3.2) is formed by bones that protect the brain and the areas associated with the special senses of sight, hearing, taste, and smell. The skull also houses the entrances for the respiratory and digestive systems – the nose and mouth, respectively. Numerous other openings (canals, fissures, and foramina) in the skull serve as conduits for the spinal cord, cranial nerves, and blood vessels (Table 3.1). The muscles of facial expression and mastication also attach to the skull.

The bones of the skull are divided into three groups (Table 3.2):

- eight cranial bones form the **neurocranium**, which protects the brain;
- 12 facial bones comprise the **viscerocranium**, which forms the substructure for the face;

- six **auditory ossicles** (malleus, incus, and stapes), three in each ear.

The total number of bones in the skull is therefore 26.

All bones of the skull, except the mandible and ear ossicles, articulate at serrated immovable sutures. They are separated by a thin layer of fibrous connective tissue, which is continuous with the periosteum. The sutures between the skull bones fuse and become less distinct with age. The plate-like bones of the neurocranium (also known as the calvaria) consist of **external** and **internal tables** of compact bone, with **diploë** (cancellous bone) between.

Treatment of skull fractures varies, depending on whether the external or internal table is damaged (see p. 12).

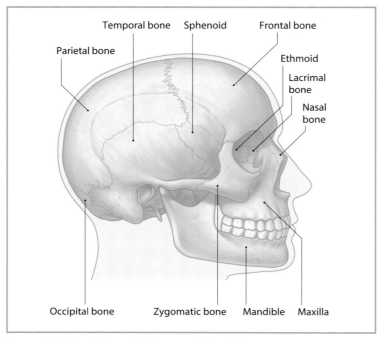

Figure 3.1 Lateral view of the bones of the skull

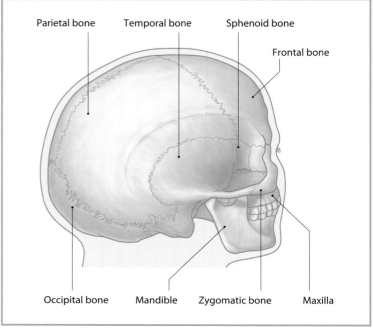

Figure 3.2 Posterolateral view of the bones of the skull

TABLE 3.1 OPENINGS IN THE SKULL		
Openings (foramina/fissures)	**Bone**	**Contents**
Optic canal	Lesser wing (of sphenoid)	Optic nerve [II] and ophthalmic artery
Superior orbital fissure	Greater and lesser wings (of sphenoid)	Lacrimal nerve [V_1], frontal nerve [V_1], trochlear nerve [IV], oculomotor nerve [III], abducent nerve [VI], nasociliary nerve [V_1], superior ophthalmic vein
Inferior orbital fissure	Greater wing (of sphenoid) and maxilla	Maxillary nerve [V_2], zygomatic nerve [V_2], inferior ophthalmic vein
Superior orbital notch/foramen	Frontal bone	Supra-orbital nerve [V_2] and vessels
Infra-orbital groove, canal, foramen	Maxilla	Infra-orbital nerve [V_2] and vessels
Zygomatico-orbital foramen	Zygomatic bone	Zygomaticotemporal and zygomaticofacial nerves [V_2]
Anterior and posterior ethmoidal foramina	Ethmoid	Anterior and posterior ethmoidal nerves [V_2] and vessels
Nasolacrimal canal	Lacrimal bone and maxilla	Nasolacrimal duct

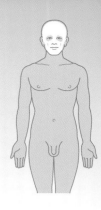

TABLE 3.2 BONES OF THE SKULL					
Cranial (neurocranium)		**Facial (viscerocranium)**		**Auditory ossicles**	
Name	**No.**	**Name**	**No.**	**Name**	**No.**
Ethmoid	1	Mandible	1	Malleus	2
Frontal	1	Vomer	1	Incus	2
Occipital	1	Inferior nasal concha	2	Stapes	2
Sphenoid	1	Maxilla	2		
Parietal	2	Nasal	2		
Temporal	2	Palatine	2		
		Zygomatic	2		
Total	**8**		**12**		**6**

NERVES

Sensory innervation of the skull is provided by the meningeal branches of several of the cranial and cervical spinal nerves.

- The anterior cranial fossa is innervated by the ophthalmic nerve $[V_1]$ – the first division of the the trigeminal nerve [V] – which originates at the trigeminal ganglion. Ethmoidal nerves branch off the ophthalmic nerve $[V_1]$ and, in turn, branch into the meningeal branches that innervate the anterior cranial fossa.
- Meningeal branches of the other two branches of the trigeminal nerve [V], the maxillary $[V_2]$ and mandibular $[V_3]$ nerves, innervate the middle cranial fossa.
- Nerve fibers from the cervical spinal nerves C2 and C3 follow the hypoglossal nerve [XII] to the oral region and upper neck, where they innervate muscles and other structures.
- C2 fibers carried by the vagus nerve [X] supply the posterior cranial fossa.

Extracranial sensory innervation of the skull is provided by periosteal branches of the three divisions of the trigeminal nerve [V] – the ophthalmic nerve $[V_1]$, maxillary nerve $[V_2]$, and the mandibular nerve $[V_3]$. These branches supply the upper, middle, and lower thirds of the face, respectively. The posterior aspect of the skull is innervated by posterior rami of the greater occipital nerve (C2) and the third occipital nerve (C3).

BRAIN AND CRANIAL NERVES
Cranial nerves

Cranial nerves arise from the brain and brainstem and are paired and numbered in a craniocaudal sequence. They innervate structures in the head and neck. The vagus nerve [X] also innervates structures in the thorax and abdomen (see Table 3.4).

Brain

The brain has three primary regions: cerebrum, cerebellum and brainstem (Figs 3.3 and 3.4). The cerebrum is made up of four lobes. The **frontal lobe** is responsible for higher mental functions such as decision making. The **parietal lobe** plays a role in receiving sensory information, initiating movement and perception of objects. The **temporal lobe** is involved in memory, hearing and speech. The **occipital lobe** is responsible for vision. Left and right hemispheres of the cerebrum are joined in the midline by the **corpus callosum**, a

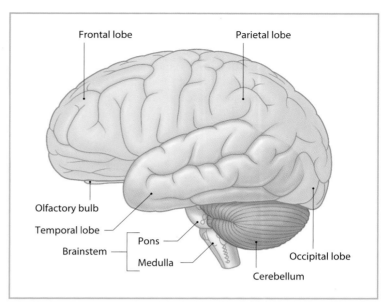

Figure 3.3 Lateral view of the brain (left side)

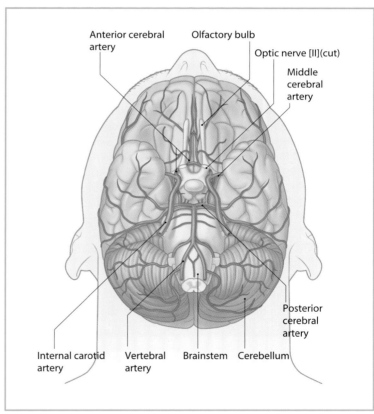

Figure 3.4 Inferior view of the arteries at the base of the brain

series of densely arranged nerve fibers that facilitate communication between hemispheres.

The **cerebellum**, a grooved region of the posterior inferior brain, is responsible for the maintenance of balance, posture and coordinated movements.

The **brainstem** is composed of the midbrain, pons and medulla oblongata. The **midbrain** is involved with coordination of eye

11

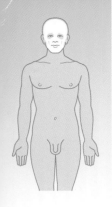

movements, hearing, and body movements. Axons from the cerebrum pass through it as they travel to areas of the body. The **pons** is anterior to the midbrain and regulates consciousness, sensory analysis and control of motor movements via the cerebellum. The most inferior part of the brainstem, the **medulla oblongata**, has a role in maintenance of vital functions such as breathing and heart rate.

ARTERIES

Blood is supplied to the meninges and bones of the neurocranium by small vessels originating from the anterior, middle, and posterior meningeal arteries:

- the **anterior meningeal artery** (Fig. 3.4) is a branch of the ophthalmic artery, which is itself a branch of the internal carotid artery;
- the **middle meningeal artery** is a branch of the maxillary artery, which supplies the middle cranial fossa and lateral wall of the neurocranium; the anterior branch of the middle meningeal artery runs deep to the pterion (the meeting point of the parietal, temporal, sphenoid and frontal bones), which is the thinnest part of the skull and the area most susceptible to trauma;
- the **posterior meningeal arteries** are derived from the occipital, ascending pharyngeal, and vertebral arteries.

The brain is supplied with blood by the two internal carotid arteries and two vertebral arteries. Within the cranial cavity, these vessels join to form the cerebral arterial circle (**circle of Willis**). The vertebral arteries contribute to the circle by ascending within the transverse foramina of the cervical vertebrae, entering the skull through the foramen magnum and uniting to form the **basilar artery**. The basilar artery divides to form two **posterior cerebral arteries** (Fig. 3.4).

The internal carotid arteries ascend through the neck and enter the skull through the carotid canal to join with the posterior cerebral arteries through the **posterior communicating artery**. Each internal carotid artery then gives off its terminal branches – the **middle cerebral** and **anterior cerebral arteries** – which form an anastomosis between the two anterior cerebral arteries through the **anterior communicating artery**, and so create the circle of Willis (Fig. 3.4). This arterial circle provides collateral circulation to the brain if one vessel becomes blocked.

VEINS AND LYMPHATICS

Venous drainage of the skull is provided by the **diploic**, **emissary**, and **meningeal veins**, which communicate with the venous dural sinuses within the cranium. These veins have no valves and can therefore conduct blood into or out of the cranial cavity, depending on the pressures within the venous sinuses of the skull. Most venous blood from the skull is returned to the internal jugular vein.

All lymph nodes and lymphatic vessels of the head and neck are extracranial; there are none within the cranial cavity.

■ CLINICAL CORRELATIONS
Skull fracture

A skull fracture may result from direct trauma to the head. If a skull fracture is diagnosed an associated brain injury must be suspected. The patient should remain still to prevent further disruption of the cranium and brain.

The first step when treating head trauma is to evaluate the patient's A, B, C:

TABLE 3.3 GLASGOW COMA SCALE				
Eye opening (E)	Score		Verbal (V)	Score
Spontaneous	4		Oriented	5
To speech	3		Confused conversation	4
To pain	2		Inappropriate words	3
No response	1		Incomprehensible sounds	2
			No response	1
Motor (M)	Score			
Obeys	6			
Localizes	5			
Withdraws	4		GCS score = E + V + M	
Flexion	3			
Extension	2			
No response	1			

- **A**irway – examine and treat the patient to ensure that the airway is open.
- **B**reathing – examine the patient to ensure that breathing is stable.
- **C**irculation – check that the patient's pulses and peripheral circulation are stable.

When evaluating and treating a patient with head trauma, a brief neurological examination such as the Glasgow Coma Scale (GCS; Table 3.3) is used to determine the level of consciousness and provide a measure of the extent of overall brain injury. This is followed by a full neurological examination.

Glasgow Coma Scale

The lowest GCS score (severe injury) is 3 and the highest GCS score (light injury) is 15. Patients with head trauma must be evaluated frequently because head and brain injuries are often unstable and the full extent of the injury does not develop fully until a few days after the initial trauma. A patient with an initial GCS score of 15 may nevertheless have significant brain injury, and subsequent GCS scores may become lower because the injury develops further.

Full examination of a patient with a suspected skull fracture includes frequent neurological examination, including GCS evaluation, and a computed tomography (CT) scan of the head to evaluate the soft (brain) and hard (bone) tissues.

Types of skull fracture

There are two relatively common types of skull fracture from direct trauma.

Depressed skull fractures usually involve the parietal or temporal regions (neurocranium). During the trauma, a piece of the internal table of bone is depressed. The edges of the fractured bone can lacerate the meninges, arteries, veins, and the brain. Treatment is usually surgical and involves elevating the depressed flap of bone.

Basilar skull fractures are linear fractures at the base of the skull. Small tears may develop in the dura mater and cause the clear CSF to leak through the ears (**CSF otorrhea**) or nose (**CSF rhinorrhea**). Bleeding can also occur into the middle ear and nose. Additional clinical characteristics of basilar skull fracture include periorbital ecchymosis (raccoon sign), retroauricular hematomas (Battle's sign), and cranial nerve deficits. Basilar skull fractures are usually stable, in that there is no depression of the fracture fragments.

Treatment is usually nonsurgical with close neurological observation. Basilar skull fractures are associated with many permanent sequelae, such as deafness and anosmia (inability to smell), because of damage to the cranial nerves.

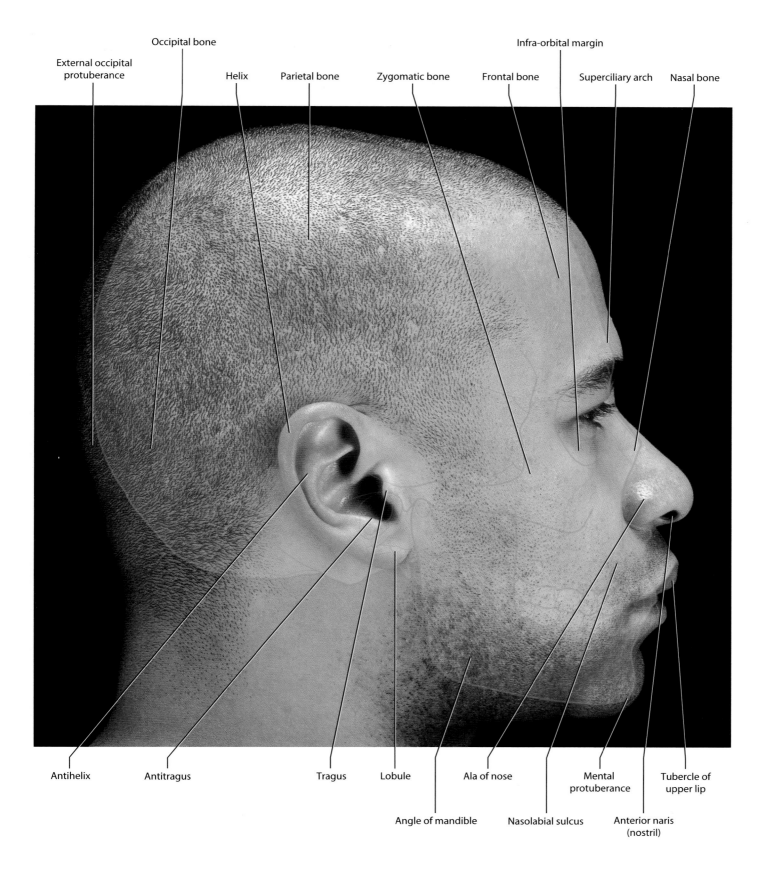

External occipital
protuberance

Occipital bone

Helix

Parietal bone

Zygomatic bone

Frontal bone

Infra-orbital margin

Superciliary arch

Nasal bone

Antihelix

Antitragus

Tragus

Lobule

Ala of nose

Mental
protuberance

Tubercle of
upper lip

Angle of mandible

Nasolabial sulcus

Anterior naris
(nostril)

Figure 3.5 Skull – surface anatomy. Lateral view of head and neck of a young male showing relevant anatomical landmarks

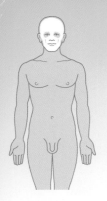

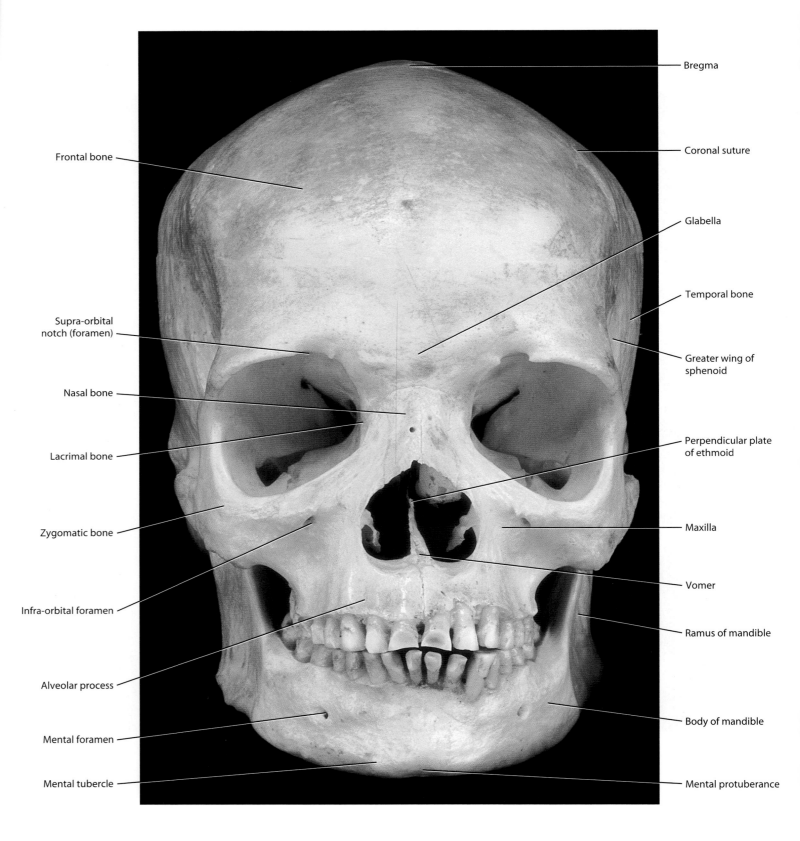

Bregma

Coronal suture

Glabella

Temporal bone

Greater wing of sphenoid

Perpendicular plate of ethmoid

Maxilla

Vomer

Ramus of mandible

Body of mandible

Mental protuberance

Frontal bone

Supra-orbital notch (foramen)

Nasal bone

Lacrimal bone

Zygomatic bone

Infra-orbital foramen

Alveolar process

Mental foramen

Mental tubercle

Figure 3.6 Skull – anterior view. Anterior view of skull (norma frontalis) showing bony relationships and relevant features. Note the worn appearance of the teeth, which resulted from grinding of the teeth and the advanced age of the individual at time of death

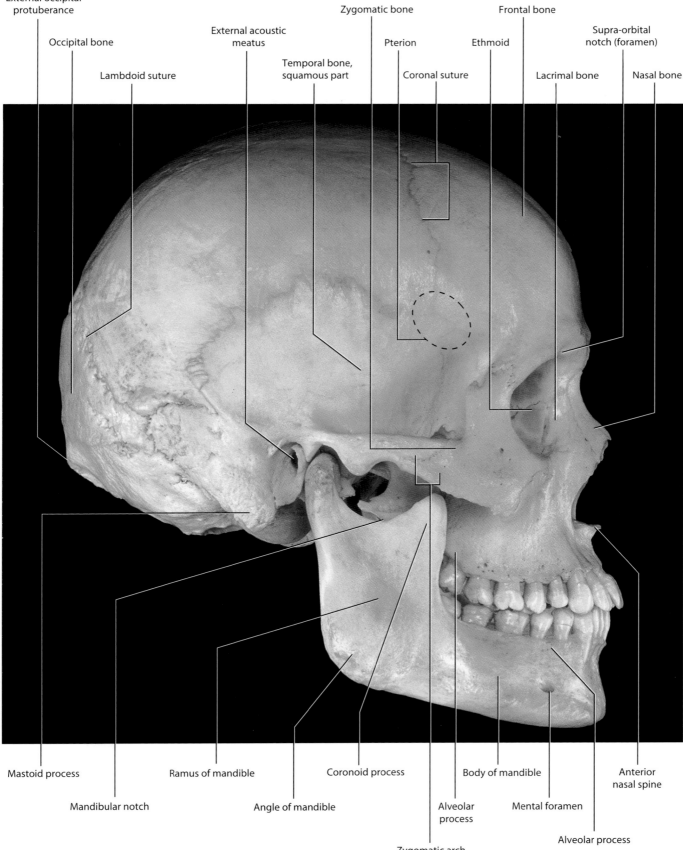

External occipital protuberance

Occipital bone

External acoustic meatus

Lambdoid suture

Temporal bone, squamous part

Zygomatic bone

Pterion

Coronal suture

Ethmoid

Frontal bone

Supra-orbital notch (foramen)

Lacrimal bone

Nasal bone

Mastoid process

Mandibular notch

Ramus of mandible

Angle of mandible

Coronoid process

Zygomatic arch

Alveolar process

Body of mandible

Mental foramen

Anterior nasal spine

Alveolar process

Figure 3.7 Skull – lateral view. Lateral view (norma lateralis) of the skull from the right side showing individual bones and their features. The skull bones are not completely fused, suggesting age at time of death to be approximately 40–60 years. Also note the presence of the third molar (wisdom tooth)

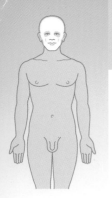

Anterior

Sagittal suture   Bregma   Frontal bone   Coronal suture   Parietal bone

Left   Right

Lambda   Occipital bone   Lambdoid suture

Posterior

Figure 3.8 Skull – superior view 1. Superior view showing major sutures of the skull. The corrugated sutures help interlock the bones of the skull and increase the strength of the entire neurocranium

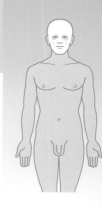

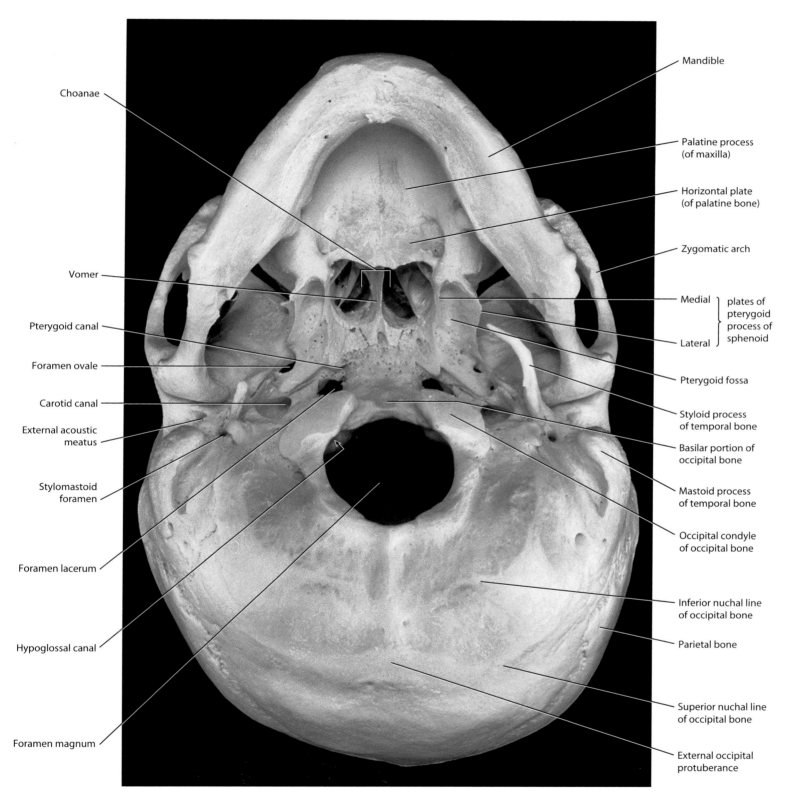

Choanae

Mandible

Palatine process
(of maxilla)

Horizontal plate
(of palatine bone)

Zygomatic arch

Vomer

Medial ⎤ plates of
⎥ pterygoid
⎥ process of
Lateral ⎦ sphenoid

Pterygoid canal

Pterygoid fossa

Foramen ovale

Carotid canal

Styloid process
of temporal bone

External acoustic
meatus

Basilar portion of
occipital bone

Stylomastoid
foramen

Mastoid process
of temporal bone

Occipital condyle
of occipital bone

Foramen lacerum

Inferior nuchal line
of occipital bone

Hypoglossal canal

Parietal bone

Superior nuchal line
of occipital bone

Foramen magnum

External occipital
protuberance

Figure 3.9 Skull – inferior view 1. Inferior view (norma basalis) of the skull with the mandible shown in its normal articulated position. Trauma has occurred to the right styloid process, which is partially broken off

17

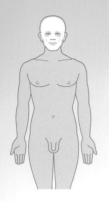

Skull   **HEAD AND NECK**

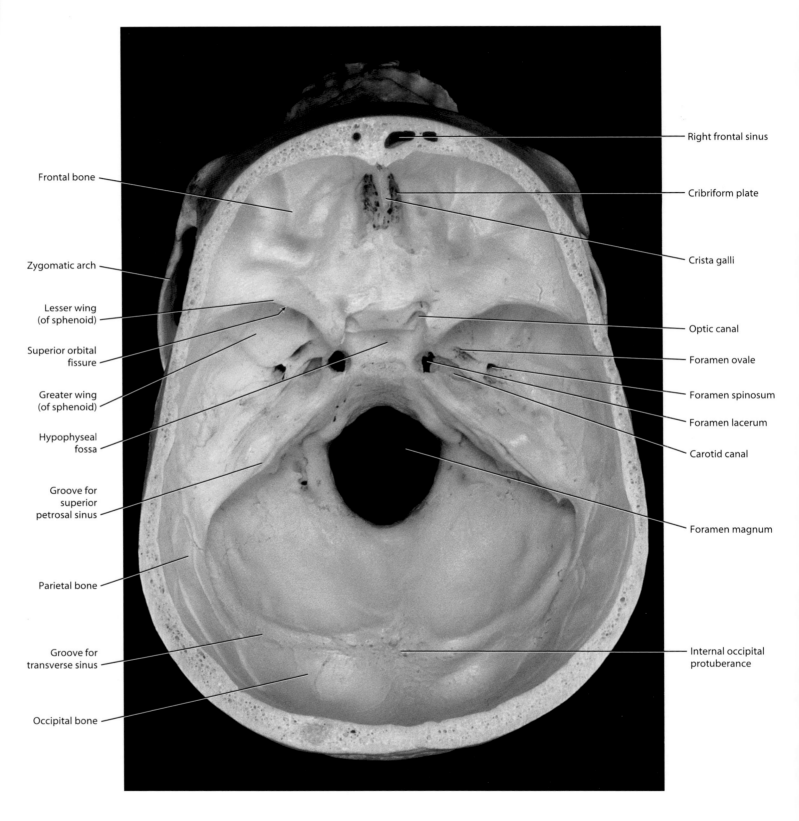

Frontal bone

Zygomatic arch

Lesser wing
(of sphenoid)

Superior orbital
fissure

Greater wing
(of sphenoid)

Hypophyseal
fossa

Groove for
superior
petrosal sinus

Parietal bone

Groove for
transverse sinus

Occipital bone

Right frontal sinus

Cribriform plate

Crista galli

Optic canal

Foramen ovale

Foramen spinosum

Foramen lacerum

Carotid canal

Foramen magnum

Internal occipital
protuberance

Figure 3.10 Skull – superior view 2. The calvarium (upper bones of the skull which cover the brain) has been removed. Note the anterior, middle, and posterior cranial fossae, which support the brain, and the absence of the left frontal sinus

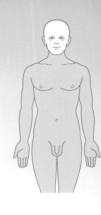

	Cranial nerve	Opening	Primary function	Symptoms of damaged nerve
		TABLE 3.4 THE CRANIAL NERVES AND THE SKULL OPENINGS THROUGH WHICH THEY PASS		
I	Olfactory	Cribriform plate	Smell	Anosmia
II	Optic	Optic canal	Vision	Visual impairment
III	Oculomotor	Superior orbital fissure	Eyeball and upper eyelid movement *Pupillary constriction, accommodation	Ptosis, external strabismus Dilated pupil and poor accommodation
IV	Trochlear	Superior orbital fissure	Superior oblique	Extortion
V	Trigeminal Ophthalmic nerve [V_1] Maxillary nerve [V_2] Mandibular nerve [V_3]	Superior orbital fissure Foramen rotundum Foraman ovale	Sensation, eyeball, anterior scalp, upper face Sensation to midface Muscles of mastication, sensation to lower third of face	Sensory loss to forehead Sensory loss to upper cheek Impaired chewing, loss of sensation to lower jaw
VI	Abducent	Superior orbital fissure	Lateral rectus	Strabismus
VII	Facial	Internal acoustic meatus – stylomastoid foramen	Muscles of facial expression. *Secretomotor to lacrimal, nasal, palatine, submandibular and sublingual glands	Facial palsy, weakness *No tearing, dry mouth Loss of taste to anterior two-thirds of tongue
VIII	Vestibulocochlear	Internal acoustic meatus	Hearing, equilibrium, position in space	Deafness and/or loss of balance
IX	Glossopharyngeal	Jugular foramen	Sensory to oropharynx, posterior one-third of tongue, carotid body and sinus Taste posterior one-third of tongue Stylopharyngeus *Parotid gland	Rarely involved Loss of taste to posterior one-third of tongue Dry mouth
X	Vagus	Jugular foramen	Sensory to mucous membrane of larynx, pharynx, trachea, lungs, esophagus, stomach, intestines, gallbladder, and skin around ear Taste: epiglottis region *Cardiac muscle, smooth muscle, and glands of foregut and midgut	Impaired cough reflex
XI	Accessory Cranial root Spinal root (C1 to C5)	Jugular foramen Foramen magnum and jugular foramen	Muscles of pharynx, larynx, and palate Muscles of pharynx, larynx, and palate Sternocleidomastoid and trapezius muscles	Impaired swallowing, hoarseness (dependent on site of lesion) Impaired head and neck movement, inability to shrug shoulder
XII	Hypoglossal	Hypoglossal canal	Tongue muscles	Impaired motor control of tongue and speech

*Parasympathetics

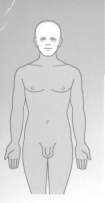

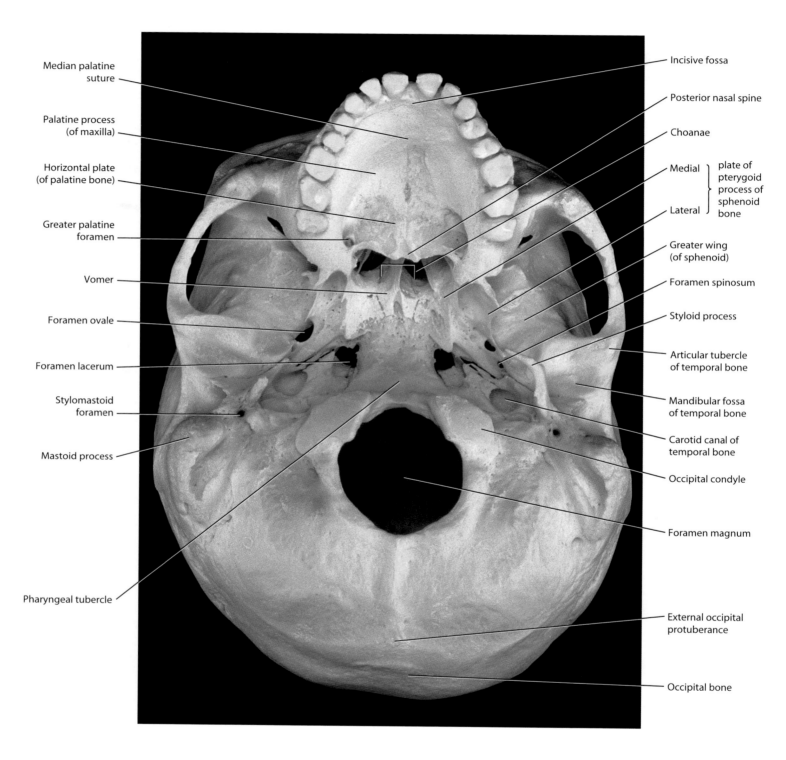

Median palatine suture

Palatine process (of maxilla)

Horizontal plate (of palatine bone)

Greater palatine foramen

Vomer

Foramen ovale

Foramen lacerum

Stylomastoid foramen

Mastoid process

Pharyngeal tubercle

Incisive fossa

Posterior nasal spine

Choanae

Medial ⎱ plate of
⎰ pterygoid
   process of
   sphenoid
Lateral ⎰ bone

Greater wing (of sphenoid)

Foramen spinosum

Styloid process

Articular tubercle of temporal bone

Mandibular fossa of temporal bone

Carotid canal of temporal bone

Occipital condyle

Foramen magnum

External occipital protuberance

Occipital bone

Figure 3.11 Skull – inferior view 2. The mandible has been removed. Observe the size of the foramen magnum, which permits passage of the spinal cord, and also the curved zygomatic bones (cheek bones)

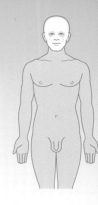

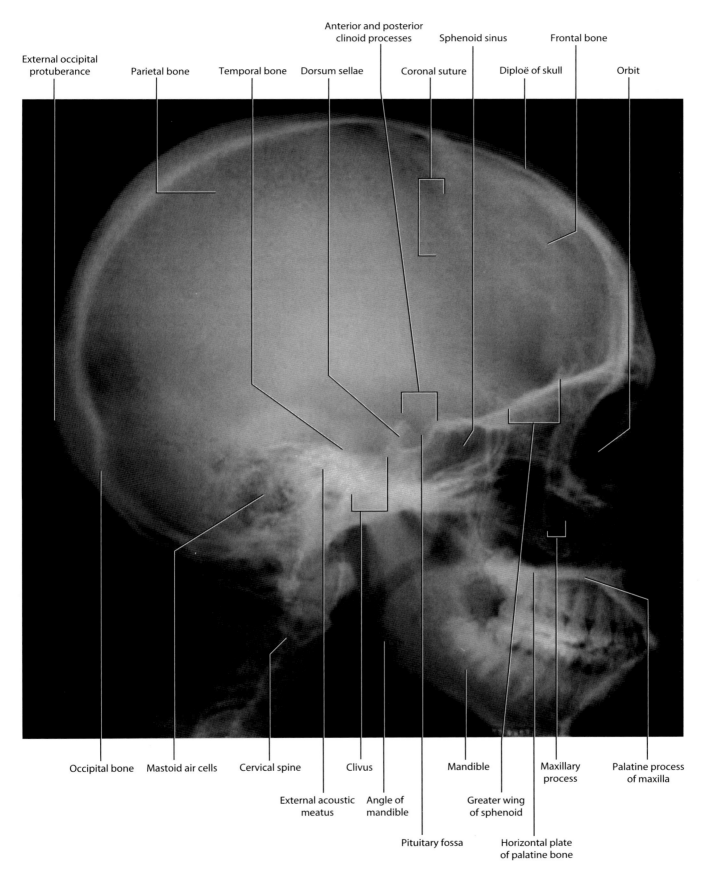

External occipital
protuberance

Parietal bone

Temporal bone

Dorsum sellae

Anterior and posterior
clinoid processes

Coronal suture

Sphenoid sinus

Diploë of skull

Frontal bone

Orbit

Occipital bone

Mastoid air cells

Cervical spine

Clivus

Mandible

Maxillary
process

Palatine process
of maxilla

External acoustic
meatus

Angle of
mandible

Greater wing
of sphenoid

Pituitary fossa

Horizontal plate
of palatine bone

Figure 3.12 Skull – lateral plain film radiograph. Bone landmarks, including those in the midline, are seen. Soft tissues are not well-visualized on skull radiographs. In this view, the bones of the calvarium are seen as having an inner and outer layer separated by the diploë

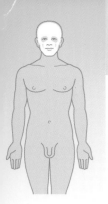

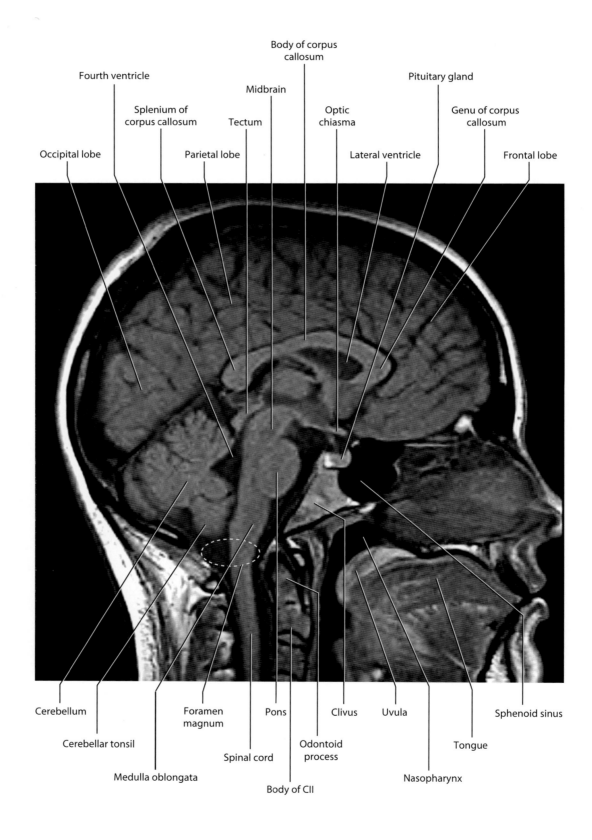

Body of corpus callosum

Fourth ventricle

Midbrain

Pituitary gland

Splenium of corpus callosum

Tectum

Optic chiasma

Genu of corpus callosum

Occipital lobe

Parietal lobe

Lateral ventricle

Frontal lobe

Cerebellum

Foramen magnum

Pons

Clivus

Uvula

Sphenoid sinus

Cerebellar tonsil

Odontoid process

Tongue

Spinal cord

Nasopharynx

Medulla oblongata

Body of CII

Figure 3.13 Skull – sagittal MRI. Note the excellent visualization of the detail of midline structures of the brain. The bones of the skull appear black, as do the sinuses

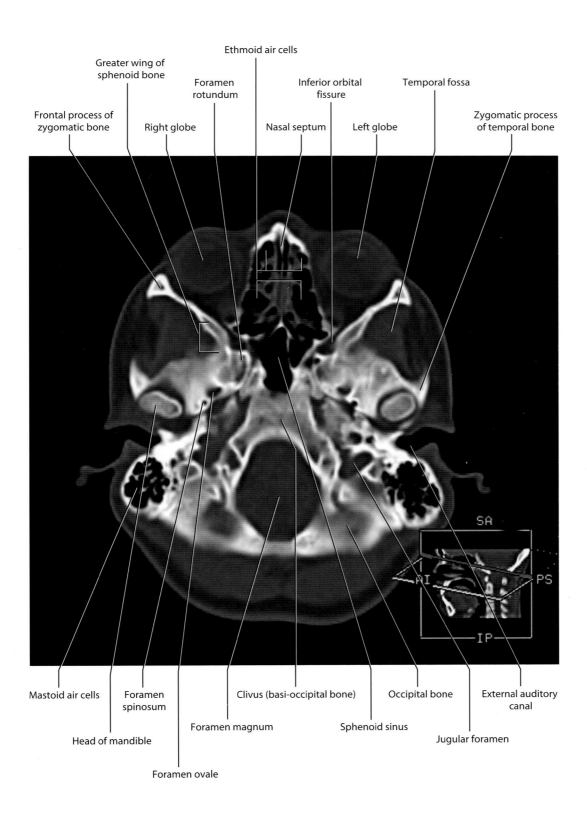

Ethmoid air cells

Greater wing of
sphenoid bone

Foramen
rotundum

Inferior orbital
fissure

Temporal fossa

Frontal process of
zygomatic bone

Right globe

Nasal septum

Left globe

Zygomatic process
of temporal bone

Mastoid air cells

Foramen
spinosum

Clivus (basi-occipital bone)

Occipital bone

External auditory
canal

Head of mandible

Foramen magnum

Sphenoid sinus

Jugular foramen

Foramen ovale

Figure 3.14 Skull – CT scan (axial view). Note the clarity of many of the foramina at the skull base. The largest is the foramen magnum, through which the spinal cord passes

4 Scalp and face

The scalp and face are two interconnected regions on the superior, lateral, and anterior surfaces of the skull. The strong, layered structure of the scalp, which includes hairbearing skin, helps protect the skull and brain.

The face is on the anterior surface of the skull. It contains openings for sight, smell, respiration, and nutrient intake through the orbits, nose, and mouth, respectively. Small changes in the muscles of facial expression of the face convey different emotions and expressions.

The scalp is supported by the bones of the neurocranium (see Chapter 3) and the face is supported by some of the smaller, more complex bones of the viscerocranium (see Chapter 3).

SCALP

The scalp extends from the supra-orbital margin of the frontal bone (**superciliary arch**) on the anterior skull (see Chapter 3) to the **superior nuchal line** on the posterior aspect of the skull (see Chapter 27). Laterally, it extends to the level of the **zygomatic arches**. The five layers of the scalp can be remembered by the acronym SCALP:

- **S**kin – containing the hair follicles, sebaceous glands, and sweat glands.
- **C**onnective tissue – a layer of strong collagen fibers mixed with small amounts of fatty tissue, and containing the blood vessels and superficial nerves.
- **A**poneurosis – a thick sheet of collagen fibers that extends between the frontalis and occipitalis muscles. These two muscles are responsible for the voluntary ability to slide the scalp back and forth across the skull and to wrinkle the forehead.
- **L**oose connective tissue ('danger zone') – a layer of collagen fibers mixed with large amounts of fatty tissue. This contains the emissary veins, which are special valveless veins that transport blood from within the skull to the veins of the scalp, so providing some of the venous drainage for the brain and allowing for the potential spread of infection.
- **P**ericranium (periosteum) – a richly innervated covering composed of dense, interweaving collagen fibers. It is loosely attached to the surface of the skull, except at the suture lines, where it passes between the skull bones, contributing to their joints. The periosteum is continuous with the periosteal layer of the dura mater within the skull.

Nerves

Motor innervation to the scalp muscles is provided by branches of the facial nerve [VII]. At the level of the ear, the sensory innervation to the scalp divides into anterior cutaneous innervation and posterior cutaneous innervation (Fig. 4.1). Anterior to the ear, the scalp is mostly innervated by branches of the divisions of the trigeminal nerve [V]:

- the **supratrochlear** and **supra-orbital nerves** (from the ophthalmic nerve [V_1]);
- the **zygomaticotemporal nerve** (from the maxillary nerve [V_2]);
- the **auriculotemporal nerve** (from the mandibular nerve [V_3]).

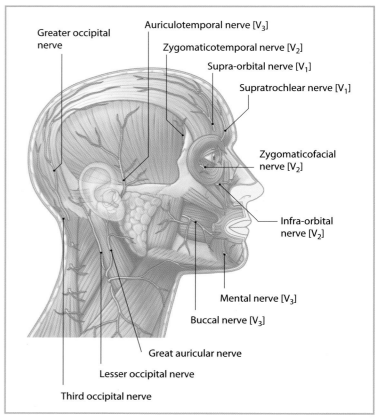

Figure 4.1 Nerves of the scalp and face (lateral view)

Posterior to the ear, the scalp receives cutaneous innervation from the spinal cutaneous nerves that originate in the neck (C2, C3):

- **greater occipital nerve** (C2),
- **lesser occipital nerve** (C2, C3), and
- **third occipital nerve** (C3).

Arteries

Blood is supplied to the scalp by four small arteries – the **supratrochlear** and **supra-orbital arteries**, which are branches of the ophthalmic artery (a branch of the internal carotid artery), and the **superficial temporal artery** and **occipital arteries**, branches of the external carotid artery.

Veins and lymphatics

Venous drainage is along the venae comitantes of the arteries:

- the **supra-orbital** and **supratrochlear veins** unite at the medial canthus of the eye to form the **facial vein**;
- the **superficial temporal vein** joins the **maxillary vein** to create the **retromandibular vein** just posterior to the neck of the mandible;
- the **posterior auricular vein** originates behind the ear and channels venous blood from the posterior scalp towards the external jugular vein.

Lymph drains from the scalp to the superficial horizontal ring of superficial lymph nodes at the junction between the head and neck. Some lymph also drains directly to the deep cervical lymph nodes (see Chapter 12).

FACE

Muscles and nerves

The face extends laterally from ear to ear, and from the chin to the hairline on the forehead. The skin of the face is thick and vascular. Beneath the skin is the subcutaneous fascia, which contains the muscles of facial expression, blood vessels, and nerves (Fig. 4.2). The face contains the organs of sight – the eyes – and the proximal portions of the respiratory and digestive systems – the nose and mouth, respectively.

The muscles of the face insert into the skin (Fig. 4.3), which allows them to move the skin of the face in complex ways. The facial nerve [VII] innervates the muscles of facial expression (Fig. 4.4). It has five main branches. From superior to inferior these branches are:

- temporal,
- zygomatic,
- buccal,
- marginal mandibular, and
- cervical.

The temporal branches extend towards the muscles around the temporal bone; the zygomatic branches extend toward the cheek bones and cheek area; the buccal branches extend to the muscles around the mouth, and cervical branches extend to the upper part of the neck (the platysma muscle).

Sensory innervation to the face is from the trigeminal nerve [V] (Fig. 4.2), which has three major divisions:

- the ophthalmic nerve [V_1] supplies the structures around the eye and orbit through its five branches (the **supratrochlear**, **supra-orbital**, **lacrimal**, **infratrochlear**, and **external nasal nerves**);

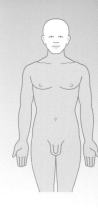

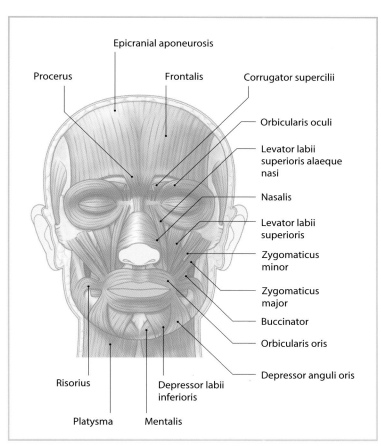

Figure 4.3 Facial muscles (anterior view)

Epicranial aponeurosis
Procerus
Frontalis
Corrugator supercilii
Orbicularis oculi
Levator labii superioris alaeque nasi
Nasalis
Levator labii superioris
Zygomaticus minor
Zygomaticus major
Buccinator
Orbicularis oris
Depressor anguli oris
Risorius
Depressor labii inferioris
Platysma
Mentalis

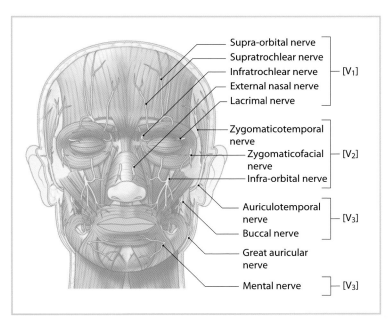

Figure 4.2 Sensory innervation of the face: trigeminal nerve [V]

Supra-orbital nerve
Supratrochlear nerve
Infratrochlear nerve — [V_1]
External nasal nerve
Lacrimal nerve
Zygomaticotemporal nerve
Zygomaticofacial nerve — [V_2]
Infra-orbital nerve
Auriculotemporal nerve — [V_3]
Buccal nerve
Great auricular nerve
Mental nerve — [V_3]

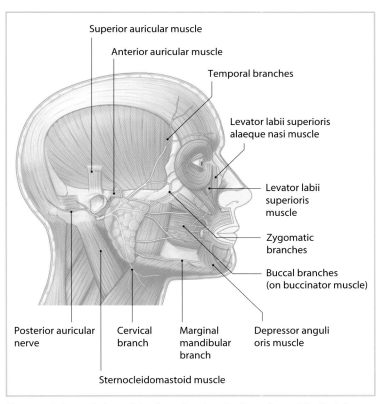

Figure 4.4 Lateral view of the face showing the branches of the facial nerve [VII]

Superior auricular muscle
Anterior auricular muscle
Temporal branches
Levator labii superioris alaeque nasi muscle
Levator labii superioris muscle
Zygomatic branches
Buccal branches (on buccinator muscle)
Posterior auricular nerve
Cervical branch
Marginal mandibular branch
Depressor anguli oris muscle
Sternocleidomastoid muscle

- the maxillary nerve [V_2] provides sensation to the central part of the face through its **infra-orbital**, **zygomaticofacial**, and **zygomaticotemporal nerve** branches;
- the mandibular nerve [V_3] provides sensation to all structures in and around the mandible through the **auriculotemporal**, **mental**, and **buccal nerves**.

Arteries

Blood is supplied to the face by branches of the internal and external carotid arteries (Fig. 4.5). The **facial artery** is a branch of the external carotid artery. It ascends across the face – from lateral to medial – ending at the medial canthus of the eye as the **angular artery**, which anastomoses with small vessels from the orbit. The second primary source of blood to the face is from the **superficial temporal artery**, which is one of the terminal branches of the external carotid artery. When the superficial temporal artery is still within the mass of the parotid gland it gives off the **transverse facial artery**, which travels toward the middle of the face just inferior to the zygomatic arches (cheek bones). The **maxillary artery** (see Fig. 2.2), the second terminal branch of the external carotid artery, supplies the structures associated with the upper and lower jaws.

Veins and lymphatics

Venous drainage of the face is through the facial vein (see Fig. 2.3), which runs alongside the facial artery, and the transverse facial vein, which likewise follows the course of its associated artery. Some small veins also communicate with the **cavernous sinus** within the skull. This connection of facial venous drainage with intracranial venous drainage accounts for the spread of some infections from the face to the brain.

Lymphatic drainage of the upper face and forehead is to the **submandibular nodes** along the inferior margin of the mandible. Lymph from the lower face and mandible also flows toward the submandibular nodes and **submental nodes** (see Fig. 2.2), from where it usually drains to the deep cervical nodes on the carotid sheath in the neck (see Chapter 12).

◼ CLINICAL CORRELATIONS
Scalp laceration

Because the scalp has five layers, lacerations can vary in depth (Fig. 4.6). The arteries of the scalp in layer 2 (the connective tissue layer) are adherent to the surrounding tissues. When a scalp artery is lacerated, the cut end of the artery cannot retract into the scalp because of its strong attachment to the surrounding connective tissue, resulting in continuous bleeding until direct pressure is applied to the wound. (In other soft tissues, such as the anterior forearm, lacerated arteries retract into the surrounding muscle tissue and contract, causing bleeding to stop.

If significant bleeding is suspected a complete blood count will reveal whether the patient has anemia secondary to blood loss. In more serious cases the patient appears pale, lethargic (very tired), and has a low blood pressure. Intravenous fluids are then needed to replace blood loss. If the complete blood count results show significant anemia, blood transfusion may be necessary. After direct pressure has been applied to the wound and any blood loss-related deficiencies have been treated (with either intravenous fluids or blood transfusion) the wound is sutured. The important clinical principles are:

- prevent further bleeding;
- then stabilize the intravascular volume;
- then treat the laceration.

Facial nerve [VII] paresis

Facial nerve [VII] paresis (weakness) is usually one-sided and can involve just the upper or lower face or the entire side of the face.

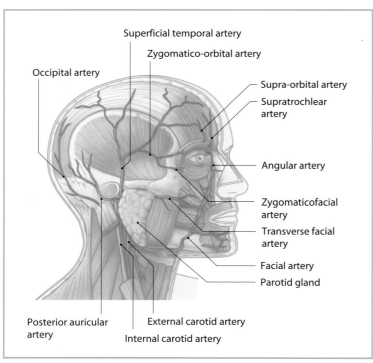

Figure 4.5 Anterolateral view of the arterial supply of the scalp and face

Occipital artery
Superficial temporal artery
Zygomatico-orbital artery
Supra-orbital artery
Supratrochlear artery
Angular artery
Zygomaticofacial artery
Transverse facial artery
Facial artery
Parotid gland
Posterior auricular artery
External carotid artery
Internal carotid artery

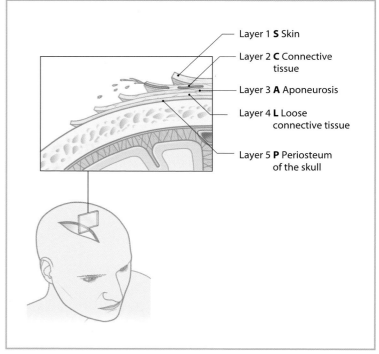

Figure 4.6 Laceration of the scalp

Layer 1 **S** Skin
Layer 2 **C** Connective tissue
Layer 3 **A** Aponeurosis
Layer 4 **L** Loose connective tissue
Layer 5 **P** Periosteum of the skull

The many causes can be grouped into three major categories – trauma, infection, and neoplasm (tumors and cancer).

The facial nerve [VII] provides motor innervation for all muscles of facial expression and the scalp muscles, and for sensory innervation to the anterior two-thirds of the tongue (including taste) and a small portion about the external acoustic meatus (of the ear). It originates from the brain and travels through the temporal bone, entering the internal acoustic meatus and lying close to the vestibulocochlear nerve [VIII]. From here the facial nerve [VII] travels inferiorly and leaves the skull through the stylomastoid foramen of the temporal bone.

Facial nerve [VII] paresis usually causes difficulty in activities such as eating. Some patients report drooling and an inability to close the eye before noticing the facial asymmetry. Other symptoms include dry eyes or increased tear secretion, blurry vision, pain around the ear, impaired taste, decreased or increased hearing ability, and difficulty swallowing.

On examination the patient will have some visible facial asymmetry, manifested by drooping of the corner of the mouth, sagging eyebrows and inferior eyelid, and an inability to close the affected eye. Sensation will be intact because it is provided by the trigeminal nerve [V]. Blood tests may be carried out to determine whether an infection is causing the paresis. If an intracranial cause of facial paresis is suspected computed tomography (CT) or magnetic resonance imaging (MRI) scans are obtained. Head CT is routine for facial nerve [VII] paresis secondary to trauma.

Traumatic facial nerve [VII] paresis is not common, but is easily diagnosed during the clinical evaluation of a patient with a head injury. The facial nerve [VII], which has a circuitous route in the skull, is easily injured in temporal bone fractures. Treatment of facial nerve [VII] paresis involves surgery only if the clinician has good reason to believe the nerve has been transected.

Bell's palsy is an idiopathic (unknown) facial nerve [VII] paralysis that is thought to have a viral cause. An illness, usually respiratory, precedes the paralysis. Facial nerve [VII] inflammation within the inflexible skull is thought to be the cause. Therefore treatment, usually with corticosteroids, aims to decrease the inflammation. Neoplasms (tumors) within or adjacent to the facial nerve [VII] can cause paresis (weakness) or paralysis. Patients are sent to the oncologist for assessment and possible surgical removal of the tumor.

In some cases of facial nerve [VII] paresis, whether caused by trauma, infection, or neoplasm, nerve function does not return.

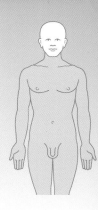

MNEMONICS	
Facial nerve branches:	**Two Zebras Bit My Calf** (**T**emporal, **Z**ygomatic, **B**uccal, **M**andibular, **C**ervical)
Layers of the scalp:	**SCALP** (**S**kin, **C**utaneous tissue, **A**poneurosis, **L**oose connective tissue, **P**ericranium)

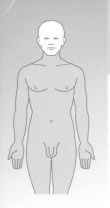

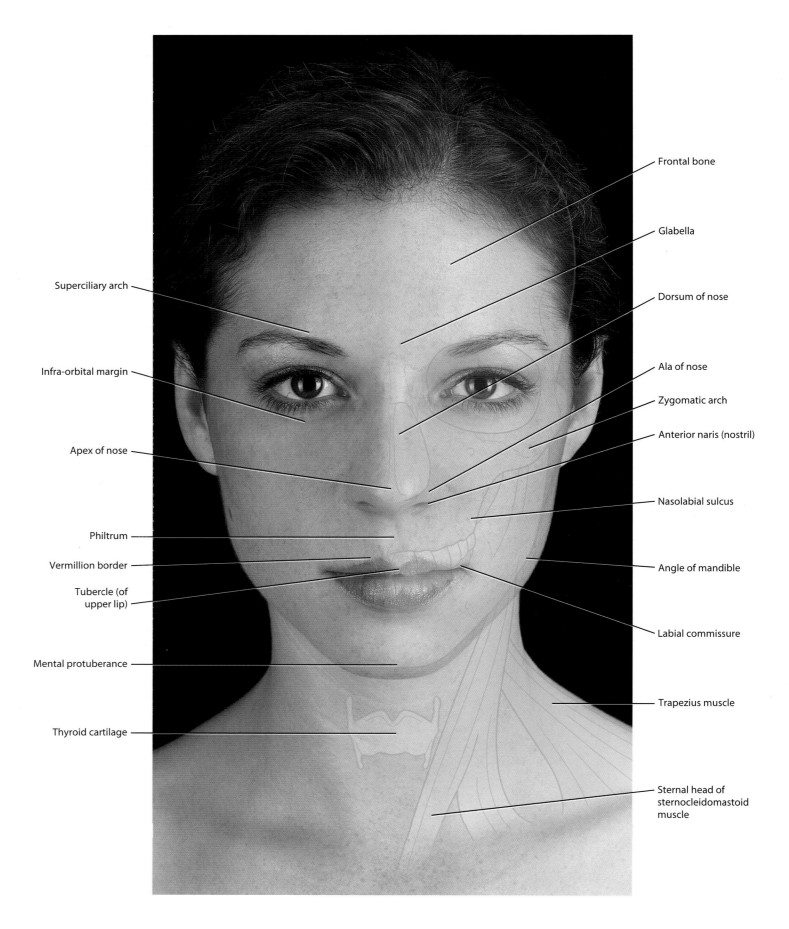

Frontal bone

Glabella

Dorsum of nose

Ala of nose

Zygomatic arch

Anterior naris (nostril)

Nasolabial sulcus

Angle of mandible

Labial commissure

Trapezius muscle

Sternal head of
sternocleidomastoid
muscle

Superciliary arch

Infra-orbital margin

Apex of nose

Philtrum

Vermillion border

Tubercle (of
upper lip)

Mental protuberance

Thyroid cartilage

Figure 4.7 Face – surface anatomy. Anterior view of the face of a female (age 25 years). Observe the border between the facial skin and upper lip known as Cupid's bow

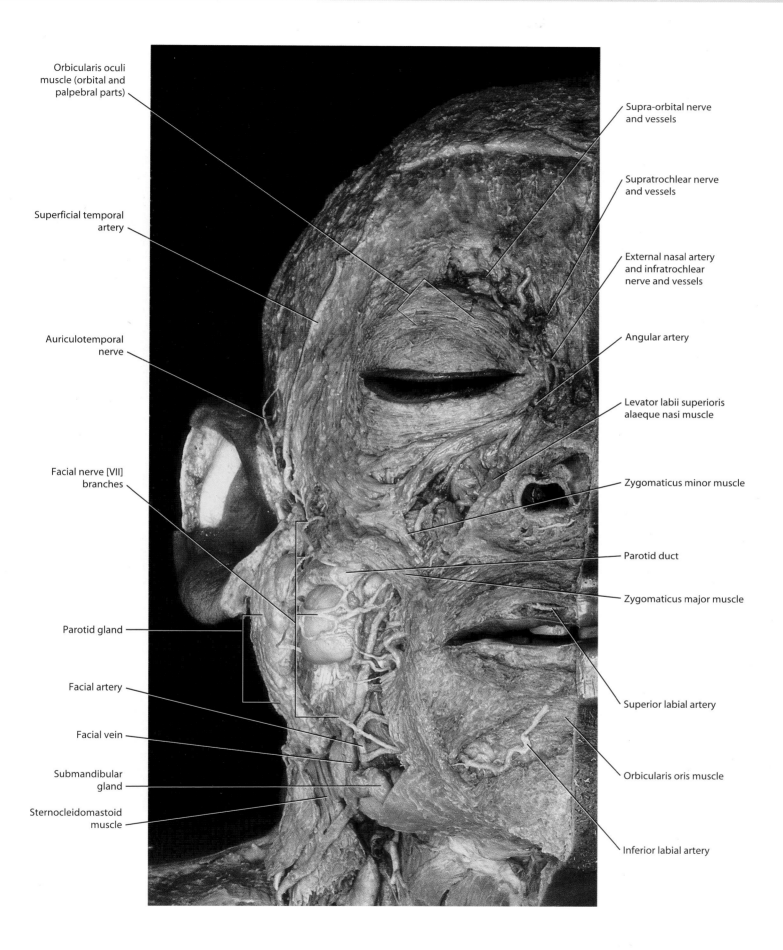

Orbicularis oculi muscle (orbital and palpebral parts)

Superficial temporal artery

Auriculotemporal nerve

Facial nerve [VII] branches

Parotid gland

Facial artery

Facial vein

Submandibular gland

Sternocleidomastoid muscle

Supra-orbital nerve and vessels

Supratrochlear nerve and vessels

External nasal artery and infratrochlear nerve and vessels

Angular artery

Levator labii superioris alaeque nasi muscle

Zygomaticus minor muscle

Parotid duct

Zygomaticus major muscle

Superior labial artery

Orbicularis oris muscle

Inferior labial artery

Figure 4.8 Face – superficial anterior dissection. Anterior view of facial muscles. This individual was approximately 40–50 years old. Observe the path of the facial artery and vein in relationship to the location of the parotid gland

29

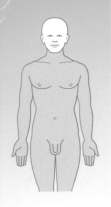

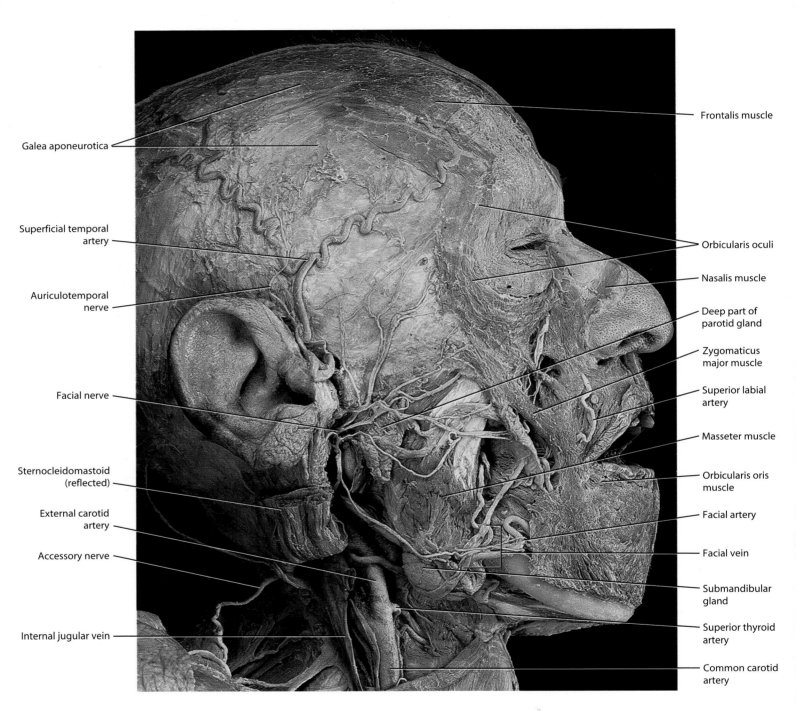

Galea aponeurotica

Superficial temporal
artery

Auriculotemporal
nerve

Facial nerve

Sternocleidomastoid
(reflected)

External carotid
artery

Accessory nerve

Internal jugular vein

Frontalis muscle

Orbicularis oculi

Nasalis muscle

Deep part of
parotid gland

Zygomaticus
major muscle

Superior labial
artery

Masseter muscle

Orbicularis oris
muscle

Facial artery

Facial vein

Submandibular
gland

Superior thyroid
artery

Common carotid
artery

30   **Figure 4.9 Face – superficial lateral dissection 1.** A portion of the parotid gland has been removed to show the branches of the facial nerve

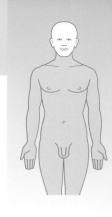

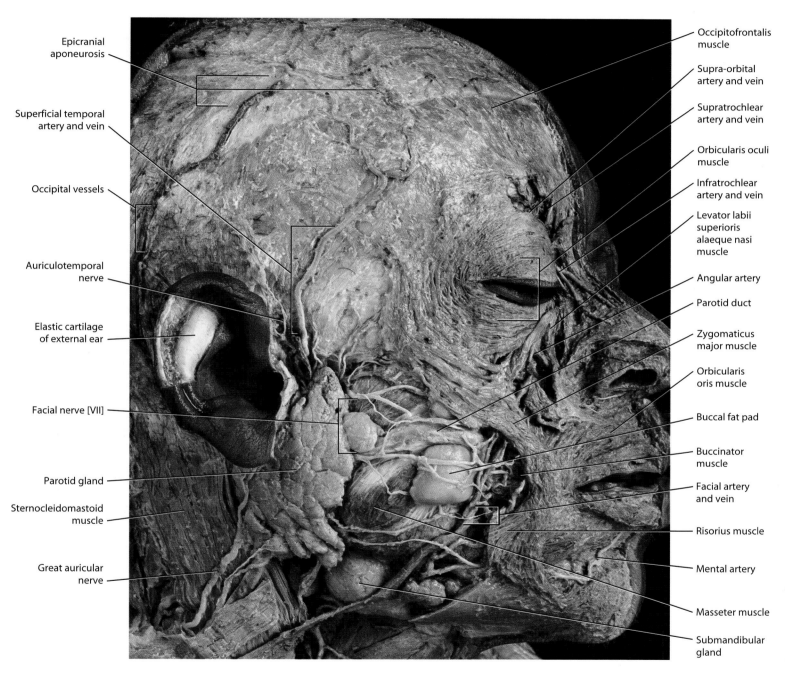

Epicranial aponeurosis

Superficial temporal artery and vein

Occipital vessels

Auriculotemporal nerve

Elastic cartilage of external ear

Facial nerve [VII]

Parotid gland

Sternocleidomastoid muscle

Great auricular nerve

Occipitofrontalis muscle

Supra-orbital artery and vein

Supratrochlear artery and vein

Orbicularis oculi muscle

Infratrochlear artery and vein

Levator labii superioris alaeque nasi muscle

Angular artery

Parotid duct

Zygomaticus major muscle

Orbicularis oris muscle

Buccal fat pad

Buccinator muscle

Facial artery and vein

Risorius muscle

Mental artery

Masseter muscle

Submandibular gland

Figure 4.10 Face – superficial lateral dissection 2. The parotid duct is visible between the buccal fat pad and zygomaticus major muscle. Also observe the relationship of the facial artery and vein to the parotid duct

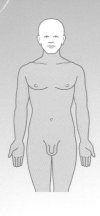

HEAD AND NECK

Scalp and face

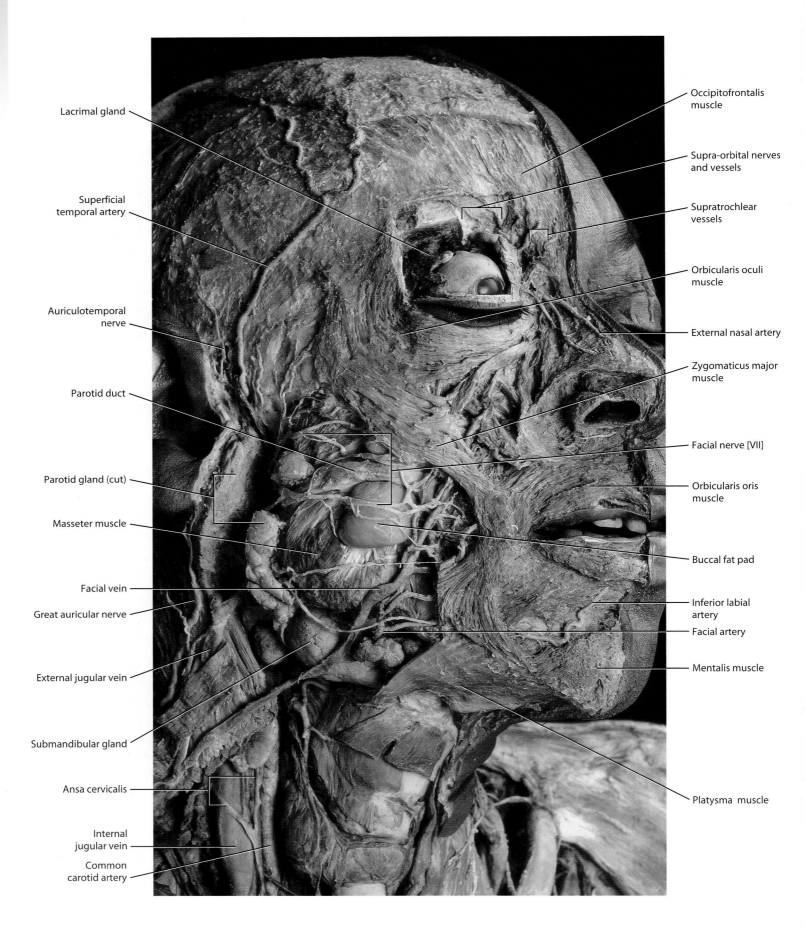

Lacrimal gland

Superficial
temporal artery

Auriculotemporal
nerve

Parotid duct

Parotid gland (cut)

Masseter muscle

Facial vein

Great auricular nerve

External jugular vein

Submandibular gland

Ansa cervicalis

Internal
jugular vein

Common
carotid artery

Occipitofrontalis
muscle

Supra-orbital nerves
and vessels

Supratrochlear
vessels

Orbicularis oculi
muscle

External nasal artery

Zygomaticus major
muscle

Facial nerve [VII]

Orbicularis oris
muscle

Buccal fat pad

Inferior labial
artery

Facial artery

Mentalis muscle

Platysma muscle

Figure 4.11 Face – superficial lateral dissection 3. This anterolateral view highlights the muscles of facial expression

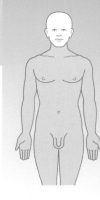

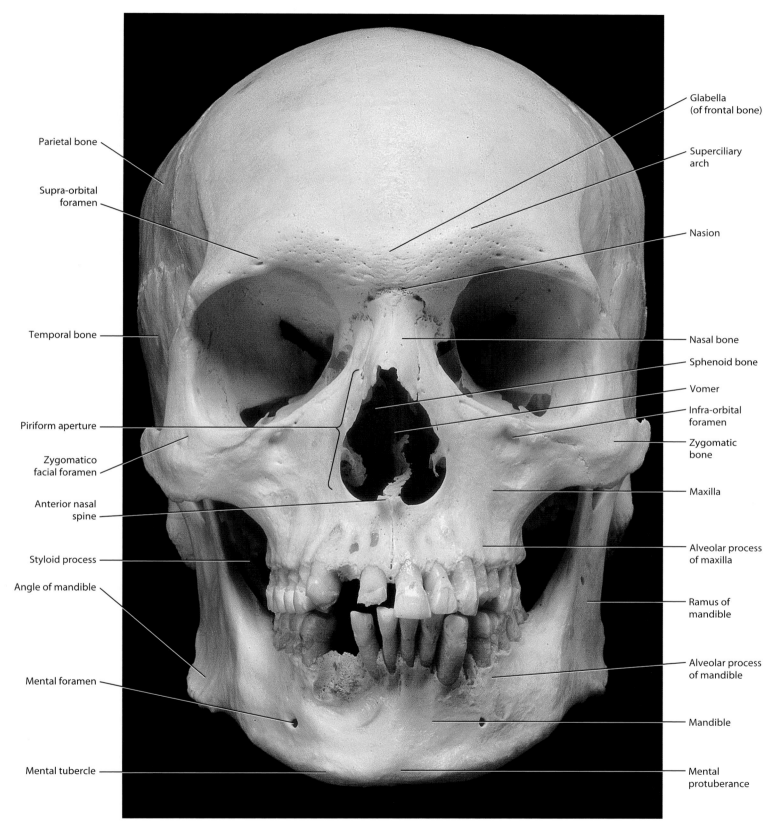

Parietal bone

Supra-orbital foramen

Temporal bone

Piriform aperture

Zygomatico facial foramen

Anterior nasal spine

Styloid process

Angle of mandible

Mental foramen

Mental tubercle

Glabella (of frontal bone)

Superciliary arch

Nasion

Nasal bone

Sphenoid bone

Vomer

Infra-orbital foramen

Zygomatic bone

Maxilla

Alveolar process of maxilla

Ramus of mandible

Alveolar process of mandible

Mandible

Mental protuberance

Figure 4.12 Face – osteology. The zygomatic (cheek) bones are prominent in this individual. Observe the location of the sphenoid bone deep within the nasal region

33

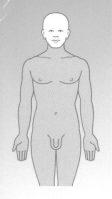

TABLE 4.1 MUSCLES OF FACIAL EXPRESSION

Muscle	Origin	Insertion	Action	Nerve supply	Blood supply
Muscles of the external ear Anterior auricular	Temporal fascia and scalp (aponeurosis)	Anterior part of medial aspect of helix	Pulls ear anteriorly	Facial nerve [VII] – temporal branches	Superficial temporal artery
Posterior auricular	Posterior surface mastoid process	Posterior, inferior medial part of auricle	Pulls ear posteriorly	Facial nerve [VII] – posterior auricular branches	Posterior auricular artery
Superior auricular	Aponeurosis of scalp and temporal fascia	Superior medial surface of auricle	Pulls ear superiorly	Facial nerve [VII] – temporal branches	Superficial temporal artery
Muscles of forehead and scalp Procerus	Nasal bone and lateral nasal cartilage	Glabellar skin	Transverse wrinkles over bridge of nose	Facial nerve [VII] – temporal, zygomatic and buccal branches	Facial artery – angular and lateral nasal branches
Corrugator	Medial aspect of supra-orbital margin	Skin of medial side of eyebrow	Pulls eyebrow down and medial, produces vertical wrinkles	Facial nerve [VII] – zygomatic and temporal branches	Superficial temporal artery
Frontalis	Aponeurosis of scalp	Skin of forehead	Elevates eyebrows, pulls scalp forward	Facial nerve [VII] – temporal branch	Superficial temporal artery – frontal branch
Occipitalis	Superior nuchal line and mastoid process	Skin of occipital region	Pulls skin posteriorly	Facial nerve [VII] – posterior auricular branch	Posterior auricular and occipital arteries
Muscles of the eye Orbicularis oculi	Orbital part – medial orbital margin	Medial palpebral ligament	Forceable closure of eyelids	Facial nerve [VII] – temporal and zygomatic branches	Superficial temporal artery and angular branch of facial artery
	Palpebral part – medial palpebral ligament	Palpebral raphe	Gentle closure of eyelids		
	Lacrimal part – lacrimal bone	Medial portion of upper and lower eyelids	Squeezes lacrimal bulb		
Muscles of the nose Nasalis	Transverse part (compressor naris) – canine eminence and incisive fossa of maxilla	Aponeurosis of nasal cartilages	Compresses nares	Facial nerve [VII] – zygomatic and buccal branches	Facial artery
	Alar part (dilator naris) – nasal notch of maxilla and minor alar cartilages	Skin of naris margin	Dilates nares		
Depressor septi nasi	Incisive fossa of maxilla	Nasal septum and posterior part of ala	Narrows nares, depresses septum	Facial nerve [VII] – zygomatic and buccal branches	Facial artery

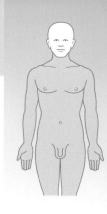

TABLE 4.1 MUSCLES OF FACIAL EXPRESSION (*Cont'd*)

Muscle	Origin	Insertion	Action	Nerve supply	Blood supply
Muscles of the mouth					
Orbicularis oris	From insertions of circumoral muscles, incisive fossae of maxilla and mandible	Skin of the lips and surrounding muscles	Compresses lips against teeth, closes oral fissure, protrudes lips	Facial nerve [VII] – zygomatic, buccal and mandibular branches	Facial artery – superior and inferior labial branches
Buccinator	Buccal alveolar processes of maxilla and mandible, pterygomandibular raphe	Upper and lower portions of orbicularis oris	Compresses cheeks against teeth, aids in mastication, sucking and blowing	Facial nerve [VII] – buccal branches	Facial and maxillary arteries
Depressor anguli oris	Oblique line of mandible	Angle of mouth into orbicularis oris and skin	Depresses angle of mouth	Facial nerve [VII] – mandibular and buccal branches	Facial artery – inferior labial branch
Levator anguli oris	Canine fossa of maxilla, inferior to infra-orbital foramen	Angle of mouth – intermingles with orbicularis oris, depressor anguli oris and zygomaticus	Elevates angle of mouth	Facial nerve [VII] – zygomatic and buccal branches	Facial artery – superior labial branch
Zygomaticus major and minor	Zygomatic portion of zygomatic arch	Angle of the mouth – orbicularis oris, levator anguli oris and depressor anguli oris	Draws angle of mouth up and back	Facial nerve [VII] – zygomatic and buccal branches	Facial artery – superior labial branch
Risorius	Fascia of parotid and masseteric regions, slips from platysma	Skin at angle of the mouth	Retracts angle of the mouth	Facial nerve [VII] – zygomatic and buccal branches	Facial artery – superior labial branch
Levator labii superioris	Angular head – frontal process of maxilla Infra-orbital head – inferior margin of orbit Zygomatic head (see zygomaticus major and minor)	Alar cartilage and skin of nose	Elevates upper lip and flares naris	Facial nerve [VII] – zygomatic and buccal branches	Facial artery – superior labial and angular branches
Depressor labii inferioris	Oblique line of mandible	Lower lip	Depresses lower lip and draws corner of mouth laterally	Facial nerve [VII] – mandibular and buccal branches	Facial artery – inferior labial branch
Mentalis	Incisive fossa of mandible	Skin of chin	Raises and protrudes lower lip	Facial nerve [VII] – mandibular branch	Facial artery – inferior labial branch
Neck					
Platysma	Pectoral and deltoid fasciae	Blends with muscles at the lower part of mouth	Depresses lower jaw and lip, tenses and ridges skin of neck	Facial nerve [VII] – cervical branch	Facial artery and submental branch of suprascapular artery

Scalp and face

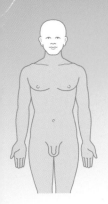

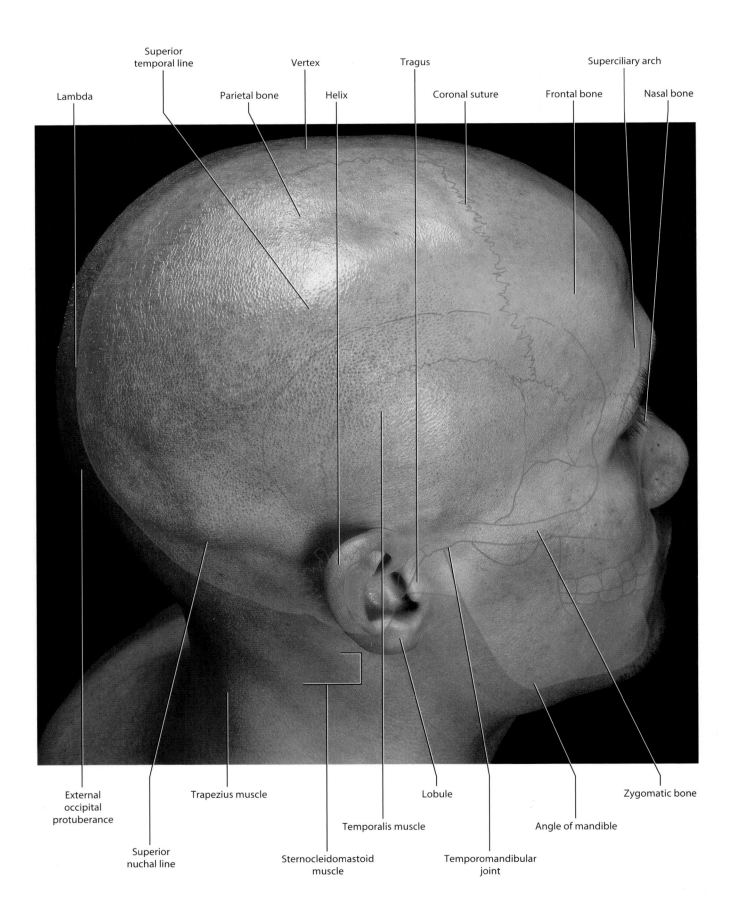

Superior
temporal line

Vertex

Tragus

Superciliary arch

Lambda

Parietal bone

Helix

Coronal suture

Frontal bone

Nasal bone

External
occipital
protuberance

Trapezius muscle

Lobule

Zygomatic bone

Superior
nuchal line

Sternocleidomastoid
muscle

Temporalis muscle

Temporomandibular
joint

Angle of mandible

36   **Figure 4.13 Scalp – surface anatomy posterolateral view.** The superior nuchal line and coronal suture are visible

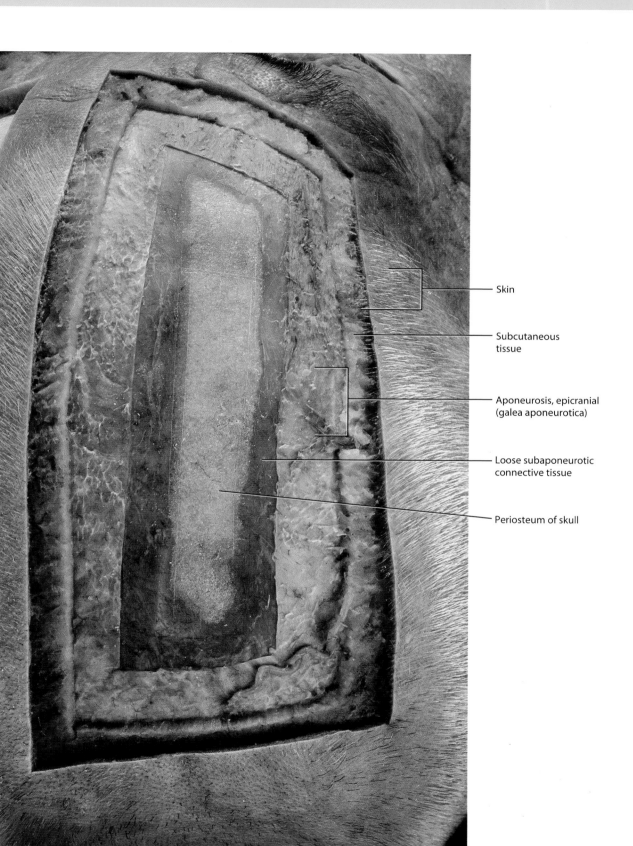

Skin

Subcutaneous
tissue

Aponeurosis, epicranial
(galea aponeurotica)

Loose subaponeurotic
connective tissue

Periosteum of skull

Figure 4.14 Scalp – layers of scalp (superior view). Observe the five layers of the scalp which have been dissected using a non-anatomic rectangular layered method: skin, cutaneous tissue, aponeurosis, loose connective tissue, pericranium (periosteum)

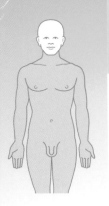

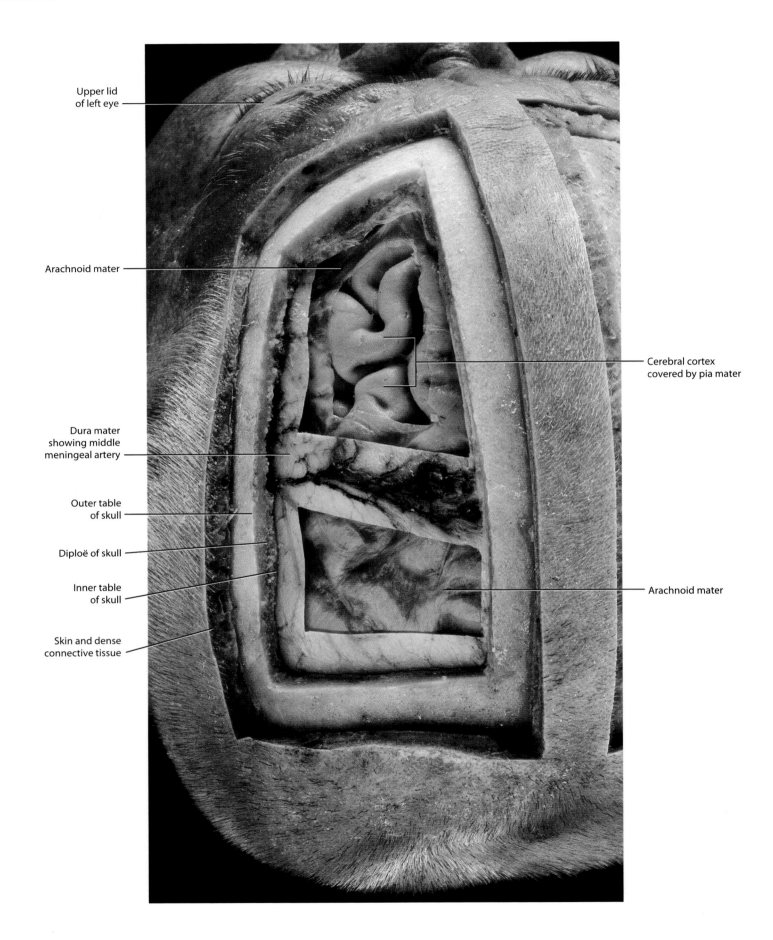

Upper lid
of left eye

Arachnoid mater

Cerebral cortex
covered by pia mater

Dura mater
showing middle
meningeal artery

Outer table
of skull

Diploë of skull

Inner table
of skull

Arachnoid mater

Skin and dense
connective tissue

Figure 4.15 Scalp – deep dissection (superior view). The layers of the meninges, as they cover the brain (dura, arachnoid, and pia mater), are shown in relationship to the scalp, skull, and brain

38

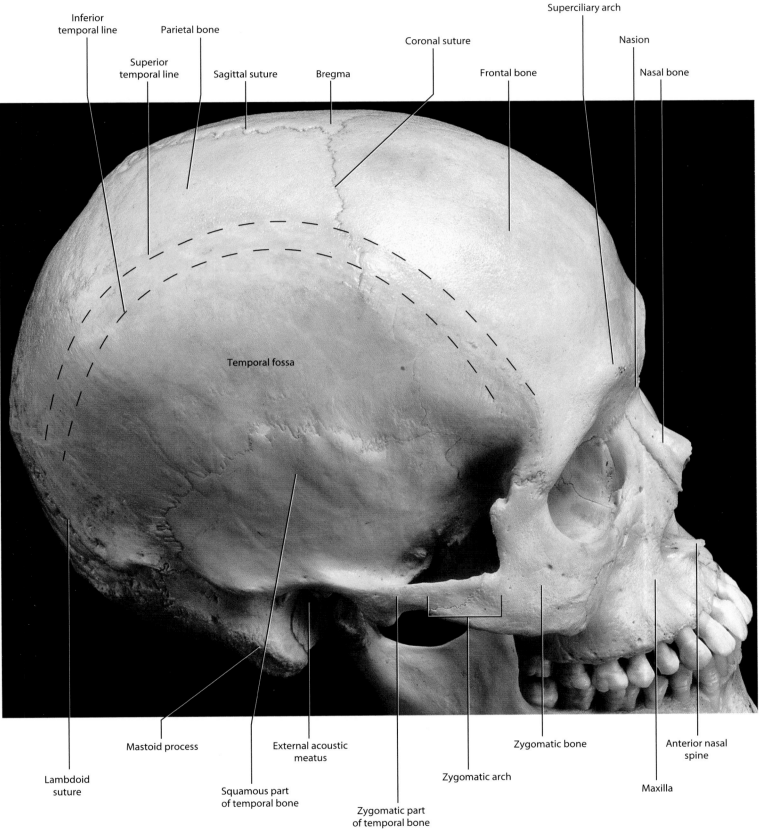

Inferior temporal line

Superior temporal line

Parietal bone

Sagittal suture

Bregma

Coronal suture

Frontal bone

Superciliary arch

Nasion

Nasal bone

Temporal fossa

Mastoid process

External acoustic meatus

Lambdoid suture

Squamous part of temporal bone

Zygomatic part of temporal bone

Zygomatic arch

Zygomatic bone

Maxilla

Anterior nasal spine

Figure 4.16 Scalp – osteology. The pterion, which is where the temporal, frontal, parietal and sphenoid bones intersect, is the thinnest part of the lateral skull

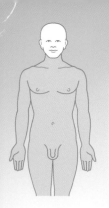

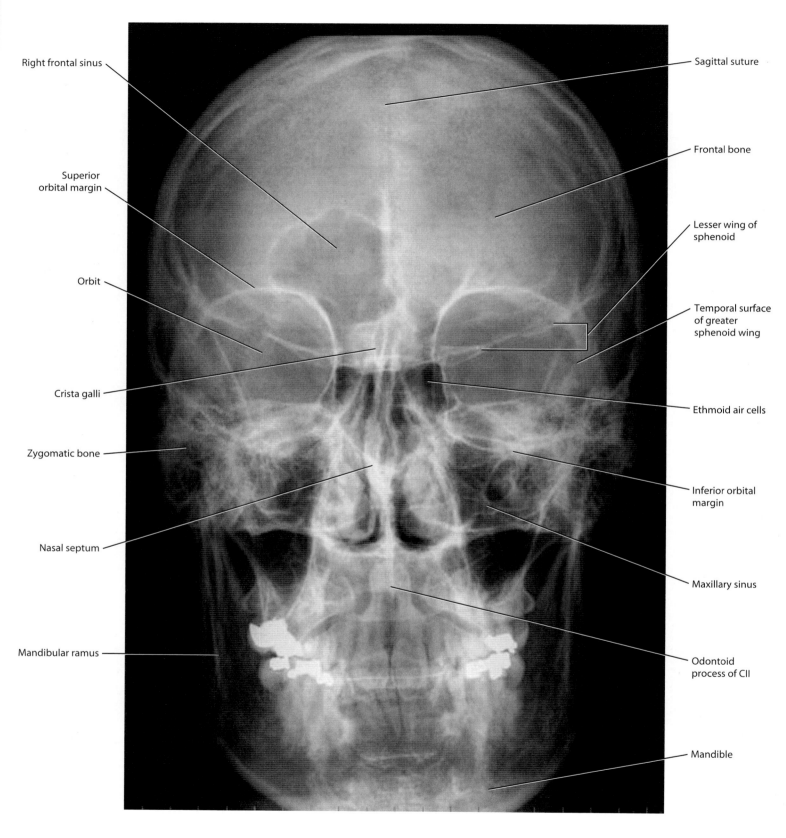

Right frontal sinus

Superior
orbital margin

Orbit

Crista galli

Zygomatic bone

Nasal septum

Mandibular ramus

Sagittal suture

Frontal bone

Lesser wing of
sphenoid

Temporal surface
of greater
sphenoid wing

Ethmoid air cells

Inferior orbital
margin

Maxillary sinus

Odontoid
process of CII

Mandible

Figure 4.17 Face – plain film radiograph (anteroposterior view). Note the arch shape of the zygomatic bones, which are commonly called the cheek bones (compare with Figure 4.12). The left frontal sinus is absent in this patient

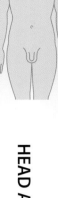

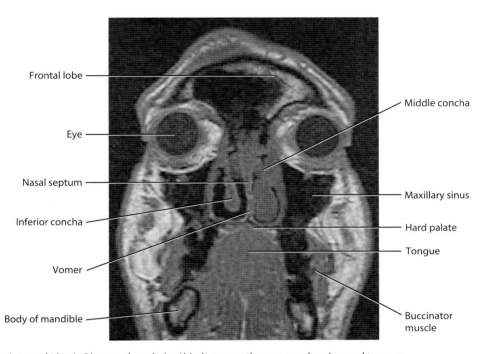

Frontal lobe

Eye

Nasal septum

Inferior concha

Vomer

Body of mandible

Middle concha

Maxillary sinus

Hard palate

Tongue

Buccinator muscle

Figure 4.18 Face – MRI scan (coronal view). Observe the relationship between the eye, nasal region and tongue

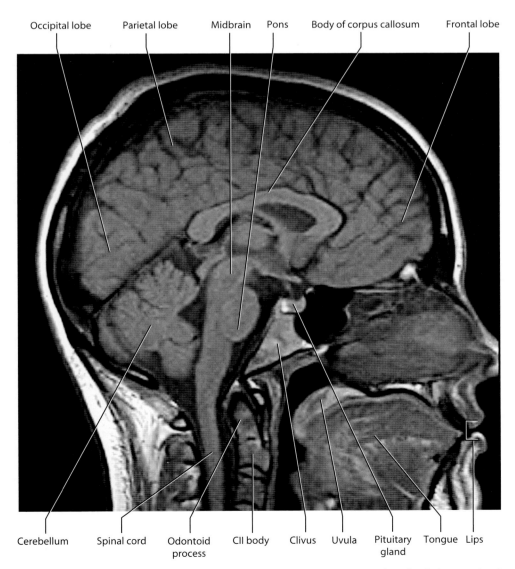

Occipital lobe   Parietal lobe   Midbrain   Pons   Body of corpus callosum   Frontal lobe

Cerebellum   Spinal cord   Odontoid process   CII body   Clivus   Uvula   Pituitary gland   Tongue   Lips

Figure 4.19 Face – MRI scan (sagittal view). The scalp appears as a thickened light colored layer surrounding the dark appearing bones. Observe the location of the lips with respect to the nasal and oral regions

5 Parotid, temporal, and pterygopalatine region

The temporal and infratemporal fossae are two anatomical areas on the lateral surface of the skull. The temporal fossa is the site of origin of the temporalis muscle and the infratemporal fossa is the site of origin of the medial and lateral pterygoid muscles. These are all muscles of mastication. The masseter muscle, the fourth muscle of mastication, is in the vicinity of the parotid gland (Fig. 5.1) on the lateral aspect of the ramus of mandible (see Chapter 4 and below). Also in the infratemporal fossa are:

- the mandibular nerve [V_3] division of the trigeminal nerve [V];
- the parasympathetic **otic ganglion**, which sends postganglionic parasympathetic nerve fibers to the parotid gland via the auriculotemporal nerve (see Chapter 4).

The temporal fossa is bounded superiorly by the **temporal lines**, laterally by the **zygomatic arch**, and inferiorly by the **infratemporal crest** (Table 5.1). It is formed by the frontal bone, the parietal bone, the greater wing of sphenoid, and the squamous part of the temporal bone. These bones unite to form an important clinical landmark – the **pterion** – which lies over the intracranial middle meningeal artery and vein and is the thinnest part of the skull; skull fracture at this site can easily cause brain damage and intracranial bleeding.

The infratemporal fossa is bounded anteriorly by the **posterior part of the maxilla**, posteriorly by the **tympanic plate** of the temporal bone, medially by the **lateral plate of the pterygoid process** of the sphenoid bone, and laterally by the **ramus** and **coronoid process of mandible** (see Table 5.1). Its roof is formed by the infratemporal surface of the **greater wing of the sphenoid**; the floor of the fossa is open.

The pterygopalatine fossa is the irregularly shaped space posterior to the maxilla and inferior and deep to the zygomatic arch. It is medial to the infratemporal fossa and its boundaries are: anteriorly, the **posterior surface of the maxilla**; posteriorly, the **lateral plate of the pterygoid process** and **greater wing** of the sphenoid; medially, the **perpendicular plate** of the palatine bone; superiorly, the **body** of the sphenoid and **orbital surface** of the palatine bone. Laterally, the pterygopalatine fossa opens through the **pterygomaxillary fissure** (see Table 5.1).

Anteriorly, the pterygopalatine fossa is closely related to the orbit through the **inferior orbital fissure**; medially it is related to the nasal cavity through the **sphenopalatine foramen**; inferiorly it is related to the oral region through the **greater** and **lesser palatine foramina**; laterally to the infratemporal fossa through the pterygomaxillary fissure; and posterosuperiorly to the middle cranial fossa, through the foramen rotundum and pterygoid canal. The pterygopalatine fossa contains the **maxillary nerve** [V_2], the **pterygopalatine ganglion**, the **nerve of pterygoid canal**, and the **third** or **pterygopalatine part of the maxillary artery** and its branches (see below). It is the contents and relationships of the pterygopalatine fossa that make an understanding of it important.

The **temporomandibular joint** and superior part of the mandible (ramus of mandible) are close to the fossae. The temporomandibular joint is a synovial joint with gliding and hinge functions, which are enhanced by the insertion of an articular disc between the head of the mandible and the mandibular fossa of the temporal bone. Major support for the temporomandibular joint is provided by the muscles of mastication (temporalis, medial pterygoid, lateral pterygoid, and masseter; see below). Additional support is provided by the **lateral**, **stylomandibular**, and **sphenomandibular ligaments**. The temporomandibular joint is innervated by the **masseteric**, **auriculotemporal**, and **deep temporal nerves**, which are all branches of the mandibular nerve [V_3].

MUSCLES

The muscles of mastication – the temporalis, masseter, medial pterygoid, and lateral pterygoid – associated with the temporal and infratemporal fossae are:

- the **temporalis** muscle is a large fan-like muscle originating from the temporal fossa, inserting inferiorly onto the coronoid process of the mandible, and acting to elevate the mandible;
- the **masseter** muscle originates from the zygomatic arch, inserts onto the ramus of mandible, and elevates the mandible;
- the **medial pterygoid** muscle originates from the tuberosity of the maxilla and palatine bone, and it inserts on the medial aspect of the mandible below the mandibular foramen, and elevates and protracts the mandible;
- the **lateral pterygoid** muscle joins the sphenoid bone to the neck of mandible and protrudes the mandible.

These four muscles are innervated by branches of the mandibular nerve [V_3] (Table 5.2).

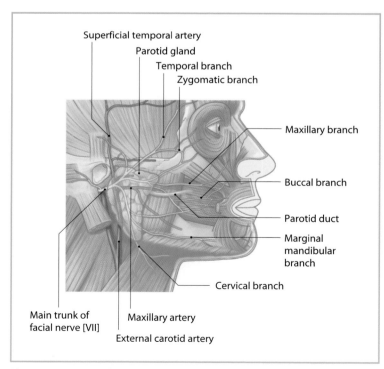

Superficial temporal artery
Parotid gland
Temporal branch
Zygomatic branch
Maxillary branch
Buccal branch
Parotid duct
Marginal mandibular branch
Cervical branch
Main trunk of facial nerve [VII]
Maxillary artery
External carotid artery

Figure 5.1 Temporal region, parotid gland and branches of the facial nerve [V]

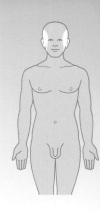

NERVES

The main nerves associated with the temporal, infratemporal, and pterygopalatine fossae are branches of the maxillary [V_2] and mandibular [V_3] nerves, which are divisions of the trigeminal nerve [V] (see Fig. 4.2).

The **maxillary nerve** [V_2] leaves the intracranial fossa through the foramen rotundum to enter the pterygopalatine fossa. It is a sensory nerve and has no motor component, and its branches provide sensation to the midsection of the face (lower orbit, nose, upper mouth, and cheek).

After entering the pterygopalatine fossa, the maxillary nerve [V_2] gives rise to the **zygomatic nerve**, two **pterygopalatine nerves**, and the **posterior superior alveolar nerves** (which supply the maxillary and the ethmoidal sinuses). The zygomatic nerve further divides into the **zygomaticofacial** and **zygomaticotemporal nerves**, which provide sensation to the respective regions of the upper lateral face (see Fig. 4.1).

The pterygopalatine nerves suspend the **pterygopalatine ganglion** (Fig. 5.2) within the pterygopalatine fossa. This ganglion receives autonomic innervation from the **nerve of pterygoid canal**, which is a combination of two nerves:

- the **parasympathetic root** (a branch of the facial nerve [VII]); and
- the **sympathetic root** (which originates from the superior cervical ganglion).

Nerves from the pterygopalatine ganglion carry parasympathetic and sympathetic fibers and sensory nerves from the maxillary nerve [V_2] to supply the lacrimal gland and the glands in the nasal and upper oropharyngeal regions.

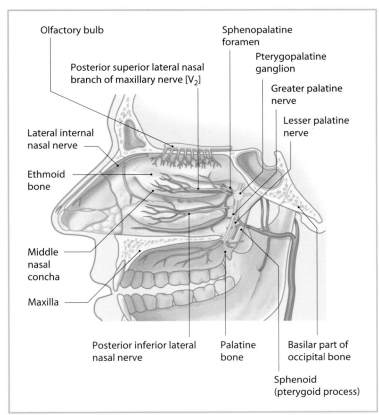

Olfactory bulb

Sphenopalatine foramen

Posterior superior lateral nasal branch of maxillary nerve [V_2]

Pterygopalatine ganglion

Greater palatine nerve

Lesser palatine nerve

Lateral internal nasal nerve

Ethmoid bone

Middle nasal concha

Maxilla

Posterior inferior lateral nasal nerve

Palatine bone

Basilar part of occipital bone

Sphenoid (pterygoid process)

Figure 5.2 Infratemporal region (hemisection)

The maxillary nerve [V_2] leaves the pterygopalatine fossa through the inferior orbital fissure. From this point it is referred to as the **infra-orbital nerve**. It enters the orbit, passes anteriorly within the infra-orbital groove and then within the infra-orbital canal, until it emerges onto the face approximately 1 cm inferior to the inferior orbital rim (see Chapter 4). The infra-orbital nerve provides sensation to the skin of the upper lip, lower eyelid, cheek, and lateral part of the nose.

The **mandibular nerve** [V_3] emerges from the skull through the foramen ovale and enters the infratemporal fossa. It carries motor fibers to the muscles of mastication and sensory fibers to the mandibular region. The sensory branches supply general sensation to the meninges, skin and mucosa of the cheeks, anterior two-thirds of the tongue, mucosa of the floor of the mouth, labial and lingual gingiva, skin of the temporal and parotid regions, and the external ear and chin.

The **mandibular nerve** [V_3] branches to form the **meningeal branch**, and the **masseteric** (motor) and **deep temporal nerves**, the **nerve to medial pterygoid** (motor), the **nerve to lateral pterygoid** (motor), and the **auriculotemporal**, **buccal**, **lingual**, and **inferior alveolar nerves**. Each of these branches innervates the muscle or region after which it is named. The four largest branches of the mandibular nerve [V_3] are the sensory auriculotemporal, buccal, lingual, and inferior alveolar nerves.

The **auriculotemporal nerve** originates from within the infratemporal fossa and travels deep to the neck of mandible and provides sensory innervation for the temporomandibular joint. It then exits the infratemporal fossa and enters the parotid gland tissue. Parasympathetic postganglionic nerve fibers traveling with the auriculotemporal nerve innervate the parotid gland. From the parotid gland the auriculotemporal nerve passes superiorly to provide sensation to the skin around the ear and lateral scalp.

After the **buccal nerve** leaves the infratemporal fossa it passes through the lateral pterygoid and temporalis muscles. It terminates to provide sensation to the skin of the cheek, buccal oral mucosa, and gingiva (gums) of the posterior mandibular teeth.

The **lingual nerve** originates in the infratemporal fossa and is joined by the **chorda tympani nerve**, which carries taste and preganglionic parasympathetic nerve fibers from the facial nerve [VII]. The adjoined nerve passes toward the tongue, where the two nerves provide sensation and taste to the anterior two-thirds of the tongue.

The **inferior alveolar nerve** descends within the infratemporal fossa along the inner surface of the upper part of the mandible. The **nerve to mylohyoid**, a branch of the inferior alveolar nerve, enters the floor of the mouth and supplies the anterior belly of the digastric and the mylohyoid muscle (see Chapter 11). The inferior alveolar nerve then enters the mandibular foramen on the medial surface of the ramus of mandible. Within the mandible, it innervates the mandibular teeth. The inferior alveolar nerve terminates in the anterior part of the mandible by branching into the **incisive** and **mental nerves**, which carry sensation from the anterior mandibular teeth and the skin around the lower lip and chin.

ARTERIES

The **maxillary artery** is the main vessel to the temporal, infratemporal, and pterygopalatine fossae (Fig. 5.3). It is a terminal branch of the external carotid artery and is divided into three regions (mandibular, pterygoid, and pterygopalatine), based on its relationship to the lateral pterygoid muscle.

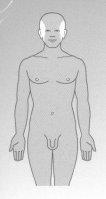

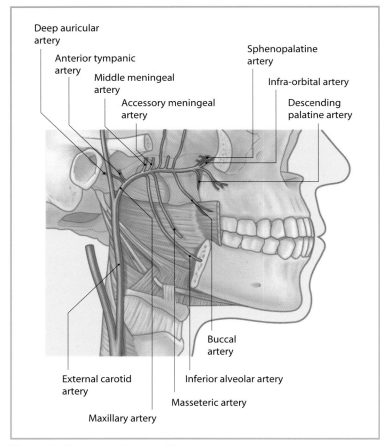

Deep auricular artery
Anterior tympanic artery
Middle meningeal artery
Accessory meningeal artery
Sphenopalatine artery
Infra-orbital artery
Descending palatine artery
Buccal artery
External carotid artery
Inferior alveolar artery
Masseteric artery
Maxillary artery

Figure 5.3 Branches of the maxillary artery

- The mandibular part of the maxillary artery is near the neck of the mandible and branches to form the **deep auricular**, **anterior tympanic**, **middle meningeal**, **accessory meningeal**, and **inferior alveolar** arteries.
- The pterygoid part of the maxillary artery is near the lateral pterygoid muscles and gives rise to **anterior deep temporal**, **posterior deep temporal**, **pterygoid**, **masseteric**, and **buccal arteries**.
- The pterygopalatine part of the maxillary artery is within the pterygopalatine fossa and branches into the **posterior superior alveolar**, **infra-orbital**, and **descending palatine arteries**, the **artery of pterygoid canal**, and **pharyngeal** and **sphenopalatine arteries**.

VEINS AND LYMPHATICS

Venous drainage of the three fossae corresponds to the branches of the maxillary arteries. The veins drain to the **pterygoid plexus** of veins within the infratemporal fossa. The pterygoid plexus communicates with the **cavernous sinus** (a dural venous sinus). It also communicates with the facial vein anteriorly. This unique series of interconnections provides a potential route for spread of superficial facial infection to the intracranial cavity.

Near the temporomandibular joint, the maxillary vein joins the superficial temporal vein to form the **retromandibular vein**. The retromandibular vein descends along the lateral face and branches into an anterior division, which empties into the **facial vein**, and a posterior division, which joins the posterior auricular vein to form the **external jugular vein**.

Lymphatic drainage of the temporal, infratemporal, and pterygopalatine fossa is to regional lymph nodes – the superficial nodes at the junction of the head and neck and the superior deep cervical nodes along the carotid sheath.

■ CLINICAL CORRELATIONS

Parotid tumors

Tumors of the parotid gland are usually well circumscribed, slow growing, and rare. They are much more common than tumors of the other major salivary glands (submandibular and sublingual glands). Smoking and increased age are two known risk factors for salivary gland tumors.

Symptoms of a parotid gland tumor may include tingling on the same side of the face, weakness or paralysis of facial muscles, numbness, trismus (spasm of the muscles that open the jaw), decreased saliva production, a lump or swelling, skin changes, pain, hearing changes, and headaches.

On examination, a mass is usually present. In some cases it is mobile, but in advanced cases it is adherent to the underlying tissue or bone. Chvostek's sign – twitching of the facial muscles when the region of the lateral face and parotid gland is tapped – is elicited in patients with hypocalcemia, but also occasionally occurs with parotid tumors. Fine-needle aspiration of the tumor aids diagnosis by providing cells for histologic analysis.

A parotid tumor can be further evaluated by computed tomography (CT) or magnetic resonance imaging (MRI). Most otolaryngologists (ear, nose, and throat specialists) prefer the sensitivity and detail afforded by MRI. In some cases, MRI reveals the presence of tumor spread.

The standard treatment and preferred diagnostic method for both malignant and nonmalignant tumors of the parotid gland is surgical excision. Care is taken to preserve the facial nerve [VII], which enters the parotid gland and divides into its terminal branches (temporal, zygomatic, buccal, marginal mandibular, and cervical). Malignant tumors can spread to nearby lymph nodes.

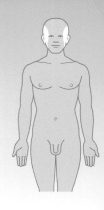

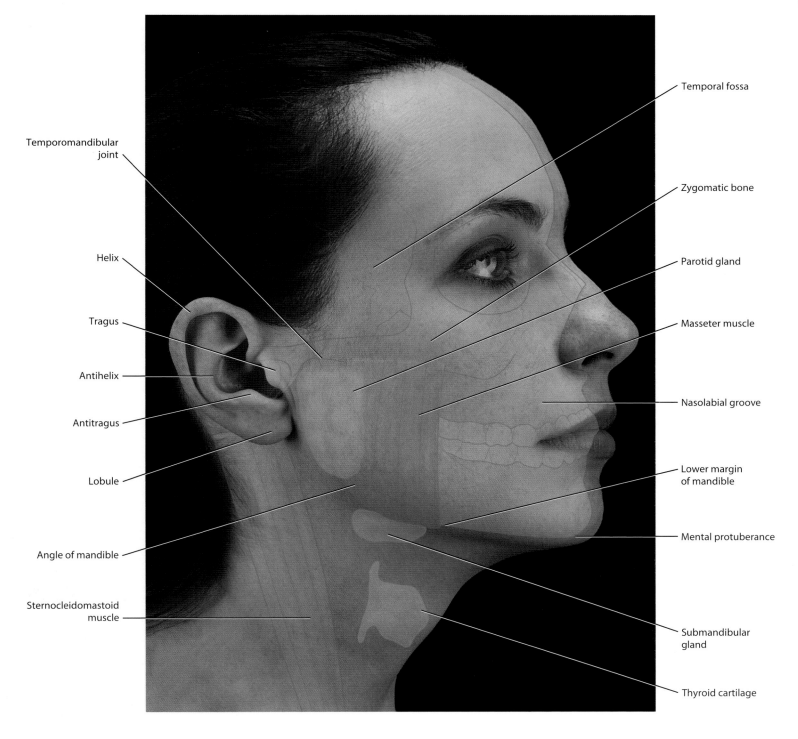

Temporomandibular joint

Helix

Tragus

Antihelix

Antitragus

Lobule

Angle of mandible

Sternocleidomastoid muscle

Temporal fossa

Zygomatic bone

Parotid gland

Masseter muscle

Nasolabial groove

Lower margin of mandible

Mental protuberance

Submandibular gland

Thyroid cartilage

Figure 5.4 Parotid and temporal region – surface anatomy. Surface landmarks of the parotid and temporal regions

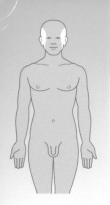

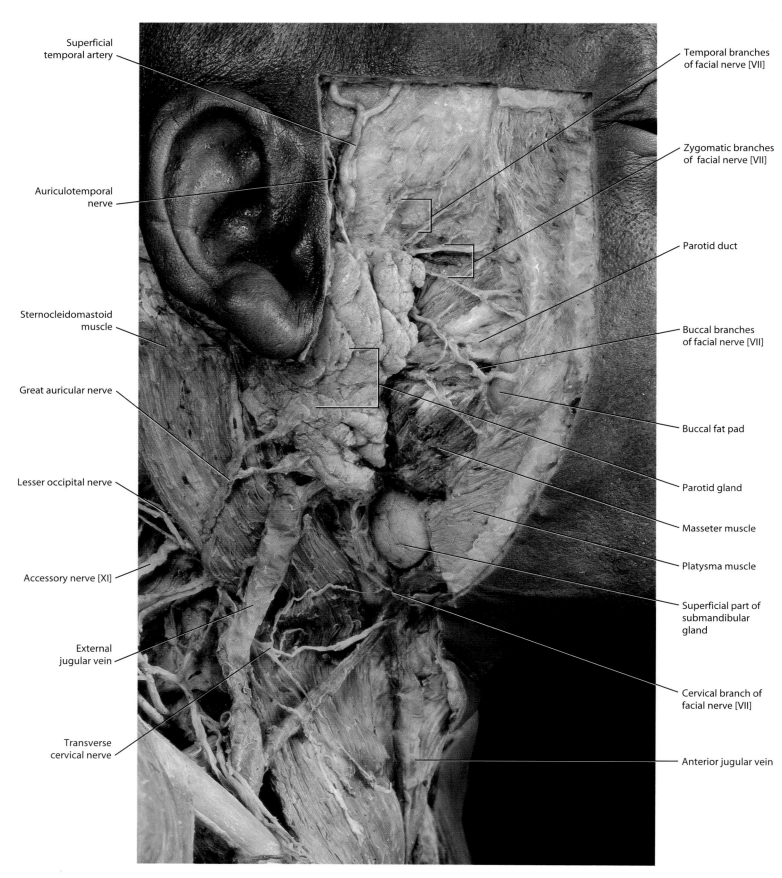

Superficial
temporal artery

Auriculotemporal
nerve

Sternocleidomastoid
muscle

Great auricular nerve

Lesser occipital nerve

Accessory nerve [XI]

External
jugular vein

Transverse
cervical nerve

Temporal branches
of facial nerve [VII]

Zygomatic branches
of facial nerve [VII]

Parotid duct

Buccal branches
of facial nerve [VII]

Buccal fat pad

Parotid gland

Masseter muscle

Platysma muscle

Superficial part of
submandibular
gland

Cervical branch of
facial nerve [VII]

Anterior jugular vein

Figure 5.5 Parotid region – superficial dissection. The facial nerve, parotid duct, and external jugular vein are visible as they emerge from the parotid gland

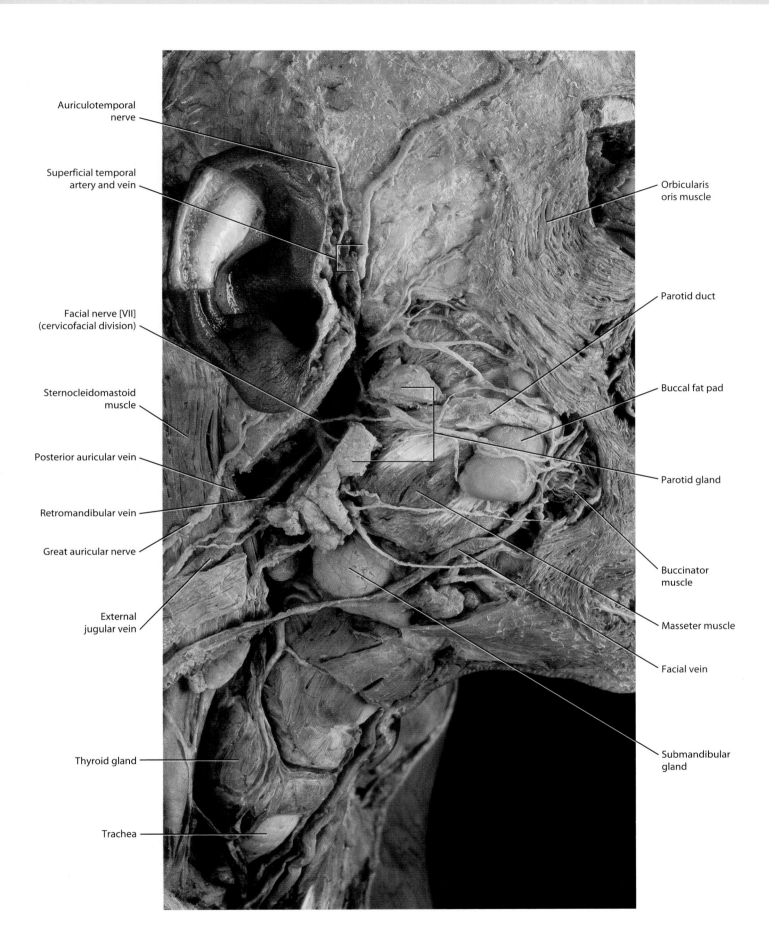

Auriculotemporal nerve

Superficial temporal artery and vein

Facial nerve [VII] (cervicofacial division)

Sternocleidomastoid muscle

Posterior auricular vein

Retromandibular vein

Great auricular nerve

External jugular vein

Thyroid gland

Trachea

Orbicularis oris muscle

Parotid duct

Buccal fat pad

Parotid gland

Buccinator muscle

Masseter muscle

Facial vein

Submandibular gland

Figure 5.6 Parotid region – intermediate dissection. Part of the parotid gland has been removed to show the origination of the external jugular vein and the branching structure of the facial nerve [VII]. Also observe the close proximity of the parotid gland to the submandibular gland

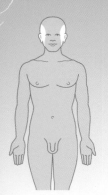

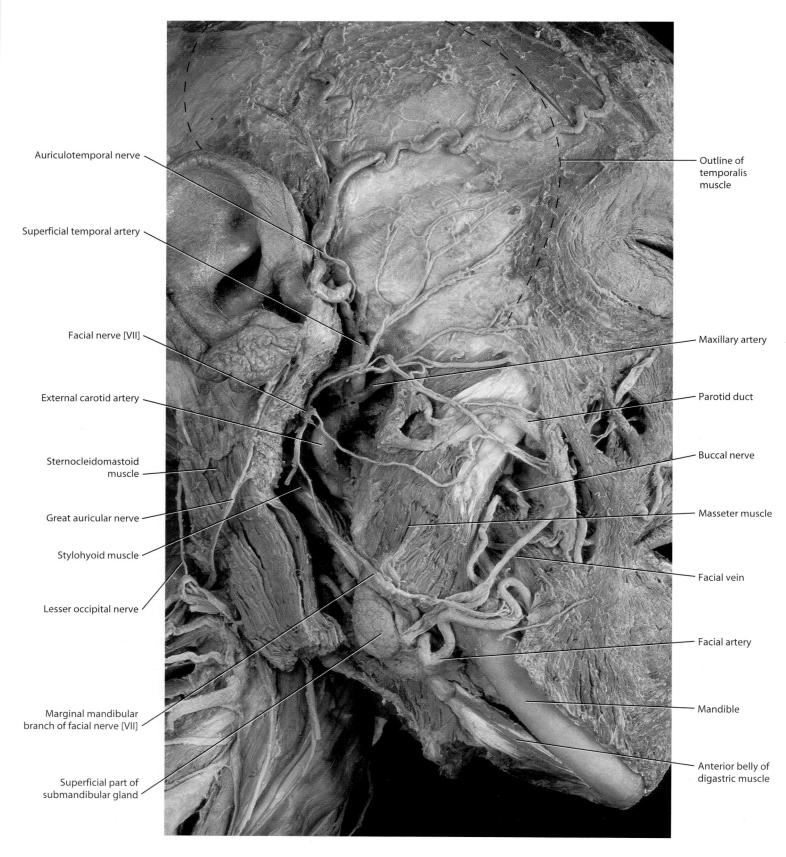

Auriculotemporal nerve

Superficial temporal artery

Facial nerve [VII]

External carotid artery

Sternocleidomastoid muscle

Great auricular nerve

Stylohyoid muscle

Lesser occipital nerve

Marginal mandibular branch of facial nerve [VII]

Superficial part of submandibular gland

Outline of temporalis muscle

Maxillary artery

Parotid duct

Buccal nerve

Masseter muscle

Facial vein

Facial artery

Mandible

Anterior belly of digastric muscle

Figure 5.7 Parotid region – deep dissection. With most of the parotid gland removed, the external carotid artery is visible in the infratemporal fossa

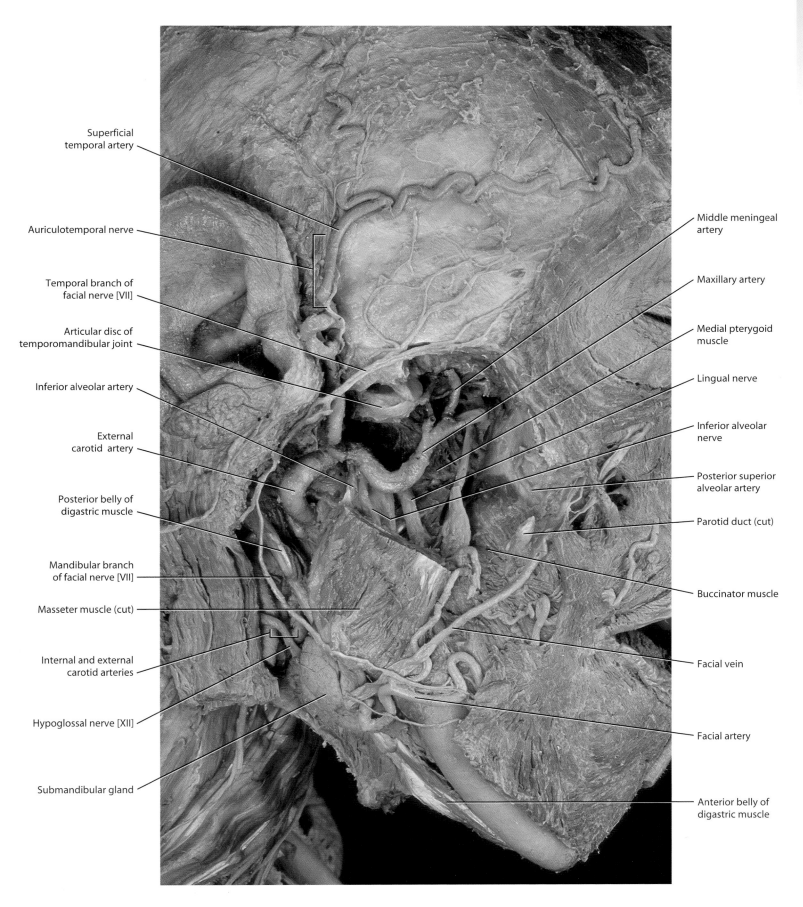

Superficial temporal artery

Auriculotemporal nerve

Temporal branch of facial nerve [VII]

Articular disc of temporomandibular joint

Inferior alveolar artery

External carotid artery

Posterior belly of digastric muscle

Mandibular branch of facial nerve [VII]

Masseter muscle (cut)

Internal and external carotid arteries

Hypoglossal nerve [XII]

Submandibular gland

Middle meningeal artery

Maxillary artery

Medial pterygoid muscle

Lingual nerve

Inferior alveolar nerve

Posterior superior alveolar artery

Parotid duct (cut)

Buccinator muscle

Facial vein

Facial artery

Anterior belly of digastric muscle

Figure 5.8 Infratemporal fossa – deep dissection. This is a continuation of the dissection in Figure 5.7. The right side of the face has been further dissected to show the branches of the maxillary artery. Small parts of the right eye and right ear are visible

49

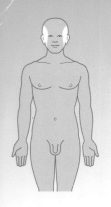

TABLE 5.1 BOUNDARIES OF THE TEMPORAL, INFRATEMPORAL, AND PTERYGOPALATINE FOSSAE

Fossa	Boundary	Components of boundary
Temporal	Lateral Superior Inferior	Zygomatic arch Temporal lines Infratemporal crest
Infratemporal	Anterior Posterior Medial Lateral Superior Inferior	Posterior part of maxilla Styloid process (of temporal bone) Lateral plate of pterygoid process (of sphenoid) Ramus and coronoid process of mandible Infratemporal surface of greater wing (of sphenoid) Open to neck
Pterygopalatine	Anterior Posterior Medial Lateral	Posterior surface of maxilla Lateral plate of pterygoid process and greater wing (of sphenoid) Perpendicular plate (of palatine bone) Open through pterygomaxillary fissure

TABLE 5.2 MUSCLES OF MASTICATION

Muscle	Origin	Insertion	Action	Nerve supply	Blood supply
Temporalis	Floor of temporal fossa and temporal fascia	Coronoid process and anterior border of ramus of mandible	Maintains resting position, elevation, retrusion, and ipsilateral excursion of mandible	Mandibular nerve [V_3] – deep temporal nerves	Superficial temporal and maxillary arteries, middle, anterior, and posterior deep temporal arteries
Masseter	Zygomatic process of maxilla and inferior aspect of zygomatic arch	Lateral aspect of ramus of mandible to angle of mandible	Elevation, protrusion, and ipsilateral excursion of mandible	Mandibular nerve [V_3] – masseter nerve	Transverses facial artery; masseteric branch of maxillary and facial arteries
Medial pterygoid	Medial aspect of lateral plate of pterygoid process of sphenoid, pyramidal process of palatine bone; tuberosity of maxilla	Medial aspect of ramus and angle of mandible	Protrudes and elevates mandible, deviates to opposite side	Mandibular nerve [V_3] – nerve to medial pterygoid	Facial and maxillary arteries
Lateral pterygoid	Infratemporal surface of greater wing of sphenoid and lateral surface of lateral plate of pterygoid process of sphenoid	Pterygoid fovea, capsule of temporomandibular joint and articular disk	Protrudes mandible, pulls disk anteriorly and deviates to opposite side	Mandibular nerve [V_3] – muscular branches from anterior division	Maxillary artery – muscular branches

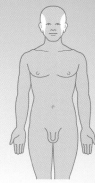

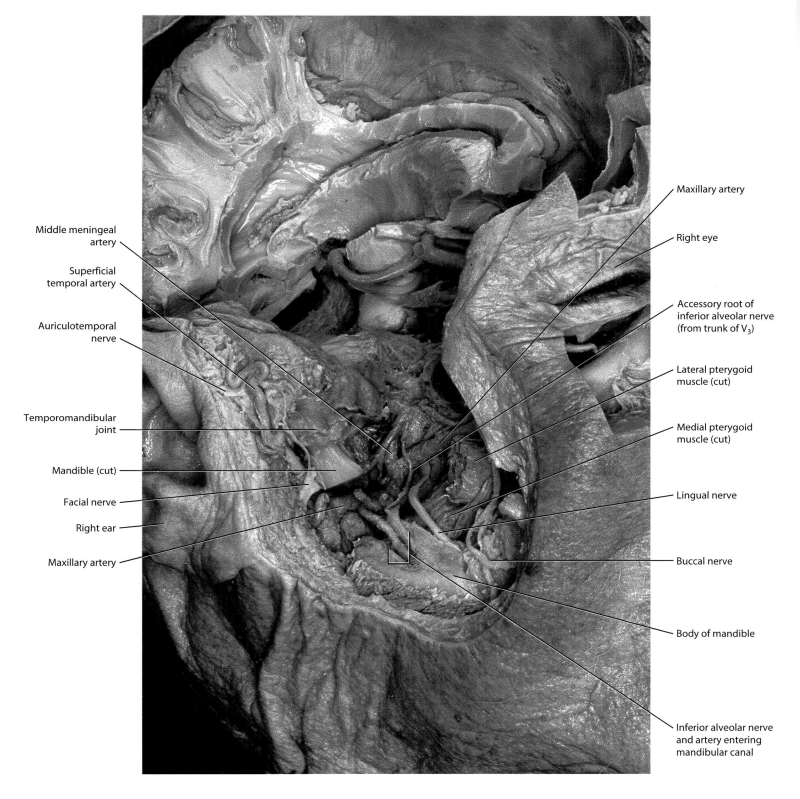

Middle meningeal artery

Superficial temporal artery

Auriculotemporal nerve

Temporomandibular joint

Mandible (cut)

Facial nerve

Right ear

Maxillary artery

Maxillary artery

Right eye

Accessory root of inferior alveolar nerve (from trunk of V₃)

Lateral pterygoid muscle (cut)

Medial pterygoid muscle (cut)

Lingual nerve

Buccal nerve

Body of mandible

Inferior alveolar nerve and artery entering mandibular canal

Figure 5.9 Infratemporal fossa – intermediate dissection. In this dissection of the infratemporal fossa the superior part of the masseter muscle has been removed to more clearly show the two terminal branches of the external carotid artery – the superficial temporal and maxillary arteries

51

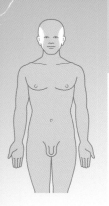

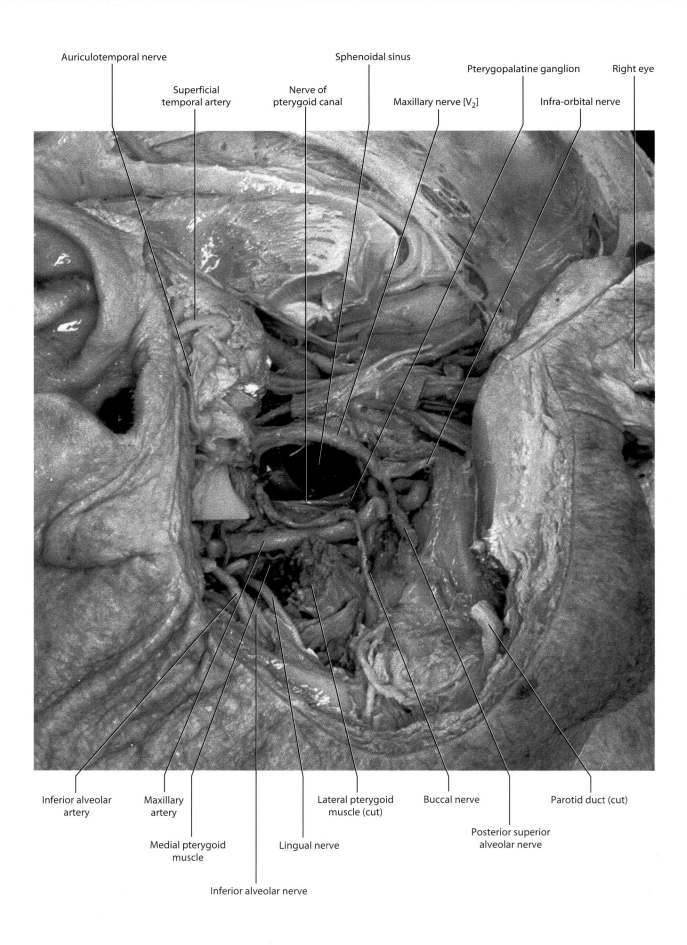

Auriculotemporal nerve

Superficial
temporal artery

Nerve of
pterygoid canal

Sphenoidal sinus

Maxillary nerve [V$_2$]

Pterygopalatine ganglion

Right eye

Infra-orbital nerve

Inferior alveolar
artery

Maxillary
artery

Medial pterygoid
muscle

Lingual nerve

Inferior alveolar nerve

Lateral pterygoid
muscle (cut)

Buccal nerve

Posterior superior
alveolar nerve

Parotid duct (cut)

Figure 5.10 Infratemporal and pterygopalatine fossae – deep dissection. The right zygomatic arch has been removed to show the maxillary artery and nerve (V$_2$). The sphenoidal sinus is visible at the deepest point in this dissection

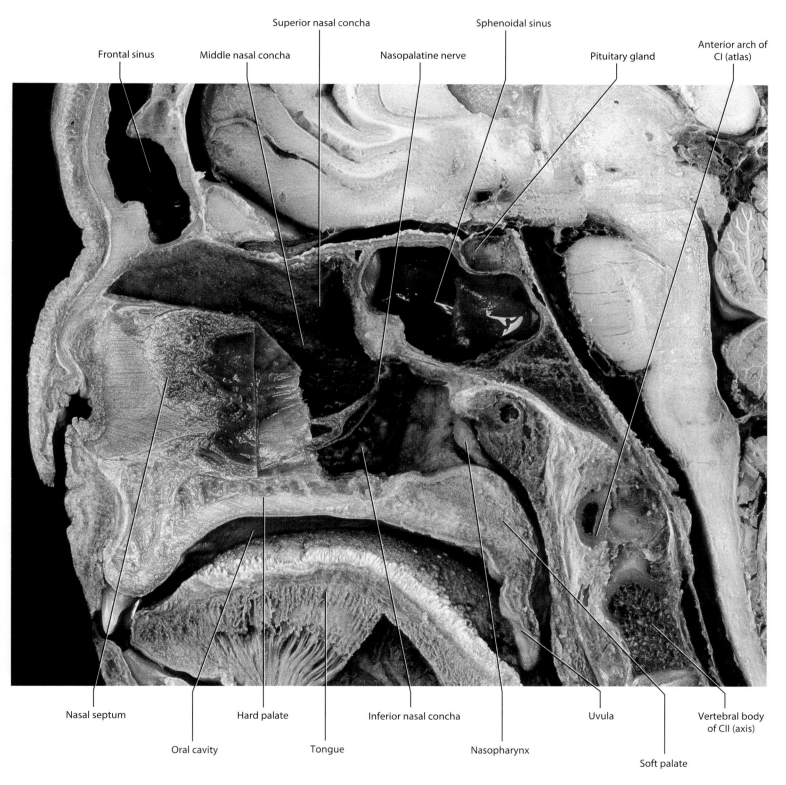

Superior nasal concha

Sphenoidal sinus

Frontal sinus

Middle nasal concha

Nasopalatine nerve

Pituitary gland

Anterior arch of CI (atlas)

Nasal septum

Hard palate

Inferior nasal concha

Uvula

Vertebral body of CII (axis)

Oral cavity

Tongue

Nasopharynx

Soft palate

Figure 5.11 Pterygopalatine fossa – median sagittal section 1. The posterior part of the nasal septum has been removed to show the right sphenoidal sinus, nasopalatine nerve, and inferior nasal concha. Observe the close proximity of the pituitary gland to the sphenoidal sinus and nasal cavity

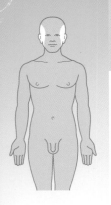

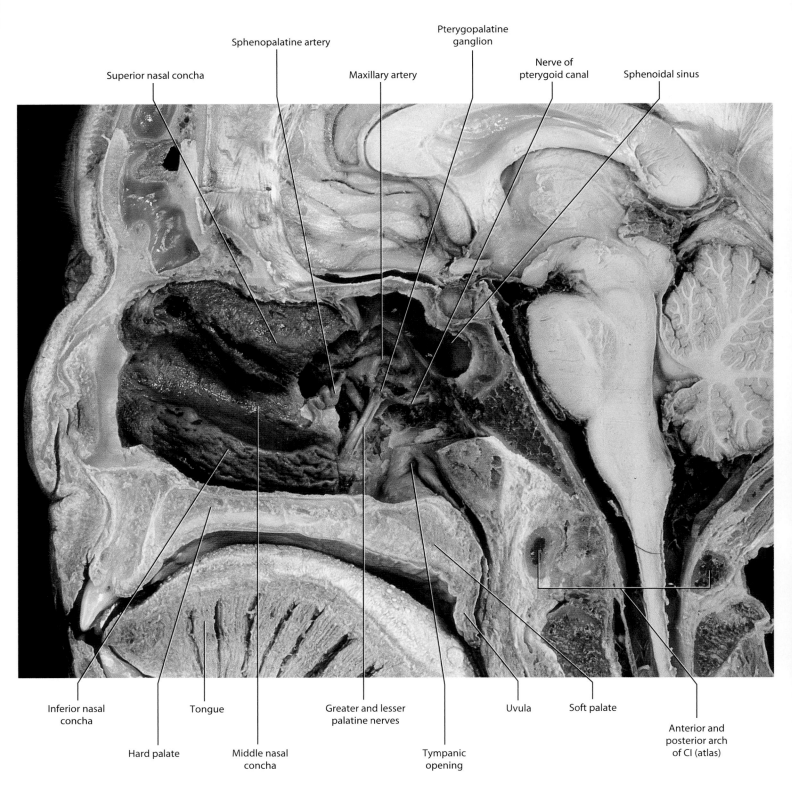

Figure 5.12 Pterygopalatine fossa – median sagittal section 2. Posterior parts of the superior and middle nasal conchae have been removed to show the two contents of the pterygopalatine fossa – the sphenopalatine artery and pterygopalatine ganglion

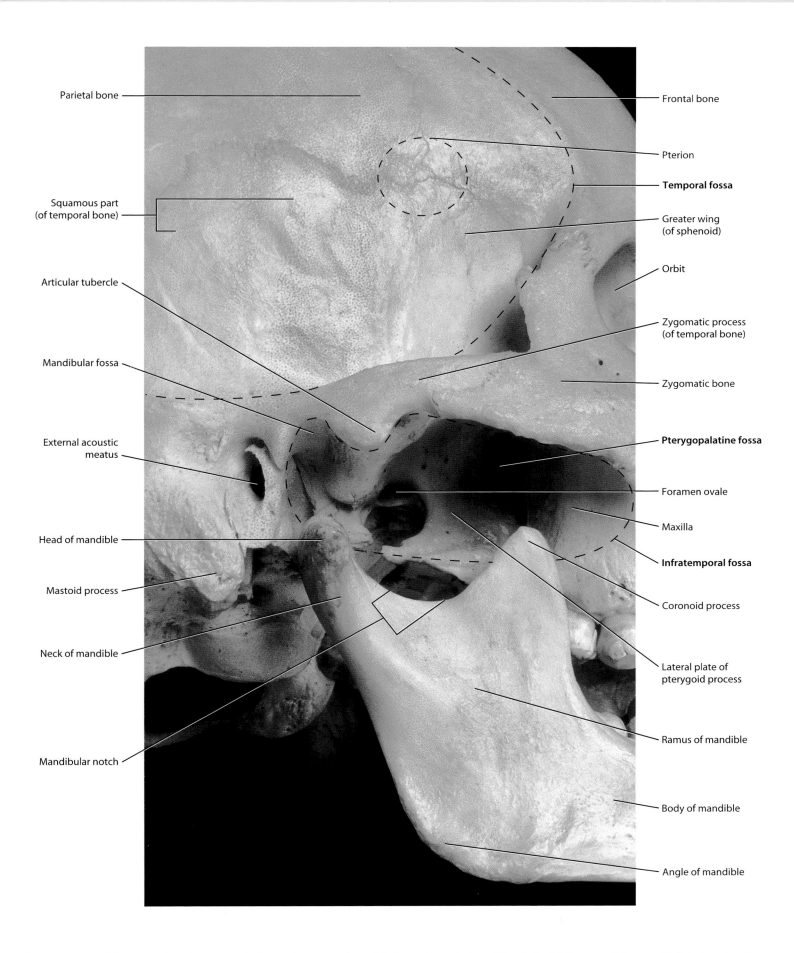

Parietal bone

Squamous part
(of temporal bone)

Articular tubercle

Mandibular fossa

External acoustic
meatus

Head of mandible

Mastoid process

Neck of mandible

Mandibular notch

Frontal bone

Pterion

Temporal fossa

Greater wing
(of sphenoid)

Orbit

Zygomatic process
(of temporal bone)

Zygomatic bone

Pterygopalatine fossa

Foramen ovale

Maxilla

Infratemporal fossa

Coronoid process

Lateral plate of
pterygoid process

Ramus of mandible

Body of mandible

Angle of mandible

Figure 5.13 Parotid, temporal, and pterygopalatine region – osteology. Inferior and lateral view of the skull with the mandible moved inferiorly out of the temporomandibular joint to show the temporal, infratemporal, and pterygopalatine fossae. The pterygopalatine fossa is deep to the infratemporal fossa

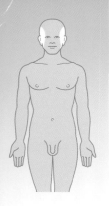

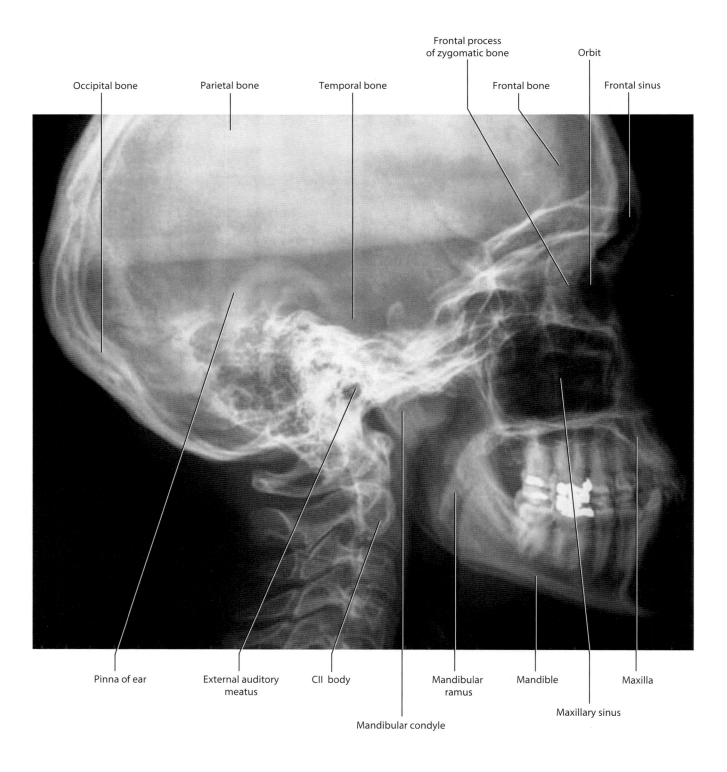

Occipital bone Parietal bone Temporal bone Frontal process of zygomatic bone Frontal bone Orbit Frontal sinus

Pinna of ear External auditory meatus CII body Mandibular ramus Mandible Maxilla

Mandibular condyle Maxillary sinus

Figure 5.14 Parotid and temporal region – plain film radiograph (lateral view). Soft tissues, such as the parotid gland, located near the region of the mandibular condyle, are not well visualized in plain film radiographs. Observe the maxillary sinus and how it is related to the external auditory meatus. On a lateral view, the temporal, infratemporal, and pterygopalatine fossae are located between these two landmarks

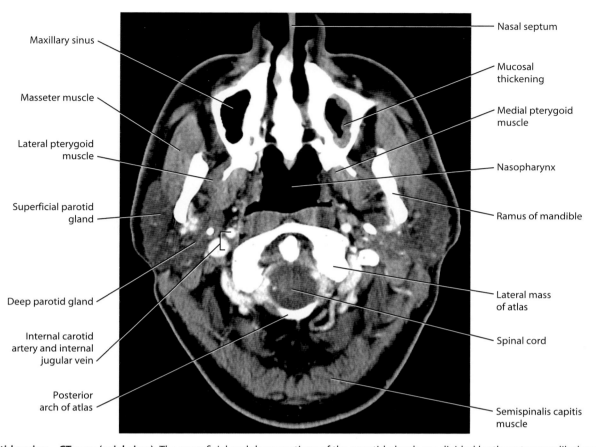

Maxillary sinus

Masseter muscle

Lateral pterygoid muscle

Superficial parotid gland

Deep parotid gland

Internal carotid artery and internal jugular vein

Posterior arch of atlas

Nasal septum

Mucosal thickening

Medial pterygoid muscle

Nasopharynx

Ramus of mandible

Lateral mass of atlas

Spinal cord

Semispinalis capitis muscle

Figure 5.15 Parotid region – CT scan (axial view). The superficial and deep portions of the parotid glands are divided by the retromandibular veins. Note that there is mucosal thickening of the left maxillary sinus because of chronic sinusitis

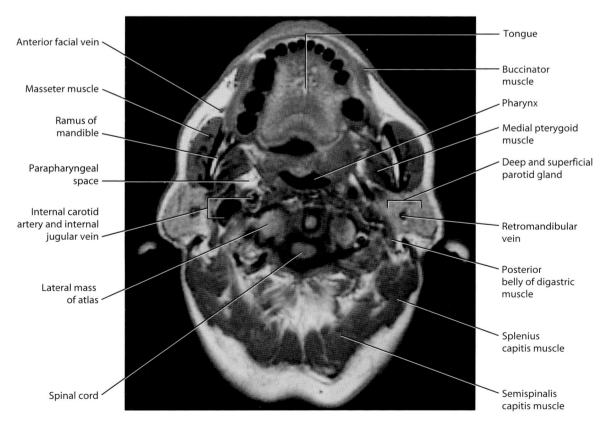

Anterior facial vein

Masseter muscle

Ramus of mandible

Parapharyngeal space

Internal carotid artery and internal jugular vein

Lateral mass of atlas

Spinal cord

Tongue

Buccinator muscle

Pharynx

Medial pterygoid muscle

Deep and superficial parotid gland

Retromandibular vein

Posterior belly of digastric muscle

Splenius capitis muscle

Semispinalis capitis muscle

Figure 5.16 Parotid region – MRI scan (axial view). Observe the relationship between the parotid gland and the masseter muscle. Also note that the internal jugular vein and internal carotid artery are located medial to the parotid gland

HEAD AND NECK Parotid, temporal, and pterygopalatine region

57

6   Eye

The eye is a complex organ that converts light entering it into a series of electrochemical signals, which the brain interprets as a visual picture of the surrounding environment (Fig. 6.1). The eye has a tough outer covering, the **sclera**, which is visible externally as the 'white' of the eye. In the central portion of the visible eye is the **cornea**, which is a transparent multilayered membrane through which light enters the eye and where preliminary focusing occurs. Abnormalities in the cornea can therefore decrease visual capacity.

Deep to the cornea is the **anterior chamber** of the eye, which contains **aqueous humor** – a clear fluid through which light passes before entering the pupil. The **pupil** is a circular aperture surrounded by the **iris**, a contractile pigmented structure that regulates the amount of light entering the eye. From the pupil, light passes through the lens, where it is focused, and then through the **vitreous humor** (a clear, gel-like substance). It finally strikes the **retina**, from where photosensitive cells send nerve impulses to the brain.

LACRIMAL APPARATUS

Tears, produced by the **lacrimal apparatus**, prevent drying of the cornea and conjunctiva, provide lubrication between the eye and eyelid, contain bactericidal enzymes, and improve the optical performance of the cornea. They supply oxygen to the avascular cornea. The lacrimal apparatus consists of the **lacrimal gland** and accessory lacrimal glands behind the upper eyelid in the superolateral angle of the orbit, and the lacrimal duct system (Fig. 6.2). Tears pass through several ducts and move across the eye in a wave-like pattern created by the upper and lower **eyelids** during blinking. Blinking also aids in removing any foreign material and bacteria.

On the medial, superior, and inferior lid margins are two openings – the **lacrimal puncta**. These collect tears that have crossed the eye and transfer them to the **lacrimal sac**. Tears are then directed into the **nasolacrimal duct**, which empties into the nasal cavity. This connection between the eye and the nasal cavity explains why people often have a runny nose (clear rhinorrhea) when crying. Sensory innervation of the lacrimal gland is from the **lacrimal nerves**, which are branches of the ophthalmic nerve [V_1]. The facial nerve [VII] provides preganglionic parasympathetic fibers, which enter the pterygopalatine ganglion. From here, nerve fibers enter the zygomatic branch of the maxillary nerve [V_2] and the lacrimal nerve (of the ophthalmic nerve [V_1]) to provide autonomic innervation.

Lymphatic drainage of the lacrimal gland is to the **parotid nodes**.

BONY ORBIT

Each eye resides within an **orbit**, which is pyramidal in shape, having an open anterior margin (or base), a posterior apex, a roof, floor, and medial and lateral walls (Fig. 6.3). The medial walls are parallel, whereas the lateral walls diverge from one another at 90°. Each orbital wall has several important adjacent relationships:

- roof – anterior cranial fossa, frontal sinus, and frontal lobes of the brain;
- floor – the maxillary sinus and infra-orbital nerves and muscles;
- medial wall – ethmoid cells, sphenoidal sinuses, and nasal cavity;
- lateral wall – temporal fossa;
- apex – middle cranial fossa, temporal lobes of brain, infratemporal fossa, and pterygopalatine fossa.

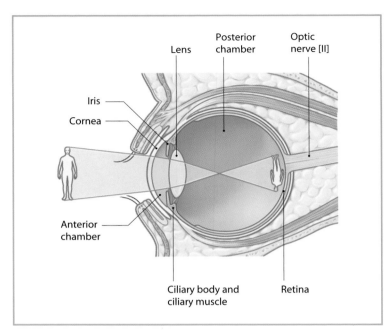

Figure 6.1 Section through the eye showing the pathway of light to the retina

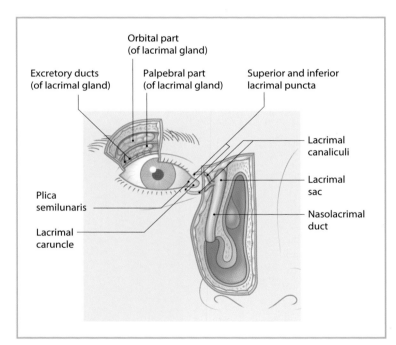

Figure 6.2 Lacrimal apparatus

The apex of the orbit is at the **optic canal**, within the lesser wing of the sphenoid and just medial to the superior orbital fissure. The **orbital margin**, made up of parts of the frontal, zygomatic, maxilla, and lacrimal bones, forms a protective rim around the edges of the orbit. The bony elements of the orbital walls are the:

- roof – **orbital plate** of frontal bone and **lesser wing** of the sphenoid;

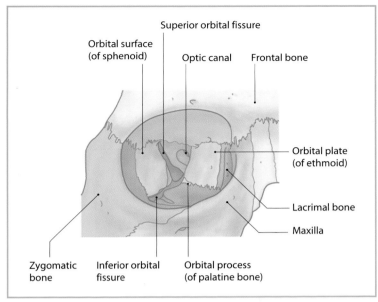

Figure 6.3 Walls of the orbit

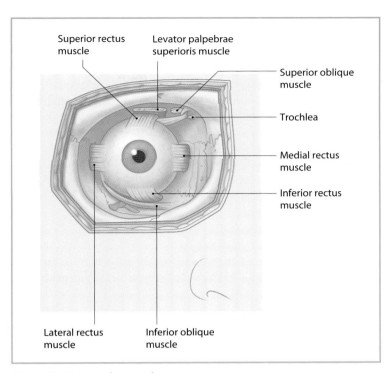

Figure 6.4 Extraocular muscles

- floor – orbital surface of the **maxilla**, and contributions from the **zygomatic** and **palatine** bones;
- lateral wall – **frontal process** of the zygomatic bone and **greater wing** of the sphenoid;
- medial wall – **orbital plate** of the ethmoid, the **lacrimal bone**, the **frontal process** of maxilla, the **body** of the sphenoid, and the **frontal bone**.

Several foramina and fissures form passageways for the vital nerves and blood vessels that support the eye, and for structures that pass through the orbit (see Fig. 6.3).

MUSCLES

Extrinsic muscles of the orbit (Table 6.1, Fig. 6.4) move the eyelids. The **levator palpebrae superioris** muscle is a sheet-like muscle that raises the superior eyelid and is innervated by the oculomotor nerve [III]. The **orbicularis oculi** muscle is innervated by the facial nerve [VII] and gently or forcefully closes the superior and inferior eyelids. It is also important in facial expression.

The remaining extrinsic muscles attach onto and elevate, depress, intort, extort, adduct, and abduct the eye. These muscles are innervated by the oculomotor nerve [III], the trochlear nerve [IV], and the abducent nerve [VI].

NERVES

Motor innervation to the orbit is from several nerves (Fig. 6.5). The **oculomotor nerve [III]** originates from the brainstem and divides into **superior** and **inferior branches**, which pass through the **superior orbital fissure** to enter the orbit. The superior division supplies the superior rectus and levator palpebrae superioris muscles. The inferior division supplies the inferior rectus, medial rectus, and inferior oblique muscles. In addition, the inferior division carries preganglionic parasympathetic nerve fibers, which synapse in the **ciliary ganglion**.

Postganglionic fibers emerge from the ciliary ganglion and travel with the short ciliary nerves of the ophthalmic nerve $[V_1]$ to supply the sphincter pupillae and ciliary muscles.

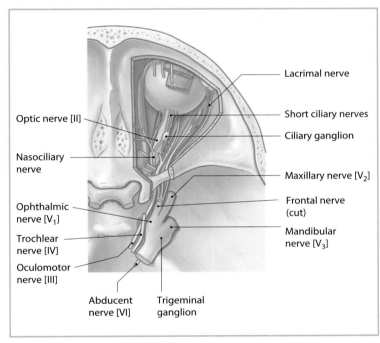

Figure 6.5 Nerve supply to the orbit (superior view of right orbit)

The **trochlear nerve [IV]** innervates the superior oblique muscle. It enters the orbit through the superior orbital fissure and enters the superior aspect of the superior oblique muscle.

The **abducent nerve [VI]** enters the orbit through the superior orbital fissure, then passes anteriorly to enter and innervate the lateral rectus muscle.

The **optic nerve [II]** carries afferent fibers from the retina. These fibers originate from the ganglion cells of the retina and converge at the posterior aspect of the eye. The optic nerve [II] runs posteriorly

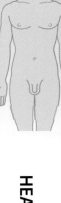

59

from the eye through the orbit to enter the **optic canal**, which enters the middle cranial fossa. Here it unites with the optic nerve [II] from the other eye to form the **optic chiasm**, where the nerve fibers reorganize so that information from the right and left visual fields of both the right and left eyes are combined into the **optic tract**. The optic tract traverses the brain to the visual cortex in the occipital lobe.

The **ophthalmic nerve [V₁]** is the first division of the trigeminal nerve [V]. It is a sensory nerve, originates from the **trigeminal ganglion** within the middle cranial fossa, and divides into the **nasociliary**, **frontal**, and **lacrimal nerves**. These three nerves pass through the superior orbital fissure to enter the orbit. Within the orbit they divide into branches that provide sensation to the eyeball, orbit and face:

- the eyeball and conjunctiva are innervated by the **long** and **short ciliary nerves**;
- the skin of the forehead, the lacrimal gland and the mucosa of frontal sinus are supplied by the **supratrochlear**, **supra-orbital**, and lacrimal nerves;
- cutaneous innervation of the superior eyelid and nose is supplied by the **infratrochlear nerve**;
- cutaneous innervation to the ethmoidal cells and superior part of nose is by the **anterior** and **posterior ethmoidal nerves**.

The **maxillary nerve [V₂]** – the second division of the trigeminal nerve [V] – leaves the trigeminal ganglion for the pterygopalatine fossa. From here it passes through the **inferior orbital fissure** to enter the orbit. The zygomatic branch of the maxillary nerve [V₂] carries postganglionic parasympathetic fibers, which originate at the pterygopalatine ganglion and run with the zygomatic nerve toward the lacrimal gland, where parasympathetic innervation stimulates tear production. After entering the orbit through the inferior orbital fissure, the maxillary nerve [V₂] becomes the **infra-orbital nerve**. This runs in the **infra-orbital groove** and **canal** within the maxilla and emerges through the **infra-orbital foramen** to provide sensory innervation to the face.

ARTERIES

Blood supply to the eye and structures of the orbit are from branches of the ophthalmic artery (Fig. 6.6), a branch of the internal carotid artery. It enters the orbit through the optic canal with the optic nerve [II]. The ophthalmic artery divides into:

- ciliary branches to the eyeball;
- muscular branches to the extraocular muscles;
- additional branches that follow the supra-orbital, supratrochlear, lacrimal, and anterior and posterior ethmoidal nerves.

A terminal branch of the ophthalmic artery forms the **central retinal artery**. This vessel is an end artery and does not anastomose with any other arteries, so if it is obstructed the retina loses its blood supply. This leads to visual field defects and, in cases of complete occlusion, possible blindness.

VEINS AND LYMPHATICS

The orbit is drained by the **superior** and **inferior ophthalmic veins** and the **infra-orbital vein**; the veins of the eyeball drain to the **vorticose veins**. The **central retinal vein** drains into the superior ophthalmic vein. These veins empty into the intracranial venous dural **cavernous sinus**.

Lymphatic drainage of the orbit is to the **parotid nodes**.

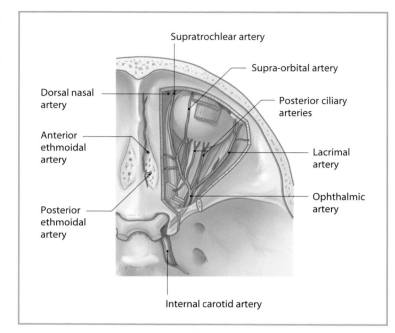

Figure 6.6 Arterial supply to the orbit

■ CLINICAL CORRELATIONS
Corneal abrasion

Corneal abrasions (Fig. 6.7) are caused by a foreign object damaging the eye. Many patients report rubbing their eyes because of the subsequent irritation or pain. They may also complain of watery eyes, blurred vision, and redness of the involved eye.

On examination, the eye is usually watering and has an irritated, erythematous (reddened) conjunctiva. A foreign body may be visible. Diagnosis is aided by applying a topical anesthetic to the eye to enable a more thorough examination. The eye can be stained with a fluorescent dye, which adheres to any abrasions on the corneal surface and is visible on inspection with ultraviolet ('black') light. A slit-lamp is used to examine the structures in the anterior segment of the eye.

Treatment of corneal abrasion aims to remove any foreign body by flushing the eye with sterile solutions, as necessary. Antibiotic eye drops are often prescribed to prevent secondary infection. Follow-up by an optometrist is also recommended.

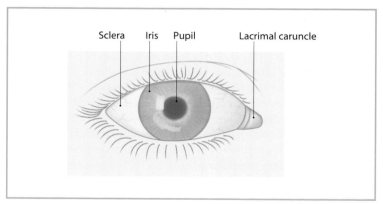

Figure 6.7 Corneal abrasion

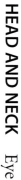

HEAD AND NECK Eye

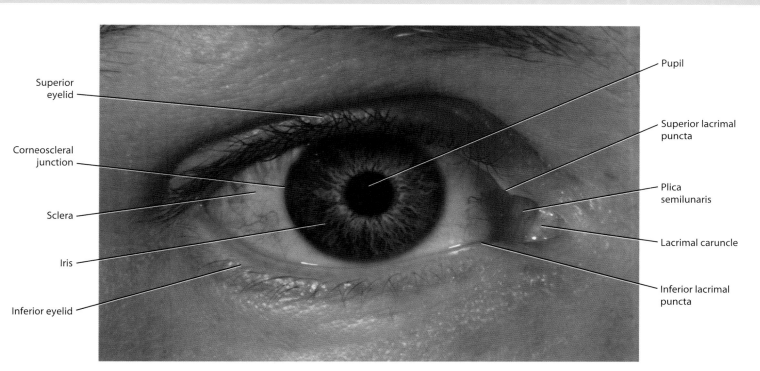

Superior eyelid

Corneoscleral junction

Sclera

Iris

Inferior eyelid

Pupil

Superior lacrimal puncta

Plica semilunaris

Lacrimal caruncle

Inferior lacrimal puncta

Figure 6.8 Eye – surface anatomy. Close-up view of right eye

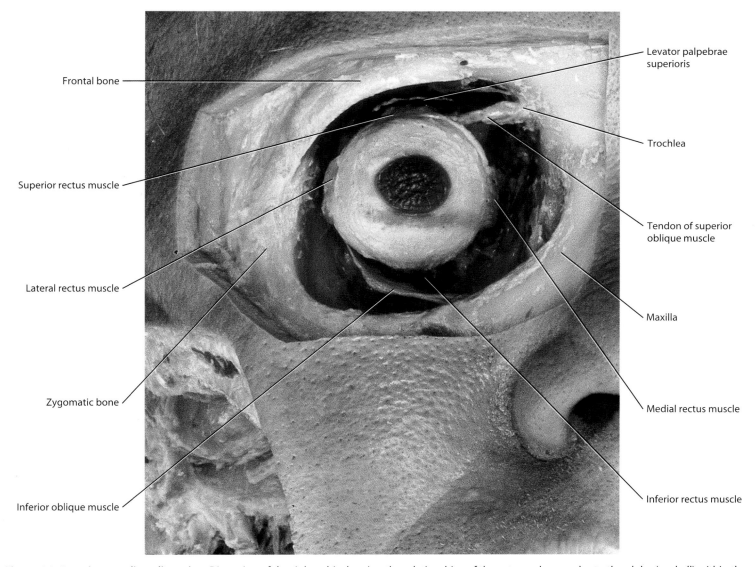

Frontal bone

Superior rectus muscle

Lateral rectus muscle

Zygomatic bone

Inferior oblique muscle

Levator palpebrae superioris

Trochlea

Tendon of superior oblique muscle

Maxilla

Medial rectus muscle

Inferior rectus muscle

Figure 6.9 Eye – intermediate dissection. Dissection of the right orbit showing the relationships of the extraocular muscles to the globe (eyeball) within the orbit. The cornea appears wrinkled and lacks its usual shiny appearance as a result of the preservation process of the cadaver. The cadaver has been modified to prevent recognition

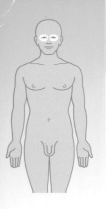

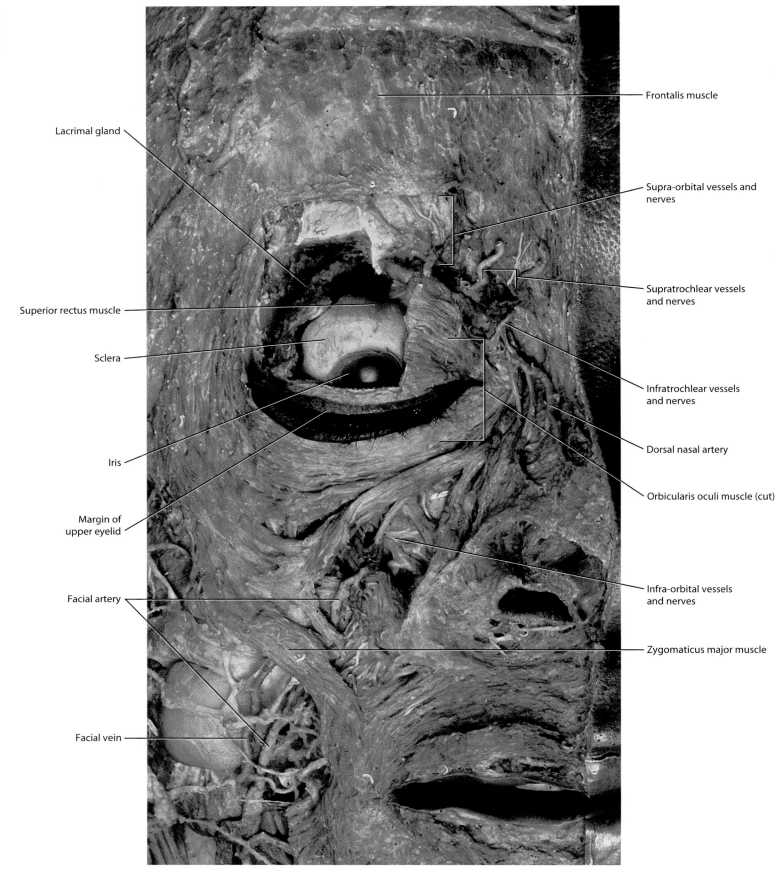

Frontalis muscle

Lacrimal gland

Supra-orbital vessels and nerves

Superior rectus muscle

Supratrochlear vessels and nerves

Sclera

Infratrochlear vessels and nerves

Iris

Dorsal nasal artery

Orbicularis oculi muscle (cut)

Margin of upper eyelid

Facial artery

Infra-orbital vessels and nerves

Zygomaticus major muscle

Facial vein

Figure 6.10 Eye – superficial dissection. Part of the right superior eyelid and levator palpebrae superioris and orbicularis oculi muscles have been removed to show the relationship of the globe (eyeball) to the surrounding muscles

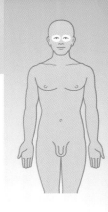

TABLE 6.1 MUSCLES OF THE EYEBALL AND EYELIDS, AND INTRINSIC MUSCLES OF THE EYE

Muscle	Origin	Insertion	Action	Nerve supply	Blood supply
Extrinsic muscles of the eyeball Superior rectus	Common tendinous ring	Superior aspect of eyeball, posterior to the corneoscleral junction	Elevates, adducts and medially rotates eyeball	Oculomotor nerve [III] – superior division	Ophthalmic artery
Inferior rectus	Common tendinous ring	Inferior aspect of eyeball, posterior to corneoscleral junction	Depresses, adducts and medially rotates eyeball	Oculomotor nerve [III] – inferior division	Ophthalmic artery
Medial rectus	Common tendinous ring	Medial aspect of eyeball, posterior to corneoscleral junction	Moves eyeball medially	Oculomotor nerve [III] – inferior division	Ophthalmic artery
Lateral rectus	Common tendinous ring	Lateral aspect of eyeball, posterior to corneoscleral junction	Moves eyeball laterally	Abducent nerve [VI]	Ophthalmic artery
Superior oblique	Body of sphenoid, above optic foramen and medial origin of superior rectus	Passes through trochlea and attaches to superior sclera between superior and lateral recti	Rotates eyeball downward and outward	Trochlear nerve [IV]	Ophthalmic artery
Inferior oblique	Anterior floor of orbit lateral to nasolacrimal canal	Lateral sclera deep to lateral rectus	Rotates eyeball upward and laterally	Oculomotor nerve [III] – inferior division	Ophthalmic artery
Muscles of eyelids Levator palpebrae superioris #	Lesser wing of sphenoid, anterior to optic canal	Superior tarsus	Raises upper eyelid	Oculomotor nerve [III] – superior division	Ophthalmic artery
# Involuntary smooth muscle part inserts into upper margin of superior tarsus innervated by postganglionic sympathetics					
Orbicularis oculi	Medial orbital margin, palpebral ligament, and lacrimal bone	Skin around orbit palpebral ligament, upper and lower eyelids	Closes eyelids	Facial nerve [VII]	Facial and superficial temporal arteries
Intrinsic muscles of the eye Sphincter pupillae (iris)	Circular smooth muscle of the iris that passes around pupil		Constricts pupil	Oculomotor nerve [III] – parasympathetics	Ophthalmic artery
Dilator pupillae (iris)	Ciliary body	Sphincter pupillae	Dilates pupil	Sympathetics	Ophthalmic artery
Ciliary	Corneoscleral junction	Ciliary body	Controls lens shape (accommodation)	Parasympathetics	Ophthalmic artery

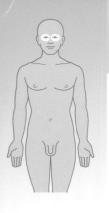

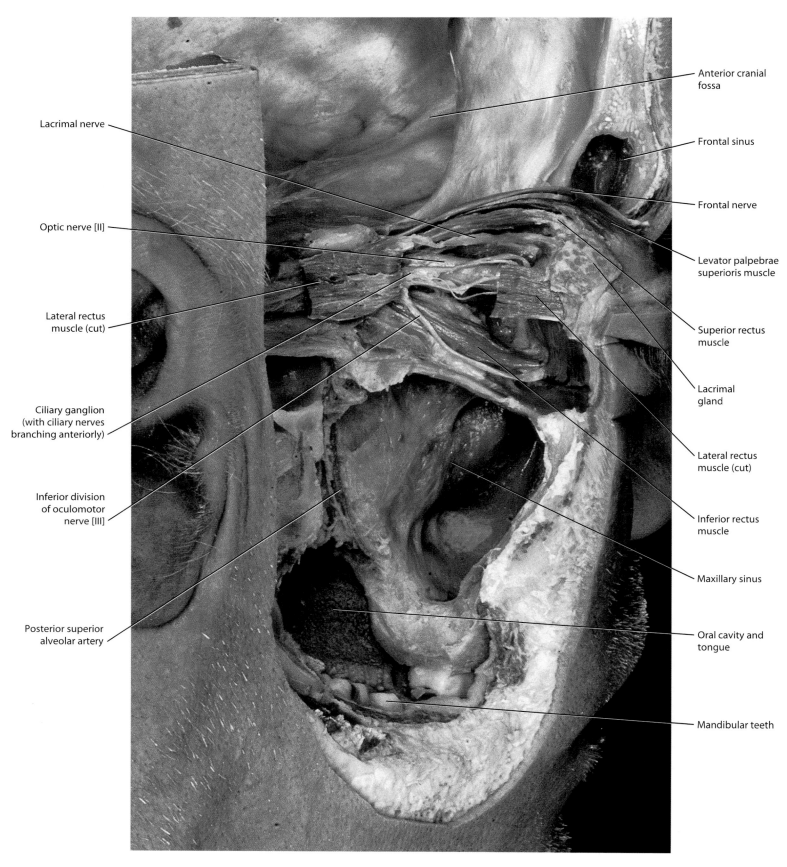

Lacrimal nerve

Optic nerve [II]

Lateral rectus
muscle (cut)

Ciliary ganglion
(with ciliary nerves
branching anteriorly)

Inferior division
of oculomotor
nerve [III]

Posterior superior
alveolar artery

Anterior cranial
fossa

Frontal sinus

Frontal nerve

Levator palpebrae
superioris muscle

Superior rectus
muscle

Lacrimal
gland

Lateral rectus
muscle (cut)

Inferior rectus
muscle

Maxillary sinus

Oral cavity and
tongue

Mandibular teeth

Figure 6.11 Orbit – deep dissection 1 (lateral view). In this dissection of the right orbit, the lateral portion of the skull has been removed to show the relationships of the extraocular muscles to the optic nerve and globe as well as the close proximity of the maxillary sinus

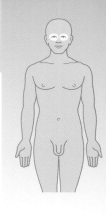

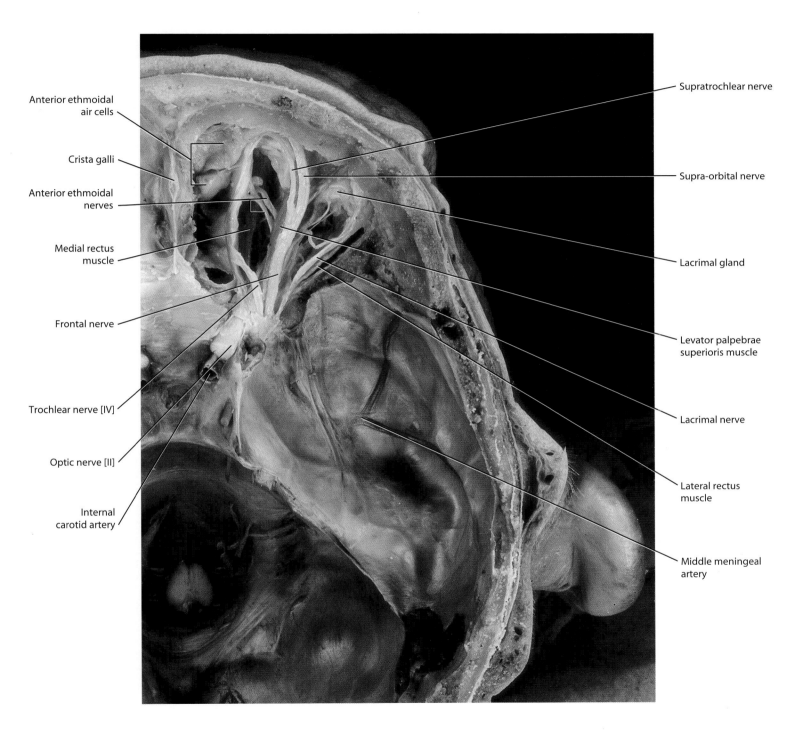

Anterior ethmoidal air cells

Crista galli

Anterior ethmoidal nerves

Medial rectus muscle

Frontal nerve

Trochlear nerve [IV]

Optic nerve [II]

Internal carotid artery

Supratrochlear nerve

Supra-orbital nerve

Lacrimal gland

Levator palpebrae superioris muscle

Lacrimal nerve

Lateral rectus muscle

Middle meningeal artery

Figure 6.12 Orbit – deep dissection 2 (superior view). The calvarium (cap-like portion of the skull), brain, and roof of the orbit (tegmentum) have been removed to reveal the structures of the orbit

65

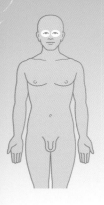

HEAD AND NECK

Eye

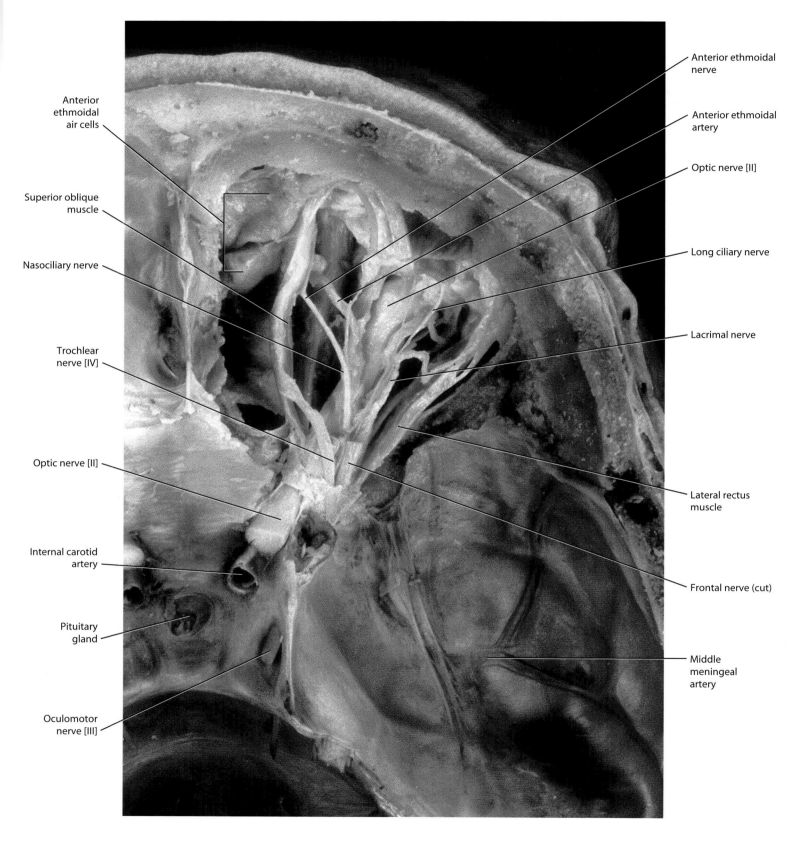

Anterior ethmoidal air cells

Superior oblique muscle

Nasociliary nerve

Trochlear nerve [IV]

Optic nerve [II]

Internal carotid artery

Pituitary gland

Oculomotor nerve [III]

Anterior ethmoidal nerve

Anterior ethmoidal artery

Optic nerve [II]

Long ciliary nerve

Lacrimal nerve

Lateral rectus muscle

Frontal nerve (cut)

Middle meningeal artery

Figure 6.13 Orbit – deep dissection 3 (superior view). A close-up view of the specimen shown in Figure 6.12. The frontal nerve has been cut to reveal deeper structures

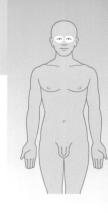

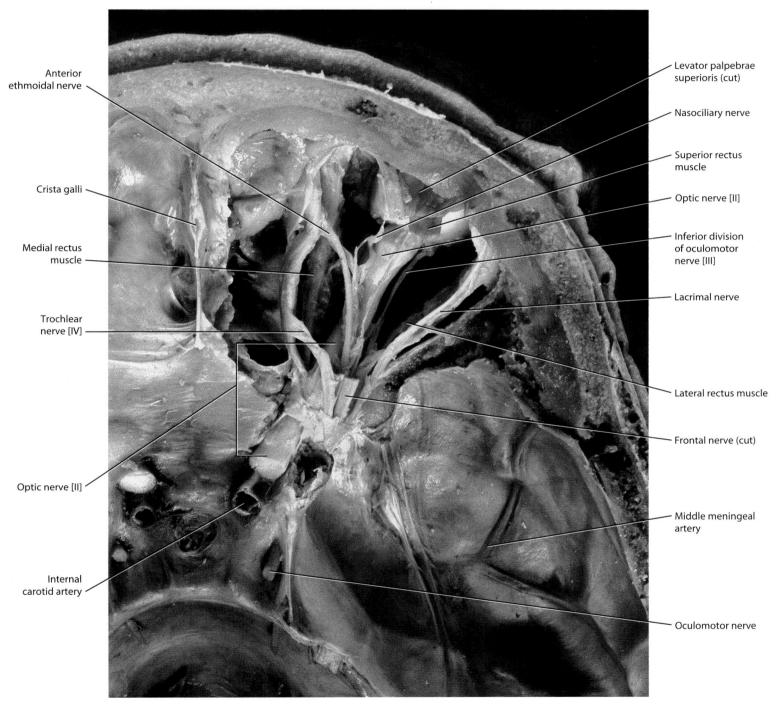

Anterior
ethmoidal nerve

Crista galli

Medial rectus
muscle

Trochlear
nerve [IV]

Optic nerve [II]

Internal
carotid artery

Levator palpebrae
superioris (cut)

Nasociliary nerve

Superior rectus
muscle

Optic nerve [II]

Inferior division
of oculomotor
nerve [III]

Lacrimal nerve

Lateral rectus muscle

Frontal nerve (cut)

Middle meningeal
artery

Oculomotor nerve

Figure 6.14 Orbit – deep dissection 4 (superior view). A close-up view of the specimen shown in Figure 6.12. The large optic nerve [II] is visible as it joins the globe (eyeball)

67

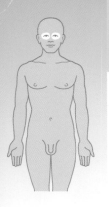

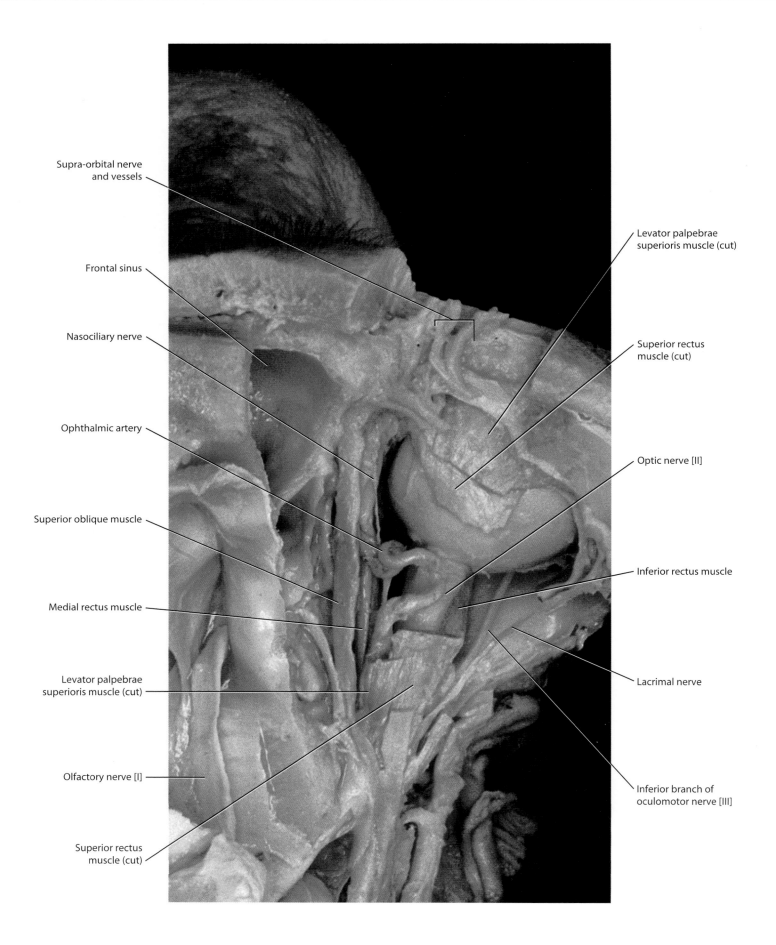

Supra-orbital nerve
and vessels

Frontal sinus

Nasociliary nerve

Ophthalmic artery

Superior oblique muscle

Medial rectus muscle

Levator palpebrae
superioris muscle (cut)

Olfactory nerve [I]

Superior rectus
muscle (cut)

Levator palpebrae
superioris muscle (cut)

Superior rectus
muscle (cut)

Optic nerve [II]

Inferior rectus muscle

Lacrimal nerve

Inferior branch of
oculomotor nerve [III]

Figure 6.15 Orbit – deep dissection 5 (superior view). The posterior part of the globe is clearly visible in relationship to the optic nerve [II] and surrounding orbital structures

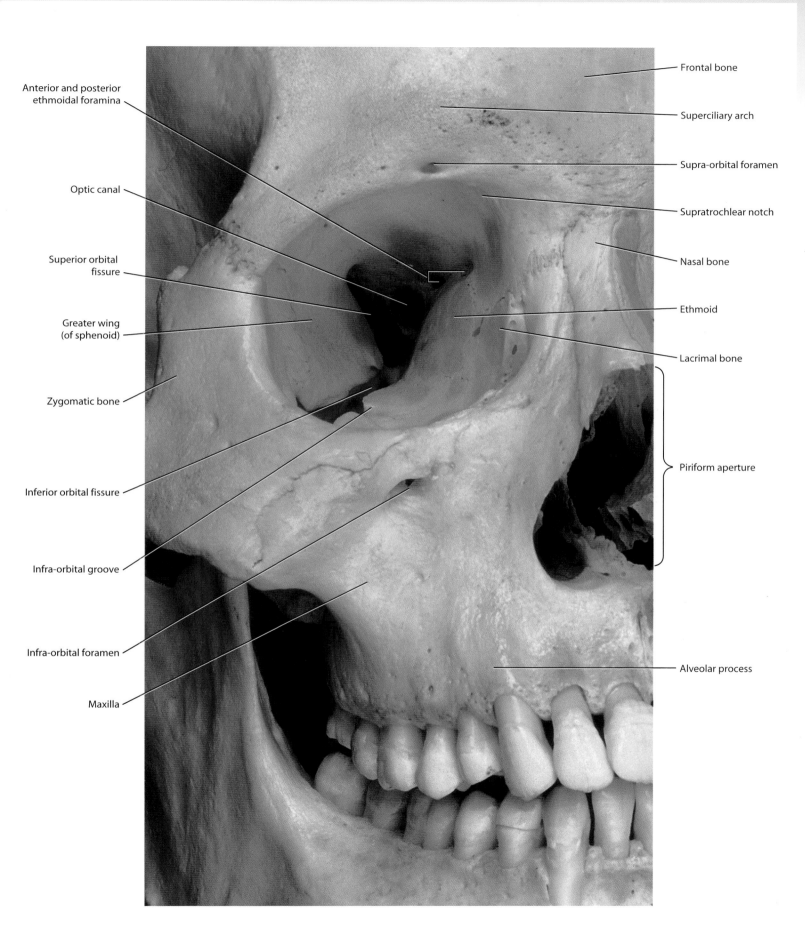

Anterior and posterior ethmoidal foramina

Optic canal

Superior orbital fissure

Greater wing (of sphenoid)

Zygomatic bone

Inferior orbital fissure

Infra-orbital groove

Infra-orbital foramen

Maxilla

Frontal bone

Superciliary arch

Supra-orbital foramen

Supratrochlear notch

Nasal bone

Ethmoid

Lacrimal bone

Piriform aperture

Alveolar process

HEAD AND NECK   Eye

Figure 6.16 Orbit – osteology. This view shows the foramina visible within the orbit (optic canal, superior orbital fissure, inferior orbital fissure, and ethmoidal foramina)

69

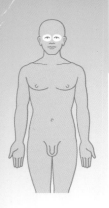

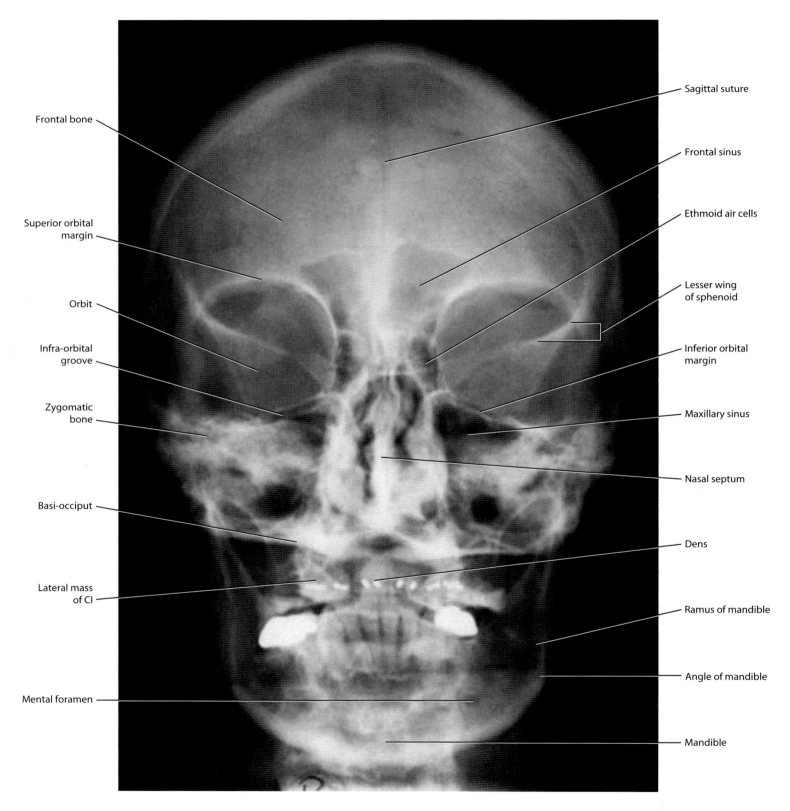

Frontal bone

Superior orbital margin

Orbit

Infra-orbital groove

Zygomatic bone

Basi-occiput

Lateral mass of CI

Mental foramen

Sagittal suture

Frontal sinus

Ethmoid air cells

Lesser wing of sphenoid

Inferior orbital margin

Maxillary sinus

Nasal septum

Dens

Ramus of mandible

Angle of mandible

Mandible

Figure 6.17 Orbit – plain film radiograph (anteroposterior view). Note the cortical definition of the osseous margin of the orbit. The infra-orbital groove is often visible in this view. Observe that the maxillary sinus is immediately inferior to the orbit

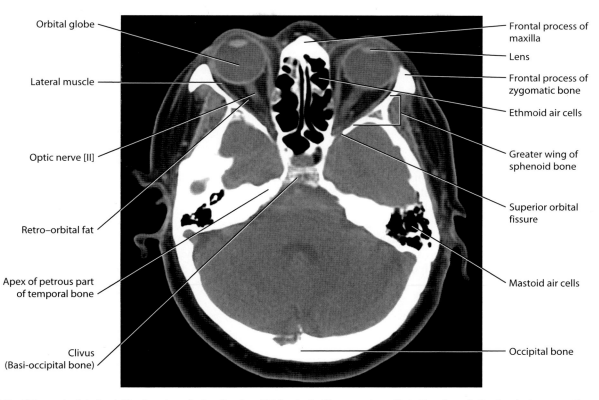

Orbital globe — Frontal process of maxilla

Lens

Lateral muscle — Frontal process of zygomatic bone

Ethmoid air cells

Optic nerve [II] — Greater wing of sphenoid bone

Superior orbital fissure

Retro–orbital fat —

Apex of petrous part of temporal bone — Mastoid air cells

Clivus (Basi-occipital bone) — Occipital bone

Figure 6.18 Orbit – CT scan (axial view). The lens is well visualized on CT due to its fibrous nature. Note the clear distinction between optic nerve and the retro-orbital fat

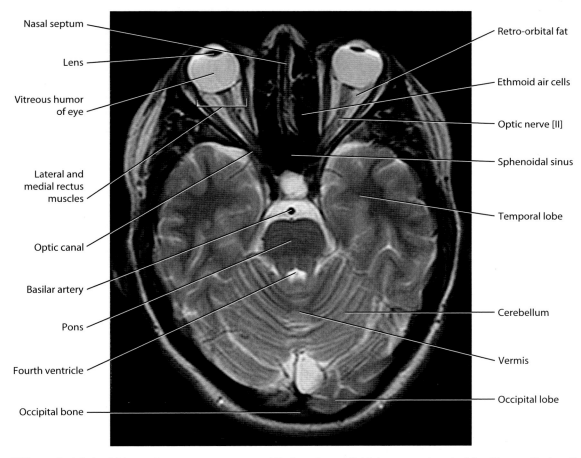

Nasal septum — Retro-orbital fat

Lens —

Vitreous humor of eye — Ethmoid air cells

Optic nerve [II]

Lateral and medial rectus muscles — Sphenoidal sinus

Optic canal — Temporal lobe

Basilar artery —

Pons — Cerebellum

Fourth ventricle — Vermis

Occipital bone — Occipital lobe

Figure 6.19 Orbit – MRI scan (axial view). The optic nerve appears gray, while the retro-orbital fat appears almost white. Observe the location of the gray extraocular muscles within the orbit

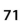

HEAD AND NECK   Eye

7 Ear

The ear is the organ of hearing and balance. It is divided into three parts – external, middle, and internal ear. Bony support for the ear is provided by the temporal bone.

EXTERNAL EAR

The external ear is composed of the **auricle** (pinna), the **external acoustic meatus** (external auditory canal), and **tympanic membrane** (Fig. 7.1).

The auricle consists of cartilage covered by thin skin and it directs sound into the external acoustic meatus. The skin over the auricle is innervated by branches of the **auriculotemporal nerve** (from the mandibular nerve [V$_3$]), **vagus nerve [X]**, **facial nerve [VII]**, and **lesser occipital nerve**. Blood is supplied to the auricle by the **superficial temporal artery** and the **posterior auricular artery**. Venous drainage is to the **external jugular vein** system; lymphatic drainage is to the **pre-** and **postauricular lymph nodes**.

EXTERNAL ACOUSTIC MEATUS

Sound directed through the auricle enters the external acoustic meatus. This canal is usually 2–3 cm in length and ends medially at the tympanic membrane (ear drum). The lateral third of the external acoustic meatus consists of cartilage, and the medial two-thirds is a channel through the temporal bone. Thin skin containing wax-producing ceruminous glands lines the osseous external acoustic meatus.

The external acoustic meatus is innervated by the auriculotemporal, vagus [X], glossopharyngeal [IX], and facial [VII] nerves. Blood is supplied by branches of the external carotid artery – the superficial temporal artery, posterior auricular artery, and deep auricular artery from the maxillary artery. Venous drainage is provided by veins that run alongside the named arteries and empty into the external jugular vein. The lymphatics drain to the pre- and postauricular nodes.

MIDDLE EAR

The tympanic membrane is a multilayered structure that forms the lateral wall of the middle ear and amplifies sound waves. It is innervated by the auriculotemporal, vagus [X], glossopharyngeal [IX], and facial [VII] nerves; irritation of one of these nerves can cause discomfort within the ear. Sound waves are transmitted from the tympanic membrane to the inner ear by the **auditory ossicles** – the **malleus** (hammer), **incus** (anvil), and **stapes** (stirrup).

The other walls of the middle ear – the roof, floor, and anterior, posterior, and medial walls – are formed by the temporal bone (Table 7.1).

The **pharyngotympanic tube** (auditory or Eustachian tube) links the middle ear to the nasopharynx, and opens on the anterior wall of the middle ear. It allows the air pressure on either side of the tympanic membrane to equalize.

Loud sounds can damage the sensitive inner ear; two small muscles in the middle ear help regulate the intensity of sound vibrations.

- The **tensor tympani** muscle is attached to the malleus and constrains its movement. It is innervated by the mandibular nerve [V$_3$]. If a very loud sound is transmitted from the tympanic membrane, the tensor tympani contracts and decreases the intensity of the vibrations.
- The **stapedius** muscle is attached to the stapes, is innervated by the facial nerve [VII], and carries out a similar protective function as the tensor tympani in response to very loud noise.

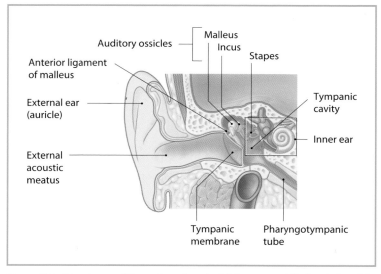

Figure 7.1 Structures of the external and middle ear, and their relationship to the inner ear

Wall or boundary	Features	Relationships
Lateral wall	Tympanic membrane, epitympanic recess ('attic'), and chorda tympani nerve	Tympanic membrane and epitympanic recess
Medial wall	Promontory (basal turn of cochlea), tympanic plexus, glossopharyngeal [IX] (parasympathetic) and corticotympanic nerves (sympathetic), round window, oval window prominences of facial nerve and lateral semicircular canal, and cochleariform process	Inner ear, facial nerve [VII]
Anterior wall	Opening of pharyngotympanic tube, semicanal for the tensor tympani muscle, internal carotid artery in its canal, and caroticotympanic canaliculus	External auditory meatus and internal carotid artery
Posterior wall	Aditus (opening) to mastoid antrum, pyramidal eminence, and facial canal	Mastoid antrum, facial nerve [VII]
Roof	Tegmen tympani	Middle cranial fossa and temporal lobe
Floor	Jugular fossa, tympanic branch of glossopharyngeal nerve [IX]	Bulb of internal jugular vein

TABLE 7.1 MIDDLE EAR (TYMPANIC CAVITY)

Sensory innervation to the middle ear is provided by the glossopharyngeal nerve [IX].

INNER EAR

The inner ear contains the auditory apparatus (the **cochlea** and **cochlear ducts**) and vestibular apparatus (Fig. 7.2). The cochlea receives vibrations from the stapes through the oval window and transmits them to liquid within the cochlear duct. Within the cochlea the vibrations are transformed into neurochemical messages, which are transported to the brain by the vestibulocochlear nerve [VIII], where they are interpreted as sound.

The vestibular apparatus is formed by fluid-filled semicircular canals (Fig. 7.3) and corresponding enlargements at the base of the canals – the utricle and saccule. These canals maintain equilibrium and balance, and contain small structures (otoliths) that move in response to changes in body position and momentum; these movements are transformed into nerve impulses, which reach the brain via the vestibulocochlear nerve [VIII].

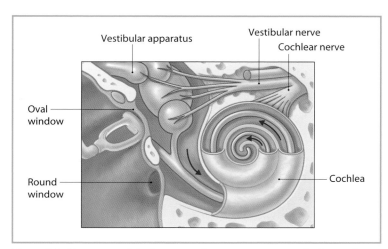

Figure 7.2 Structures of the inner ear. Arrows represent path of sound

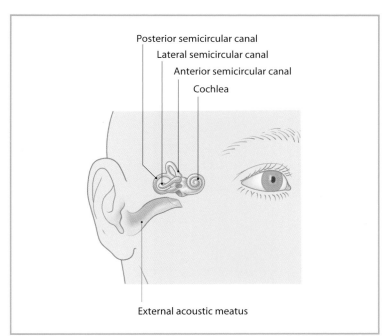

Figure 7.3 Orientation of the vestibular canals

Blood is supplied to the inner ear by the **labyrinthine artery**, a branch of the basilar artery, and the **stylomastoid artery**, a branch of the posterior auricular artery. Venous drainage is through veins that lie alongside the arteries and flow toward the **cavernous sinus** within the brain. Lymphatic drainage is to the pre- and postauricular lymph node groups.

■ CLINICAL CORRELATIONS
Otitis media

Otitis media is infection and inflammation in the middle ear. In children the pharyngotympanic tube is oriented horizontally and is usually less than 2 cm in length; in adults it is more vertical and longer. These differences have been cited as the reason for the higher incidence of otitis media in children. In advanced stages the tympanic membrane may rupture, causing otorrhea (discharge of pus from the external acoustic meatus).

On examination, the light reflex (a cone of light reflected from the tympanic membrane, and seen through an otoscope, Fig. 7.4) is usually decreased; this is a sign of infection. In addition, the membrane may be yellow or darkened in color, and it is sometimes erythematous. Insufflation of the tympanic membrane reflects immobility, a hallmark of otitis media.

Otitis externa

Otitis externa is infection and inflammation of the external acoustic meatus. The wax from the cerumen-producing glands in the lining of the canal creates a protective water-resistant layer in the external acoustic meatus. However, trauma, prolonged exposure to water, or submersion can breach this protective layer, allowing infectious agents to enter the external acoustic meatus.

Otitis externa usually causes itching and pain within the external acoustic meatus, which may swell and become edematous with continuing infection. The external ear and auricle are tender to the touch. Any manipulation that also causes movement of the auditory canal is very painful. Otoscopic examination reveals an edematous and swollen external acoustic meatus, which can also be erythematous. Purulent discharge within the canal can obstruct visualization of the tympanic membrane.

Treatment is directed at cleansing the external acoustic meatus by irrigation. For mild infections this is usually followed by topical antibiotic drops for several days. Follow-up examination is necessary to ensure that the infection resolves.

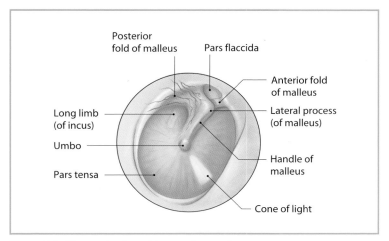

Figure 7.4 Otoscopic view of tympanic membrane

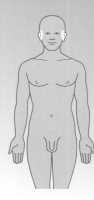

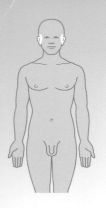

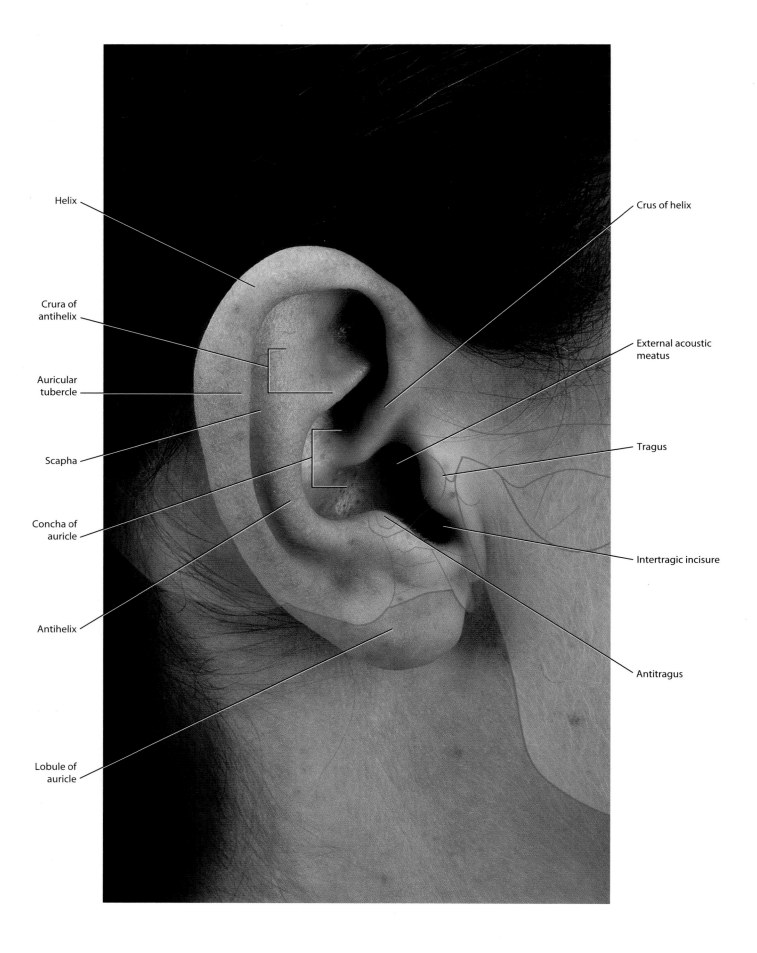

Helix

Crura of
antihelix

Auricular
tubercle

Scapha

Concha of
auricle

Antihelix

Lobule of
auricle

Crus of helix

External acoustic
meatus

Tragus

Intertragic incisure

Antitragus

Figure 7.5 Ear – surface anatomy. Right ear of a young woman. Observe the external acoustic meatus

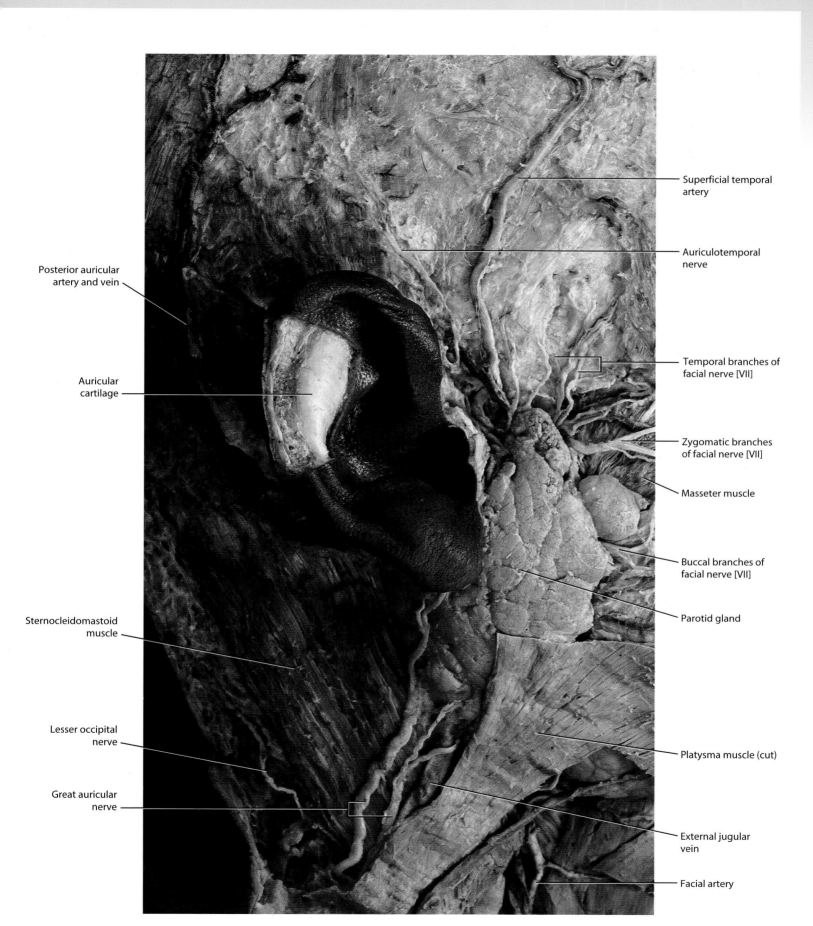

Superficial temporal artery

Auriculotemporal nerve

Temporal branches of facial nerve [VII]

Zygomatic branches of facial nerve [VII]

Masseter muscle

Buccal branches of facial nerve [VII]

Parotid gland

Platysma muscle (cut)

External jugular vein

Facial artery

Posterior auricular artery and vein

Auricular cartilage

Sternocleidomastoid muscle

Lesser occipital nerve

Great auricular nerve

Figure 7.6 Ear – superficial dissection. Part of the skin covering the right ear has been removed to show the underlying cartilage. Also observe the close proximity of the parotid gland to the external acoustic meatus

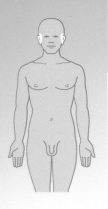

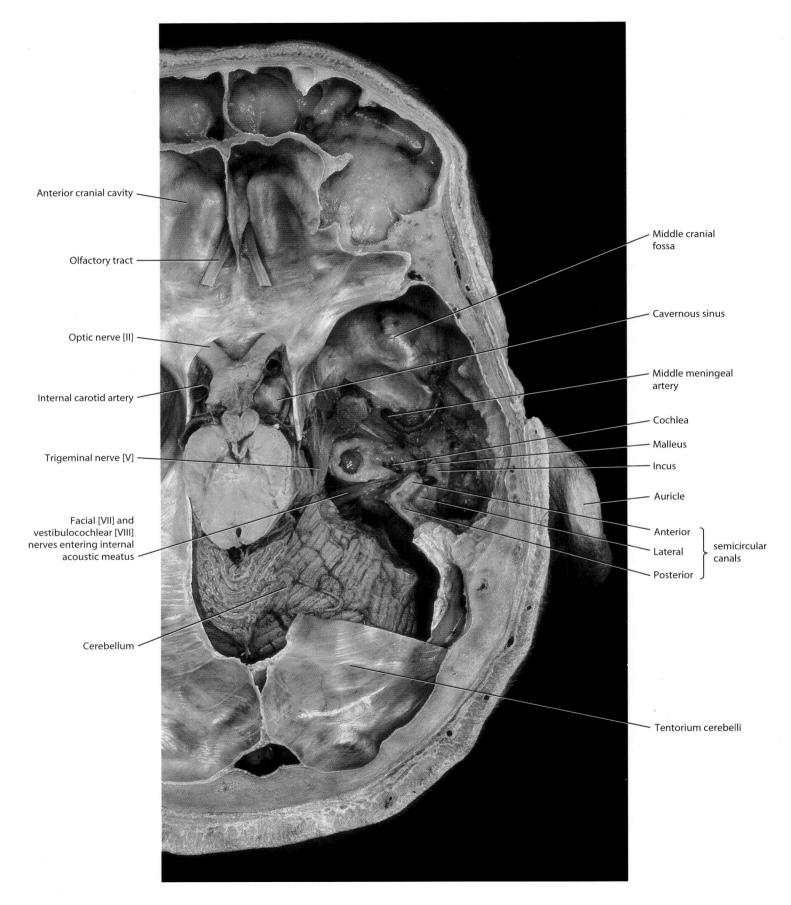

Anterior cranial cavity

Olfactory tract

Optic nerve [II]

Internal carotid artery

Trigeminal nerve [V]

Facial [VII] and
vestibulocochlear [VIII]
nerves entering internal
acoustic meatus

Cerebellum

Middle cranial
fossa

Cavernous sinus

Middle meningeal
artery

Cochlea

Malleus

Incus

Auricle

Anterior
Lateral } semicircular
canals
Posterior

Tentorium cerebelli

Figure 7.7 Ear – transverse section. Superior view of a transverse skull section. The calvarium has been removed. The roof of the middle and inner ear formed by the temporal bone has also been removed to show the cochlea, semicircular canals, and middle ear ossicles

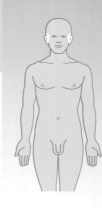

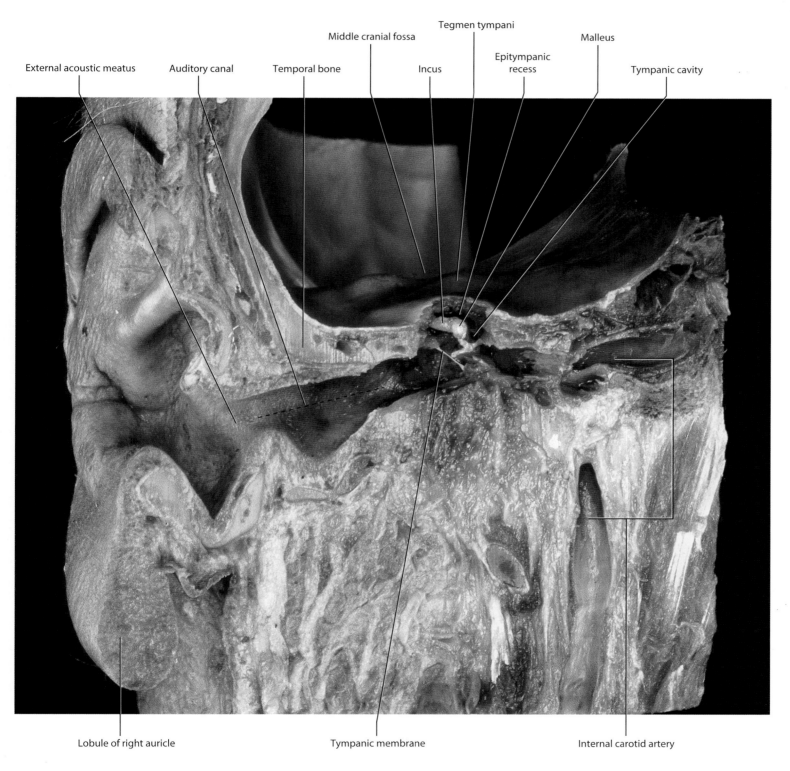

Tegmen tympani

Middle cranial fossa

Malleus

External acoustic meatus

Auditory canal

Temporal bone

Incus

Epitympanic recess

Tympanic cavity

Lobule of right auricle

Tympanic membrane

Internal carotid artery

Figure 7.8 Ear – coronal section. A section through the skull to show the external acoustic meatus, tympanic membrane, and middle ear cavity of the right ear

77

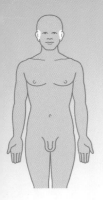

TABLE 7.2 STRUCTURE AND FUNCTION OF THE EAR

	Structure	Function	Cranial nerves
Outer ear			
Auricle (pinna)	Cartilage (except most inferior portion, lobule)		Trigeminal [V]
External acoustic meatus (EAM)	Lateral third to half: cartilage containing modified sebaceous and ceruminous glands and hairs (cilia) Medial portion: squamous and tympanic portions of temporal bone	Protects middle and inner ear; directs sound to middle ear	Trigeminal [V] Facial [VII] Vagus [X] Glossopharyngeal [IX]
Middle ear			
Tympanic membrane (TM)	Cone-shaped; displaced inward near center by approximately 2mm Three layers: thin cutaneous layer continuous with EAM; fibrous middle layer; internal layer of serous membrane	Conducts sound to ossicles	Facial [VII] Glossopharyngeal [IX] Vagus [X]
Ossicles			
Malleus	Head projects upward, occupies half of epitympanic recess; handle of malleus attaches to TM forming umbo of tympanic ring; head attaches to body of incus		
Incus	Body attaches to head of malleus, long limb to head of stapes	Conducts sound from TM to cochlea	
Stapes	Head attaches to long limb of incus; footplate occupies round window		
Muscles			
Tensor tympani	Origin: bony semicanal running parallel to pharyngotympanic tube Insertion: handle of malleus 25mm long	Increases tension of TM; partial protection from loud noise	Mandibular division of trigeminal [V_3]
Stapedius	Origin: bony canal running parallel to facial nerve canal Insertion: head of stapes via tendon 6mm long	Draws stapedius posteriorly at 90° to movement of ossicular chain; partial protection from loud noise	Facial [VII]
Auditory tube	Osseous (12mm), cartilaginous (18–24mm), and membranous portions	Communication between middle ear and nasopharynx: equalizes middle ear pressure, drainage	Glossopharyngeal [IX]
Inner ear			
Auditory apparatus			
Cochlea	Spiral canal (3 channels: scala media, vestibuli and tympani) making $2\frac{3}{4}$ turns around bony modiolus, which houses nerves and blood supply	Sensory mechanism of hearing: base receives high- and apex receives low-frequency sounds	
Organ of Corti	Sensory epithelium, lined with sensory hair cells, between scala media and tympani	Sensory hair cells receive vibration and send information to brain	
Vestibular apparatus			
Semicircular canals	Three fluid-filled canals within fluid-containing bony labyrinth, each containing ampullary crest (sensory area)	Detect rotational movements	Vestibulocochlear [VIII]
Utricle and saccule	Utricle at base of semicircular canal, saccule between utricle and scala vestibuli Lined with macula, sensory epithelium covered by gelatinous material containing otoliths (crystals)	Maculae respond to linear acceleration Macula of utricle senses gravity and body/head tilt	

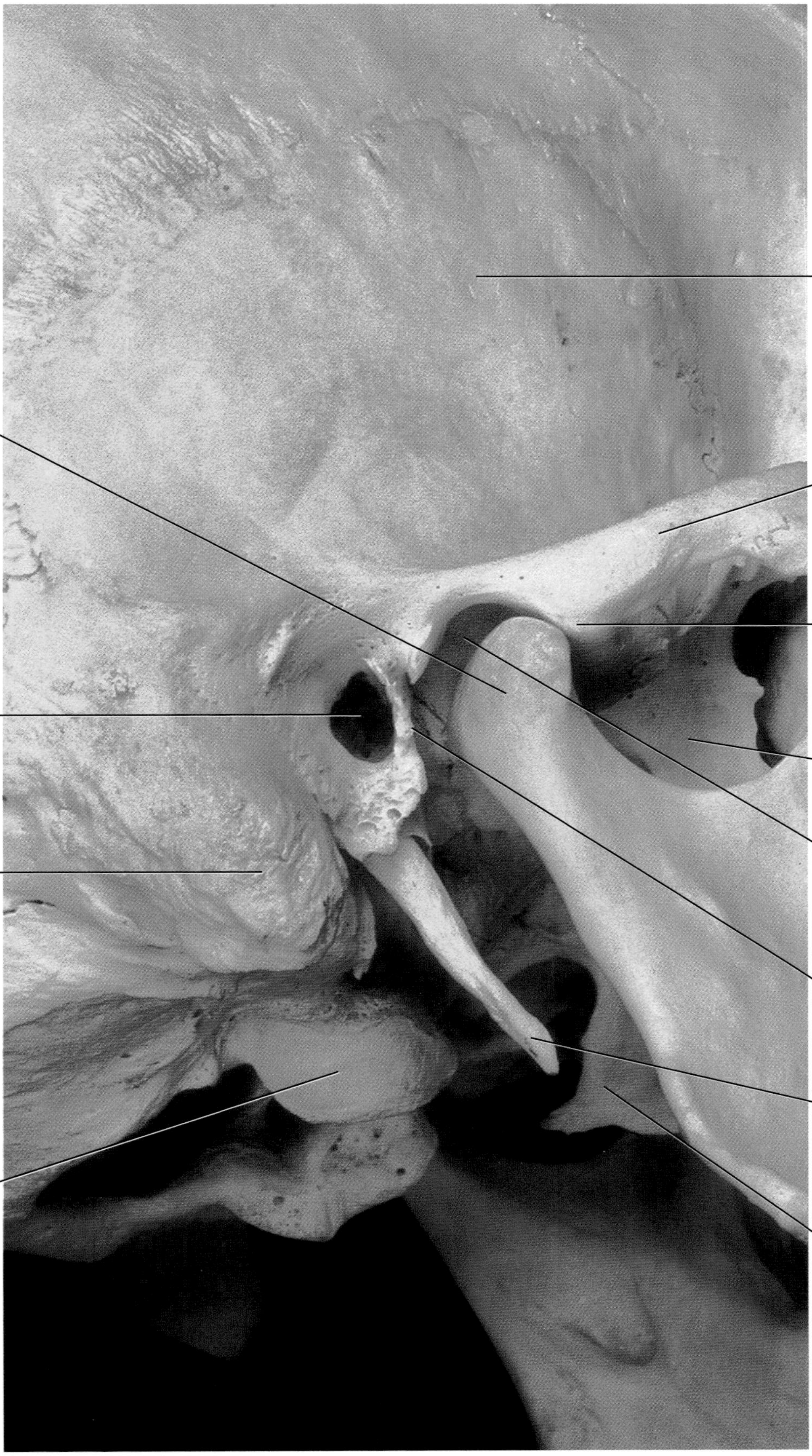

Squamous part
(of temporal bone)

Head of mandible

Zygomatic process
(of temporal bone)

Articular tubercle

External acoustic
meatus

Right lateral plate of
pterygoid process

Mastoid process

Mandibular fossa

Tympanic plate

Styloid process

Condylar process
(of occipital bone)

Left lateral plate of
pterygoid process

Figure 7.9 Ear – osteology. A view of the right side of the skull which shows the external acoustic meatus and its relationship to the temporomandibular joint

79

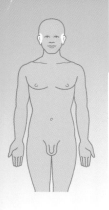

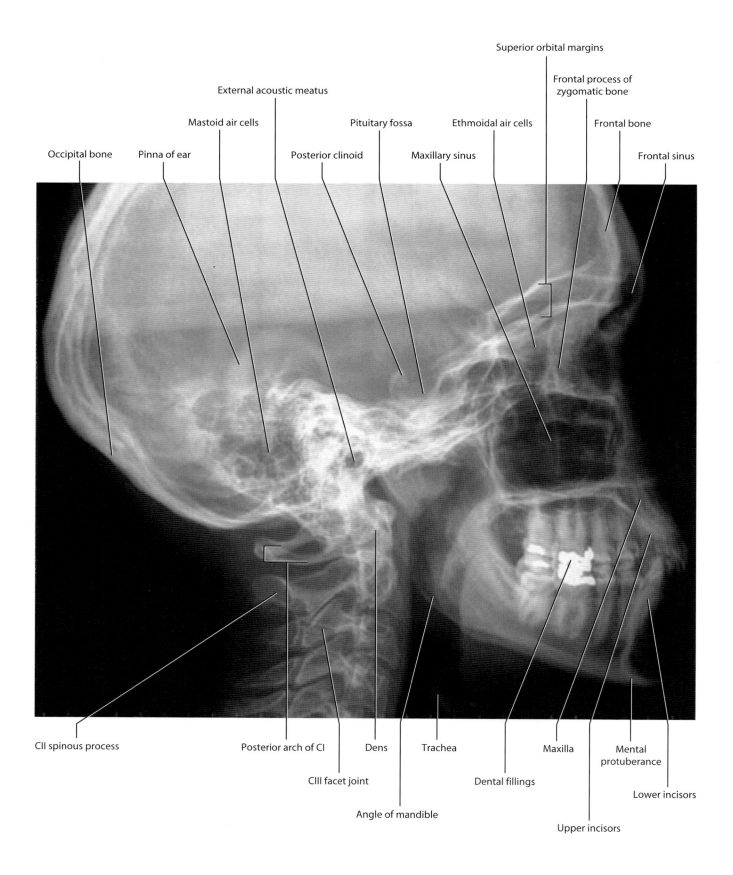

Superior orbital margins

Frontal process of
zygomatic bone

External acoustic meatus

Mastoid air cells

Pituitary fossa

Ethmoidal air cells

Frontal bone

Occipital bone

Pinna of ear

Posterior clinoid

Maxillary sinus

Frontal sinus

CII spinous process

Posterior arch of CI

Dens

Trachea

Maxilla

Mental
protuberance

CIII facet joint

Dental fillings

Lower incisors

Angle of mandible

Upper incisors

Figure 7.10 Ear – plain film radiograph (lateral view). The soft tissues of the pinna and the external acoustic meatus are visible on plain film radiographs. For visualization of the middle and inner ear, however, CT and MRI are superior. Observe the relationship between the external acoustic meatus and the first cervical vertebra (CI)

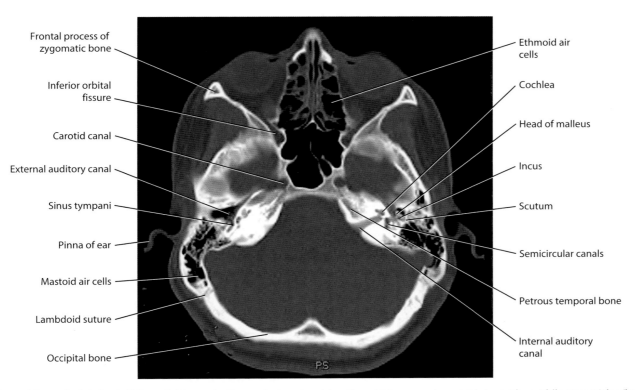

Frontal process of zygomatic bone
Inferior orbital fissure
Carotid canal
External auditory canal
Sinus tympani
Pinna of ear
Mastoid air cells
Lambdoid suture
Occipital bone

Ethmoid air cells
Cochlea
Head of malleus
Incus
Scutum
Semicircular canals
Petrous temporal bone
Internal auditory canal

Figure 7.11 Ear – CT scan (axial view). CT is useful for evaluating pathology involving the middle ear and mastoid sinus. The middle ear ossicles (bones) are visible in this view. Observe how they are located lateral to the cochlea

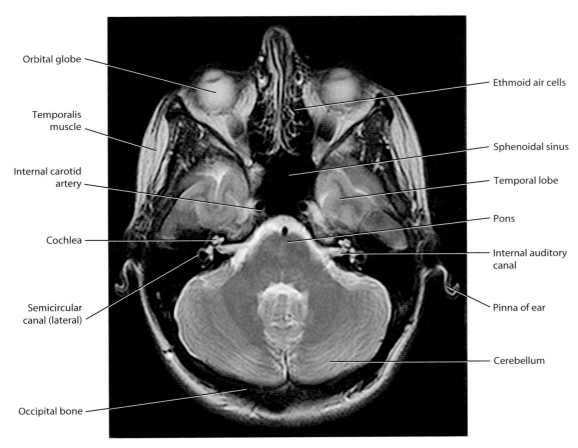

Orbital globe
Temporalis muscle
Internal carotid artery
Cochlea
Semicircular canal (lateral)
Occipital bone

Ethmoid air cells
Sphenoidal sinus
Temporal lobe
Pons
Internal auditory canal
Pinna of ear
Cerebellum

Figure 7.12 Ear – MRI scan (axial view). Note that osseous detail is not well visualized using MRI, so the bones of the middle ear are not seen. The fluid-filled lateral semicircular canal is well visualized in this view

81

8 Nose

The nasal region includes the nose, nasal cavity, and paranasal sinuses. Air is filtered, humidified, and warmed in this region before entering the respiratory tract. The nasal cavity contains the specialized olfactory mucosa responsible for the sense of smell.

EXTERNAL NOSE

The superior portion of the external nose is bony and is composed of **paired nasal bones** and the **frontal processes of the maxillae**. The inferior expanded portion of the nose is cartilaginous and is formed by the **major** and **minor alar cartilages** and a variable number of **accessory cartilages** (Fig. 8.1).

The triangular shape created by the nasal cartilages is an architecturally stable structure that creates and maintains an open airway. The skin covering the nose is freely movable over the nasal bones but is firmly attached over the cartilages. The external nose has two **nares** (nostrils) into which air flows during inspiration.

Attached to the external nose are muscles for dilating and flattening the nose – the dilator and compressor muscles, respectively – which are innervated by the facial nerve [VII].

Sensory innervation of the external nose is provided by branches of the **ophthalmic [V₁]** and **maxillary [V₂] nerve** divisions of the trigeminal nerve [V]. Blood is supplied by branches of the **ophthalmic artery** (a branch of the internal carotid artery) and the **facial artery** (a branch of the external carotid artery). Venous drainage is important clinically because it is to the **facial** and **ophthalmic veins,** which communicate with the **cavernous sinus** within the cranial cavity; this presents a potential route for infection from the superficial face to the brain and intracranial structures.

NASAL CAVITY

The nasal cavity extends from the vestibule of the nose to the **choanae** (the posterior nasal apertures) (Table 8.1, p. 84). The nasal cavity has a floor, roof, two lateral walls, and a midline **nasal septum** that divides it in half. The walls of the nasal cavity are covered with respiratory epithelium. Olfactory epithelium, involved in the sense of smell, is present on the superior part of the nasal septum and superior conchae.

The roof of the nasal cavity is narrow, arched, and inferior to the anterior cranial fossa. From anterior to posterior it is formed by the nasal cartilages, the nasal and frontal bones, the **cribriform plate** of the ethmoid, and the body of the sphenoid.

Paired **horizontal plates** of the palatine bones and the **palatine processes** of the maxillae form the floor of the nasal cavity and roof of the oral cavity. Foramina for the greater and lesser palatine nerves and vessels are located posteriorly, with the incisive foramen located anteriorly for the nasopalatine nerve.

The nasal septum is formed anteriorly by the septal cartilage. Posterior to this is the **perpendicular plate** of ethmoid and the **vomer** bone. The lateral walls of the nasal cavity are complex, with three horizontally oriented bony medial projections – the **superior, middle,** and **inferior nasal conchae** (or turbinates) – which increase the nasal surface area (Fig. 8.2).

The area posterior to the superior concha is the **spheno-ethmoidal recess** and the space inferior to each concha is a nasal meatus. The **middle nasal meatus** has a bulge (the **ethmoidal bulla**), which contains the paranasal **middle ethmoidal cells.**

Below the ethmoidal bulla is a half-moon-shaped opening, the **semilunar hiatus.** There are openings here for the frontal and

Frontal process (of maxilla)

Nasal bone

Lateral process
(of septal nasal cartilage)

Septal nasal cartilage

Lateral and medial crura
(of major alar cartilage)

Anterior nasal spine
(of maxilla)

Alar fibrofatty tissue

Infra-orbital foramen

Figure 8.1 Nose (anterolateral view)

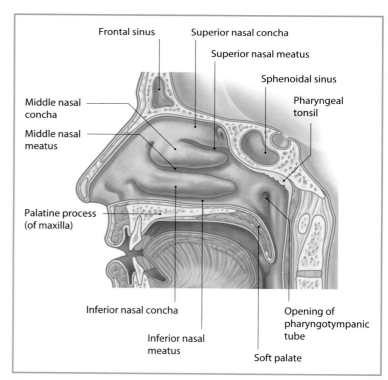

Frontal sinus

Superior nasal concha

Superior nasal meatus

Sphenoidal sinus

Middle nasal
concha

Pharyngeal
tonsil

Middle nasal
meatus

Palatine process
(of maxilla)

Inferior nasal concha

Opening of
pharyngotympanic
tube

Inferior nasal
meatus

Soft palate

Figure 8.2 Internal anatomy of the nose

maxillary sinuses, and anterior ethmoidal cells. The sphenoidal sinus opens into the spheno-ethmoidal recess and the posterior ethmoidal cells open into the **superior nasal meatus**. Each of the paranasal sinuses therefore opens into the nasal cavity on its lateral wall.

Tears from the lacrimal gland drain to the **inferior nasal meatus** through the **nasolacrimal duct**.

NERVES

The nerves providing sensory innervation of the nasal cavity are branches of the ophthalmic [V_1] and maxillary [V_2] nerve divisions of the trigeminal nerve [V] (Fig. 8.3). The anterior upper quadrant of the lateral wall is supplied by the **anterior ethmoidal nerve** (a branch of the ophthalmic nerve [V_1]). The posterior upper quadrant of the lateral wall is supplied by the **posterior superior lateral nasal nerve** (a branch of the maxillary nerve [V_2]). The nasal septum is innervated by the anterior ethmoidal, **anterior superior alveolar**, and **nasopalatine nerves**. The olfactory epithelium in the roof of the nasal cavity is innervated by the olfactory nerve [I].

ARTERIES

The **ophthalmic artery** (a branch of the internal carotid artery) and the **sphenopalatine artery** (a branch of the maxillary artery) supply blood to the nasal cavity (see Fig. 5.3).

VEINS AND LYMPHATICS

The veins draining the nasal cavity flow to the **pterygoid plexus** of veins within the infratemporal fossa and to the **facial veins** of the face. Lymphatic drainage of the posterior nasal cavity is to the **retropharyngeal nodes**; the anterior nasal cavity drains to the **submandibular nodes**.

PARANASAL SINUSES

The paranasal sinuses are ingrowths into the maxillary, ethmoid, frontal, and sphenoid bones. They are small at birth; they grow slowly and continuously during childhood and rapidly during adolescence, to reach their adult size. There are four pairs – the maxillary, frontal, and sphenoidal sinuses, and the ethmoidal cells (Fig. 8.4, Table 8.2).

The paranasal sinuses are lined with respiratory epithelium in which cilia move secretions toward their openings on the lateral walls of the nasal cavity. It has been suggested that the sinuses perform the following functions:

- aid vocal resonance;
- reduce the weight of the skull;
- protect intracranial structures;
- increase surface area for additional mucus secretions.

Clinically they are important because they are often the site of infection.

■ CLINICAL CORRELATIONS
Nosebleed (epistaxis)

Nosebleeds are common in children, and their frequency decreases with age. Most occur in the anterior part of the nasal cavity. Patients usually report trauma to the nose, such as prolonged nose-blowing, a direct blow, or even overenthusiastic nose-picking. If bleeding does not stop readily, emergency medical treatment is usually sought. The most common site of bleeding is the anterior nasal mucosa.

Direct pressure to both sides of the cartilaginous part of the nose for 15–20 minutes usually resolves the nosebleed. If it does not, and there is bleeding within the deeper parts of the nose, advanced treatment such as nasal packing may be required. However, most patients do not require this and should be advised to avoid further nasal trauma, such as picking or blowing the nose. Medications that increase bleeding, and prolonged coughing or abdominal straining,

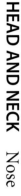

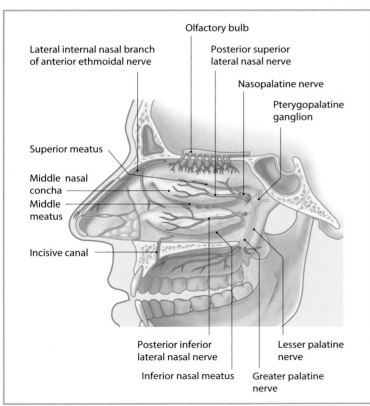

Figure 8.3 Nerves and vessels of the nasal region

Olfactory bulb
Lateral internal nasal branch of anterior ethmoidal nerve
Posterior superior lateral nasal nerve
Nasopalatine nerve
Pterygopalatine ganglion
Superior meatus
Middle nasal concha
Middle meatus
Incisive canal
Posterior inferior lateral nasal nerve
Lesser palatine nerve
Inferior nasal meatus
Greater palatine nerve

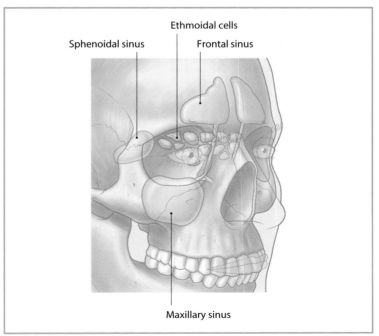

Figure 8.4 Paranasal sinuses

Ethmoidal cells
Sphenoidal sinus
Frontal sinus
Maxillary sinus

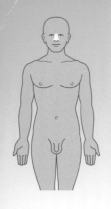

should be avoided. Topical antibiotics and a humidifier to keep the nasal mucosa moist are also recommended.

Sinusitis

Sinusitis is an inflammation of at least one of the paranasal sinuses (i.e. ethmoidal cells or maxillary, frontal, or sphenoidal sinus). The paranasal sinuses are hollow spaces within the facial bones after which they are named. They communicate with the nasal cavity through small openings (ostia). Each sinus is lined with a specialized layer of cells (mucosa), which possesses cilia and produces mucus. Under normal conditions, mucus produced within the sinus captures small inhaled particles, transferring them to the nasal cavity and then to the oropharynx for removal by coughing, sneezing, or swallowing. The sinuses also decrease the weight of the skull and are said to increase resonance during speaking.

Anything that disrupts the internal milieu of a sinus can result in sinusitis. One of the most common causes of acute sinusitis is viral upper respiratory tract infection, which can block the outflow of mucus through the ostia, thus trapping infectious agents (virus or bacteria) in the sinus.

On examination, there is tenderness to percussion over the involved sinus. In addition, thick yellow (mucopurulent) nasal secretions, and erythema and edema of the nasal mucosa are usually evident on nasal examination. Placing the patient in a supine position commonly worsens the pain within the affected sinus. Cultures are taken to aid diagnosis from patients with chronic sinusitis. Plain film radiography or a CT scan can aid diagnosis, but are typically reserved for more severe cases, and may show an air–fluid level within the affected sinus or thickening of the mucosa (usually seen best with CT images).

TABLE 8.1 WALLS OF THE NASAL CAVITY

Walls	Components	Relationships
Roof	Nasal cartilages, nasal and frontal bones, cribriform plate of the ethmoid, body of sphenoid, and parts of the vomer and palatine bones	Anterior cranial fossa, olfactory nerves [I] and bulb, and sphenoidal sinus
Floor	Palatine process of maxilla and horizontal plate of palatine bones	Lies between the nasal and oral cavities
Medial wall/septum	Septal cartilage, perpendicular plate of the ethmoid and the vomer	Separates the two nasal cavities
Lateral walls	Nasal bone, the maxilla, lacrimal, ethmoid (labyrinth and conchae), inferior nasal concha, palatine (perpendicular plate) and sphenoid bones (medial plate of pterygoid process; 3 nasal conchae and their underlying nasal meatuses and the spheno-ethmoidal recess	Medial to the orbits, the ethmoidal cells and maxillary sinuses and the pterygopalatine fossa

TABLE 8.2 PARANASAL SINUSES

Sinus	Relationships	Drainage site	Nerve and blood supply
Frontal	Superior to the orbit and anterior to the anterior cranial fossa	Directly to the middle nasal meatus or via frontonasal duct	Supra-orbital nerve and artery
Maxillary	Lateral to nasal cavity, contributes to floor of the orbit, maxillary teeth are inferior, infratemporal and pterygopalatine fossae are posterior	Middle nasal meatus via the semilunar hiatus high drainage site	Anterior, middle, and posterior superior alveolar nerves and arteries
Ethmoidal (cells) Anterior	Lateral to the nasal cavity, medial to the orbit, and inferior to the anterior cranial fossa	Anterior part of semilunar hiatus	Anterior and posterior ethmoidal nerves and arteries
Middle		Ethmoidal bulla	
Posterior		Superior nasal meatus	
Sphenoidal	Anterior to the pons and the basilar artery. Inferior to the optic chiasm, optic nerves [VII] and pituitary gland. Posterior to the nasal cavity. Superior to the nasal cavity and nasopharynx. Medial to the cavernous sinus and its contacts (internal carotid artery, ophthalmic [V_1] maxillary [V_2], trochlear [IV], abducent [VI], and oculomotor [III] nerves)	Spheno-ethmoidal recess	Lateral posterior superior nasal nerve, posterior ethmoidal nerve and artery

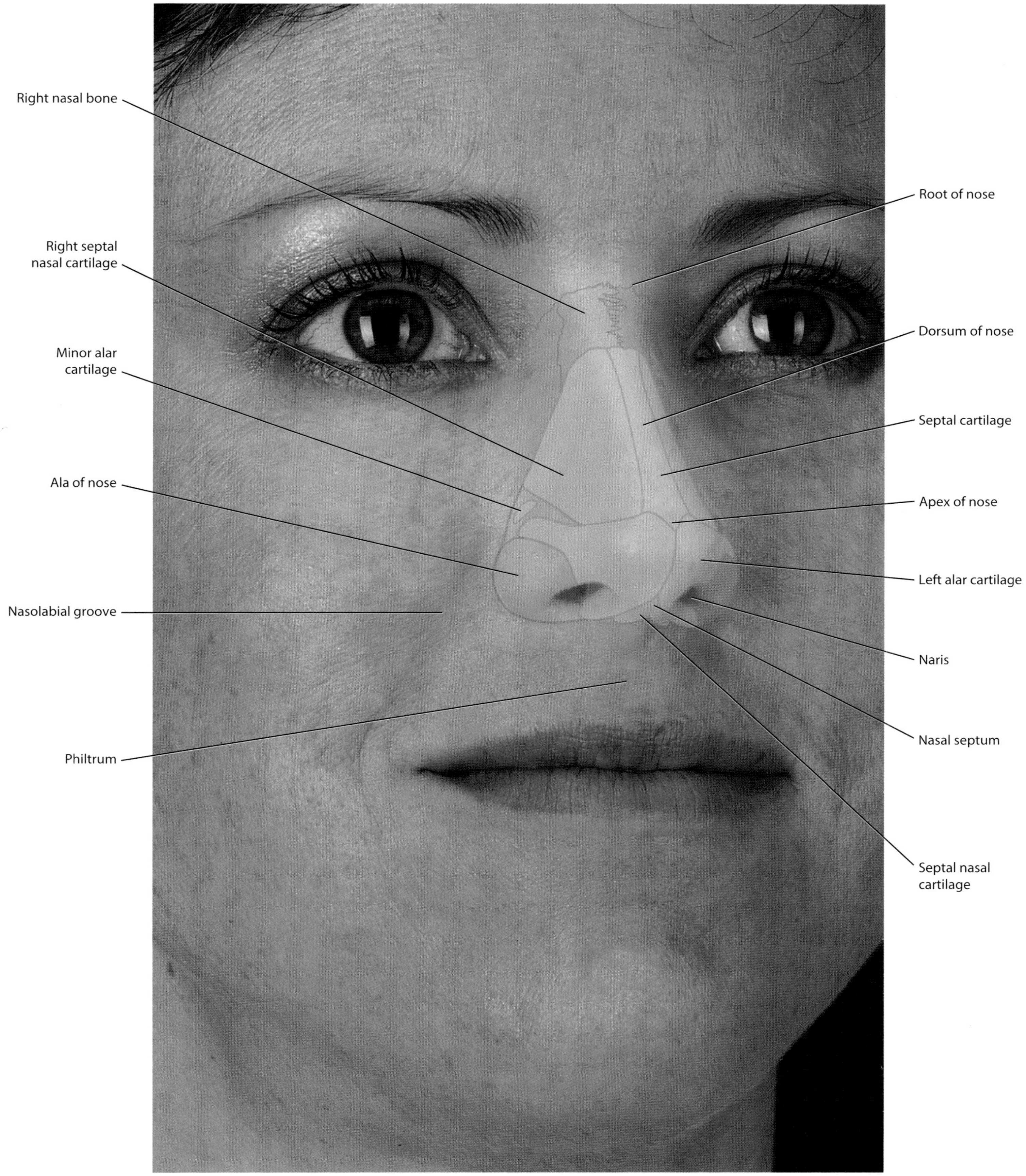

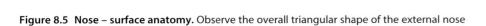

Right nasal bone

Right septal
nasal cartilage

Minor alar
cartilage

Ala of nose

Nasolabial groove

Philtrum

Root of nose

Dorsum of nose

Septal cartilage

Apex of nose

Left alar cartilage

Naris

Nasal septum

Septal nasal
cartilage

Figure 8.5 Nose – surface anatomy. Observe the overall triangular shape of the external nose

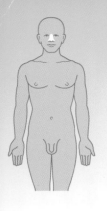

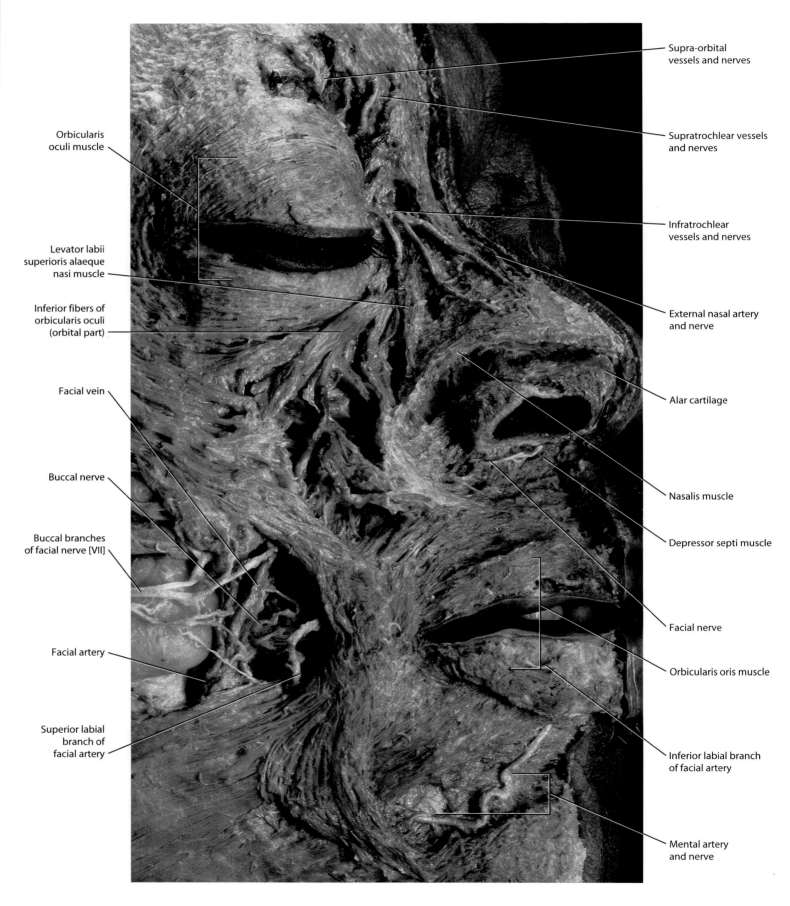

Orbicularis
oculi muscle

Levator labii
superioris alaeque
nasi muscle

Inferior fibers of
orbicularis oculi
(orbital part)

Facial vein

Buccal nerve

Buccal branches
of facial nerve [VII]

Facial artery

Superior labial
branch of
facial artery

Supra-orbital
vessels and nerves

Supratrochlear vessels
and nerves

Infratrochlear
vessels and nerves

External nasal artery
and nerve

Alar cartilage

Nasalis muscle

Depressor septi muscle

Facial nerve

Orbicularis oris muscle

Inferior labial branch
of facial artery

Mental artery
and nerve

Figure 8.6 Nose – superficial dissection. Lateral view of right side of nose. Observe the alar cartilage of the nose and the external nasal artery and nerve

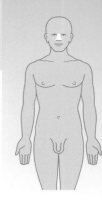

Frontal sinus

Nasal bone

Septal nasal cartilage

Apex of nose

Palate (floor of
nasal cavity)

Ethmoid

Perpendicular plate
(of ethmoid)

Sphenoidal sinus

Vomer

Choana

Opening of
pharyngotympanic tube

Epiglottis

Epiglottic vallecula

Hyoid bone

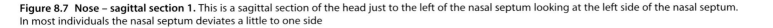

Figure 8.7 Nose – sagittal section 1. This is a sagittal section of the head just to the left of the nasal septum looking at the left side of the nasal septum.
In most individuals the nasal septum deviates a little to one side

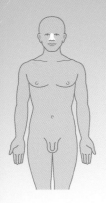

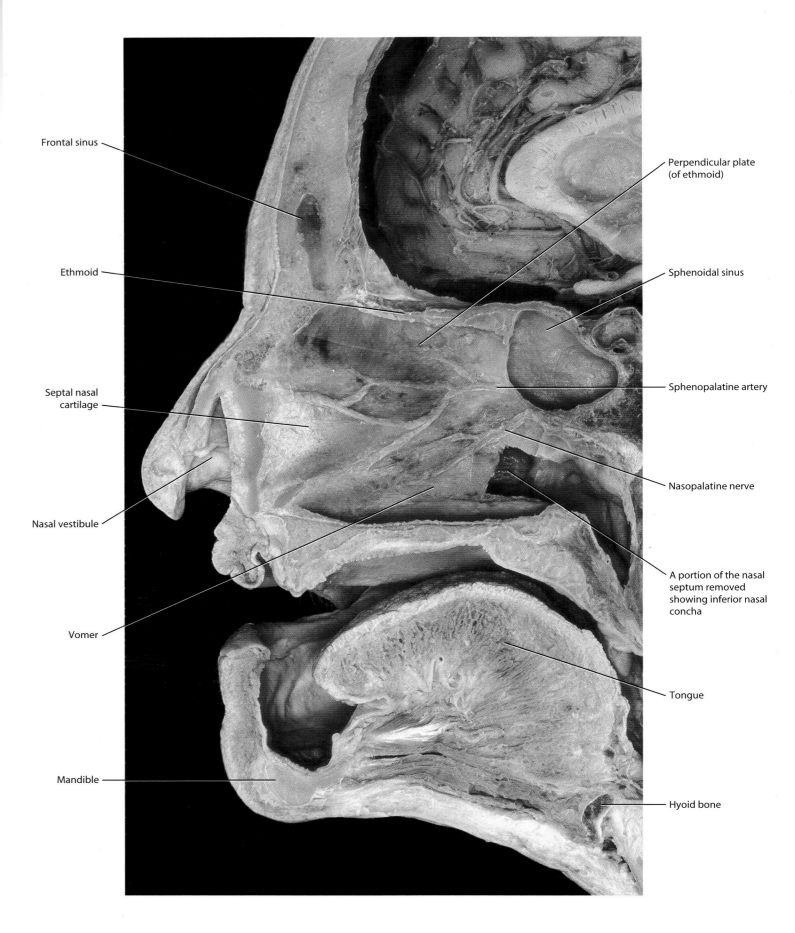

Frontal sinus

Ethmoid

Septal nasal
cartilage

Nasal vestibule

Vomer

Mandible

Perpendicular plate
(of ethmoid)

Sphenoidal sinus

Sphenopalatine artery

Nasopalatine nerve

A portion of the nasal
septum removed
showing inferior nasal
concha

Tongue

Hyoid bone

Figure 8.8 Nose – sagittal section 2. This is a continuation of the dissection in Figure 8.7, to reveal the sphenopalatine artery on the nasal septum. A part of the posterior nasal septum has been removed to show the inferior nasal concha

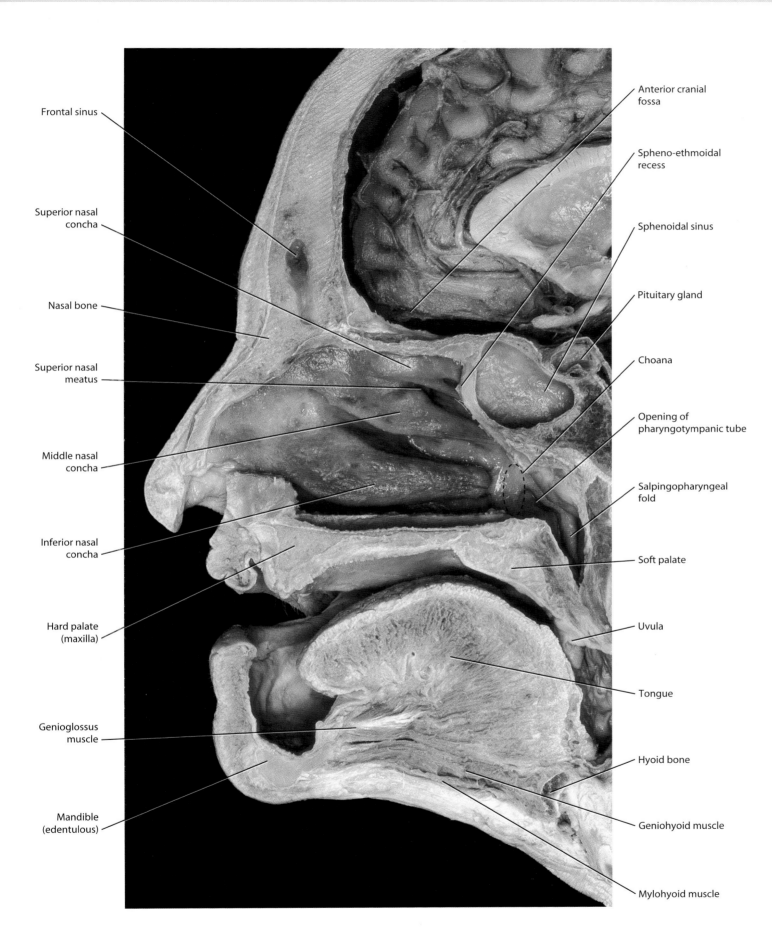

Frontal sinus

Superior nasal
concha

Nasal bone

Superior nasal
meatus

Middle nasal
concha

Inferior nasal
concha

Hard palate
(maxilla)

Genioglossus
muscle

Mandible
(edentulous)

Anterior cranial
fossa

Spheno-ethmoidal
recess

Sphenoidal sinus

Pituitary gland

Choana

Opening of
pharyngotympanic tube

Salpingopharyngeal
fold

Soft palate

Uvula

Tongue

Hyoid bone

Geniohyoid muscle

Mylohyoid muscle

Figure 8.9 Nose – sagittal section 3. The nasal septum has been removed to show the superior, middle and inferior nasal conchae. Also observe the opening of the pharyngotympanic tube, which connects the nasopharynx with the middle ear cavity

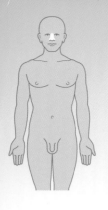

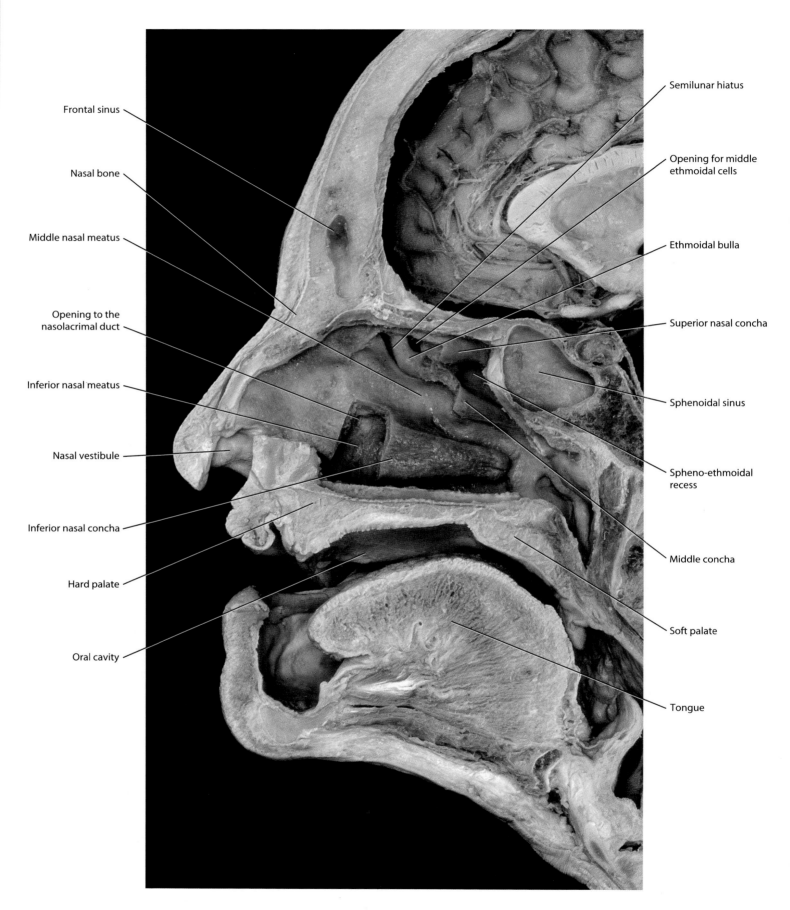

Frontal sinus

Nasal bone

Middle nasal meatus

Opening to the
nasolacrimal duct

Inferior nasal meatus

Nasal vestibule

Inferior nasal concha

Hard palate

Oral cavity

Semilunar hiatus

Opening for middle
ethmoidal cells

Ethmoidal bulla

Superior nasal concha

Sphenoidal sinus

Spheno-ethmoidal
recess

Middle concha

Soft palate

Tongue

Figure 8.10 Nose – sagittal section 4. The nasal septum and anterior part of the inferior nasal concha have been removed to reveal the opening of the
nasolacrimal duct

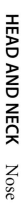

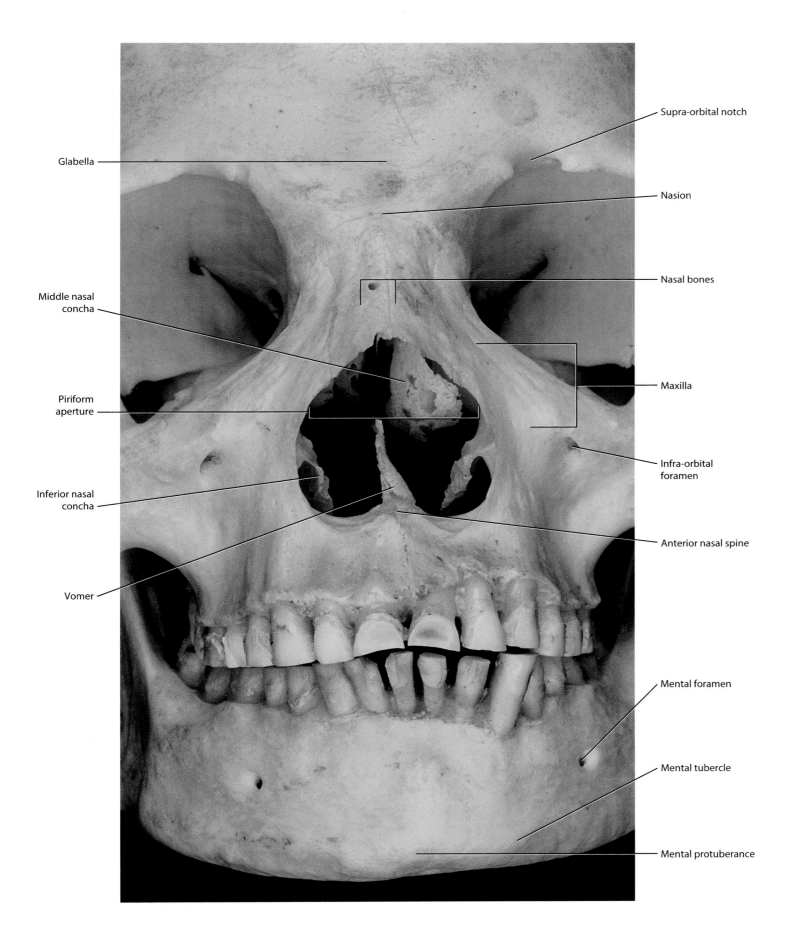

Glabella

Supra-orbital notch

Nasion

Nasal bones

Middle nasal concha

Piriform aperture

Maxilla

Inferior nasal concha

Infra-orbital foramen

Vomer

Anterior nasal spine

Mental foramen

Mental tubercle

Mental protuberance

Figure 8.11 Nose – osteology. Anterior view of piriform aperture (opening in skull to nasal cavity). Observe the middle and inferior nasal conchae

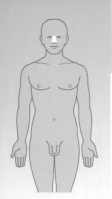

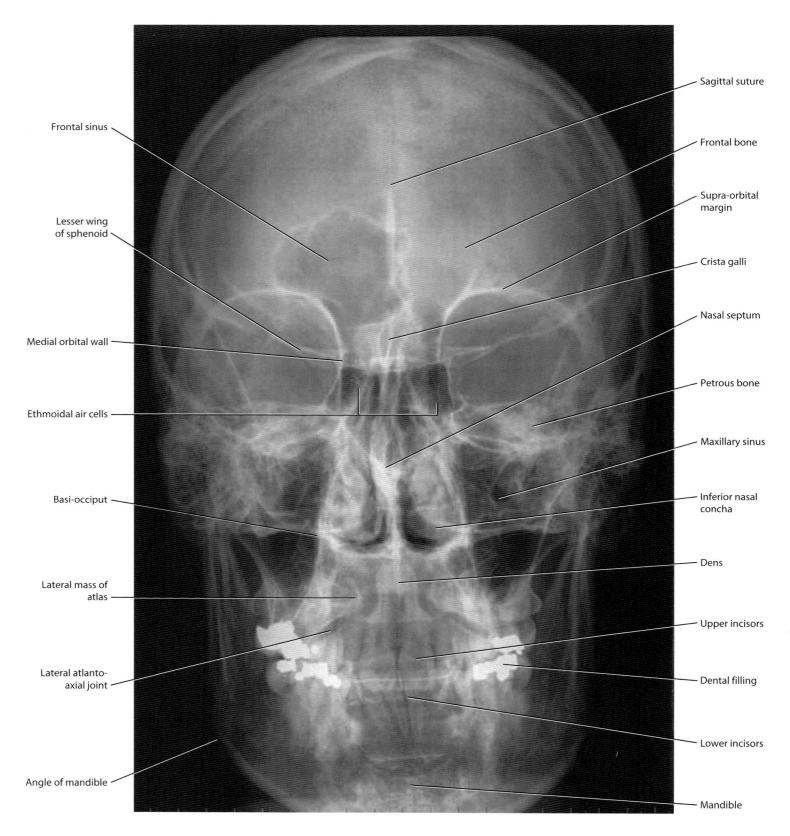

Frontal sinus

Lesser wing
of sphenoid

Medial orbital wall

Ethmoidal air cells

Basi-occiput

Lateral mass of
atlas

Lateral atlanto-
axial joint

Angle of mandible

Sagittal suture

Frontal bone

Supra-orbital
margin

Crista galli

Nasal septum

Petrous bone

Maxillary sinus

Inferior nasal
concha

Dens

Upper incisors

Dental filling

Lower incisors

Mandible

Figure 8.12 Nose – plain film radiograph (anteroposterior view). Osseous detail of the nose can be seen; in this example the septum is deviated to the right. Note the location of the inferior nasal concha and compare this view with Figure 8.11

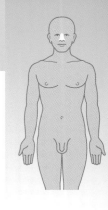

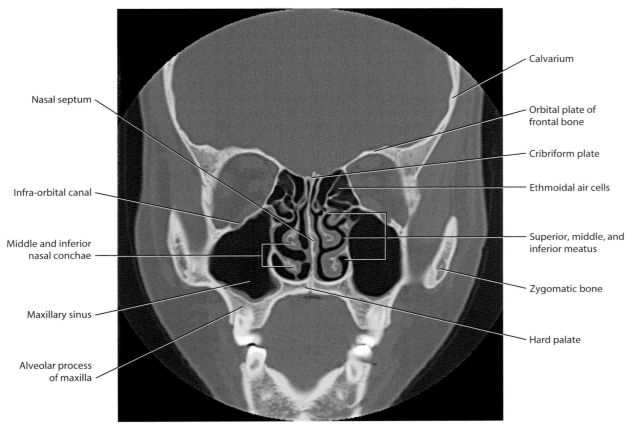

Calvarium

Orbital plate of frontal bone

Cribriform plate

Ethmoidal air cells

Superior, middle, and inferior meatus

Zygomatic bone

Hard palate

Nasal septum

Infra-orbital canal

Middle and inferior nasal conchae

Maxillary sinus

Alveolar process of maxilla

Figure 8.13 Nose and sinuses – CT scan (coronal view). The osseous and soft tissue of the nasal conchae are clearly seen. Note that the mucosae of the conchae are thicker on the patient's left side. This normal physiologic mucosal thickening alternates from left to right and varies with time, to facilitate primary air flow through one side of the nasal cavity at a time

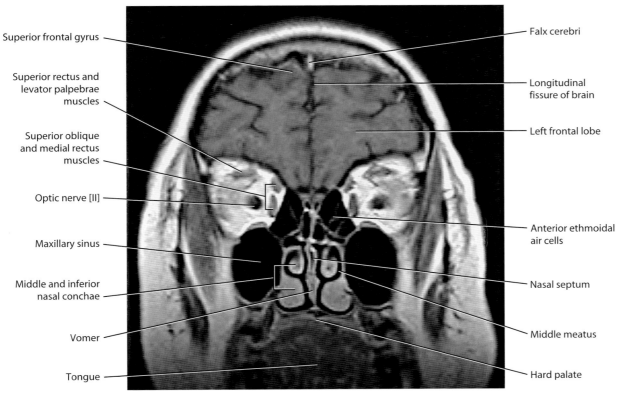

Superior frontal gyrus

Superior rectus and levator palpebrae muscles

Superior oblique and medial rectus muscles

Optic nerve [II]

Maxillary sinus

Middle and inferior nasal conchae

Vomer

Tongue

Falx cerebri

Longitudinal fissure of brain

Left frontal lobe

Anterior ethmoidal air cells

Nasal septum

Middle meatus

Hard palate

Figure 8.14 Nose and sinuses – MRI scan (coronal view). Observe how the nasal cavity is closely related to the ethmoid air cells and maxillary sinus

93

The digestive tract starts in the **oral cavity** (Figs 9.1 and 9.2). It extends from the lips to the posterior **oropharynx** and is defined by the **palate** and **cheeks**, which form the roof and walls, respectively, and the floor of the oral cavity. The oral cavity provides an entry point for food into the digestive tract and a conduit for respiration and speech.

Bony support to the oral region is provided by the mandible and bones of the viscerocranium (see Chapter 3). The **hard palate** – part of the roof of the oral cavity – is formed from the palatine processes of the maxillae and the horizontal plates of the palatine bones.

The **soft palate** is suspended from the posterior edge of the hard palate and moves posteriorly against the pharynx during swallowing to prevent material entering the nasal cavity. Anterior and lateral support to the oral region is from the maxillae and mandible. The floor of the oral region is occupied by the tongue, which is supported by the muscles of the submandibular region (see Chapter 11).

MUSCLES

The **orbicularis oris** and **buccinator** muscles are muscles of facial expression and they support the lips and cheeks, respectively. They have a secondary role in mastication. They are innervated by the facial nerve [VII] (see Chapter 4).

Five pairs of muscles support the soft palate and aid swallowing (Table 9.1). The tongue is a complex set of muscles, covered by mucous membrane, that rests on the floor of the oral cavity. It is attached to the hyoid bone and mandible and is supported by the **geniohyoid** and **mylohyoid** muscles. The muscles of the tongue are divided into extrinsic and intrinsic groups (Table 9.2).

NERVES

Developmentally, the maxilla and mandible are innervated by divisions of the trigeminal nerve [V]. The upper lip is innervated by **labial branches** of the **infra-orbital nerve**, from the maxillary nerve [V_2] division, and the lower lip is innervated by the **mental branch** of the **inferior alveolar nerve**, from the mandibular nerve [V_3] division. The hard and soft palates receive sensory innervation from the **nasopalatine** and **greater** and **lesser palatine nerves**, which are derived from the pterygopalatine portion of the maxillary nerve [V_2]. The teeth of the upper jaw are innervated by the **anterior**, **middle**, and **posterior superior alveolar branches** of the maxillary nerve [V_2]. The teeth of the lower jaw are innervated by the inferior alveolar nerve and **incisive branches** of the mandibular nerve [V_3].

General sensation to the anterior two-thirds of the tongue is provided by the **lingual nerve**, from the mandibular nerve [V_3]; the **glossopharyngeal nerve [IX]** supplies the posterior one-third. The taste buds on the anterior two-thirds of the tongue are innervated by the **facial nerve [VII]** (**chorda tympani**), and the taste buds on the posterior one-third are supplied by the glossopharyngeal nerve [IX]. Motor innervation to the tongue is provided by the hypoglossal nerve [XII], except for the palatoglossus muscle, which is innervated by the accessory nerve [XI] via the vagus [X].

ARTERIES

The blood supply to the oral region is primarily through branches of the **external carotid artery**.

The hard and soft palates receive blood from the **sphenopalatine** and **descending palatine arteries**, which are branches of the third part of the **maxillary artery** (see Fig. 5.3).

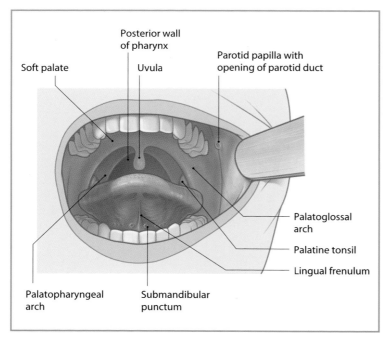

Figure 9.1 Oral cavity – surface features

- Soft palate
- Posterior wall of pharynx
- Uvula
- Parotid papilla with opening of parotid duct
- Palatoglossal arch
- Palatine tonsil
- Lingual frenulum
- Palatopharyngeal arch
- Submandibular punctum

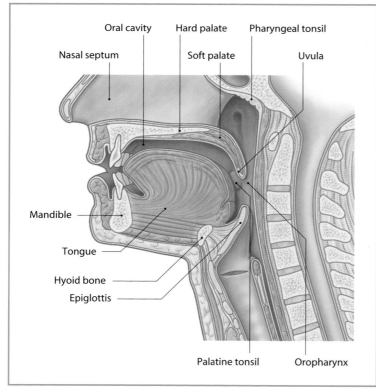

Figure 9.2 Oral cavity – hemisected sagittal specimen

- Oral cavity
- Hard palate
- Pharyngeal tonsil
- Nasal septum
- Soft palate
- Uvula
- Mandible
- Tongue
- Hyoid bone
- Epiglottis
- Palatine tonsil
- Oropharynx

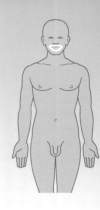

The **superior** and **inferior alveolar arteries** (branching from the maxillary artery – see Fig. 5.3) supply blood to the maxillary and mandibular teeth. Blood supply to the buccal region (i.e. the cheeks), is provided by the **transverse facial artery** (from the maxillary artery), and the **facial** and **buccal arteries** (from the external carotid artery – see Fig. 5.3).

The **lingual artery** is the primary artery to the tongue.

VEINS AND LYMPHATICS

The veins draining the oral region parallel the arteries (see Fig. 2.3). Vessels that drain along the path of the maxillary artery return blood to the pterygoid plexus of veins within the infratemporal fossa. From here, blood drains to the internal jugular vein or common facial vein. Blood from the buccal region drains to the facial vein. The tongue is drained by the **deep lingual veins**, which empty into the **internal jugular vein**.

SALIVARY GLANDS

There are three, paired, **major salivary glands** – the parotid, submandibular, and sublingual glands (Fig. 9.3). There are also many **minor salivary glands** in the oral cavity – the lingual, palatal, buccal, and labial glands. Secretions from these glands moisten the mouth, initiate digestion, and assist in chewing, swallowing, and phonation.

The **parotid gland** is the largest major salivary gland, and is between the mandible and mastoid process of temporal bone (see Chapter 4). The **submandibular gland**, in the floor of the mouth, is divided into superficial and deep portions, which wrap around the posterior aspect of the mylohyoid muscle. A duct arises from the deep portion of the gland and passes anteriorly between the hyoglossus and mylohyoid muscles to enter the oral cavity lateral to the midline frenulum of the tongue. The **sublingual gland** is deep to the sublingual mucosa and secretes saliva directly into the floor of the mouth.

The submandibular and sublingual glands are innervated by postganglionic sympathetic fibers that arise from the **superior cervical ganglion** and run alongside the lingual and facial arteries. Venous drainage is to the lingual and facial veins, and lymphatic drainage is to small vessels that empty into the **submandibular nodes**.

■ CLINICAL CORRELATIONS

Tonsillitis

Tonsillitis is an inflammation of the **palatine tonsil**. It causes a prodrome of upper respiratory symptoms – nasal congestion, headache, fever, myalgia, and cough – which may precede or follow the pharyngitis (sore throat), or be absent depending on the infecting agent.

Patients who have frequent infections or enlargement of the tonsils causing partial airway obstruction, are generally referred to a general surgeon or otorhinolaryngologist for evaluation and treatment. If necessary, the palatine tonsil can be removed surgically.

Sialadenitis

Sialadenitis is an inflammation of the salivary gland caused by infection and obstruction of the gland by bacteria, viruses, or calculi (stones). Active infection causes pain and swelling of the involved gland, and fever. The most common causes of infectious sialadenitis are staphylococcal bacteria and the mumps virus. Bacterial infections can be treated with antibiotics. Other causes of sialadenitis are managed by oral hydration and sialogogues (medication or food that stimulates saliva secretion). If sialadenitis does not respond to conservative management, it might be necessary to remove the gland surgically.

Sialolithiasis

Sialolithiasis occurs when a calculus (stone) is lodged within a salivary duct. The most common location for a sialolith (salivary duct calculus) is in the submandibular duct. Sialolithiasis usually causes pain and swelling in the affected duct during eating. Diagnosis is usually made by plain radiography because approximately 90% of stones in the submandibular duct are radiopaque. Ultrasound and computed tomography (CT) can also be used for diagnosis.

Treatment of sialolithiasis is aimed at increasing the flow of saliva through the duct by oral rehydration or sialogogues. The stone is removed surgically in chronic sialolithiasis.

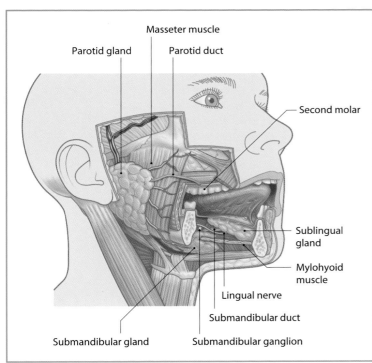

Figure 9.3 Major salivary glands

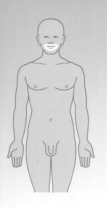

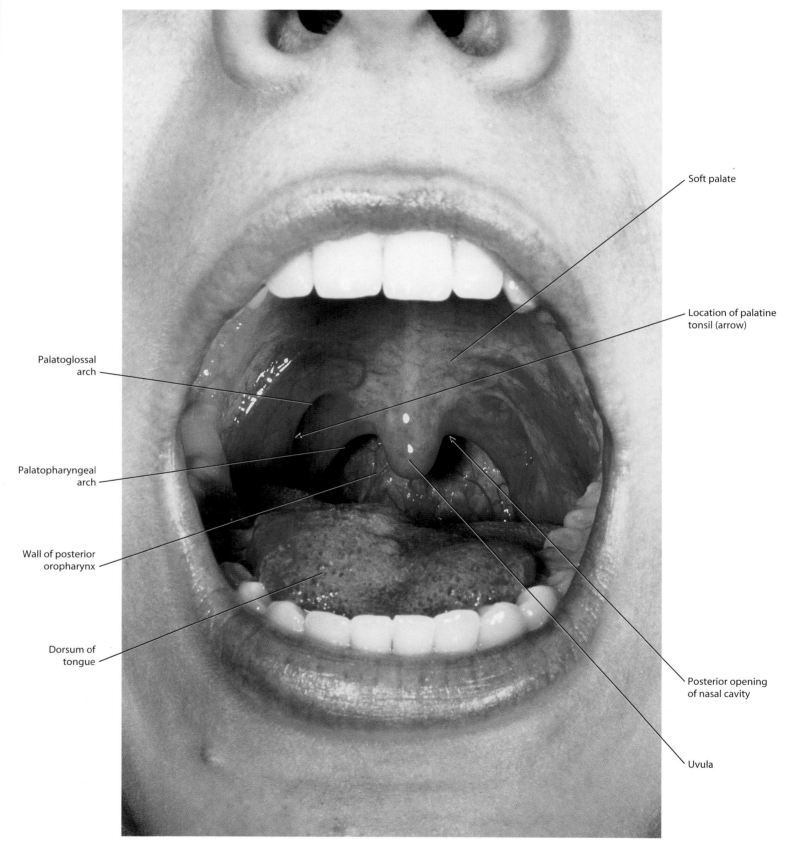

Soft palate

Location of palatine tonsil (arrow)

Palatoglossal arch

Palatopharyngeal arch

Wall of posterior oropharynx

Dorsum of tongue

Posterior opening of nasal cavity

Uvula

Figure 9.4 Oral region – surface anatomy. Observe the palatal arches created by the palatoglossus and palatopharyngeus muscles. In healthy individuals the palatine tonsils are usually not enlarged and therefore are not seen in this view

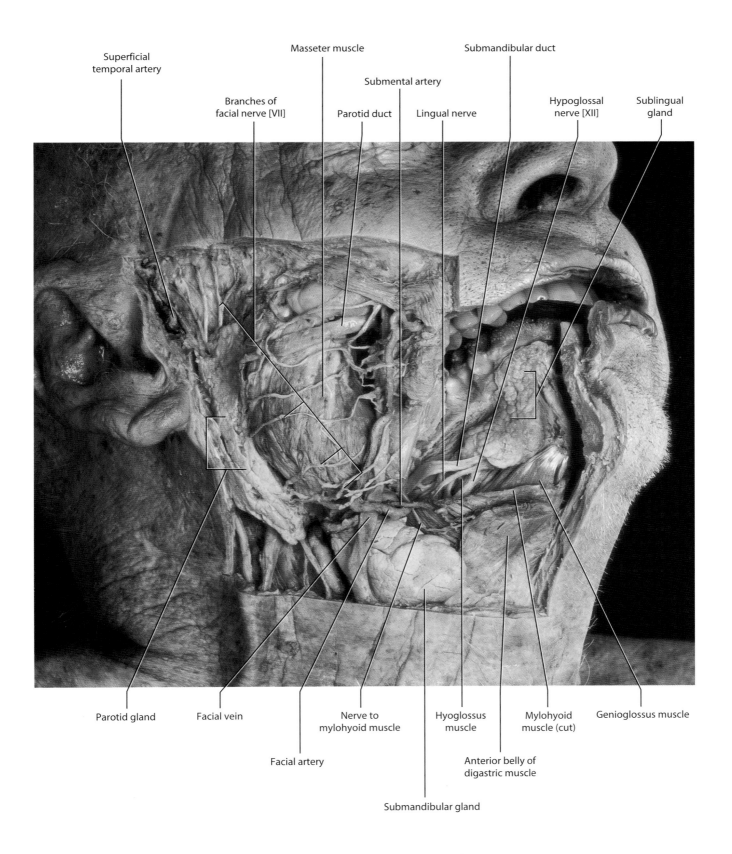

Superficial
temporal artery

Masseter muscle

Submandibular duct

Submental artery

Branches of
facial nerve [VII]

Parotid duct

Lingual nerve

Hypoglossal
nerve [XII]

Sublingual
gland

Parotid gland

Facial vein

Nerve to
mylohyoid muscle

Hyoglossus
muscle

Mylohyoid
muscle (cut)

Genioglossus muscle

Facial artery

Anterior belly of
digastric muscle

Submandibular gland

Figure 9.5 Oral cavity – sagittal section 1. Removal of the mandible reveals the relationships between the parotid, submandibular, and sublingual salivary glands

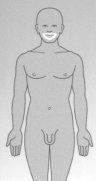

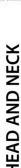

TABLE 9.1 MUSCLES OF THE SOFT PALATE

Muscle	Origin	Insertion	Innervation	Action	Blood supply
Levator veli palatini	Petrous part of temporal bone, cartilage of pharyngotympanic tube	Palatine aponeurosis	Accessory nerve [XI] via the vagus [X]	Elevates the soft palate	Ascending palatine artery (branch of facial artery); descending palatine artery (branch of maxillary artery)
Tensor veli palatini	Scaphoid fossa and spine of sphenoid, cartilage of pharyngotympanic tube	Palatine aponeurosis	Nerve to medial pterygoid, mandibular nerve [V$_3$]	Tenses and elevates soft palate	Ascending palatine artery (branch of facial artery); descending palatine artery (branch of maxillary artery)
Musculus uvulae	Posterior nasal spine, palatine aponeurosis	Mucous membrane of uvula	Accessory nerve [XI] via the vagus [X]	Raises uvula	Ascending palatine artery (branch of facial artery); descending palatine artery (branch of maxillary artery)
Palatoglossus	Inferior aspect of palatine aponeurosis	Lateral aspect of the tongue	Accessory nerve [XI] via the vagus [X]	Narrows oropharyngeal isthmus, elevates pharynx	Palatine branches from facial, maxillary, and ascending pharyngeal arteries
Palatopharyngeus	Bony palate and palatine aponeurosis	Posterior border of thyroid cartilage	Accessory nerve [XI] via the vagus [X]	Elevates pharynx and larynx	Ascending palatine artery (branch of facial artery); descending palatine artery (branch of maxillary artery)

TABLE 9.2 MUSCLES OF THE TONGUE

Muscle	Origin	Insertion	Innervation	Action	Blood supply
Extrinsic muscles of the tongue					
Genioglossus	Superior mental tubercle of mandible	Body of hyoid bone, radiates throughout tongue posterior to anterior	Hypoglossal nerve [XII]	Protrudes, retracts, and depresses tongue	Sublingual and submental arteries
Hyoglossus	Body and greater horn of hyoid bone	Lateral aspect of tongue	Hypoglossal nerve [XII]	Depresses and retracts tongue	Sublingual and submental arteries
Styloglossus	Anterior aspect of styloid process	Sides of the tongue, mingles with hyoglossus	Hypoglossal nerve [XII]	Retracts and elevates tongue	Sublingual artery
Intrinsic muscles of the tongue					
Superior longitudinal	Posterior aspect of tongue (submucosa)	Tip of tongue, unites with opposite muscle	Hypoglossal nerve [XII]	Shortens tongue, turns tip upward	Deep lingual and facial arteries
Inferior longitudinal	Between genioglossus and hyoglossus	Tip of tongue, blends with styloglossus	Hypoglossal nerve [XII]	Shortens tongue, turns tip downwards	Deep lingual and facial arteries
Transverse	Median fibrous septum	Dorsum and side of tongue	Hypoglossal nerve [XII]	Narrows and elongates tongue	Deep lingual and facial arteries
Vertical	Dorsum of tongue	Dorsum (superior) to inferior tongue	Hypoglossal nerve [XII]	Flattens and broadens tongue	Deep lingual and facial arteries

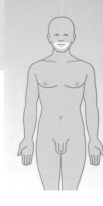

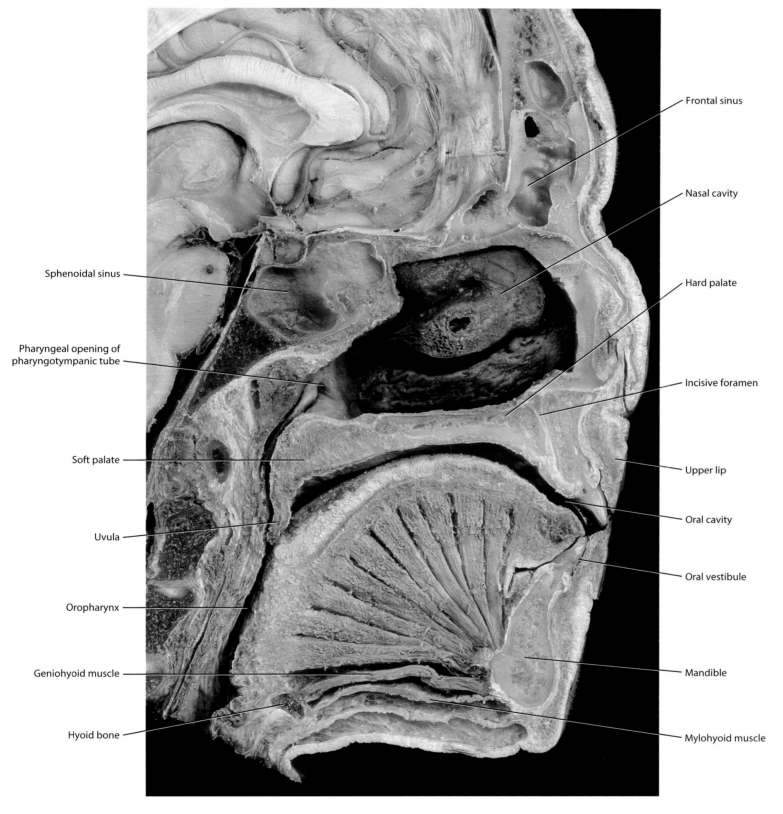

Frontal sinus

Nasal cavity

Hard palate

Incisive foramen

Upper lip

Oral cavity

Oral vestibule

Mandible

Mylohyoid muscle

Sphenoidal sinus

Pharyngeal opening of pharyngotympanic tube

Soft palate

Uvula

Oropharynx

Geniohyoid muscle

Hyoid bone

Figure 9.6 Oral cavity – sagittal section 2. Looking at the left side of a hemisected cadaver, the relationships of the tongue and hard and soft palate are visible. The fan-like grooves on the cut surface of the tongue have been added to give perspective on its size

99

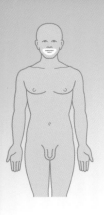

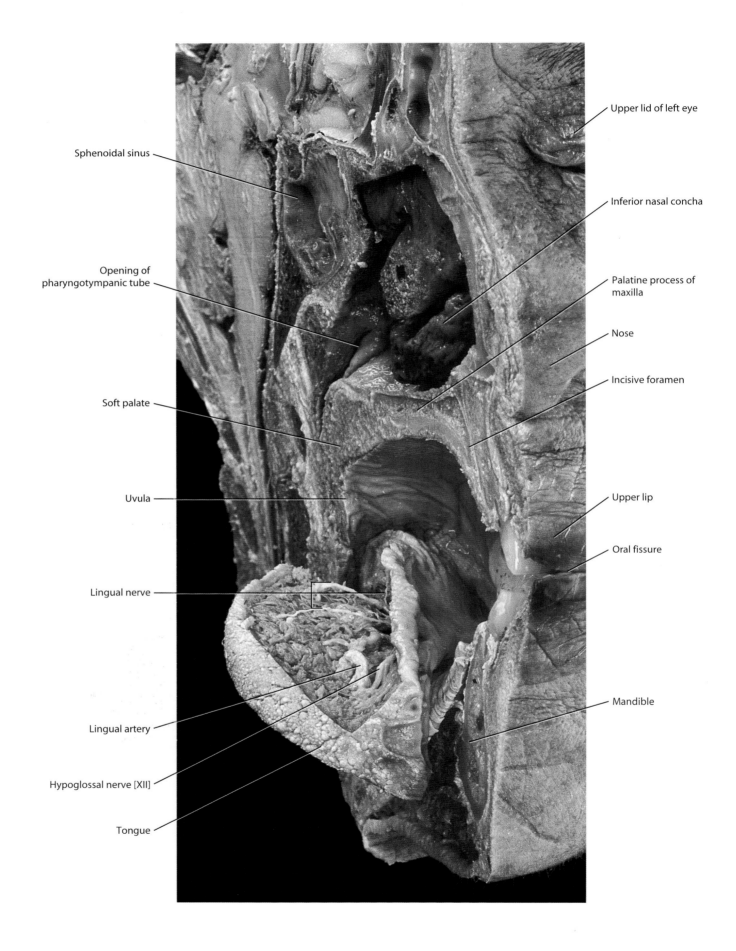

Sphenoidal sinus

Opening of
pharyngotympanic tube

Soft palate

Uvula

Lingual nerve

Lingual artery

Hypoglossal nerve [XII]

Tongue

Upper lid of left eye

Inferior nasal concha

Palatine process of
maxilla

Nose

Incisive foramen

Upper lip

Oral fissure

Mandible

Figure 9.7 **Oral cavity – sagittal section 3.** The complex relationships between the teeth, tongue, oral region, and hard and soft palate are seen here

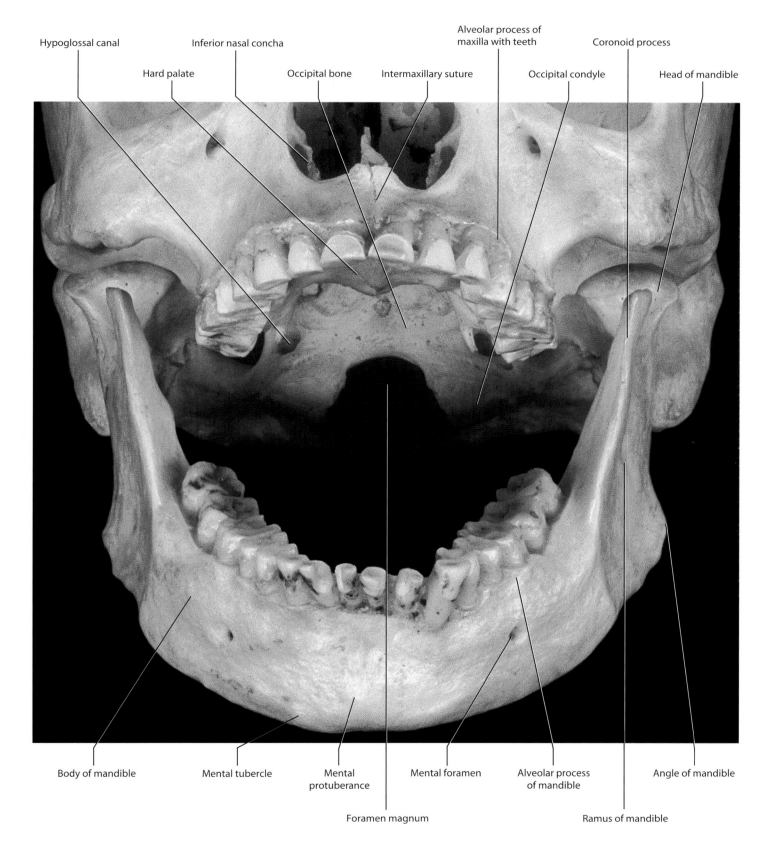

Hypoglossal canal

Inferior nasal concha

Hard palate

Occipital bone

Intermaxillary suture

Alveolar process of maxilla with teeth

Occipital condyle

Coronoid process

Head of mandible

Body of mandible

Mental tubercle

Mental protuberance

Mental foramen

Alveolar process of mandible

Angle of mandible

Foramen magnum

Ramus of mandible

Figure 9.8 Oral cavity – osteology. In this open mouth view observe that the foramen magnum is immediately posterior to the oral region

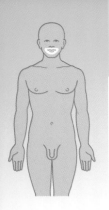

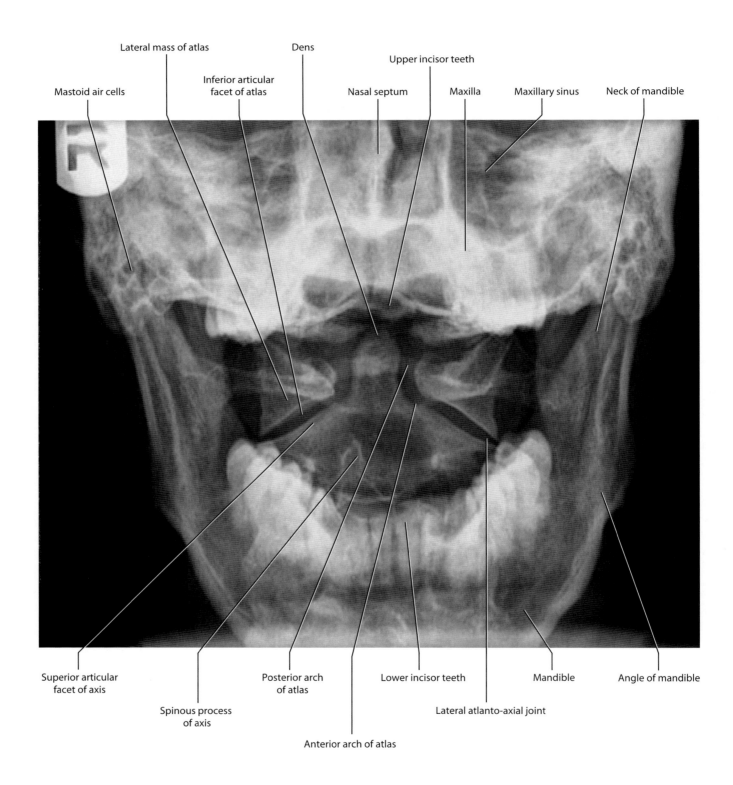

Lateral mass of atlas

Dens

Upper incisor teeth

Mastoid air cells

Inferior articular facet of atlas

Nasal septum

Maxilla

Maxillary sinus

Neck of mandible

Superior articular facet of axis

Posterior arch of atlas

Lower incisor teeth

Mandible

Angle of mandible

Spinous process of axis

Lateral atlanto-axial joint

Anterior arch of atlas

Figure 9.9 Oral region – plain film radiograph (anteroposterior view). This open-mouth view demonstrates the cervical spine with respect to the mouth. Note that the radiographic technician places a mark on the radiograph to guide the clinician in determining which is the right and which the left side. This is especially useful if a fracture or other abnormality is observed

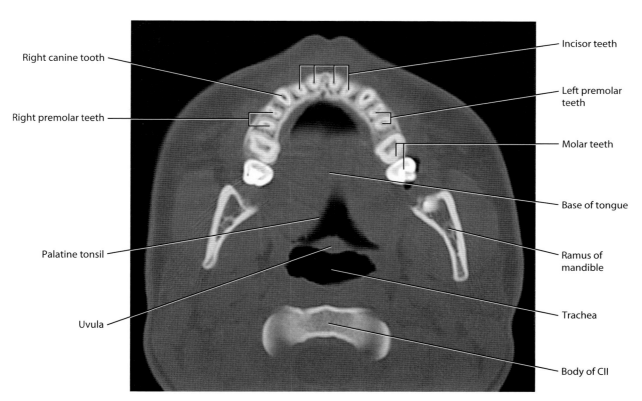

Right canine tooth

Right premolar teeth

Palatine tonsil

Uvula

Incisor teeth

Left premolar teeth

Molar teeth

Base of tongue

Ramus of mandible

Trachea

Body of CII

Figure 9.10 Oral region – CT scan (axial view). Observe the relationship between the second cervical vertebra, trachea and the mandibular teeth

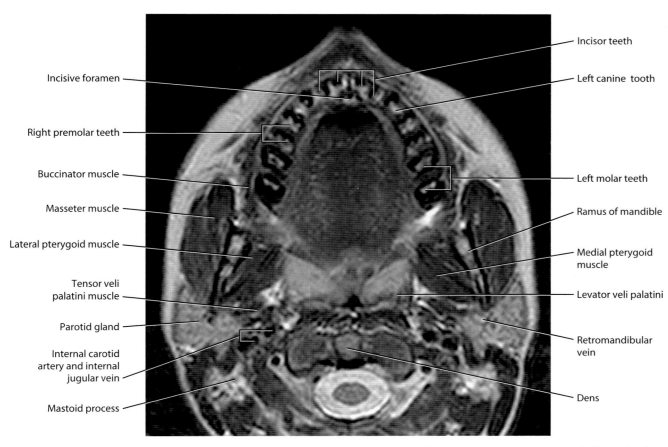

Incisive foramen

Right premolar teeth

Buccinator muscle

Masseter muscle

Lateral pterygoid muscle

Tensor veli palatini muscle

Parotid gland

Internal carotid artery and internal jugular vein

Mastoid process

Incisor teeth

Left canine tooth

Left molar teeth

Ramus of mandible

Medial pterygoid muscle

Levator veli palatini

Retromandibular vein

Dens

Figure 9.11 Oral region – MRI scan (axial view). Observe the soft tissues at the level of the maxilla. Also note that the spinal cord is located a short distance posterior to the oral cavity

103

10 Pharynx and larynx

The pharynx and larynx are tube-like structures in the upper neck. The **pharynx** is part of the digestive system and is a pathway for food and air; the **larynx** connects the lower part of the pharynx to the trachea. Commonly referred to as the 'windpipe', the **trachea** channels air into the lungs.

PHARYNX

The pharynx is a fibromuscular tube that connects the nasal cavity, oral cavity, and larynx. Accordingly, it is subdivided into the nasopharynx, oropharynx, and laryngopharynx (Fig. 10.1). The pharynx extends from the base of the skull to the level of the cricoid cartilage (at vertebral level CVI) where the pharynx joins the esophagus. Structural support is provided by bony, cartilaginous, and ligamentous elements associated with the skull, hyoid bone, and laryngeal cartilages. The pharynx is a channel for swallowing and respiration.

The **nasopharynx** – the superior part of the pharynx – communicates anteriorly with the nasal cavity through the choanae and extends inferiorly to the soft palate. The pharyngeal opening for the pharyngotympanic tube is visible next to the **torus tubarius**, a cartilaginous elevation on the lateral wall of the pharynx. The pharyngotympanic tube connects the nasopharynx to the middle ear and equalizes air pressure on both sides of the tympanic membrane (see Chapter 7). This can be a route for the spread of infection from the nasopharynx to the middle ear. The **pharyngeal tonsil** (adenoid) is on the posterior wall of the nasopharynx.

The **oropharynx** lies between the soft palate and tip of the epiglottis. It communicates anteriorly with the oral cavity through the **oropharyngeal isthmus**, which is formed by the tongue inferiorly and the **palatoglossal** and **palatopharyngeal arches** laterally. The palatoglossal (anterior) and palatopharyngeal

(posterior) folds on the lateral walls of the oropharynx are formed by the palatoglossus and palatopharyngeus muscles, respectively.

The palatine tonsil lies between the palatoglossal and palatopharyngeal folds. Throat infections in children often result in enlarged palatine tonsils, which can interfere with breathing and speech (see Chapter 9). The palatine tonsil is innervated by branches of the glossopharyngeal nerve [IX]. Blood is supplied by **tonsillar branches** of the facial, ascending palatine, lingual, descending palatine, and ascending pharyngeal arteries. Venous drainage is to the **pharyngeal plexus** of veins. Lymphatic drainage is mainly to the **jugulodigastric node** of the deep cervical lymph node group (see Chapter 12).

The **laryngopharynx** extends from the tip of the epiglottis to the level of the cricoid cartilage (vertebral level CVI), where it joins the esophagus. Anteriorly, it communicates with the larynx through the **laryngeal inlet** (aditus). During swallowing, the **epiglottis** bends posteriorly and the laryngeal structures are pulled superiorly. As a result the laryngeal inlet is partially closed by the epiglottis, which prevents food from entering the trachea. The piriform fossae are on both sides of the laryngeal inlet and channel swallowed substances to the esophagus.

Muscles

The muscular layer of the pharynx (Figs 10.2 and 10.3) comprises the semicircular **superior**, **middle**, and **inferior constrictor** muscles, and the longitudinal **palatopharyngeus**, **salpingopharyngeus**, and **stylopharyngeus** muscles. The constrictors propel food toward the esophagus; the longitudinal muscles elevate the pharynx and larynx during swallowing and phonation.

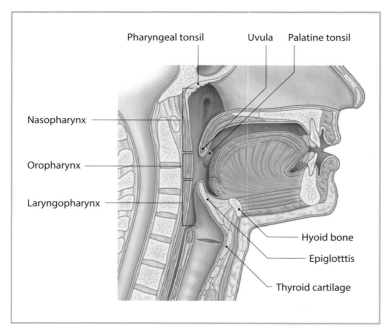

Figure 10.1 Divisions of the pharynx

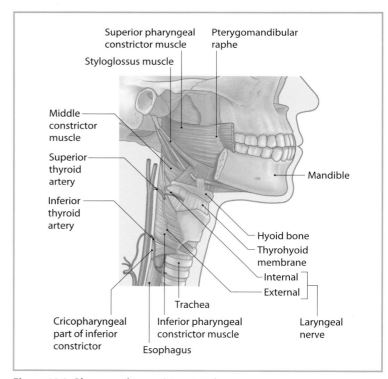

Figure 10.2 Pharyngeal constrictor muscles

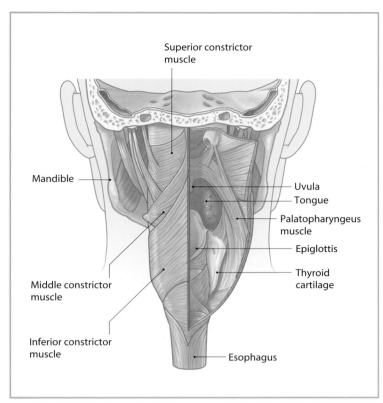

Figure 10.3 Posterior view of the pharynx

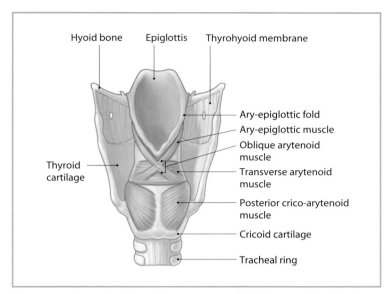

Figure 10.4 Posterior view of the structures of the larynx and epiglottis

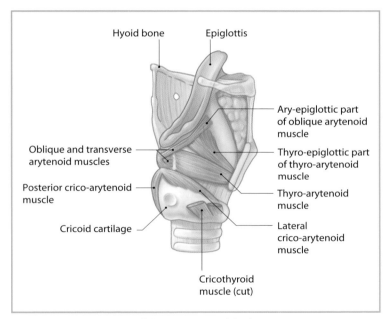

Figure 10.5 Lateral view of the structures of the larynx

Nerves

Sensory and motor innervation to the pharynx originates from the **pharyngeal plexus** on the posterior aspect of the pharyngeal constrictors. This plexus is formed by pharyngeal branches of the vagus [X] and glossopharyngeal [IX] nerves, and postganglionic sympathetic nerve fibers from the superior cervical ganglion.

Motor fibers in the plexus are from the cranial part of the accessory nerve [XI], which runs with the vagus nerve [X] and supplies all muscles of the pharynx, larynx, and soft palate except for the tensor veli palatini and stylopharyngeus muscles, which are innervated by the trigeminal [V] and glossopharyngeal [IX] nerves, respectively.

Sensory innervation to the pharynx is from the glossopharyngeal nerve [IX] . The maxillary [V$_2$] and vagus [X] nerves also carry sensation from a small part of the pharynx.

Arteries

Blood supply to the pharynx is by branches of the ascending pharyngeal, superior thyroid, lingual, facial, and maxillary arteries.

Veins and lymphatics

Venous drainage of the pharynx is through the **pharyngeal plexus** on the posterior aspect of the pharynx. Blood drains from here to the internal jugular vein. Lymphatic drainage is to the retropharyngeal and deep cervical nodes.

LARYNX

The larynx (Figs 10.4 and 10.5) is inferior to the nasopharynx and superior to the trachea. It is approximately 8 cm long and is anterior to the prevertebral fascia and prevertebral muscles, which are anterior to cervical vertebrae CIII–CVI. It is supported by nine cartilages, which also provide attachment for muscles and ligaments. There are **three single cartilages** (the epiglottis and thyroid and cricoid cartilages), and **three paired cartilages** (the arytenoid, corniculate, and cuneiform cartilages). The ligamentous **thyrohyoid membrane** and **cricothyroid ligament** (**cricovocal membrane**) attach the cartilages after which they are named. The hyoid bone also provides support for the thyrohyoid membrane. The **vocal folds** (true vocal cords) and **vestibular folds** (false vocal cords) are between the thyroid and arytenoid cartilages within the laryngeal canal deep to the mucous membrane lining the respiratory pathway.

Muscles

The larynx has **extrinsic** and **intrinsic muscles**. The attachment points of the **extrinsic muscles** are outside the larynx.

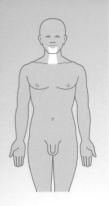
These muscles move the larynx as a whole. The larynx is elevated by the thyrohyoid, stylohyoid, mylohyoid, digastric, stylopharyngeus, and palatopharyngeus muscles; it is depressed by the omohyoid, sternohyoid, and sternothyroid muscles (see Chapter 12).

The **intrinsic laryngeal muscles** have attachment points within the larynx. They move and support the laryngeal cartilages, so modulating the sounds produced during phonation (Table 10.1). They are therefore sometimes referred to as the vocal muscles. These are the **transverse** and **oblique arytenoid**, **thyro-arytenoid**, **lateral** and **posterior crico-arytenoid**, and **cricothyroid** muscles.

Nerves

Nerve supply to the larynx is from the vagus [X] and accessory [XI] nerves. The **internal branch** of the **superior laryngeal nerve** arises from the vagus nerve [X] and pierces the thyrohyoid membrane to provide sensation to the mucosa of the larynx superior to the vocal folds (see Fig. 10.2). Sensory innervation to the mucosa below the vocal folds is provided by the **recurrent laryngeal nerve**, which also supplies all muscles of the larynx except the cricothyroid muscle, which is innervated by the **external branch** of the superior laryngeal nerve.

Arteries

Blood is supplied to the larynx by laryngeal branches of the **superior** and **inferior laryngeal arteries**, which are branches of the external carotid artery and thyrocervical trunk, respectively (see Fig. 10.2).

Veins and lymphatics

Veins draining from the larynx follow the route of the laryngeal arteries. The **superior laryngeal vein** drains to the superior thyroid vein, which empties into the internal jugular vein. The **inferior laryngeal vein** drains to the inferior thyroid vein and to the left brachiocephalic vein.

Lymphatic drainage of the larynx superior to the vocal ligaments is to the superior deep cervical nodes. Drainage inferior to the vocal folds is to the paratracheal and pretracheal nodes, which ultimately drain to the inferior deep cervical nodes.

■ CLINICAL CORRELATIONS
Viral croup

Croup is an infection and inflammation of the **glottis** and laryngeal regions. It is usually caused by the parainfluenza virus and affects children between 6 months and 5 years of age.

The typical clinical course of croup involves upper respiratory symptoms (e.g. runny nose, nasal congestion, mild fever) with rapid progression to a 'barking' cough, which is usually worse at night. In more severe cases, there may be inspiratory and expiratory stridor (a 'wheezing' sound caused by air rushing across a narrowed laryngeal inlet). Children with these symptoms should be evaluated and a diagnosis made based on the history and clinical examination.

Management of croup is aimed at decreasing the inflammation in the glottic and laryngeal regions by using cold air or cool mist, corticosteroids, and other medications as needed. Croup usually resolves within a few days.

Epiglottitis

Epiglottitis is an infection of the epiglottis, usually by *Haemophilus influenzae* type B bacteria. Children between 1 and 5 years of age are at highest risk, but epiglottitis can also occur in adults.

Symptoms of epiglottitis may begin as an upper respiratory infection and progress to a high fever accompanied by severe throat pain. Respiratory distress can occur as the infection progresses. Classically patients lean forward, drooling from the mouth and trying to breathe through the mouth, with severe inspiratory stridor. Leaning forward is an instinctive response that causes the epiglottis to tilt forward, opening the airway to facilitate breathing. Lateral neck radiographs show the classic 'thumbprint' sign – the epiglottis, which is usually a thin structure, swells and looks like a thumb.

Treatment of epiglottitis is aimed at maintaining a stable open airway because progressive epiglottic swelling will cause the airway to close and result in asphyxiation. Urgent surgical consultation and concurrent antibiotics and corticosteroids are necessary to maintain a stable airway. Depending on the severity of the disease, a surgical airway (tracheostomy) may be needed. With prompt treatment, epiglottitis usually resolves in several days.

Pharyngitis

Although most cases of pharyngitis (sore throat) are caused by viruses and cannot be treated with antibiotics, some are caused by bacteria. A common cause of bacterial pharyngitis in children in the US is group A β-hemolytic streptococcus. Depending on the severity of infection, the pharyngotympanic tubes may become occluded, predisposing the patient to otitis media (see Chapter 7).

The hallmark symptom of pharyngitis is throat pain, which is worse on swallowing. Occasionally, the pain radiates to the ears because they have several nerves in common. Patients with streptococcal pharyngitis usually complain of a painful sore throat and fever. Examination reveals an erythematous posterior oropharynx and, usually, tender cervical adenopathy (palpable lymph nodes). Diagnosis is based on culture obtained from swabbing the posterior oropharynx and tonsil.

Treatment of pharyngitis is directed at treating the symptoms. A soft diet of bland foods is recommended, and antipyretics as needed. Antibiotics are added to the treatment regimen for bacterial pharyngitis.

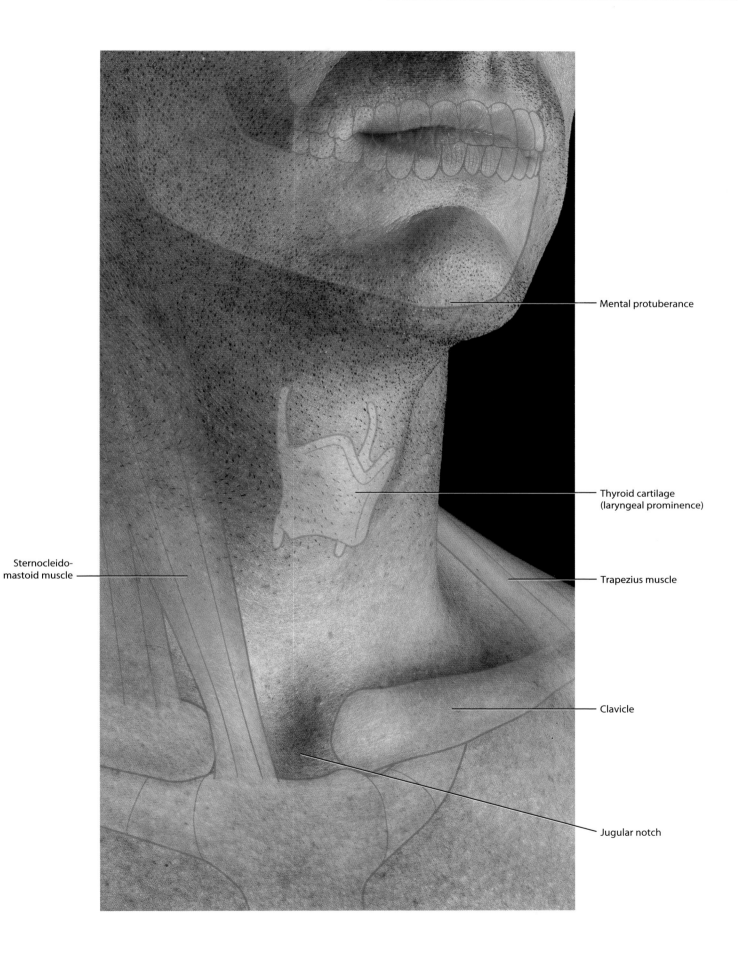

Mental protuberance

Thyroid cartilage
(laryngeal prominence)

Sternocleido-
mastoid muscle

Trapezius muscle

Clavicle

Jugular notch

Figure 10.6 Pharynx and larynx – surface anatomy. This photograph shows the right side of the lower face and neck. Observe the laryngeal prominence

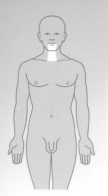

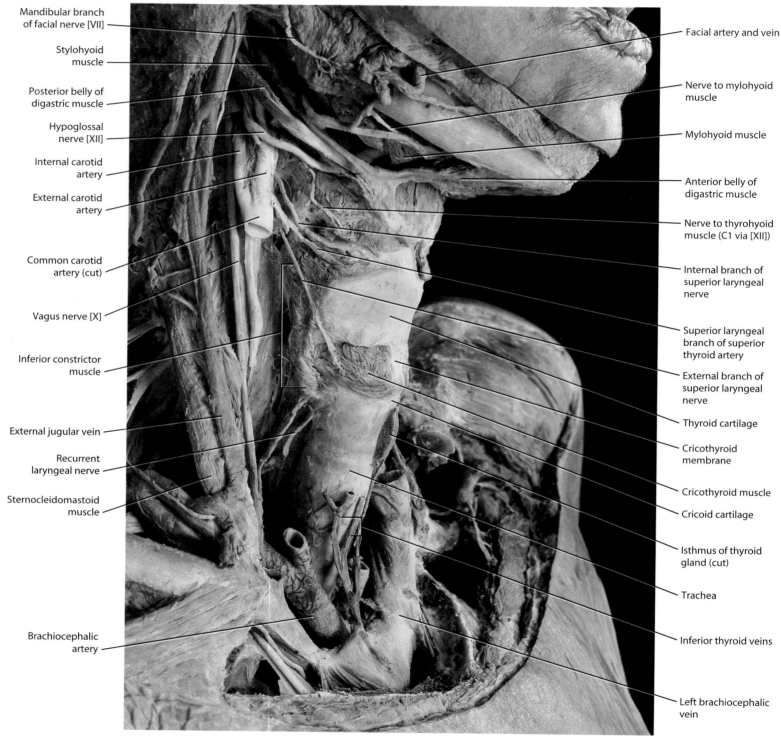

Mandibular branch of facial nerve [VII]

Stylohyoid muscle

Posterior belly of digastric muscle

Hypoglossal nerve [XII]

Internal carotid artery

External carotid artery

Common carotid artery (cut)

Vagus nerve [X]

Inferior constrictor muscle

External jugular vein

Recurrent laryngeal nerve

Sternocleidomastoid muscle

Brachiocephalic artery

Facial artery and vein

Nerve to mylohyoid muscle

Mylohyoid muscle

Anterior belly of digastric muscle

Nerve to thyrohyoid muscle (C1 via [XII])

Internal branch of superior laryngeal nerve

Superior laryngeal branch of superior thyroid artery

External branch of superior laryngeal nerve

Thyroid cartilage

Cricothyroid membrane

Cricothyroid muscle

Cricoid cartilage

Isthmus of thyroid gland (cut)

Trachea

Inferior thyroid veins

Left brachiocephalic vein

Figure 10.7 Pharynx and larynx – superficial dissection. View of the right side of the neck showing parts of the larynx and pharynx. Observe the cricothyroid membrane, which is a small fibrous connection between the thyroid and cricoid cartilages

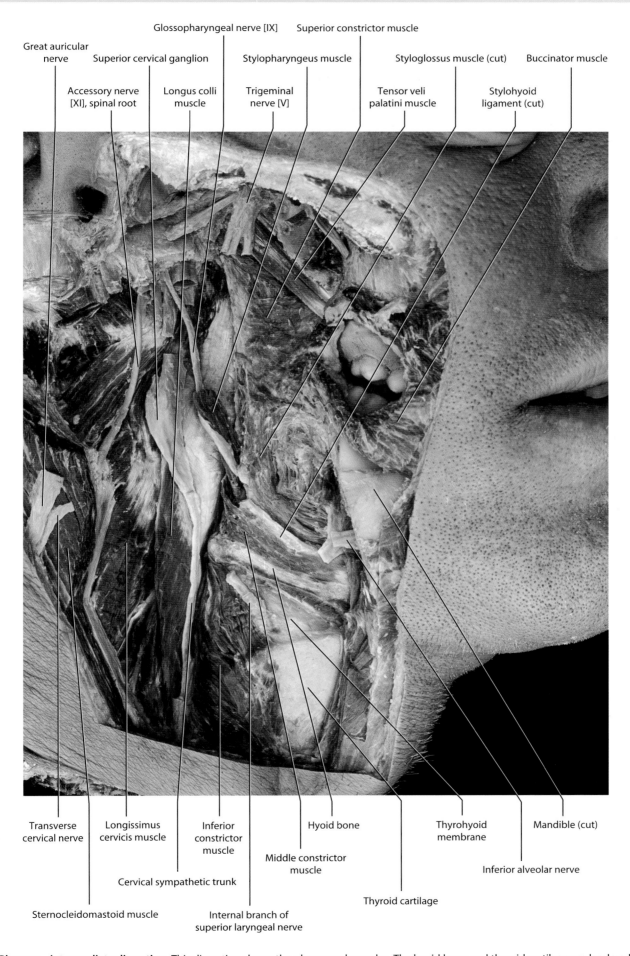

Great auricular nerve

Accessory nerve [XI], spinal root

Superior cervical ganglion

Longus colli muscle

Glossopharyngeal nerve [IX]

Trigeminal nerve [V]

Stylopharyngeus muscle

Superior constrictor muscle

Tensor veli palatini muscle

Styloglossus muscle (cut)

Stylohyoid ligament (cut)

Buccinator muscle

Transverse cervical nerve

Longissimus cervicis muscle

Inferior constrictor muscle

Hyoid bone

Thyrohyoid membrane

Mandible (cut)

Middle constrictor muscle

Inferior alveolar nerve

Cervical sympathetic trunk

Thyroid cartilage

Sternocleidomastoid muscle

Internal branch of superior laryngeal nerve

Figure 10.8 Pharynx – intermediate dissection. This dissection shows the pharyngeal muscles. The hyoid bone and thyroid cartilage are landmarks in this region

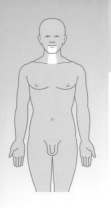

Pharynx and larynx **HEAD AND NECK**

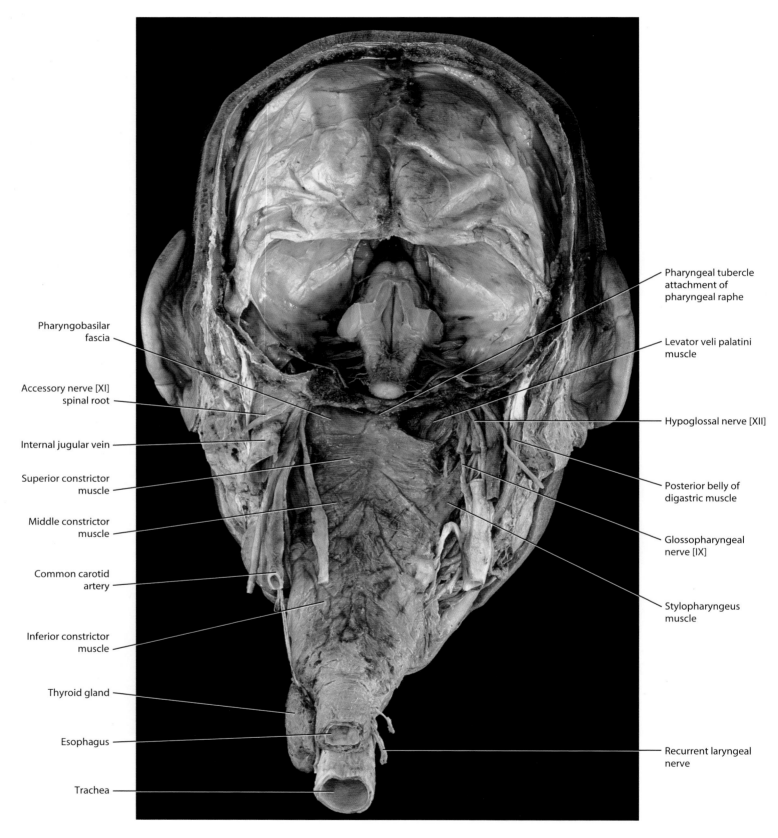

Pharyngobasilar fascia

Accessory nerve [XI] spinal root

Internal jugular vein

Superior constrictor muscle

Middle constrictor muscle

Common carotid artery

Inferior constrictor muscle

Thyroid gland

Esophagus

Trachea

Pharyngeal tubercle attachment of pharyngeal raphe

Levator veli palatini muscle

Hypoglossal nerve [XII]

Posterior belly of digastric muscle

Glossopharyngeal nerve [IX]

Stylopharyngeus muscle

Recurrent laryngeal nerve

Figure 10.9 Pharynx – deep dissection 1. This deep dissection provides a posterior view of the pharynx with the neck muscles and cervical vertebrae removed. Observe the relationships of the spinal cord, esophagus, and trachea to the pharynx

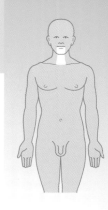

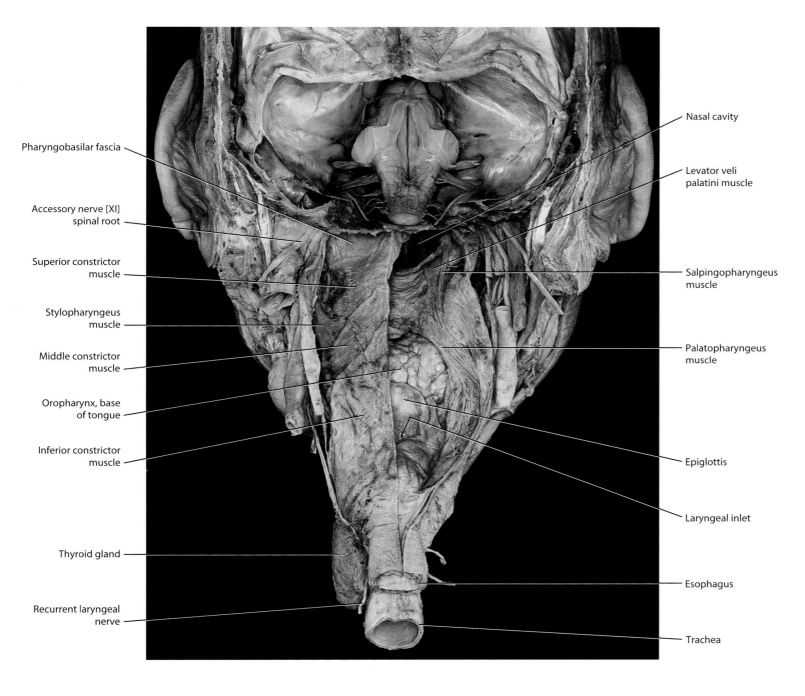

Pharyngobasilar fascia

Accessory nerve [XI] spinal root

Superior constrictor muscle

Stylopharyngeus muscle

Middle constrictor muscle

Oropharynx, base of tongue

Inferior constrictor muscle

Thyroid gland

Recurrent laryngeal nerve

Nasal cavity

Levator veli palatini muscle

Salpingopharyngeus muscle

Palatopharyngeus muscle

Epiglottis

Laryngeal inlet

Esophagus

Trachea

Figure 10.10 Pharynx – deep dissection 2. Posterior view of the pharynx. The pharyngeal muscles have been cut in the midline and reflected to show the posterior part of the tongue and the epiglottis

111

Pharynx and larynx   **HEAD AND NECK**

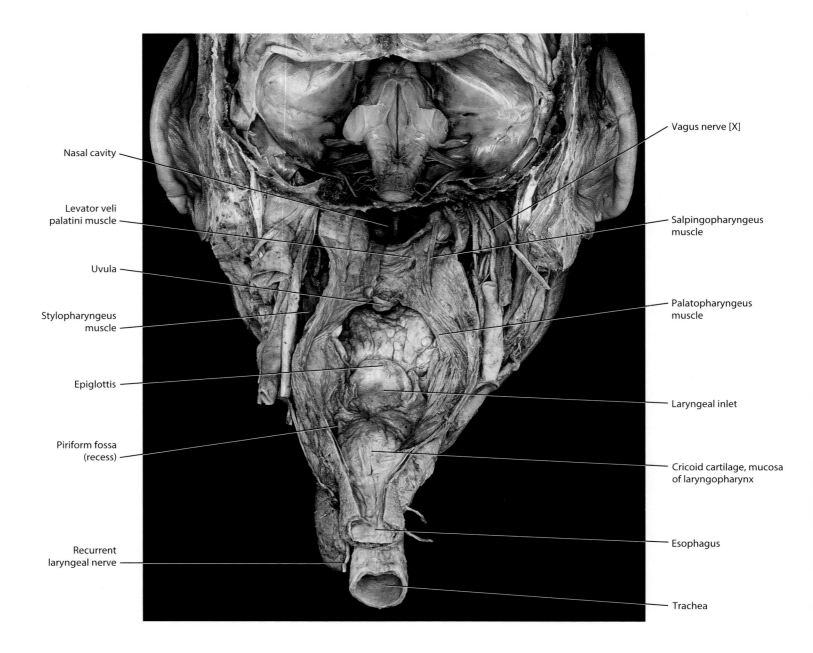

Nasal cavity

Levator veli
palatini muscle

Uvula

Stylopharyngeus
muscle

Epiglottis

Piriform fossa
(recess)

Recurrent
laryngeal nerve

Vagus nerve [X]

Salpingopharyngeus
muscle

Palatopharyngeus
muscle

Laryngeal inlet

Cricoid cartilage, mucosa
of laryngopharynx

Esophagus

Trachea

Figure 10.11 Pharynx – deep dissection 3. Posterior view of the pharynx. The pharyngeal muscles have been reflected bilaterally. Observe the posterior nasal cavity as it relates to the posterior oral region and tongue

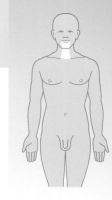

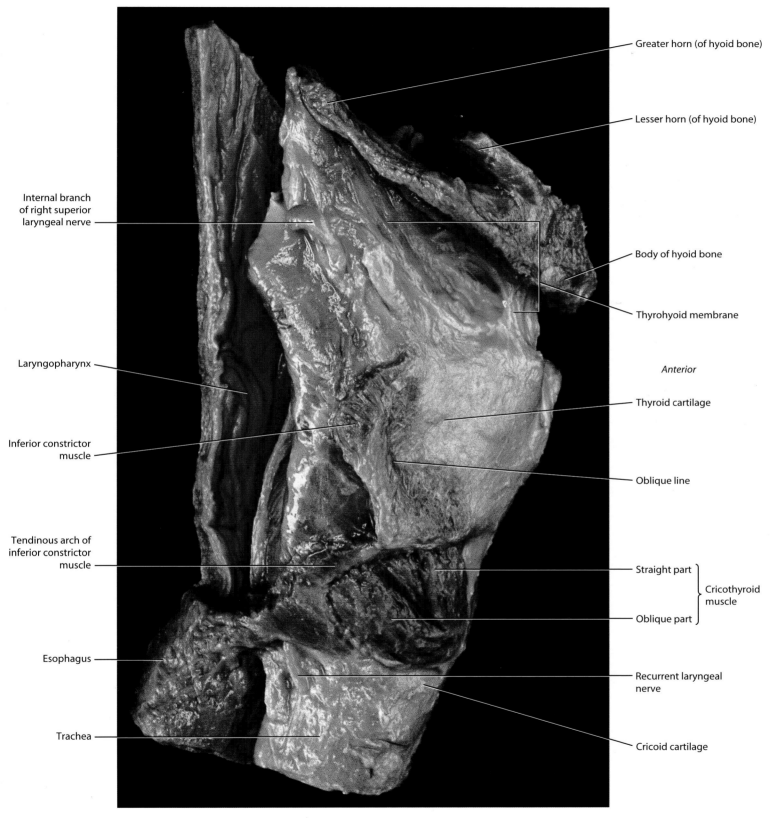

Greater horn (of hyoid bone)

Lesser horn (of hyoid bone)

Internal branch of right superior laryngeal nerve

Body of hyoid bone

Thyrohyoid membrane

Laryngopharynx

Anterior

Thyroid cartilage

Inferior constrictor muscle

Oblique line

Tendinous arch of inferior constrictor muscle

Straight part ⎫
⎬ Cricothyroid muscle
Oblique part ⎭

Esophagus

Recurrent laryngeal nerve

Trachea

Cricoid cartilage

Figure 10.12 Larynx – isolated 1. This is a view looking onto the right side of the larynx. The larynx has been removed from the cadaver to show its structures. Note the greater and lesser horns of the hyoid bone

113

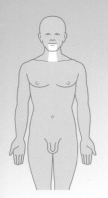

Pharynx and larynx **HEAD AND NECK**

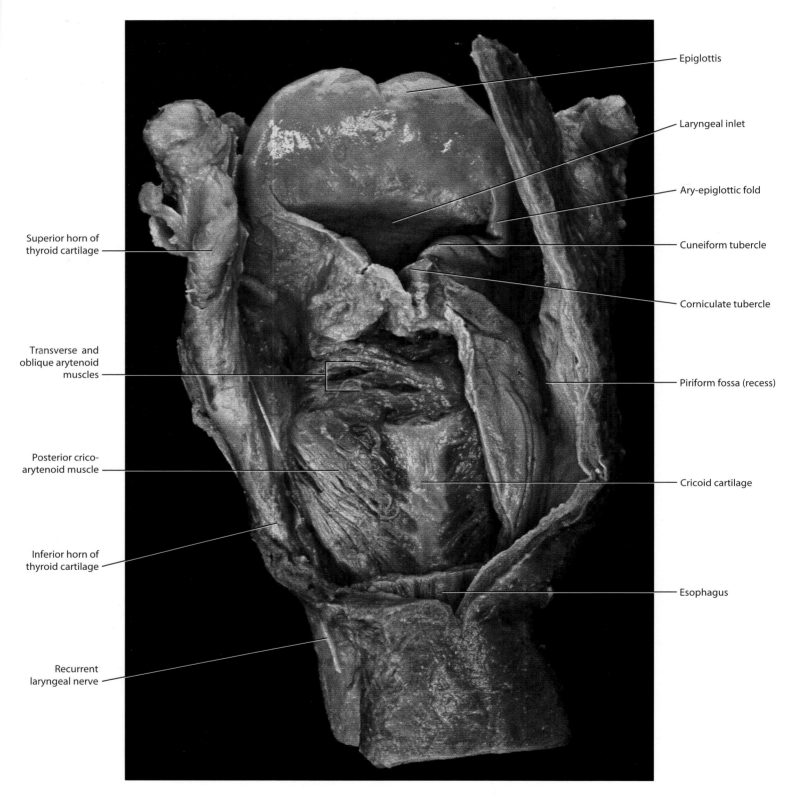

Epiglottis

Laryngeal inlet

Ary-epiglottic fold

Cuneiform tubercle

Superior horn of thyroid cartilage

Corniculate tubercle

Transverse and oblique arytenoid muscles

Piriform fossa (recess)

Posterior crico-arytenoid muscle

Cricoid cartilage

Inferior horn of thyroid cartilage

Esophagus

Recurrent laryngeal nerve

Figure 10.13 Larynx – isolated 2. The posterior wall of the pharyngeal muscles has been opened to show the epiglottis and laryngeal muscles. Observe the transverse and oblique arytenoid muscles

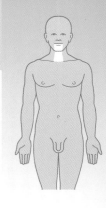

TABLE 10.1 INTRINSIC MUSCLES OF THE LARYNX

Muscle	Origin	Insertion	Innervation	Action	Blood supply
Cricothyroid	Arch of cricoid cartilage	Inferior border of thyroid cartilage and its inferior horn	External branch of superior laryngeal nerve	Lengthens and tenses vocal ligaments	Superior and inferior thyroid arteries
Posterior crico-arytenoid	Lamina of cricoid cartilage	Muscular process of arytenoid cartilage	Recurrent laryngeal nerve	Abducts vocal cords	Superior and inferior thyroid arteries
Lateral crico-arytenoid	Arch of cricoid cartilage	Muscular process of arytenoid cartilage	Recurrent laryngeal nerve	Adducts vocal cords	Superior and inferior thyroid arteries
Thyro-arytenoid	Posterior aspect of thyroid cartilage	Muscular process of arytenoid cartilage	Recurrent laryngeal nerve	Shortens and relaxes vocal cords	Superior and inferior thyroid arteries
*Vocalis	Vocal process of arytenoid cartilage	Vocal ligament	Recurrent laryngeal nerve	Increases or decreases tension on vocal ligament	
*Thyro-epiglottic				Supports quadrangular membrane	
Transverse and oblique arytenoids	Posterior aspect of arytenoid cartilage	Opposite arytenoid cartilage	Recurrent laryngeal nerve	Closes rima glottidis, intercartilaginous portion	Superior and inferior thyroid arteries

*Subsidiary muscles of the thyro-arytenoid muscle.

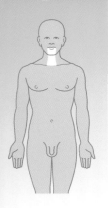

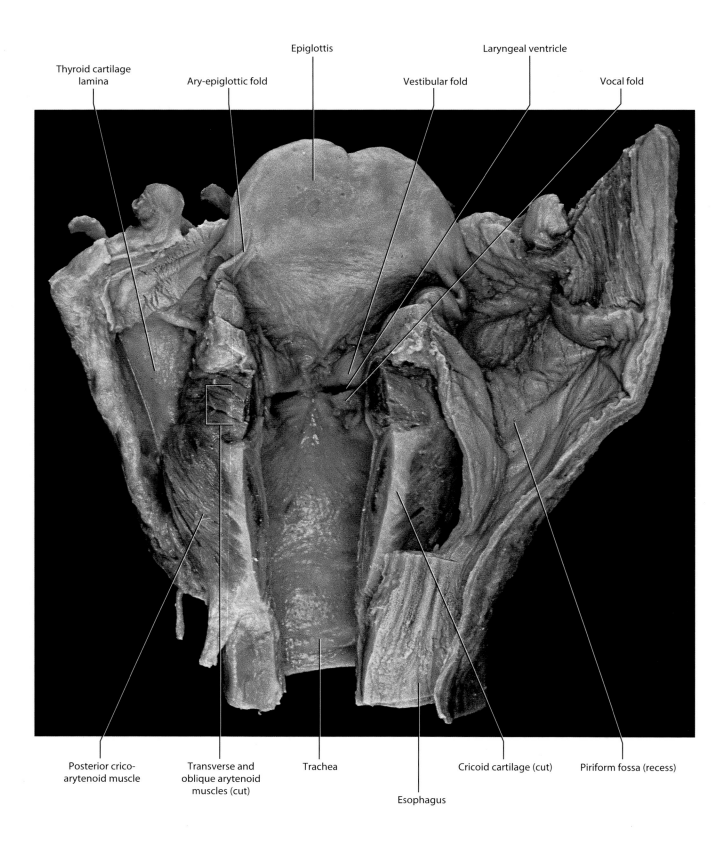

Thyroid cartilage lamina

Ary-epiglottic fold

Epiglottis

Vestibular fold

Laryngeal ventricle

Vocal fold

Posterior crico-arytenoid muscle

Transverse and oblique arytenoid muscles (cut)

Trachea

Esophagus

Cricoid cartilage (cut)

Piriform fossa (recess)

116   Figure 10.14 The larynx – isolated 3. The posterior wall of the larynx has been opened to show the false and true vocal folds (vocal cords)

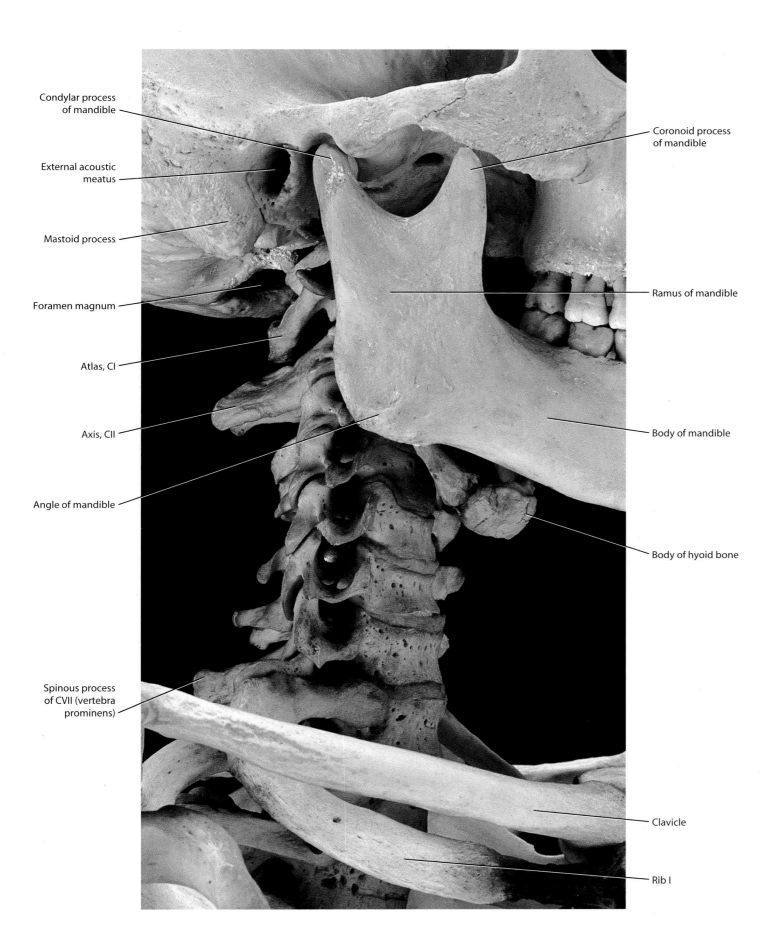

Condylar process
of mandible

External acoustic
meatus

Mastoid process

Foramen magnum

Atlas, CI

Axis, CII

Angle of mandible

Spinous process
of CVII (vertebra
prominens)

Coronoid process
of mandible

Ramus of mandible

Body of mandible

Body of hyoid bone

Clavicle

Rib I

HEAD AND NECK Pharynx and larynx

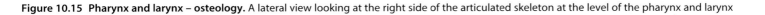

Figure 10.15 Pharynx and larynx – osteology. A lateral view looking at the right side of the articulated skeleton at the level of the pharynx and larynx

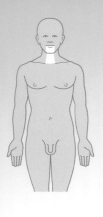

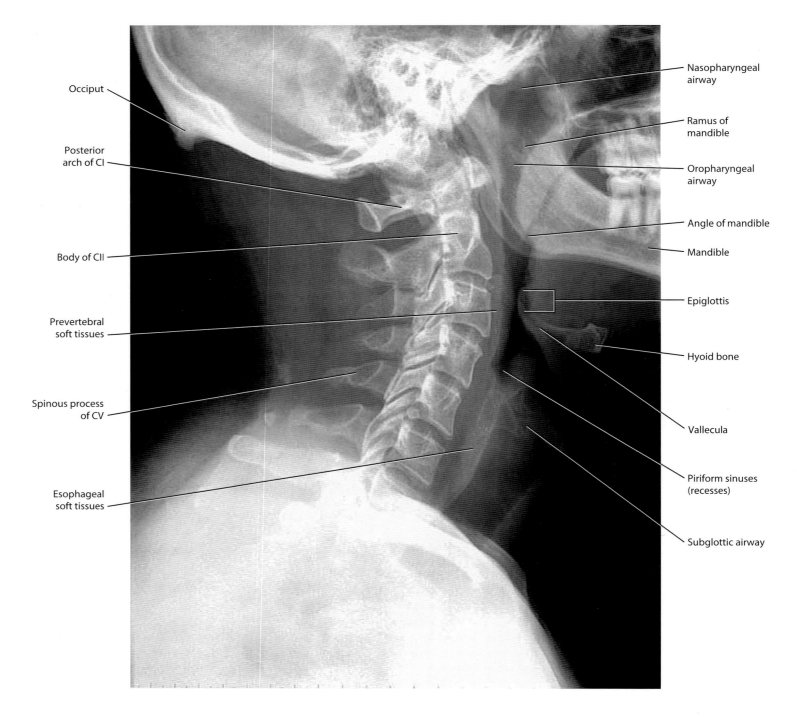

Occiput

Posterior arch of CI

Body of CII

Prevertebral soft tissues

Spinous process of CV

Esophageal soft tissues

Nasopharyngeal airway

Ramus of mandible

Oropharyngeal airway

Angle of mandible

Mandible

Epiglottis

Hyoid bone

Vallecula

Piriform sinuses (recesses)

Subglottic airway

Figure 10.16 Pharynx and larynx – plain film radiograph (lateral view). The epiglottis and epiglottic folds are well seen. Note that the airway, which appears dark, is located anterior to the esophagus (esophageal soft tissues)

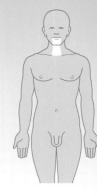

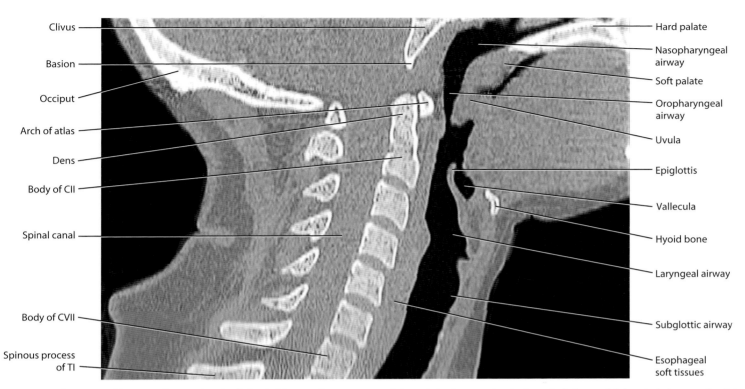

Clivus

Basion

Occiput

Arch of atlas

Dens

Body of CII

Spinal canal

Body of CVII

Spinous process
of TI

Hard palate

Nasopharyngeal
airway

Soft palate

Oropharyngeal
airway

Uvula

Epiglottis

Vallecula

Hyoid bone

Laryngeal airway

Subglottic airway

Esophageal
soft tissues

Figure 10.17 Pharynx and larynx – CT scan (sagittal view). Observe the structures of the epiglottis; note that its base (inferior part) is located at approximately the same level as the hyoid bone

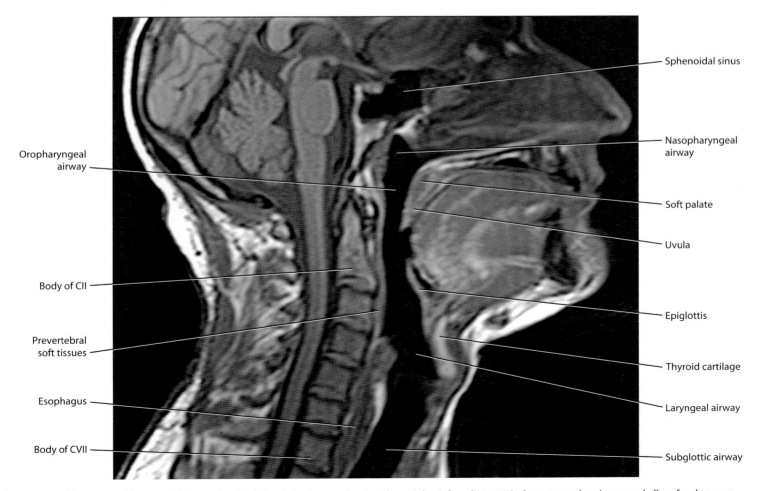

Oropharyngeal
airway

Body of CII

Prevertebral
soft tissues

Esophagus

Body of CVII

Sphenoidal sinus

Nasopharyngeal
airway

Soft palate

Uvula

Epiglottis

Thyroid cartilage

Laryngeal airway

Subglottic airway

Figure 10.18 Pharynx and larynx – MRI scan (sagittal view). During swallowing the epiglottis bends posteriorly to cover the airway and allow food to pass into the esophagus

11 Submandibular region

The submandibular region lies between the mandible and hyoid bones and is formed by the **submental** and **submandibular triangles**. It contains the submandibular gland. Skeletal support is provided by the mandible and hyoid bones. The mandible is the site of attachment for some of the **suprahyoid muscles** and all **muscles of mastication**. In the adult the mandible, which normally contains 16 permanent teeth, articulates with the temporal bone of the skull through the **temporomandibular joint**.

The hyoid bone is at the level of vertebra CIII, does not articulate with other bones, and is suspended by ligaments and the suprahyoid and infrahyoid muscles. It is linked to the **thyroid cartilage** through the **thyrohyoid membrane**. The hyoid muscles therefore move the larynx both superiorly and inferiorly during swallowing and speech.

MUSCLES

The most superficial muscle of the submandibular region is the **digastric muscle** (Table 11.1), which has two bellies (anterior and posterior) connected by an intermediate tendon attached to the hyoid bone by a 'fascial pulley' (Fig. 11.1). The **stylohyoid muscle** extends from the styloid process of the temporal bone to the hyoid

bone. The stylohyoid muscle is perforated by the tendon of the digastric muscle at the hyoid bone to create the fascial pulley.

The **mylohyoid muscle** is deep to the anterior belly and superior to the posterior belly of the digastric muscle, and forms the floor of the mouth; it is a sheet-like muscle that extends from the mylohyoid line of the mandible to the hyoid bone. Lymph nodes and neurovascular structures of the submandibular region are superficial to the mylohyoid muscle.

In the midline, and deep to the mylohyoid muscle, the **geniohyoid muscle** emerges from the internal surface of the mandible and attaches to the hyoid bone (Fig. 11.2). Just lateral and posterior to the geniohyoid, the **hyoglossus muscle** attaches the hyoid bone to the base of the tongue.

NERVES

Several cranial nerves and their branches are associated with the submandibular region. The mandibular nerve [V$_3$] division of the trigeminal nerve [V] gives off two nerves to this area:

- the first branch – the **nerve to mylohyoid** (from the inferior alveolar nerve) – passes along the mylohyoid groove on the medial surface of the mandible and innervates the mylohyoid muscle and the anterior belly of the digastric muscle.
- the second branch – the **lingual nerve** – passes anteriorly and inferiorly from its origin in the head towards the tongue, carries general sensation from the anterior two-thirds of the tongue, the mucosa of the floor of the mouth, and the mandibular lingual

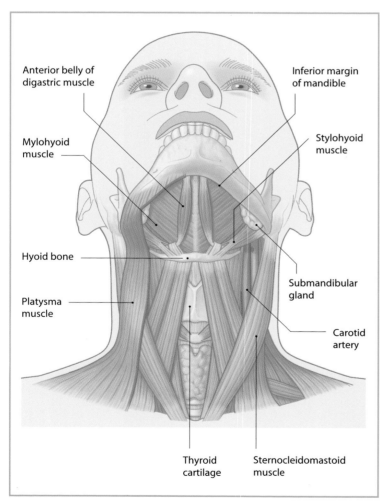

Figure 11.1 Submandibular region and its major muscles

Labels: Anterior belly of digastric muscle; Inferior margin of mandible; Mylohyoid muscle; Stylohyoid muscle; Hyoid bone; Submandibular gland; Platysma muscle; Carotid artery; Thyroid cartilage; Sternocleidomastoid muscle

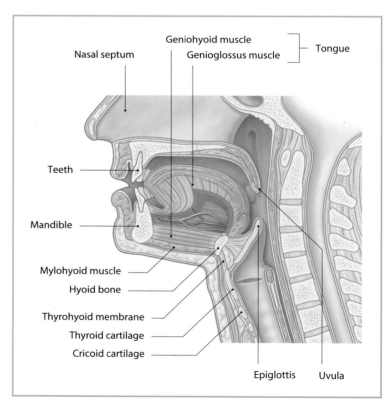

Figure 11.2 Major structures of the submandibular region in a hemisected specimen

Labels: Nasal septum; Geniohyoid muscle; Genioglossus muscle; Tongue; Teeth; Mandible; Mylohyoid muscle; Hyoid bone; Thyrohyoid membrane; Thyroid cartilage; Cricoid cartilage; Epiglottis; Uvula

gingiva, and also contains taste and preganglionic parasympathetic nerve fibers from the facial nerve [VII] via the **chorda tympani nerve**.

The **hypoglossal nerve [XII]** (see Fig. 12.2) passes between the carotid arterial plane and the deep aspect of the digastric and mylohyoid muscles to enter the submandibular region. It runs between the mylohyoid and hyoglossus muscles and provides motor innervation to all tongue muscles, except the palatoglossus muscle, which is innervated by the **accessory nerve [XI]**, and runs with the vagus nerve [X]. The hypoglossal nerve [XII] also carries fibers from the C1 spinal nerve, to innervate the geniohyoid muscle.

The facial nerve [VII] innervates the stylohyoid muscle and the posterior belly of the digastric muscle (see Chapter 5).

The **submandibular ganglion** (Fig. 11.3) in the submandibular region lateral to the hyoglossus muscle supplies autonomic parasympathetic innervation to the tongue. The submandibular ganglion is suspended from the lingual nerve. The ganglion receives preganglionic fibers from the facial nerve [VII] (chorda tympani) and sends postganglionic secretomotor nerve fibers to the sublingual and submandibular salivary glands.

ARTERIES
The arteries in the submandibular region arise from branches of the external carotid artery (see Fig. 12.3). The **lingual artery** arises from the external carotid artery at the level of the greater horn of the hyoid bone. It supplies blood to the tongue, palatine tonsil, and structures in the floor of the mouth.

The **facial artery** is usually the third branch of the external carotid

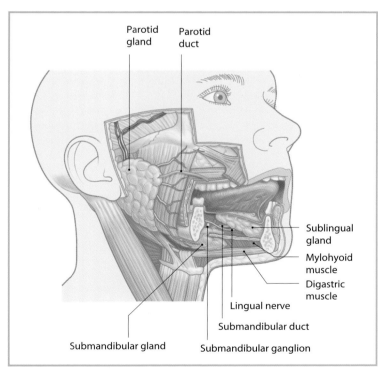

Parotid gland
Parotid duct
Sublingual gland
Mylohyoid muscle
Digastric muscle
Lingual nerve
Submandibular duct
Submandibular gland
Submandibular ganglion

Figure 11.3 Major structures of the submandibular region

artery. It passes anteriorly from its origin deep to the stylohyoid muscle and gives off branches to the palatine tonsil, palate, and submandibular gland. As it reaches the edge of the mandible, the facial artery gives off a small **submental branch** before passing around the edge of the mandible to enter the face just anterior to the masseter muscle.

VEINS AND LYMPHATICS
Most of the major arteries in the submandibular region have accompanying veins (venae comitantes). These come together to drain into either the **external** or **internal jugular veins** (see Fig. 2.3). Occasionally, a large nerve, such as the hypoglossal nerve [XII], also has venae comitantes. The venae comitantes of the hypoglossal nerve [XII] arise in the tongue, follow the course of the hypoglossal nerve [XII], and empty into the internal jugular veins.

Lymph vessels from the submandibular region also follow the named arteries and drain first to the **mental** and **submandibular nodes** (see Fig. 12.5). From here, lymph empties to the deep cervical nodes alongside the internal jugular vein.

SUBMANDIBULAR GLAND
The submandibular gland is a combined mucous and serous salivary gland at the posterior border of the mylohyoid muscle (Fig. 11.3). It wraps around the posterior mylohyoid muscle and therefore has superficial and deep parts. The **submandibular duct**, which is approximately 5 cm long, arises from the deep part and opens into the oral cavity on both sides of the frenulum of tongue. The submandibular gland is innervated by postganglionic parasympathetic fibers from the submandibular ganglion. Saliva is produced when these nerves are stimulated. Blood is supplied by branches of the facial artery.

■ CLINICAL CORRELATIONS
Mandibular fracture
Mandibular fractures are usually accompanied by edema (swelling), ecchymosis (bruising), and wounds on the face, but some patients have few such symptoms.

The cardinal symptoms of a mandibular fracture are malocclusion (inability of the maxillary and mandibular teeth to meet in normal fashion), pain, and drooling. On examination, intraoral lacerations and hematomas may be seen.

By definition, all mandible fractures are open fractures because of the close apposition of the oral mucosa to the mandible. It is therefore common practice to use antibiotics to prevent infection.

The most common sites of mandibular fracture are the condylar region, the angle of mandible, and body and symphysis of mandible. Because of the location of the muscles of mastication (see Chapter 5), some mandibular fractures are considered favorable and others unfavorable. A favorable fracture is one in which the fracture line will spontaneously reduce when the patient closes the mouth. In unfavorable fractures, the fracture lines do not spontaneously close with contraction of the muscles of mastication. These and more complex fractures require surgical repair.

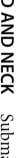

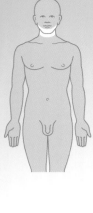

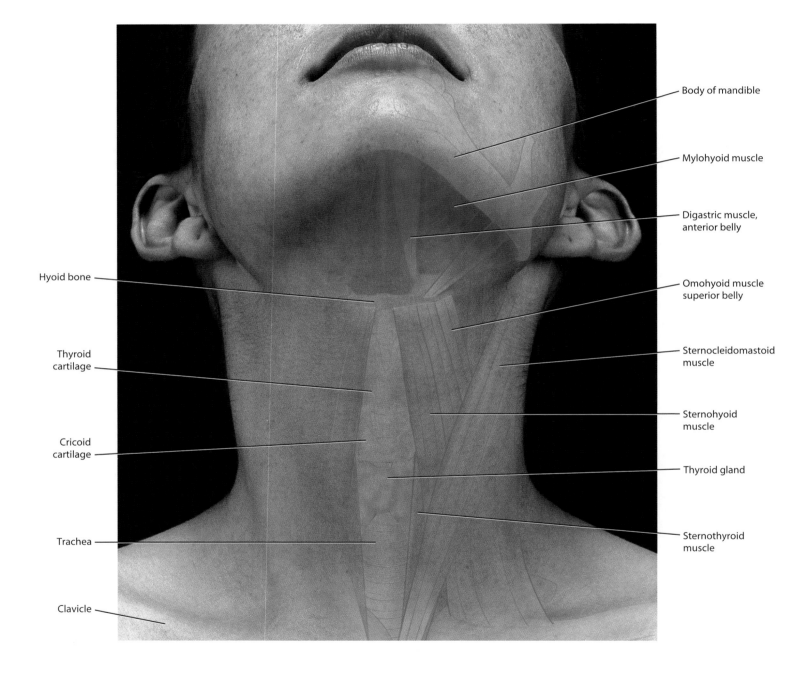

Body of mandible

Mylohyoid muscle

Digastric muscle,
anterior belly

Hyoid bone

Omohyoid muscle
superior belly

Thyroid
cartilage

Sternocleidomastoid
muscle

Sternohyoid
muscle

Cricoid
cartilage

Thyroid gland

Trachea

Sternothyroid
muscle

Clavicle

Figure 11.4 Submandibular region – surface anatomy. Inferior view of the submandibular region and neck of a young woman. Observe the sternocleidomastoid muscles, which span the distance between the mastoid process of the temporal bone and the medial part of the sternum and clavicle

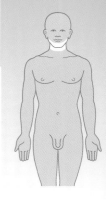

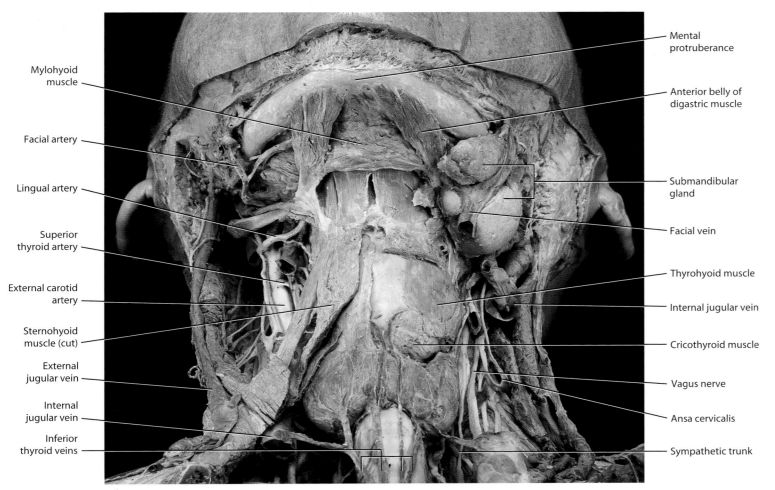

Mylohyoid muscle

Facial artery

Lingual artery

Superior thyroid artery

External carotid artery

Sternohyoid muscle (cut)

External jugular vein

Internal jugular vein

Inferior thyroid veins

Mental protruberance

Anterior belly of digastric muscle

Submandibular gland

Facial vein

Thyrohyoid muscle

Internal jugular vein

Cricothyroid muscle

Vagus nerve

Ansa cervicalis

Sympathetic trunk

Figure 11.5 Submandibular region – superficial dissection. This dissection shows the submandibular gland and its relationship to the anterior belly of the digastric muscle and the mylohyoid muscle

TABLE 11.1 MUSCLES OF THE SUBMANDIBULAR REGION (SUPRAHYOID MUSCLES)					
Muscle	**Origin**	**Insertion**	**Action**	**Nerve supply**	**Blood supply**
Digastric – anterior belly	Digastric fossa of mandible	Intermediate tendon through fibrous loop that attaches to greater horn and body of the hyoid bone	Elevates hyoid bones and base of tongue, fixes hyoid bone, depresses mandible	Nerve to mylohyoid from mandibular nerve (V$_3$)	Submental artery
Digastric – posterior belly	Mastoid notch of temporal bone	"	"	Facial nerve [VII]	Muscular branches of occipital and posterior auricular arteries
Stylohyoid	Styloid process of temporal bone	Hyoid bone at junction of body	Retracts hyoid bone and base of tongue	Facial nerve [VII]	Muscular branches of facial and occipital arteries
Mylohyoid	Mylohyoid line on medial surface of mandible	Median mylohyoid raphe	Elevates floor of mouth and hyoid bone, and depresses mandible	Nerve to mylohyoid from mandibular nerve (V$_3$)	Mylohyoid branch of inferior alveolar artery, submental branch of facial artery, and sublingual branch of lingual artery
Geniohyoid	Inferior mental spine, symphysis of mandible	Anterior aspect of body of hyoid bone	Protrudes hyoid bone and tongue	Branch of C1 through hypoglossal nerve [XII]	Sublingual branch of lingual artery

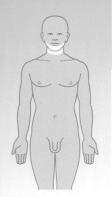

HEAD AND NECK

Submandibular region

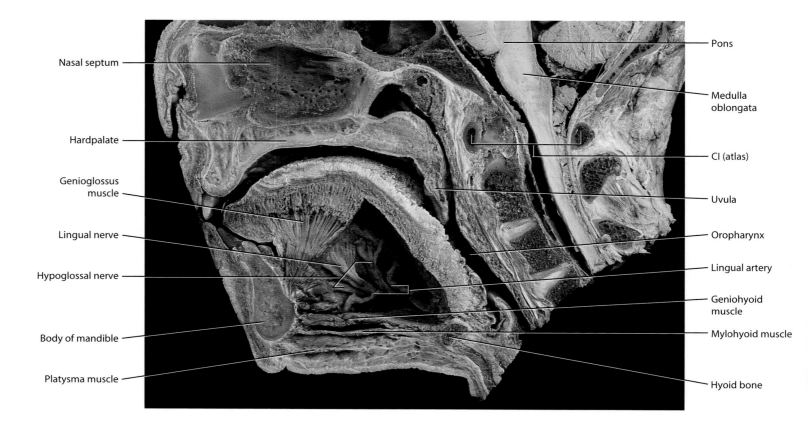

Nasal septum

Hardpalate

Genioglossus
muscle

Lingual nerve

Hypoglossal nerve

Body of mandible

Platysma muscle

Pons

Medulla
oblongata

CI (atlas)

Uvula

Oropharynx

Lingual artery

Geniohyoid
muscle

Mylohyoid muscle

Hyoid bone

Figure 11.6 Submandibular region – sagittal section. A window has been cut into the tongue of this hemisected cadaver to show the lingual artery and nerve, hypoglossal nerve [XII], and submandibular duct

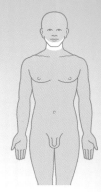

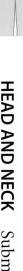

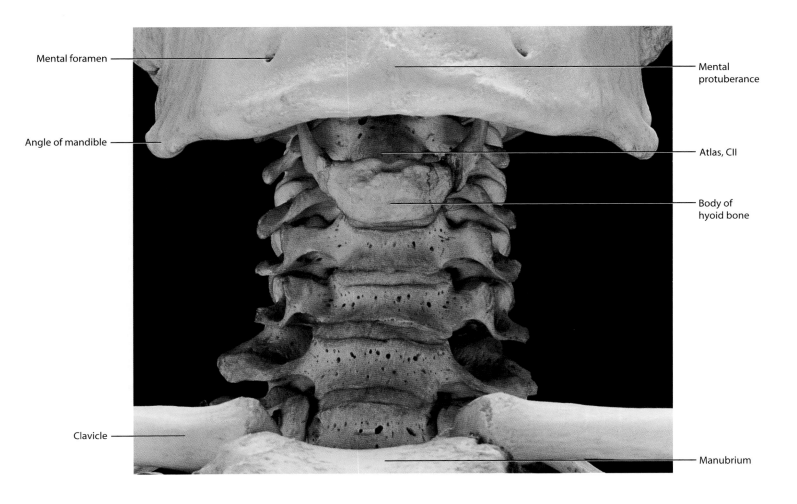

Mental foramen

Mental protuberance

Angle of mandible

Atlas, CII

Body of hyoid bone

Clavicle

Manubrium

Figure 11.7 Submandibular region – osteology. Observe the hyoid bone as it would be found suspended by muscles and tendons in the submandibular region

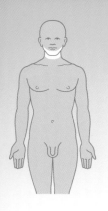

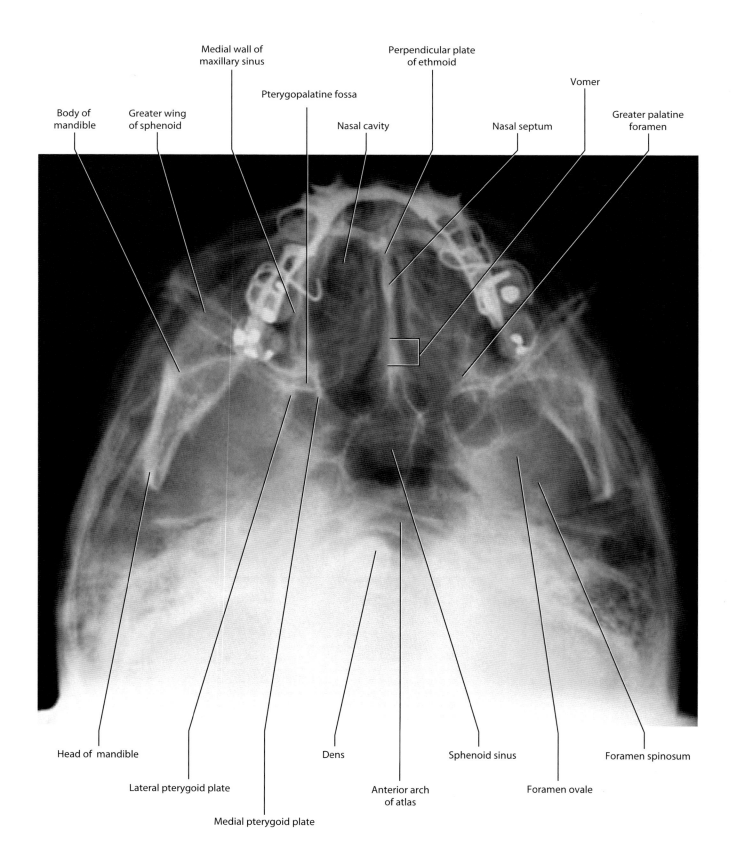

Body of
mandible

Greater wing
of sphenoid

Medial wall of
maxillary sinus

Pterygopalatine fossa

Nasal cavity

Perpendicular plate
of ethmoid

Nasal septum

Vomer

Greater palatine
foramen

Head of mandible

Lateral pterygoid plate

Medial pterygoid plate

Dens

Anterior arch
of atlas

Sphenoid sinus

Foramen ovale

Foramen spinosum

Figure 11.8 Submandibular region – plain film radiograph (submental view). This radiograph shows the relationship between the superimposed maxillary and mandibular arches, and the maxillary and sphenoidal sinuses. In addition, the dens of CII is visible in a similar coronal plane as the head of the mandible. The extensive dental work is radio-opaque and illustrates the arch-like arrangement of the teeth as seen from this perspective

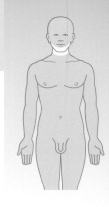

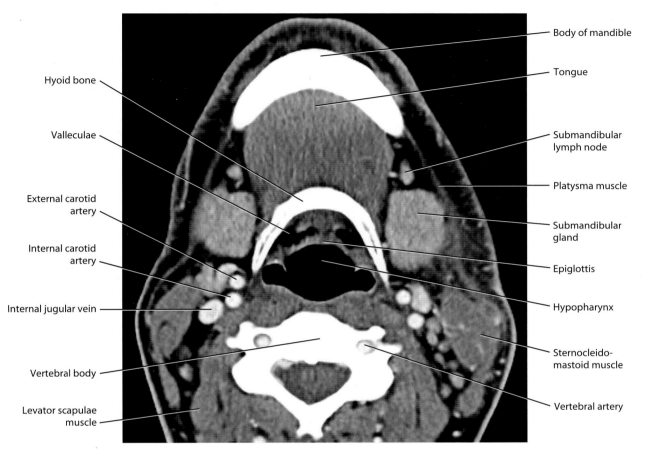

Body of mandible

Tongue

Submandibular lymph node

Platysma muscle

Submandibular gland

Epiglottis

Hypopharynx

Sternocleido-mastoid muscle

Vertebral artery

Hyoid bone

Valleculae

External carotid artery

Internal carotid artery

Internal jugular vein

Vertebral body

Levator scapulae muscle

Figure 11.9 Submandibular region – CT scan (axial view). The submandibular glands are defined by the surrounding submandibular fat (which appears dark). Submandibular lymph nodes may be enlarged and demonstrate abnormal enhancement in infectious and neoplastic disease of the neck

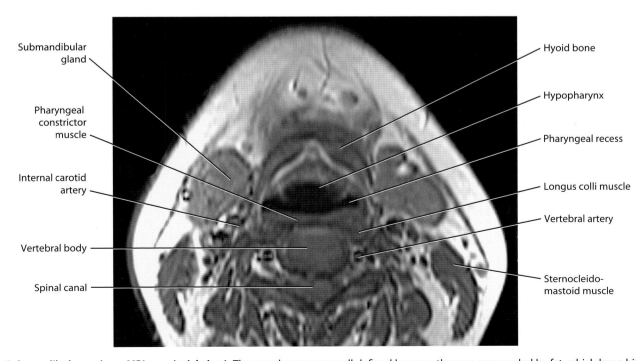

Submandibular gland

Pharyngeal constrictor muscle

Internal carotid artery

Vertebral body

Spinal canal

Hyoid bone

Hypopharynx

Pharyngeal recess

Longus colli muscle

Vertebral artery

Sternocleido-mastoid muscle

Figure 11.10 Submandibular region – MRI scan (axial view). The muscles are very well defined because they are surrounded by fat, which has a high signal intensity in MRI scans. For this reason, MRI is better than CT for the evaluation of soft tissue tumors

12 Anterior triangle of the neck

The anterior triangle of the neck is formed by the anterior border of the sternocleidomastoid muscle, inferior border of the mandible, and the midline of the neck (Fig. 12.1). It is further subdivided by the superior belly of the omohyoid muscle and the anterior and posterior bellies of the digastric muscle into the **submandibular**, **submental**, **carotid**, and **muscular triangles**. These arbitrary subdivisions of the anterior neck help compartmentalize and assist with the localization of important anatomical structures.

The anterior triangle contains the **platysma** muscle, which is a thin, sheet-like muscle within the superficial cervical fascia that spreads out over the neck and shoulders. Also located superficially are the cervical branches of the facial nerve [VII], cutaneous nerves from the cervical plexus, and superficial veins. Airway structures can be palpated in the midline:

- the hyoid bone – vertebral level CIII;
- the thyroid cartilage – vertebral level CIV–CV;
- the cricoid cartilage – vertebral level CVI;
- the tracheal rings – vertebral level CVI to TIV/TV.

At the inferior border of the anterior triangle of the neck is the jugular notch (vertebral level TII/TIII).

Bony support for the anterior neck comes from the seven cervical vertebrae, the base of the skull, bones of the upper thorax, and the pectoral girdle. An additional point of bony support is the **hyoid bone**, which is suspended below the mandible by the suprahyoid and infrahyoid muscles. The hyoid bone has a pair of greater horns extending posteriorly from the body of the hyoid bone, giving it a three-dimensional 'U'-shape. The lesser horns project superiorly and are additional points of muscle attachment.

MUSCLES

The **sternocleidomastoid** muscle divides the neck into the anterior and posterior triangles. It originates from the sternum and clavicle, ascends to insert onto the mastoid process of the skull, and rotates and flexes the head. It is innervated by the accessory nerve [XI] and the anterior rami of spinal nerves C2 and C3.

The infrahyoid muscles (the sternohyoid, sternothyroid, thyrohyoid, and omohyoid muscles) are deep to the platysma, cutaneous nerves, and superficial veins. These muscles attach to the structures after which they are named and, as a group, contract to depress the hyoid bone and larynx, except the thyrohyoid muscle, which elevates the larynx (Table 12.1).

NERVES

The infrahyoid muscles are innervated by the **cervical plexus**, which is a network of nerves formed by the anterior rami (nerve roots) of the first four cervical spinal nerves (Fig. 12.2). The cervical plexus lies on the middle scalene muscle just posterior to the carotid sheath (a fascial structure that encloses the internal jugular veins, carotid arteries, vagus nerves [X], and part of the ansa cervicalis). The **great auricular**, **lesser occipital**, **transverse cervical**, and **supraclavicular nerves** originate from the cervical plexus to innervate the skin of the neck (Table 12.2). The **ansa cervicalis** is a motor loop that arises from spinal roots C1 to C3 and innervates the infrahyoid muscles.

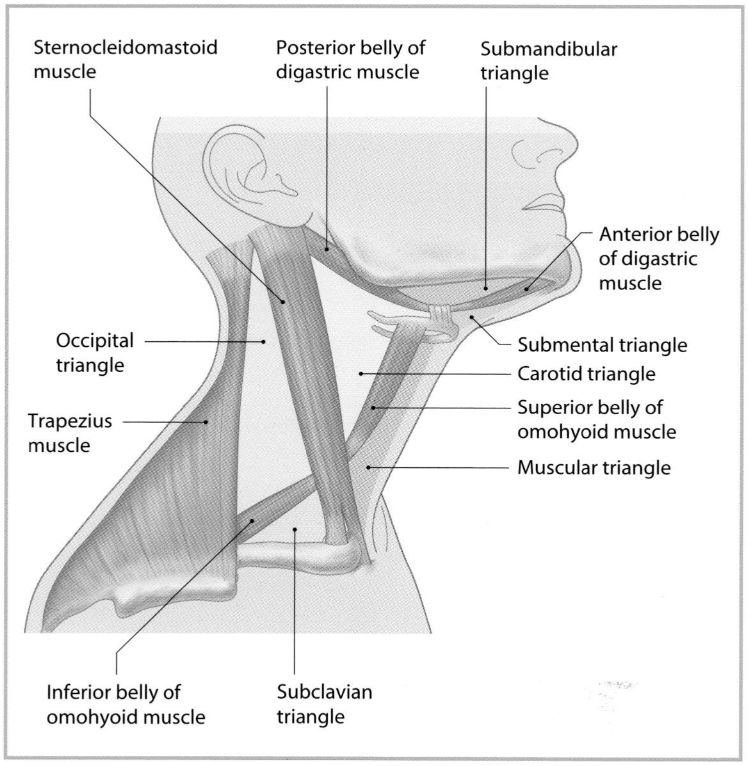

Figure 12.1 The anterior triangle of the neck and its descriptive subdivisions

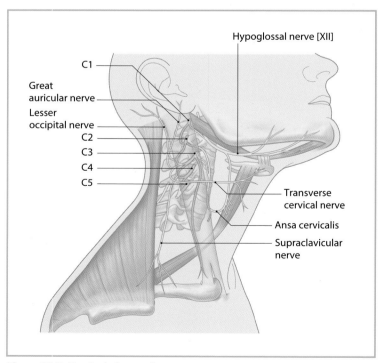

Figure 12.2 Cervical plexus of nerves

The **vagus nerve [X]** is a major structure in the anterior triangle of the neck. It leaves the jugular foramen at the base of the skull and descends into the neck within the carotid sheath with the internal and external carotid arteries and internal jugular vein. During its passage through the neck, the vagus nerve [X] innervates several deeper neck structures:

- **pharyngeal branches** pass to the pharynx;
- **cardiac branches** convey parasympathetic innervation to the heart (cardiac plexus);
- the **superior laryngeal nerve** branch divides into internal and external branches, which then pass to the laryngeal region and cricothyroid muscle.

The **left** and **right recurrent laryngeal nerve** branches of the vagus nerve [X] are located in the anterior neck. They recur around the subclavian artery (on the right) and the arch of the aorta (on the left), and then ascend to the larynx. The recurrent laryngeal nerves provide sensation to the larynx inferior to the vocal folds. They supply all intrinsic muscles of the larynx except the cricothyroid muscle (see Chapter 10).

ARTERIES

Blood is supplied to the anterior triangle of the neck by branches of the common carotid and subclavian arteries (Fig. 12.3). The left common carotid artery arises from the arch of the aorta whereas the right common carotid artery arises from the brachiocephalic trunk. The common carotid arteries ascend superiorly in the neck within the carotid sheaths on each side of the neck. At the upper margin of the thyroid cartilage (vertebral level CIII), the common carotid arteries divide into internal and external branches. Two important structures at this level are the carotid sinus and carotid body:

- the **carotid sinus** is a dilation in the wall of the root of the internal carotid artery that responds to changes in blood pressure and transmits information to the central nervous system;
- the **carotid body** is a small, pea-like structure that responds to changes in the concentration of oxygen and carbon dioxide in the blood. It is located in the notch created by the bifurcation of the common carotid artery.

Both the carotid sinus and carotid body are innervated by branches of the **glossopharyngeal nerve [IX]** and **vagus nerve [X]**, and by **sympathetic nerves**.

The **internal carotid artery** ascends from its point of origin to the head to supply more cranial structures; the **external carotid artery** has eight branches to supply structures in the neck (Table 12.3). As it continues superiorly in the neck, the external carotid artery passes through the parotid gland and then divides into its terminal branches – the **maxillary artery** and the **superficial temporal artery** (see Chapter 5).

VEINS AND LYMPHATICS

The **internal jugular veins** are the largest veins in the head and neck (see Fig. 2.3). They originate at the jugular foramen of the skull as a continuation of the sigmoid sinus (an intracranial dural venous channel) and run inferiorly through the neck within the carotid sheaths. Along their route, the internal jugular veins are lateral and superficial to the carotid arteries. This relationship is clinically significant when placing a central venous catheter into the vein.

Lymphatic drainage from the anterior triangle of the neck is to a horizontal ring of **deep nodes**, which are divided into three main groups according to the region they drain (see Fig. 12.5).

THYROID GLAND

The thyroid gland is an H-shaped endocrine organ that consists of two lateral **lobes** joined by an **isthmus**. The isthmus is usually at the level of the second and third tracheal rings. Occasionally, there is an additional **pyramidal lobe**, which extends superiorly from the isthmus. The thyroid is enclosed in pretracheal fascia. It produces hormones (thyroid hormone and calcitonin), which regulate growth and help maintain chemical homeostasis.

Sympathetic innervation to the thyroid gland is by postganglionic fibers from the sympathetic **cervical ganglia** (see Chapter 13), which travel with arteries that supply the gland. The **external branch** of the **superior laryngeal nerve**, a branch from the vagus nerve [X], is closely associated with the superior thyroid artery.

Blood is supplied to the thyroid gland by the **superior thyroid artery**, which originates from the external carotid artery, and the **inferior thyroid artery**, a branch from the thyrocervical trunk. The recurrent laryngeal nerve, which supplies the intrinsic muscles of the larynx, is close to the inferior thyroid artery. Rarely, there is a third arterial supply to the thyroid gland from the **thyroid ima** artery, which is a direct branch of the aorta or brachiocephalic arteries.

Venous drainage of the thyroid gland is by the **superior** and **middle thyroid veins**, which empty into the internal jugular vein, and **inferior thyroid veins**, which drain into the left brachiocephalic vein.

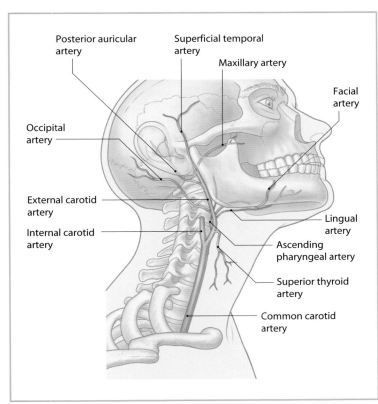

Figure 12.3 Carotid artery and its branches in the neck

Posterior auricular artery
Superficial temporal artery
Maxillary artery
Facial artery
Occipital artery
External carotid artery
Internal carotid artery
Lingual artery
Ascending pharyngeal artery
Superior thyroid artery
Common carotid artery

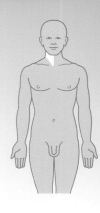

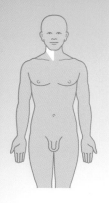

Lymphatic drainage of the thyroid gland is to the **prelaryngeal**, **pretracheal**, **paratracheal**, and **deep cervical nodes**. The paratracheal nodes communicate with the mediastinal lymph nodes and so can provide a route for the spread of infection or cancer to the thorax.

PARATHYROID GLANDS

There are usually four parathyroid glands, a **superior** and an **inferior** pair. They are posterior to the lateral lobe of the thyroid gland within a capsule. Each gland is about the size of a lentil and is yellow–brown in color. They are innervated by branches of the sympathetic trunk or from the superior and middle cervical sympathetic ganglia, and their blood supply is mainly from the inferior thyroid arteries, with some supplied by the superior thyroid arteries. Lymphatic drainage is to the deep cervical and paratracheal nodes.

■ CLINICAL CORRELATIONS

Thyroid mass or nodules

The thyroid gland has a bosselated surface but a homogeneous interior, within which masses or nodules may develop (Fig. 12.4). Most thyroid nodules are benign, but a small percentage are malignant. Solitary nodules are more likely to be malignant than multiple nodules, but approximately 80% of solitary thyroid tumors are benign. Commonly a thyroid mass is investigated by fine-needle aspiration – a procedure that involves placing a needle (on a syringe) into the mass and aspirating (withdrawing) a small amount of tissue or fluid from the mass for analysis. The most common form of thyroid cancer is papillary thyroid cancer.

Treatment of thyroid cancer is total thyroidectomy, during which the surgeon must take great care not to damage the recurrent laryngeal nerve. A 'breathy voice' after thyroidectomy may be diagnostic of unilateral recurrent laryngeal nerve injury, which usually resolves, at least partially, depending on the severity of damage. Rarely, bilateral recurrent laryngeal nerve injury presents with shortness of breath or inspiratory stridor because the laryngeal muscles are unable to abduct. Surgical treatment may then be necessary to establish an airway.

Damage to the superior laryngeal nerve during surgery can make it impossible to increase voice pitch because the cricothyroid muscle is unable to increase the tension of the vocal folds.

Neck mass or nodule

Neck masses or nodules can occur at any age. In young patients a neck mass is usually indicative of an inflammatory or congenital problem, such as a branchial cleft cyst, and can be removed surgically. In older patients, especially those in risk groups such as smokers, tobacco chewers, and alcohol drinkers, there is a much higher risk that such a mass is malignant.

Sometimes a very small tumor in the neck causes ear pain. This referred pain results from the extensive innervation of the neck and ear by branches of the vagus [X] and glossopharyngeal [IX] nerves. If the vagus nerve [X] is 'irritated' in one area it can 'refer' the irritation and pain to another of the areas it supplies.

Patients with cancer of the neck usually present with a lump in the neck or problems related to swallowing or speaking. Treatment of neck cancers is primarily surgical removal accompanied by radio- or chemotherapy.

Smaller neck nodules are commonly the result of lymph node enlargement. Lymph nodes that are enlarged because of infection are usually tender and painful to touch; those enlarged by cancer are usually firm and painless. Lymph nodes up to 2 cm in diameter can be considered within the normal range, but nevertheless they should be examined by a physician.

Figure 12.5 shows the major lymph node groups of the head and neck. A palpable node in a labeled region is likely to be draining material from the area shown.

Figure 12.4 Thyroid mass

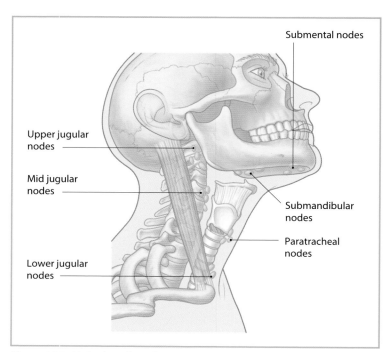

Figure 12.5 Major lymph node groups in the neck

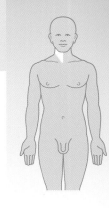

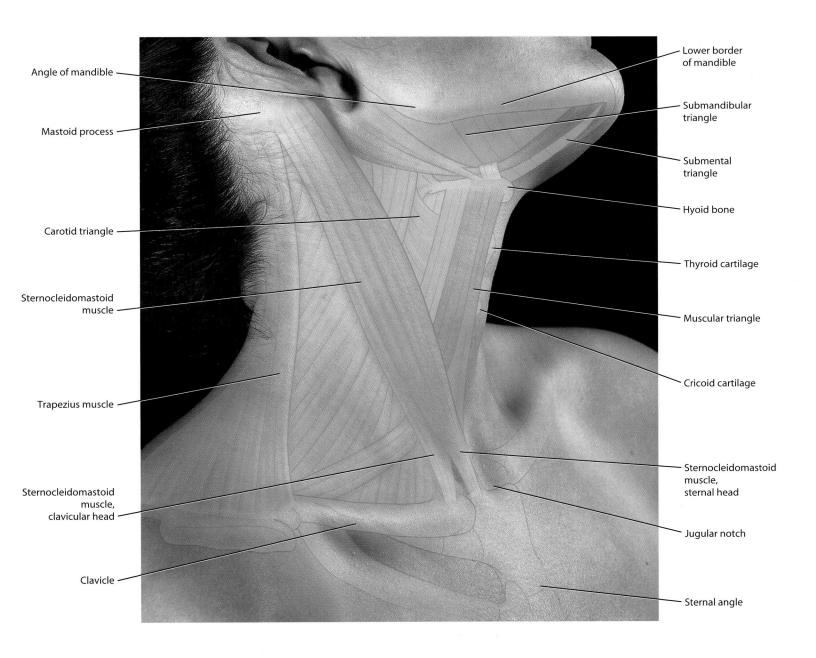

Angle of mandible

Mastoid process

Carotid triangle

Sternocleidomastoid muscle

Trapezius muscle

Sternocleidomastoid muscle, clavicular head

Clavicle

Lower border of mandible

Submandibular triangle

Submental triangle

Hyoid bone

Thyroid cartilage

Muscular triangle

Cricoid cartilage

Sternocleidomastoid muscle, sternal head

Jugular notch

Sternal angle

Figure 12.6 Anterior triangle of the neck – surface anatomy.

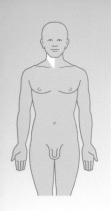

Anterior triangle of the neck

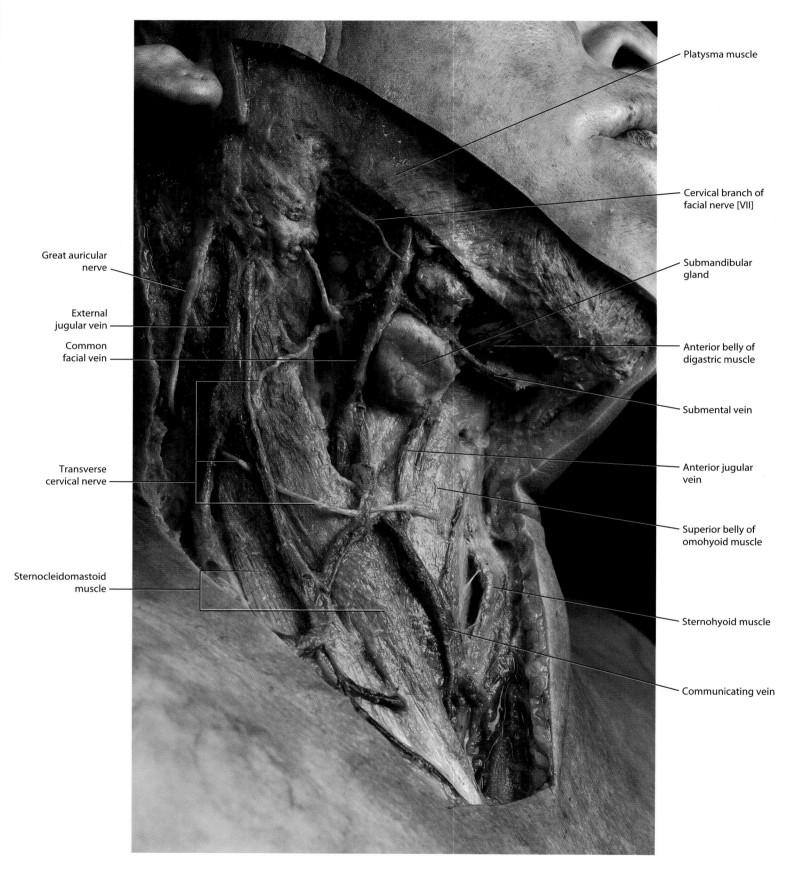

Platysma muscle

Cervical branch of
facial nerve [VII]

Submandibular
gland

Anterior belly of
digastric muscle

Submental vein

Anterior jugular
vein

Superior belly of
omohyoid muscle

Sternohyoid muscle

Communicating vein

Great auricular
nerve

External
jugular vein

Common
facial vein

Transverse
cervical nerve

Sternocleidomastoid
muscle

Figure 12.7 Anterior triangle of the neck – superficial dissection.

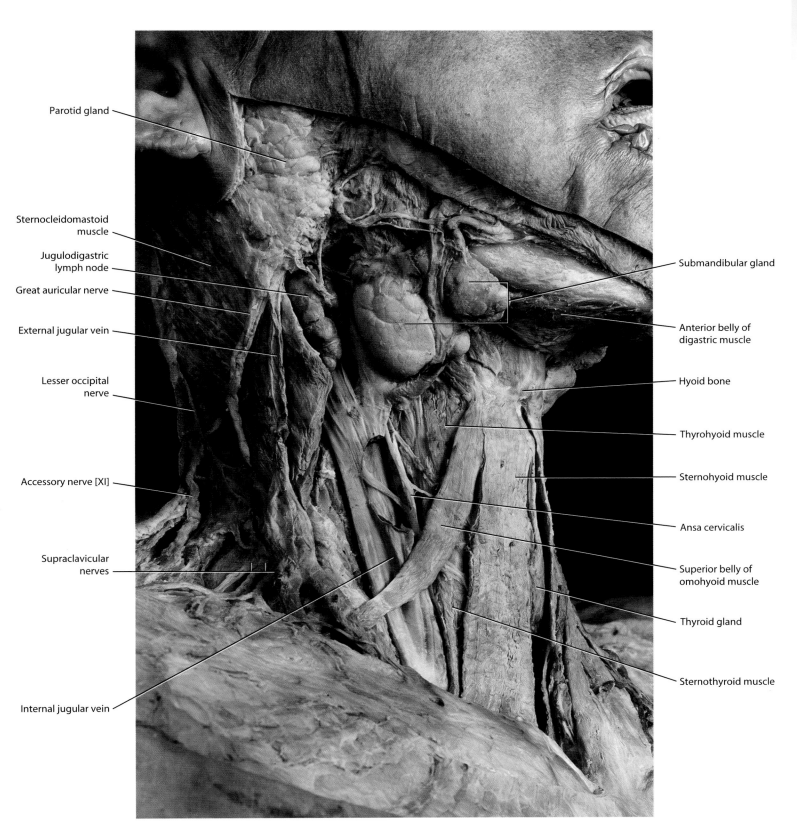

Parotid gland

Sternocleidomastoid muscle

Jugulodigastric lymph node

Great auricular nerve

External jugular vein

Lesser occipital nerve

Accessory nerve [XI]

Supraclavicular nerves

Internal jugular vein

Submandibular gland

Anterior belly of digastric muscle

Hyoid bone

Thyrohyoid muscle

Sternohyoid muscle

Ansa cervicalis

Superior belly of omohyoid muscle

Thyroid gland

Sternothyroid muscle

HEAD AND NECK Anterior triangle of the neck

Figure 12.8 Anterior triangle of the neck – intermediate dissection 1.

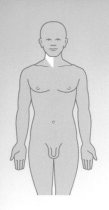

TABLE 12.1 MUSCLES OF THE ANTERIOR TRIANGLE OF THE NECK

Muscle	Origin	Insertion	Innervation	Action	Blood supply
Platysma	Fascia and skin over the upper part of the deltoid and pectoralis major muscles	Lower border of the mandible and muscles of the lips	Cervical branch of the facial nerve [VII]	Anterior part depresses the mandible, draws down lower lip, and angles mouth down on each side	Submental branch of facial artery, suprasternal branch of suprascapular artery (thyrocervical trunk)
Sternocleidomastoid	Sternum and medial third of clavicle	Mastoid process of temporal bone and superior nuchal line	Accessory nerve [XI], spinal root	Acting alone it bends the head to the same side as the muscle and rotates it so face is turned to opposite side. The two muscles, acting together, flex the neck; if neck is kept extended by post-vertebral muscles, sternocleidomastoid muscles act together to raise sternum and assist forced inspiration	Posterior auricular, superior thyroid, occipital, suprascapular arteries
Trapezius (cervical part)	Medial part of superior nuchal line, external occipital protuberance, ligamentum nuchae, and spine of CVII	Lateral third of clavicle, acromion and spine of scapula	Accessory nerve [XI], spinal root	Elevates the tip of shoulder, draws scapula medially and braces the shoulder backward	Transverse cervical and suprascapular arteries
Digastric – anterior belly	Digastric fossa, medial aspect of mandible near symphysis	Intermediate tendon	Nerve to mylohyoid – inferior alveolar branch of mandibular nerve [V₃]	Both bellies act together to raise the hyoid bone during swallowing. Acting with infrahyoid strap muscles, they fix the hyoid bone, providing support for tongue movement	Branches of submental artery
Digastric – posterior belly	Digastric notch, medial to mastoid process	Intermediate tendon	Facial nerve [VII]		Muscular branches of posterior auricular and occipital arteries
Stylohyoid	Styloid process of temporal bone	Hyoid bone splits to embrace intermediate tendon of digastric muscles	Facial nerve [VII]	Pulls hyoid bone upward and backward during swallowing	Muscular branches of facial and occipital arteries
Omohyoid – superior belly	Body and horn of hyoid bone	Intermediate tendon	Ansa cervicalis (C1 to C3)	These muscles depress the larynx and hyoid bone after being elevated by the pharynx during swallowing and speech; they also can: 1. depress hyoid bone or when acting with suprahyoid muscles they furnish a stable base for the tongue; 2. elevate the larynx in the first phase of swallowing; 3. depress the larynx during second phase of swallowing.	Suprahyoid branch of lingual artery
Omohyoid – inferior belly	Lateral and superior border of scapula	Intermediate tendon	Ansa cervicalis (C1 to C3)		Superior thyroid artery
Sternohyoid	Posterior aspect of manubrium of sternum and medial end of clavicle	Body of hyoid bone	Ansa cervicalis (C1 to C3)		Hyoid branches of superior thyroid and lingual arteries
Sternothyroid	Posterior aspect of manubrium of sternum and first costal cartilage	Oblique line on thyroid cartilage	Ansa cervicalis (C1 to C3)		Cricothyroid branch of superior thyroid artery
Thyrohyoid	Oblique line of thyroid cartilage	Lower aspect of the greater horn of hyoid bone	C1		Infrahyoid branch of superior thyroid artery

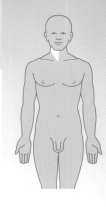

TABLE 12.2 NERVES

Nerves	Spinal roots (anterior rami)	Structures supplied and areas of innervation
Cutaneous nerves		
Lesser occipital	C2 (C3)	Skin of posterolateral aspect of neck
Great auricular	C2, C3	Skin of ear and parotid region
Transverse cervical	C2, C3	Skin of anterior and lateral aspect of the neck
Supraclavicular anterior (medial, intermediate, lateral)	C3, C4	Skin of shoulder and upper chest
Motor branches		
Ansa cervicalis*	C1 to C3	Infrahyoid muscles
Segmental and other muscular branches	C1 to C5	Prevertebral muscles, parts of the scalene, levator scapulae, trapezius, and sternocleidomastoid muscles
Phrenic	C3 to C5	Descends through the neck and thorax to supply motor and sensory fibers to the diaphragm; sensory fibers from pericardium and mediastinum

*Fibers from C1 accompany the hypoglossal nerve [XII] to the thyrohyoid and geniohyoid muscles. They also form the superior root of the ansa cervicalis. The superior root descends on the internal and common carotid arteries and forms a loop, the ansa cervicalis, with the inferior root (C2, 3) which descends on the internal jugular vein

TABLE 12.3 BRANCHES OF THE EXTERNAL CAROTID ARTERY

Artery	Distribution
1. Superior thyroid artery	Thyroid gland, larynx, pharynx, and infrahyoid muscles
2. Lingual artery	Tongue, suprahyoid muscles, tonsil, soft palate, sublingual and submandibular glands
3. Facial artery	Tonsil, soft palate, submandibular gland, upper and lower lips, and facial musculature
4. Ascending pharyngeal artery	Pharynx, tonsil, soft palate, pharyngotympanic tube
5. Occipital artery	Upper posterior neck, back of scalp to vertex
6. Posterior auricular artery	Auricle and adjacent scalp
7. Maxillary artery	Enters the infratemporal and pterygopalatine fossae and is distributed with branches of the maxillary [V$_2$] and mandibular [V$_3$] divisions of the trigeminal nerve [V]
8. Superficial temporal artery	Parotid gland, masseter muscle, lateral and anterior scalp

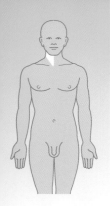

Anterior triangle of the neck   **HEAD AND NECK**

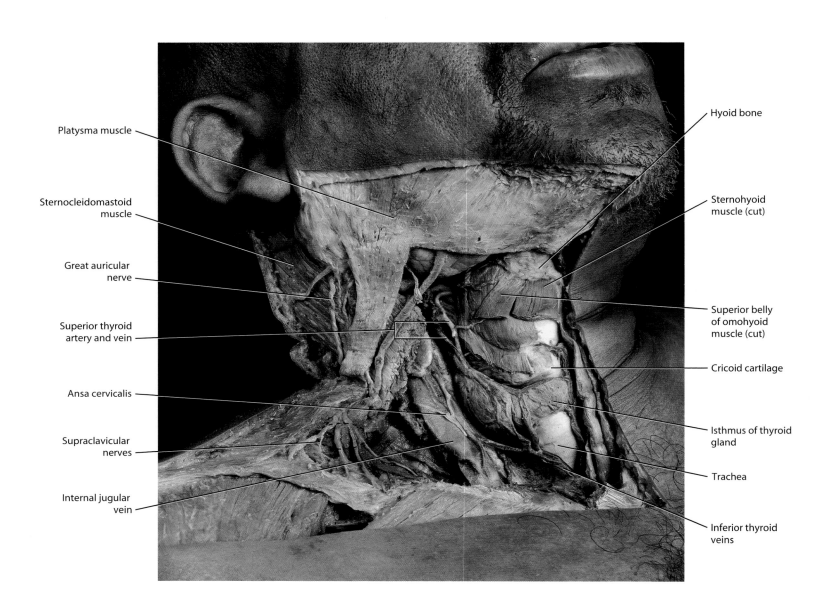

Platysma muscle

Sternocleidomastoid muscle

Great auricular nerve

Superior thyroid artery and vein

Ansa cervicalis

Supraclavicular nerves

Internal jugular vein

Hyoid bone

Sternohyoid muscle (cut)

Superior belly of omohyoid muscle (cut)

Cricoid cartilage

Isthmus of thyroid gland

Trachea

Inferior thyroid veins

136   Figure 12.9 Anterior triangle of the neck – intermediate dissection 2.

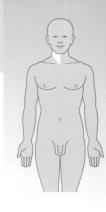

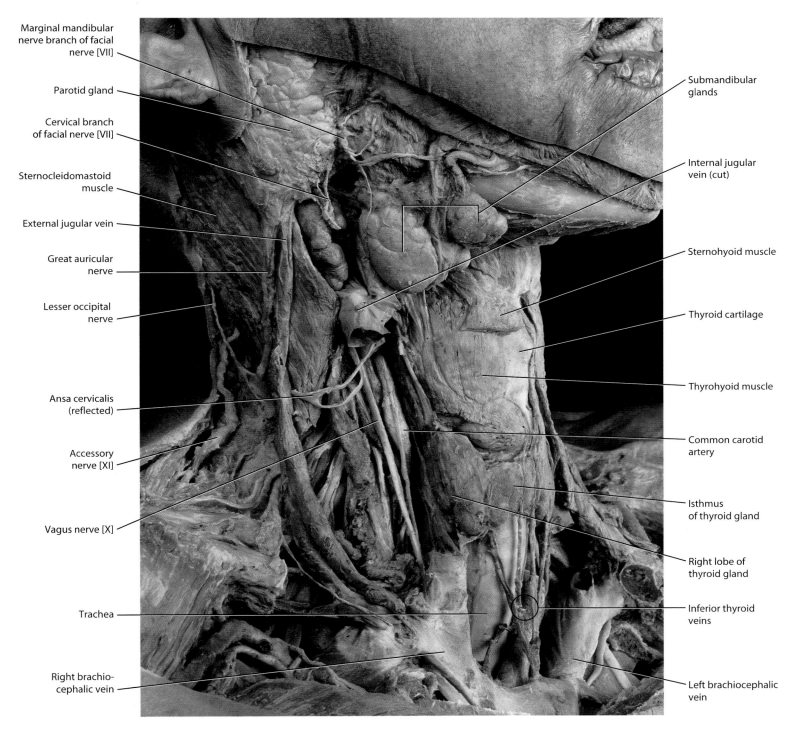

Marginal mandibular nerve branch of facial nerve [VII]

Parotid gland

Cervical branch of facial nerve [VII]

Sternocleidomastoid muscle

External jugular vein

Great auricular nerve

Lesser occipital nerve

Ansa cervicalis (reflected)

Accessory nerve [XI]

Vagus nerve [X]

Trachea

Right brachio-cephalic vein

Submandibular glands

Internal jugular vein (cut)

Sternohyoid muscle

Thyroid cartilage

Thyrohyoid muscle

Common carotid artery

Isthmus of thyroid gland

Right lobe of thyroid gland

Inferior thyroid veins

Left brachiocephalic vein

Figure 12.10 Anterior triangle of the neck – deep dissection 1.

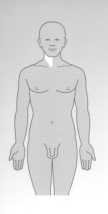

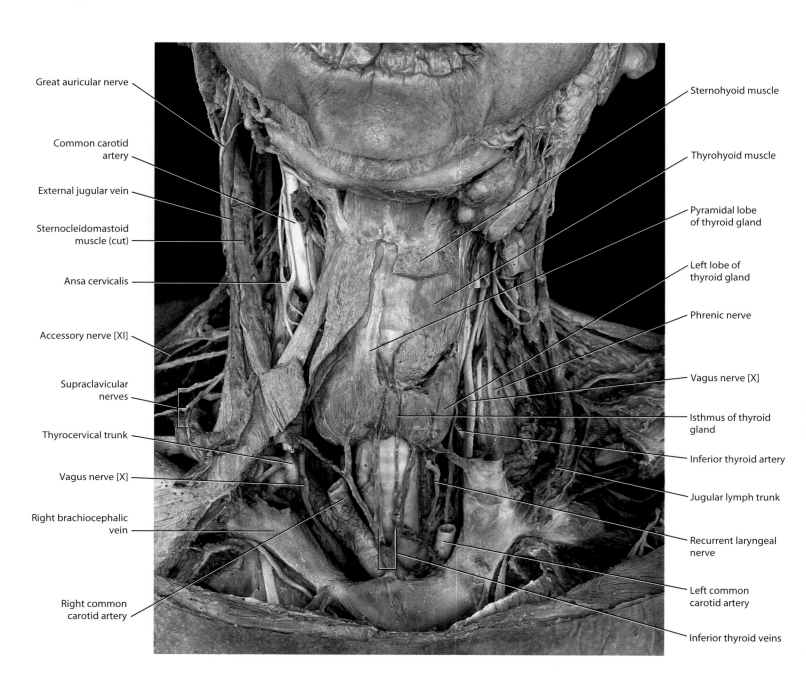

Great auricular nerve

Common carotid artery

External jugular vein

Sternocleidomastoid muscle (cut)

Ansa cervicalis

Accessory nerve [XI]

Supraclavicular nerves

Thyrocervical trunk

Vagus nerve [X]

Right brachiocephalic vein

Right common carotid artery

Sternohyoid muscle

Thyrohyoid muscle

Pyramidal lobe of thyroid gland

Left lobe of thyroid gland

Phrenic nerve

Vagus nerve [X]

Isthmus of thyroid gland

Inferior thyroid artery

Jugular lymph trunk

Recurrent laryngeal nerve

Left common carotid artery

Inferior thyroid veins

Figure 12.11 Anterior triangle of the neck – deep dissection 2.

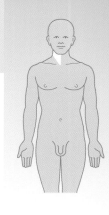

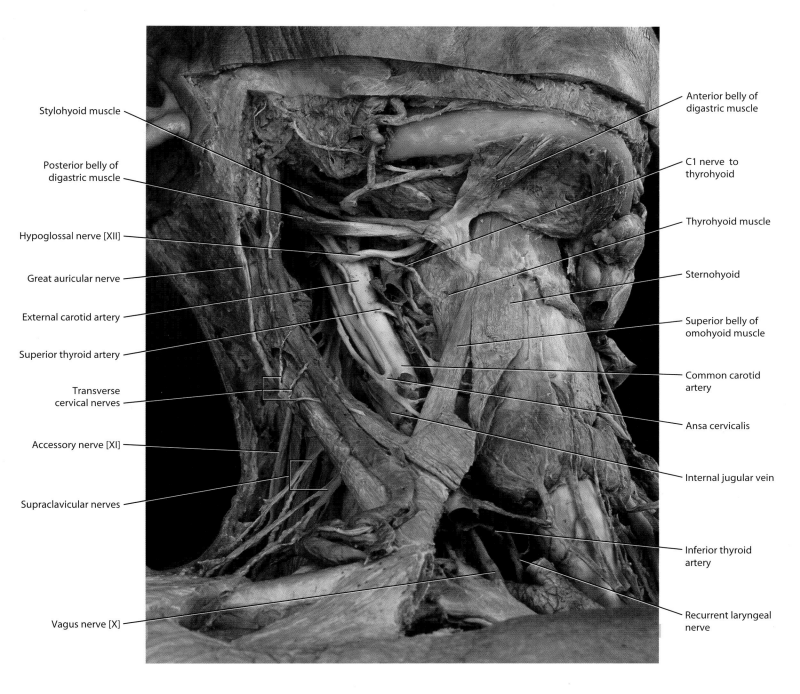

Stylohyoid muscle

Posterior belly of
digastric muscle

Hypoglossal nerve [XII]

Great auricular nerve

External carotid artery

Superior thyroid artery

Transverse
cervical nerves

Accessory nerve [XI]

Supraclavicular nerves

Vagus nerve [X]

Anterior belly of
digastric muscle

C1 nerve to
thyrohyoid

Thyrohyoid muscle

Sternohyoid

Superior belly of
omohyoid muscle

Common carotid
artery

Ansa cervicalis

Internal jugular vein

Inferior thyroid
artery

Recurrent laryngeal
nerve

HEAD AND NECK   Anterior triangle of the neck

Figure 12.12 Anterior triangle of the neck – deep dissection 3.

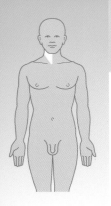

HEAD AND NECK

Anterior triangle of the neck

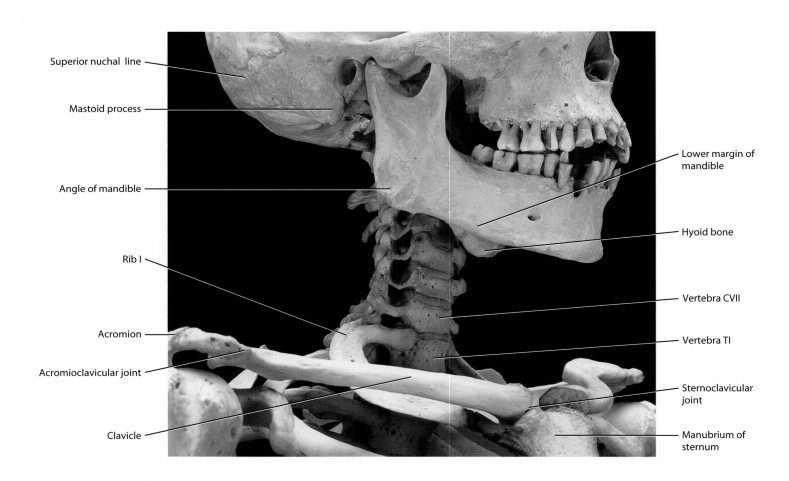

Superior nuchal line

Mastoid process

Angle of mandible

Rib I

Acromion

Acromioclavicular joint

Clavicle

Lower margin of mandible

Hyoid bone

Vertebra CVII

Vertebra TI

Sternoclavicular joint

Manubrium of sternum

Figure 12.13 Anterior triangle of the neck – osteology. Anterolateral view of the bony framework for the anterior triangle of the neck

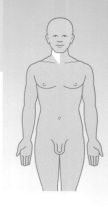

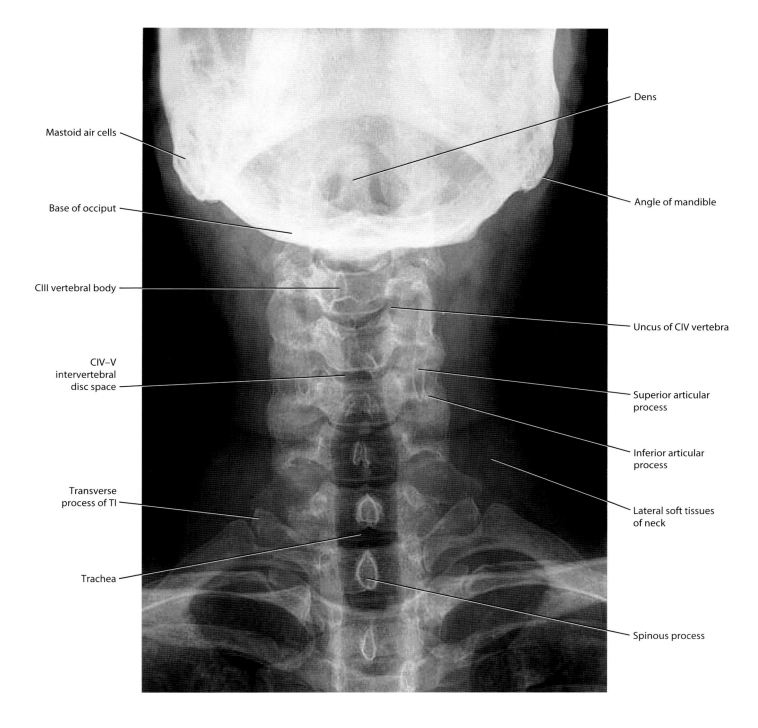

Mastoid air cells

Base of occiput

CIII vertebral body

CIV–V
intervertebral
disc space

Transverse
process of TI

Trachea

Dens

Angle of mandible

Uncus of CIV vertebra

Superior articular
process

Inferior articular
process

Lateral soft tissues
of neck

Spinous process

Figure 12.14 Anterior triangle of the neck – plain film radiograph (anteroposterior view). The trachea is visible as a darker area in the middle of this radiograph. Deviation of the trachea to one side can be observed in patients with life-threatening tension pneumothorax

141

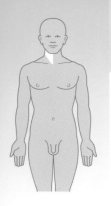

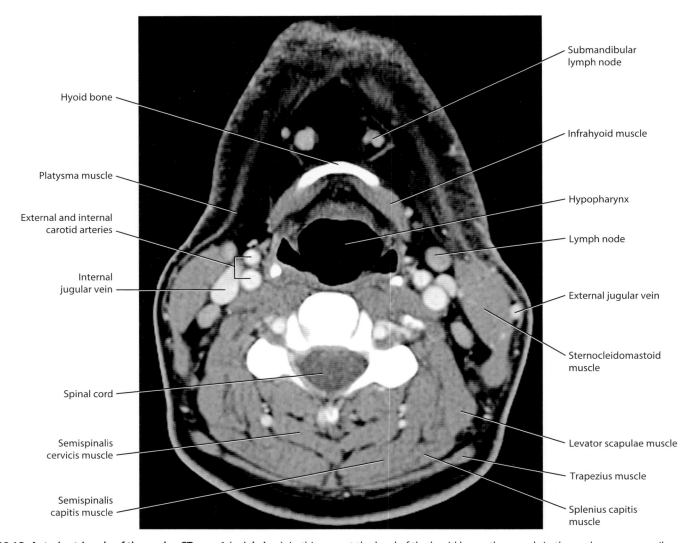

Hyoid bone

Platysma muscle

External and internal carotid arteries

Internal jugular vein

Spinal cord

Semispinalis cervicis muscle

Semispinalis capitis muscle

Submandibular lymph node

Infrahyoid muscle

Hypopharynx

Lymph node

External jugular vein

Sternocleidomastoid muscle

Levator scapulae muscle

Trapezius muscle

Splenius capitis muscle

Figure 12.15 Anterior triangle of the neck – CT scan 1 (axial view). In this scan at the level of the hyoid bone, the vessels in the neck are more easily distinguishable from lymph nodes because of the use of intravenous contrast, which enhances the vessels

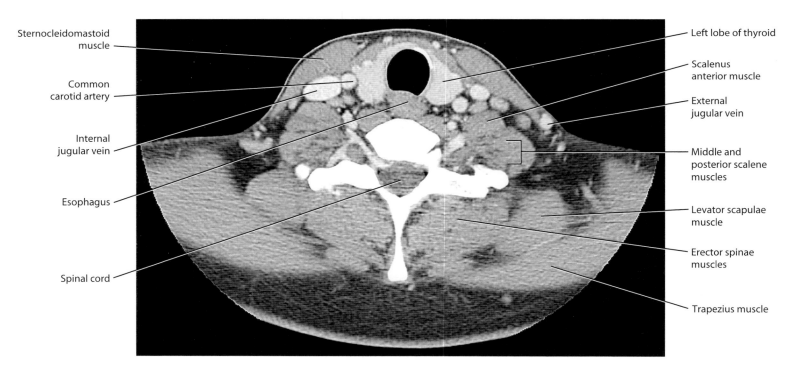

Sternocleidomastoid muscle

Common carotid artery

Internal jugular vein

Esophagus

Spinal cord

Left lobe of thyroid

Scalenus anterior muscle

External jugular vein

Middle and posterior scalene muscles

Levator scapulae muscle

Erector spinae muscles

Trapezius muscle

Figure 12.16 Anterior triangle of the neck – CT scan 2 (axial view). This scan is at the level of the thyroid gland. Observe that the esophagus is located immediately posterior to the trachea

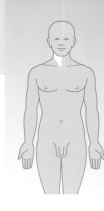

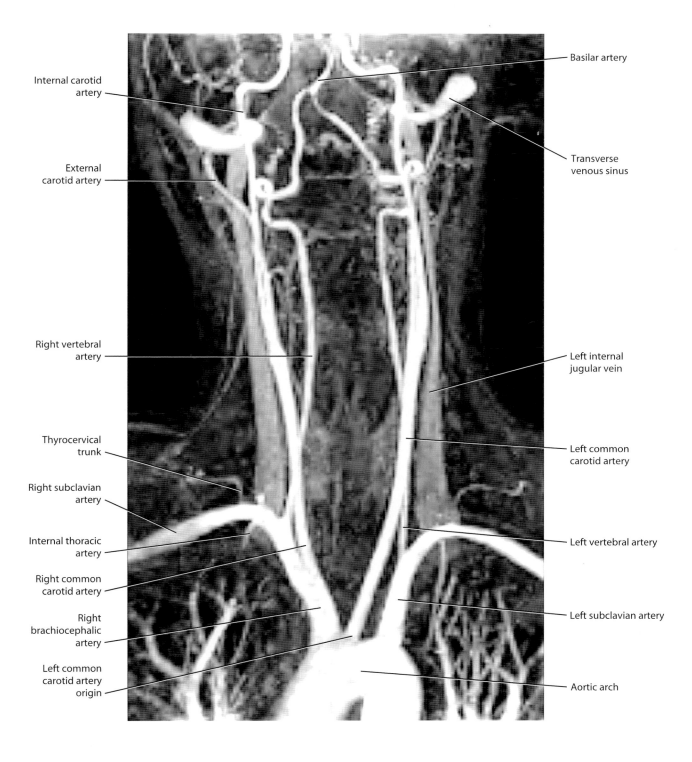

Internal carotid artery

External carotid artery

Right vertebral artery

Thyrocervical trunk

Right subclavian artery

Internal thoracic artery

Right common carotid artery

Right brachiocephalic artery

Left common carotid artery origin

Basilar artery

Transverse venous sinus

Left internal jugular vein

Left common carotid artery

Left vertebral artery

Left subclavian artery

Aortic arch

Figure 12.17 Anterior triangle of the neck – MRA scan (coronal view). Magnetic resonance angiograms (MRA) have the advantage of visualizing the veins at the same time as the arteries, whereas conventional angiography usually shows only the arteries or only the veins

13 Posterior triangle of the neck and deep neck

The posterior triangle of the neck (Fig. 13.1) is bounded by:

- the middle one-third of the clavicle inferiorly;
- the trapezius muscle posteriorly;
- the posterior border of the sternocleidomastoid muscle anteriorly.

The investing cervical fascia and the broad thin platysma muscle form the roof. The floor of the posterior triangle contains several muscles covered by prevertebral fascia. From superior to inferior these muscles are splenius capitis, levator scapulae, the middle scalene, the posterior scalene, and the first digitations of serratus anterior muscle.

The inferior belly of the omohyoid muscle crosses the inferior part of the posterior triangle, creating two minor triangles – the occipital and subclavian.

The posterior triangle contains the accessory nerve [XI] (Fig. 13.2), cutaneous nerve branches from the cervical plexus, the phrenic nerve, roots of the brachial plexus, the third part of the subclavian artery and lymph nodes. Many structures are common to both the deep neck and prevertebral regions.

The deep neck structures communicate with the thoracic cavity and upper limb (Fig. 13.3).

MUSCLES

An overview of the muscles of the deep neck and the posterior triangle is given in Table 13.1. The **sternocleidomastoid** muscle divides the neck into anterior and posterior triangles and covers the

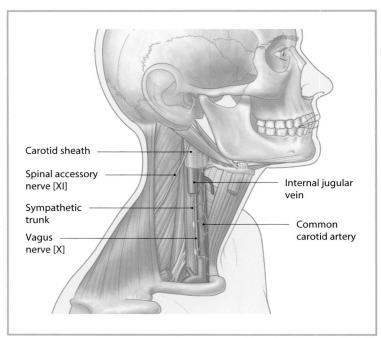

Figure 13.2 Removal of sternocleidomastoid from Fig. 13.1 reveals major vessels and nerves to and from the head

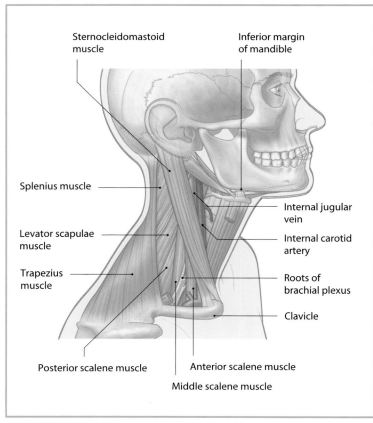

Figure 13.1 Major muscles of deep neck and posterior triangle of the neck

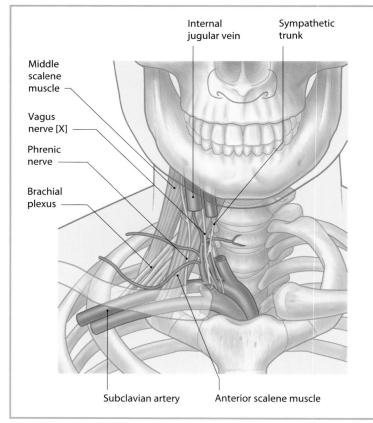

Figure 13.3 Structures of the deep neck visible at the thoracic inlet

carotid sheath and cervical plexus of nerves. It is partly covered by the platysma and the external jugular vein, and cutaneous nerves emerge from its posterior border. The sternocleidomastoid muscle flexes and rotates the head, and spasms can produce wry neck (torticollis). It is closely related to the **trapezius** muscle, which is a superficial back and neck muscle (see Chapter 28). Both sternocleidomastoid and trapezius muscles are innervated by the spinal accessory nerve [XI]. The anterior rami of cervical nerves C2 to C4 provide additional motor innervation and proprioception.

The **anterior**, **middle**, and **posterior scalene** muscles are in the deep neck and attach the cervical vertebrae to the upper two ribs. They are important because of their relationship to the brachial plexus, phrenic nerve, and subclavian vessels. Their main action is to elevate the first and second ribs during deep inspiration; they are also responsible for lateral bending of the neck. The scalene muscles are innervated by the anterior rami of cervical nerves C3 to C8.

The rest of the deep neck muscles are on the anterior surface of the cervical and thoracic vertebrae. The **longus capitis** and **longus colli** muscles arise from the transverse processes of the lower cervical vertebrae and insert into vertebra CI (the atlas) and the occipital bone. They support the natural posture of the neck, flex and rotate the head and neck, and are innervated by segmental anterior rami from cervical nerves C2 to C8 and C1 to C4, respectively.

The **rectus capitis anterior** and **rectus capitis lateralis** muscles are anterior vertebral muscles that originate from CI and insert onto the occipital bone. They are postural muscles that flex and rotate the head and are innervated by cervical nerves C1 and C2.

NERVES

The **spinal accessory nerve [XI]** enters the posterior triangle of the neck by piercing the middle portion of the sternocleidomastoid to innervate it and the trapezius muscle. It has a superficial subcutaneous course in the posterior triangle and can be damaged during surgery or trauma.

The **cervical plexus** of nerves (anterior rami of C1 to C4) is deep to the sternocleidomastoid muscle. Several cutaneous nerves arise from this plexus to innervate the regions after which they are named – the **lesser occipital**, **great auricular**, **transverse cervical**, and **supraclavicular nerves**. All emerge onto the superficial neck at the posterior border of the sternocleidomastoid.

The **phrenic nerve** (C3 to C5) arises from cervical nerves and lies on the anterior surface of the anterior scalene muscle. It enters the thoracic cavity between the subclavian artery and vein. Running anterior to the hilum of each lung, it innervates the diaphragm. Sensory fibers of the phrenic nerve are important clinically because pain originating from the diaphragmatic area is sometimes referred to the shoulder because the phrenic nerves share the same spinal levels as the supraclavicular nerves.

The roots and trunks of the brachial plexus are in the root of the neck, between the anterior and middle scalene muscles. The rest of the brachial plexus is within the axilla (see Chapter 16).

The **dorsal scapular nerve** arises from the anterior ramus of C5. It pierces and innervates the middle scalene muscle, descends deep to levator scapulae, and, finally, innervates the rhomboid muscles (see Chapter 17).

The **vagus nerves [X]** lie within the carotid sheath in the deep neck. They provide motor (via the accessory nerve [XI]) and sensory innervation to the pharynx and larynx. From the deep neck, the vagus nerves [X] enter the thorax, on both sides of the trachea, and provide parasympathetic innervation to the heart and structures of the upper gastrointestinal tract as far as the left colic flexure of the colon. In the thorax, the left and right vagus nerves [X] pass anteriorly and posteriorly to the esophagus, respectively.

ARTERIES

The blood supply to the posterior triangle of the neck and deep neck is from branches of the external carotid and subclavian arteries (Fig. 13.4). The **superior thyroid artery**, the first branch of the external carotid artery, supplies the larynx and thyroid gland. The **occipital artery** ascends through the apex of the posterior triangle to supply the posterior aspect of the scalp (see Chapter 27).

The **subclavian artery** enters the deep neck between the anterior and middle scalene muscles, and branches several times to supply the head, neck, and thorax. It divides into three groups of arteries, each with a different relationship to the anterior scalene muscle:

- the **vertebral** and **internal thoracic arteries**, and **thyrocervical trunk** are medial to the the anterior scalene;
- the **costocervical** trunk is posterior to it;
- the **dorsal scapular artery** is lateral to the anterior scalene.

The vertebral artery also arises from the subclavian artery and ascends within the transverse foramina of the cervical vertebrae to segmentally supply the neck, the brain, and intracranial structures.

The internal thoracic artery descends into the chest and supplies the breast and anterior chest wall.

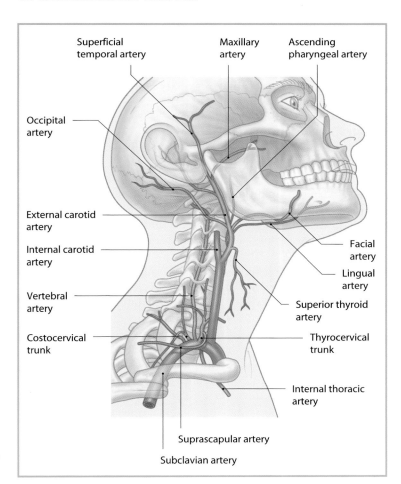

Labels: Superficial temporal artery, Maxillary artery, Ascending pharyngeal artery, Occipital artery, External carotid artery, Internal carotid artery, Vertebral artery, Costocervical trunk, Facial artery, Lingual artery, Superior thyroid artery, Thyrocervical trunk, Internal thoracic artery, Suprascapular artery, Subclavian artery

Figure 13.4 Arteries of the deep neck and posterior triangle

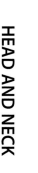

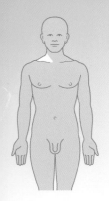

The third branch of the subclavian artery is the thyrocervical trunk, which itself has three branches named after the areas they supply – the **suprascapular**, **transverse cervical**, and **inferior thyroid** arteries. The suprascapular and transverse cervical arteries travel through the deep neck and supply structures in the posterior neck and shoulder region. The inferior thyroid artery and its main branch (the **ascending cervical artery**) run superiorly in the neck to supply the thyroid glands, parathyroid glands, cervical vertebrae, and spinal cord.

The costocervical trunk has two branches – the **deep cervical** and **superior intercostal arteries** – which supply the deep neck muscles and the upper posterior chest wall. The **dorsal scapular artery** is usually the last branch off the subclavian artery and its origin is variable. It contributes to the arterial anastomoses around the scapula (see Chapter 17).

VEINS AND LYMPHATICS

Venous drainage of the posterior triangle of the neck begins superiorly with the **external jugular vein**. Formed by the union of the **posterior retromandibular vein** and **posterior auricular vein**, the external jugular vein descends superficially to the sternocleidomastoid muscle to drain into the **subclavian vein**.

The **suprascapular**, **transverse cervical**, and **anterior jugular veins** empty into the external jugular vein.

The subclavian vein is anterior to the anterior scalene muscle, and provides venous drainage for the upper limb and neck. The subclavian and internal jugular veins join in the deep neck to form the **brachiocephalic vein**.

Lymphatic drainage of the posterior triangle of the neck is to the groups of deep cervical nodes along the carotid sheath. The lymphatic vessels follow the course of the arteries and small unnamed veins in the neck. Lymphatic drainage of the deep neck structures is to the **mediastinal** or **axillary nodes**.

■ CLINICAL CORRELATIONS

Penetrating neck trauma

For penetrating trauma to the neck, surgeons divide the neck into three zones (Fig. 13.5):

- zone I extends from the jugular (suprasternal) notch to the cricoid cartilage;
- zone II extends from the cricoid cartilage to the angle of mandible;
- zone III extends from the angle of mandible up to the head.

Initial management of patients with penetrating injuries to the neck, such as stab or bullet wounds, is to establish and maintain a stable airway. Sometimes this requires endotracheal intubation. After this, most surgeons take patients with zone II injuries directly to the operating room for surgical exploration; patients with zone I or zone III injuries are sent to the radiology department for an angiogram of the neck vessels. The four major vessels to the neck (left and right common carotid and left and right vertebral arteries) and major branches of the aorta must be visualized to exclude major vessel damage. Many surgeons believe that any neck injury penetrating the platysma muscle warrants surgical exploration.

Thoracic outlet syndrome

Thoracic outlet syndrome is a collection of signs and symptoms caused by compression of the neurovascular bundle that emerges from the mediastinum at the level of rib I (subclavian arteries,

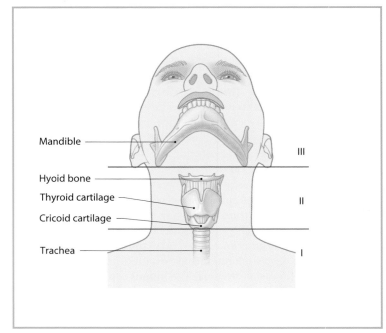

Figure 13.5 Surgical zones of the neck for evaluating penetrating neck trauma

subclavian veins, and roots of brachial plexus). It can be caused by congenital abnormalities, such as a cervical rib, or by trauma (clavicular fracture or fracture of rib I).

Most patients with thoracic outlet syndrome present with brachial plexus compression symptoms, usually of the ulnar nerve, complaining of paresthesiae of the neck, shoulder, arm, and hand. Weakness or coolness of the involved extremity is also common. On examination, the involved limb has a weak radial pulse and a lower blood pressure than the uninvolved limb. There may also be edema or atrophy of muscles and soft tissues on the affected side. Tinel's test – tapping the supraclavicular fossa of the affected limb – is positive if it initiates paresthesia in the limb.

Treatment of thoracic outlet syndrome is primarily nonsurgical and involves physical therapy to improve mobility and posture. If this is not successful, surgery will be required to remove the cervical rib (if present) or repair a fracture (if necessary).

Placement of a central line (venous catheter)

Patients who have had major trauma and some who require close monitoring may need a central line. Occasionally, a central line is placed when intravenous access cannot be obtained using a peripheral intravenous line.

Central line placement is commonly carried out through the subclavian vein. First, a syringe with a large-bore needle is placed into anesthetized skin, usually inferior to the middle of the clavicle. Dark venous blood flows into the syringe on accessing the subclavian vein. Using the Seldinger technique, a large-bore intravenous catheter is then placed into the subclavian vein over a guide-wire. The tip of the catheter is placed at the level of the superior vena cava.

Chest radiography is carried out after placement to make sure that the central line is well positioned and to rule out a pneumothorax (see Chapter 31). The latter may occur because the upper part of the lung is close to the ideal position for a central line and therefore it is sometimes injured during the placement. Central line placement should only be carried out by a trained professional.

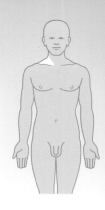

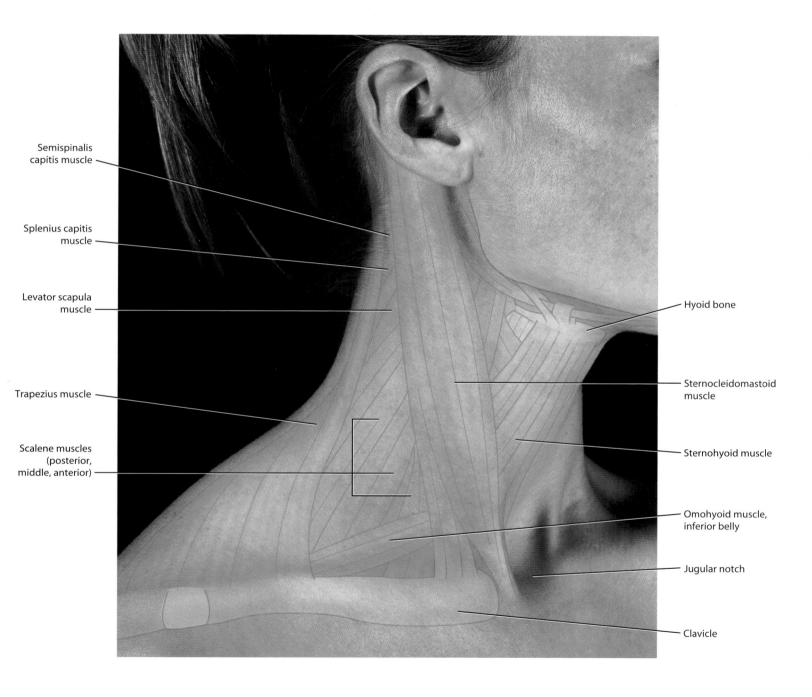

Semispinalis
capitis muscle

Splenius capitis
muscle

Levator scapula
muscle

Trapezius muscle

Scalene muscles
(posterior,
middle, anterior)

Hyoid bone

Sternocleidomastoid
muscle

Sternohyoid muscle

Omohyoid muscle,
inferior belly

Jugular notch

Clavicle

Figure 13.6 Posterior neck – surface anatomy. Observe how the sternocleidomastoid muscle divides the neck into anterior and posterior triangles

147

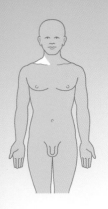

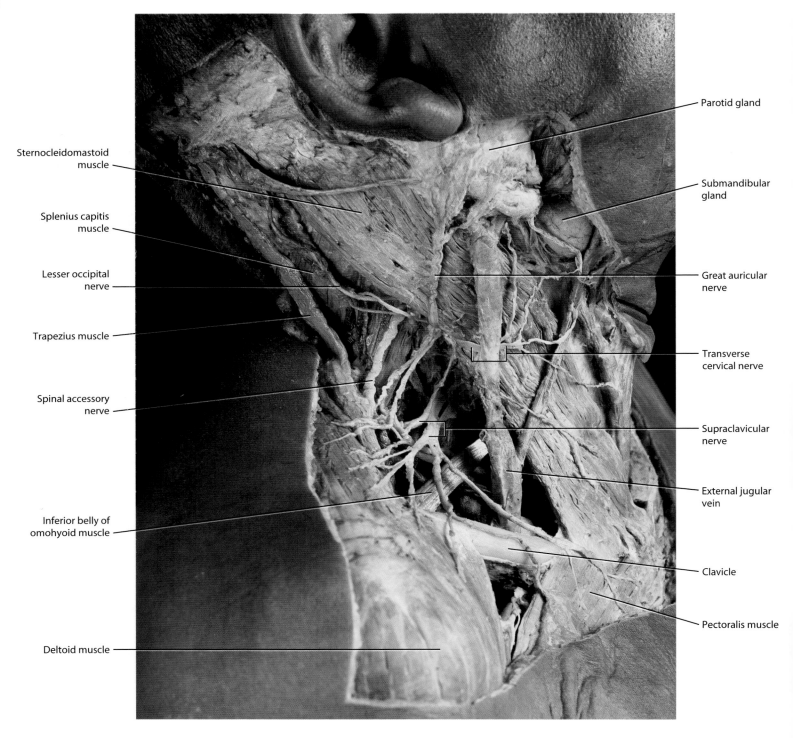

Parotid gland

Submandibular gland

Sternocleidomastoid muscle

Splenius capitis muscle

Lesser occipital nerve

Trapezius muscle

Spinal accessory nerve

Inferior belly of omohyoid muscle

Deltoid muscle

Great auricular nerve

Transverse cervical nerve

Supraclavicular nerve

External jugular vein

Clavicle

Pectoralis muscle

Figure 13.7 Posterior triangle of the neck – superficial dissection. This photograph was taken using special lighting techniques to enhance the three-dimensional perspective of the location of the omohyoid muscle and its relationships to the nerves and other structures

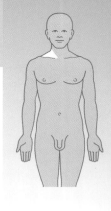

TABLE 13.1 MUSCLES OF THE POSTERIOR TRIANGLE OF THE NECK					
Muscle	Origin	Insertion	Innervation	Action	Blood supply
Anterior scalene	Anterior tubercles of transverse processes of CIII to CVI	Scalene tubercle upper surface of rib I	Anterior rami C5 to C8	Elevates rib I, flexes and rotates vertebral column	Ascending cervical branch of inferior thyroid artery
Middle scalene	Posterior tubercles of transverse processes of CII to CVII	Upper surface of rib I behind subclavian groove	Anterior rami C3, C4	Elevates rib I; together, flexes neck; individually flexes cervical column laterally	Muscular branches of ascending cervical artery
Posterior scalene	Posterior tubercles of transverse processes of CIV to CVI	Superior aspect of rib II	Anterior rami C5 to C8	Elevates rib II; together, flex neck; individually flexes cervical column laterally	Ascending cervical of thyrocervical trunk; superficial branch of transverse cervical
Levator scapulae	Transverse processes of CI to CIV	Superior aspect of vertebral border of scapula	Dorsal scapular nerve C3, C4	Elevate and rotate scapulae	Dorsal scapular artery
Splenius capitis	Ligamentum nuchae, lower cervical spinous processes	Superior nuchal line and mastoid process	Posterior rami C7, C8	Together extend and laterally flex the head and neck and slightly rotate the head	Occipital and transverse cervical arteries
Semispinalis capitis	Transverse processes CVII, TI to TVI	Occipital bones between superior and inferior nuchal lines	Posterior rami C1 to C6	Extension and lateral flexion of column; extension of head	Posterior intercostal arteries, occipital artery, costocervical trunk
Omohyoid	Inferior belly: upper border of scapula and suprascapular ligament	Intermediate tendon			
	Superior belly: intermediate tendon	Lower border of body of hyoid bone	C1 to C3	Stabilizes hyoid bone, depresses and retracts hyoid and larynx	Lingual and superior thyroid arteries
Serratus anterior	Lateral surfaces of upper 8 ribs	Anterior aspect of medial border of scapula	Long thoracic nerve C5 to C7	Rotates, protracts, and holds scapula against thoracic wall	Scapular anastomosis
Longus colli	Vertical part vertebral bodies, CV to CVII and TI to TIII	Vertebral bodies	C2 to C4		
	Inferior oblique part bodies of TI to TIII	Anterior tubercle transverse processes CV and CVI	C2 to C8	Flexes and rotates neck and head, flexes column laterally	Ascending pharyngeal, ascending cervical and vertebral arteries
	Superior oblique part anterior tubercles of transverse processes CIII to CV	Anterior tubercle of atlas			
Longus capitis	Anterior tubercles of transverse processes CIII to CVI	External, inferior surface of basilar part occipital bone	C1 to C4	Flexes and rotates neck and head	Inferior thyroid, ascending pharyngeal, and vertebral arteries
Rectus capitis anterior	Atlas	Base of occipital bone anterior to foramen magnum	C1 to C2	Flexes and rotates the head	Vertebral and ascending pharyngeal arteries
Rectus capitis lateralis	Transverse process of atlas	Jugular process of occipital bone	C1 to C2	Flexes head laterally	Vertebral, occipital, and ascending pharyngeal arteries

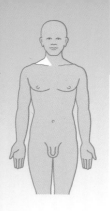

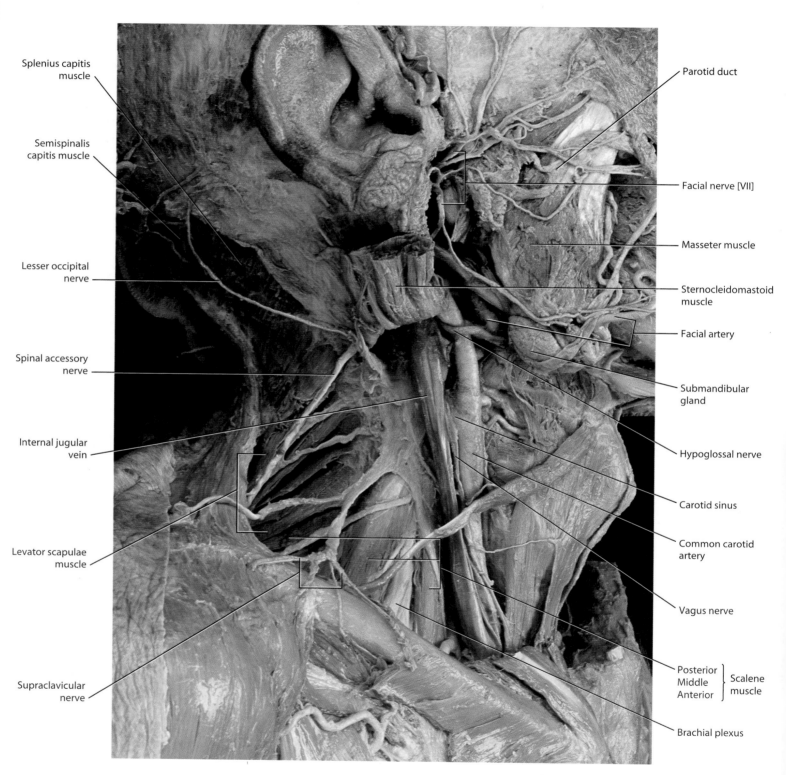

Splenius capitis muscle

Semispinalis capitis muscle

Lesser occipital nerve

Spinal accessory nerve

Internal jugular vein

Levator scapulae muscle

Supraclavicular nerve

Parotid duct

Facial nerve [VII]

Masseter muscle

Sternocleidomastoid muscle

Facial artery

Submandibular gland

Hypoglossal nerve

Carotid sinus

Common carotid artery

Vagus nerve

Posterior
Middle   Scalene
Anterior muscle

Brachial plexus

Figure 13.8 Posterior triangle of neck – intermediate dissection 1. In this lateral view the sternocleidomastoid muscle has been cut and reflected to show the carotid artery, internal jugular vein, and vagus nerve [X]

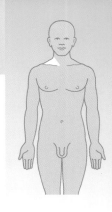

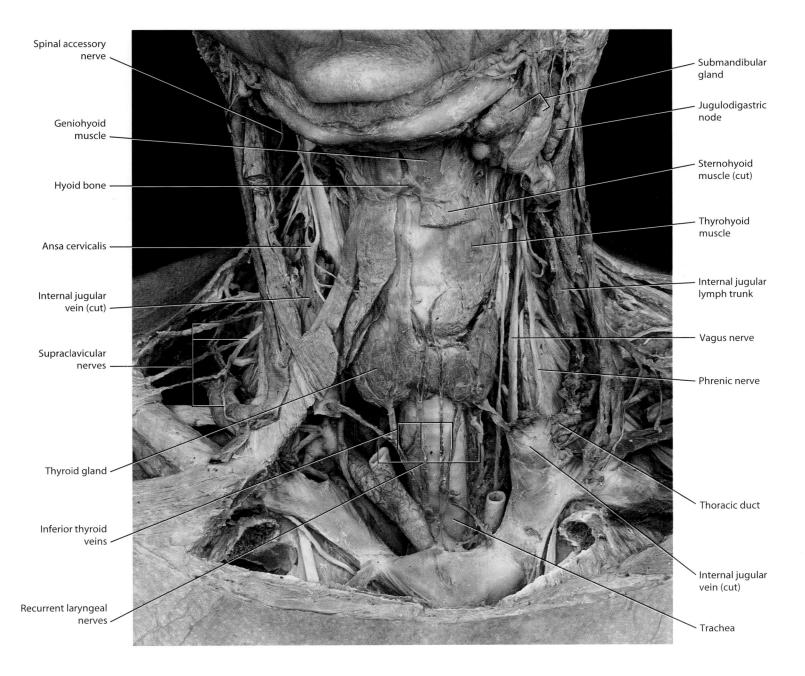

Spinal accessory nerve

Geniohyoid muscle

Hyoid bone

Ansa cervicalis

Internal jugular vein (cut)

Supraclavicular nerves

Thyroid gland

Inferior thyroid veins

Recurrent laryngeal nerves

Submandibular gland

Jugulodigastric node

Sternohyoid muscle (cut)

Thyrohyoid muscle

Internal jugular lymph trunk

Vagus nerve

Phrenic nerve

Thoracic duct

Internal jugular vein (cut)

Trachea

HEAD AND NECK Posterior triangle of the neck and deep neck

Figure 13.9 Posterior triangle of the neck – intermediate dissection 2. The infrahyoid muscles have been removed to show the thyroid cartilage, thyroid gland, and trachea

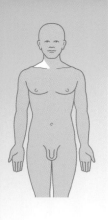

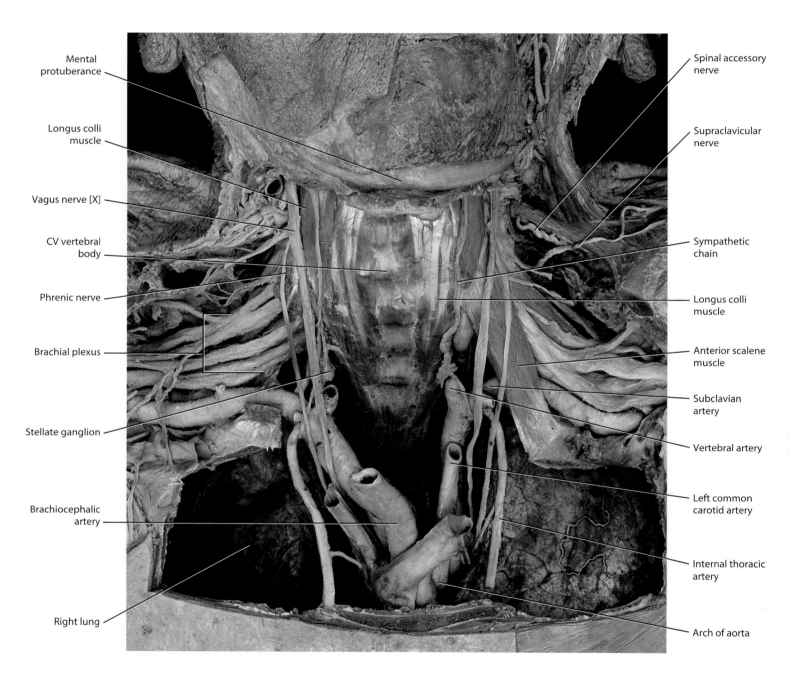

Mental protuberance

Longus colli muscle

Vagus nerve [X]

CV vertebral body

Phrenic nerve

Brachial plexus

Stellate ganglion

Brachiocephalic artery

Right lung

Spinal accessory nerve

Supraclavicular nerve

Sympathetic chain

Longus colli muscle

Anterior scalene muscle

Subclavian artery

Vertebral artery

Left common carotid artery

Internal thoracic artery

Arch of aorta

Figure 13.10 Deep neck – intermediate dissection 1. An anterior view of the prevertebral muscles. The trachea and thyroid gland have been removed to show the prevertebral muscles as well as the upper part of the sternum and medial part of the clavicles. The lungs and their relationship to the region are easily appreciated

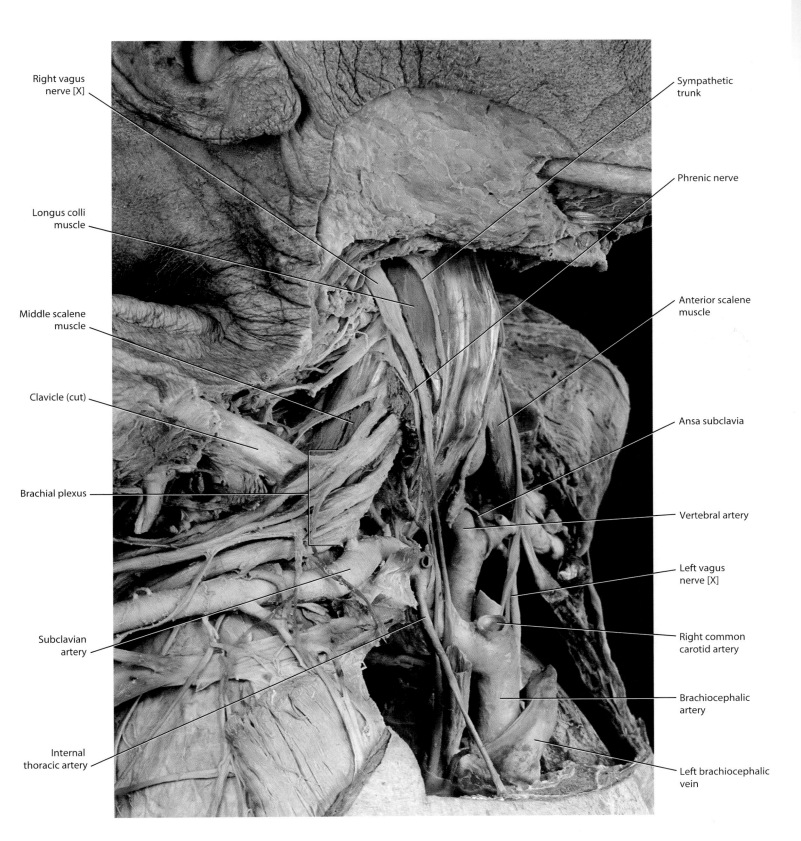

Right vagus
nerve [X]

Longus colli
muscle

Middle scalene
muscle

Clavicle (cut)

Brachial plexus

Subclavian
artery

Internal
thoracic artery

Sympathetic
trunk

Phrenic nerve

Anterior scalene
muscle

Ansa subclavia

Vertebral artery

Left vagus
nerve [X]

Right common
carotid artery

Brachiocephalic
artery

Left brachiocephalic
vein

Figure 13.11 Deep neck – intermediate dissection 2. This is a lateral view of Figure 13.10 to aid understanding of the location of the prevertebral muscles and how they are related to the lower jaw and the upper mediastinum

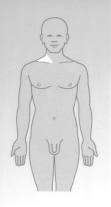

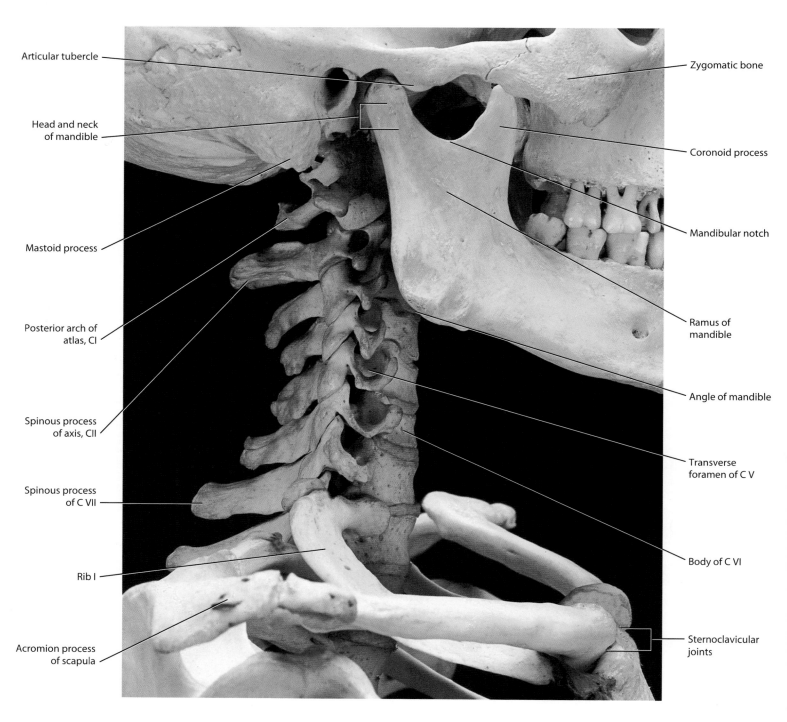

Articular tubercle

Head and neck of mandible

Mastoid process

Posterior arch of atlas, CI

Spinous process of axis, CII

Spinous process of C VII

Rib I

Acromion process of scapula

Zygomatic bone

Coronoid process

Mandibular notch

Ramus of mandible

Angle of mandible

Transverse foramen of C V

Body of C VI

Sternoclavicular joints

Figure 13.12 Posterior neck – osteology – articulated skeleton. Lateral view of the right side of the head and neck bones shows the relationships of the skull to the cervical spine and upper ribs and clavicle

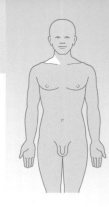

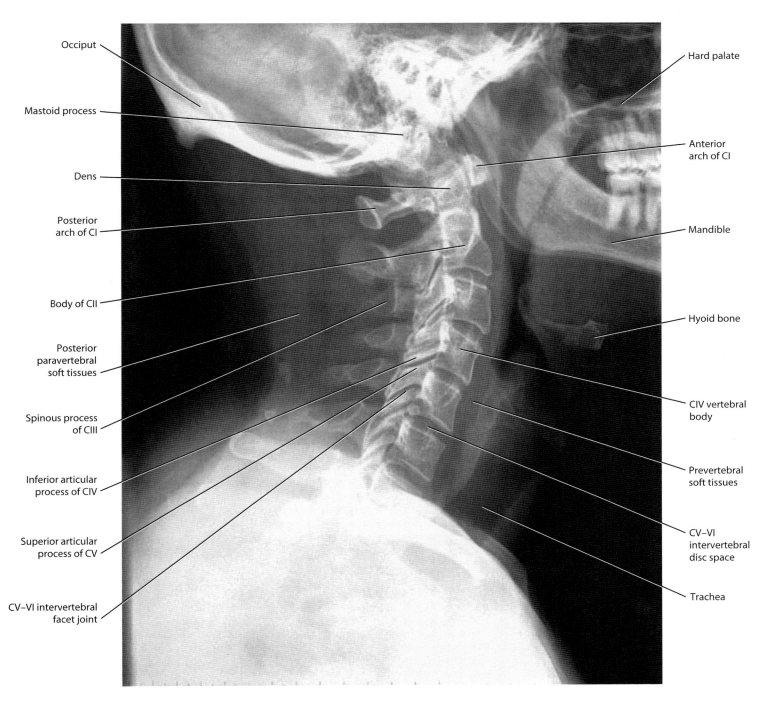

Occiput

Mastoid process

Dens

Posterior arch of CI

Body of CII

Posterior paravertebral soft tissues

Spinous process of CIII

Inferior articular process of CIV

Superior articular process of CV

CV–VI intervertebral facet joint

Hard palate

Anterior arch of CI

Mandible

Hyoid bone

CIV vertebral body

Prevertebral soft tissues

CV–VI intervertebral disc space

Trachea

Figure 13.13 Posterior triangle of the neck – plain film radiograph (lateral view). The prevertebral soft tissues include the prevertebral longus colli muscles of the deep neck. Note the location of the hyoid bone, inferior to the mandible

155

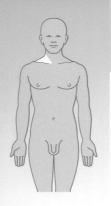

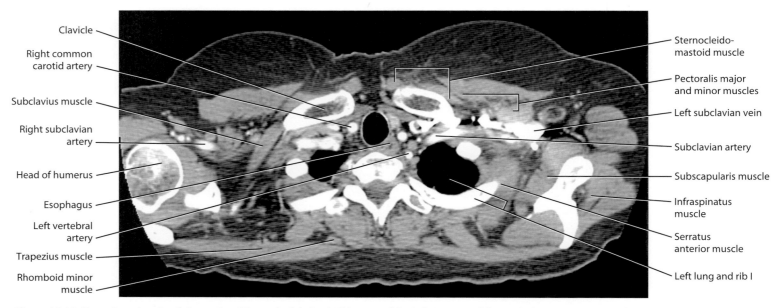

Clavicle
Right common carotid artery
Subclavius muscle
Right subclavian artery
Head of humerus
Esophagus
Left vertebral artery
Trapezius muscle
Rhomboid minor muscle

Sternocleido-mastoid muscle
Pectoralis major and minor muscles
Left subclavian vein
Subclavian artery
Subscapularis muscle
Infraspinatus muscle
Serratus anterior muscle
Left lung and rib I

Figure 13.14 Posterior triangle of the neck – CT scan (axial view). This scan of the inferior part of the neck shows upper parts of the lungs. Observe how the clavicle, rib I, and first thoracic vertebrae protect the carotid and vertebral arteries

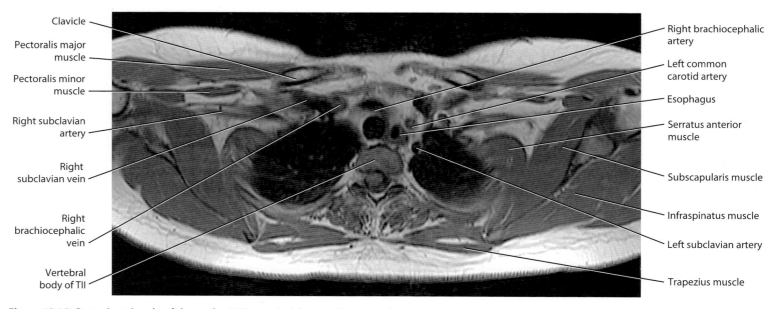

Clavicle
Pectoralis major muscle
Pectoralis minor muscle
Right subclavian artery
Right subclavian vein
Right brachiocephalic vein
Vertebral body of TII

Right brachiocephalic artery
Left common carotid artery
Esophagus
Serratus anterior muscle
Subscapularis muscle
Infraspinatus muscle
Left subclavian artery
Trapezius muscle

Figure 13.15 Posterior triangle of the neck – MRI scan (axial view). This scan of the lower neck demonstrates the major vessels that pass to and from the heart anterior to the vertebral body of TII

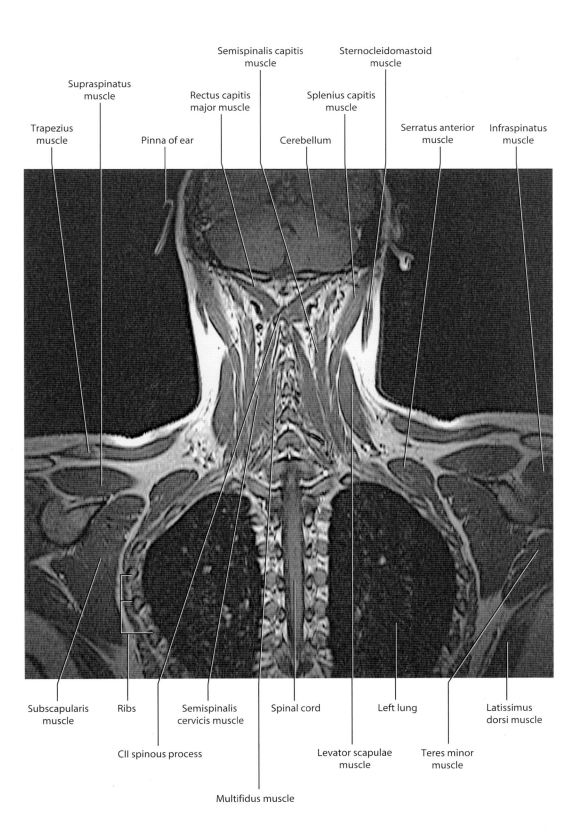

Semispinalis capitis muscle

Sternocleidomastoid muscle

Supraspinatus muscle

Rectus capitis major muscle

Splenius capitis muscle

Trapezius muscle

Pinna of ear

Cerebellum

Serratus anterior muscle

Infraspinatus muscle

Subscapularis muscle

Ribs

Semispinalis cervicis muscle

Spinal cord

Left lung

Latissimus dorsi muscle

CII spinous process

Levator scapulae muscle

Teres minor muscle

Multifidus muscle

Figure 13.16 Posterior triangle of the neck – CT scan (coronal view). This scan demonstrates the muscles that support the neck. Whiplash injuries due to hyperextension of the neck can damage muscles in this region

157

Introduction to the upper limb

The upper limb is attached to the **pectoral girdle** (shoulder girdle), which comprises the **scapula** and **clavicle** articulating at the **acromioclavicular joint**. The only bony point of contact between the upper limb and the pectoral girdle and chest is at the **sternoclavicular joint**. All other attachments to the upper limb and pectoral girdle are muscular.

The **axilla** (armpit) is a fat-filled, pyramid-shaped region between the chest wall and upper limb. It contains the **brachial plexus**, **axillary artery** and **vein**, and **lymph nodes**, and acts as a funnel for neurovascular structures to pass to and from the neck region. The rest of the upper limb is segmented into the **arm**, between the shoulder and the elbow, the **forearm**, from the elbow to the wrist, and and the **hand**, which joins the forearm at the wrist.

The upper limb is highly mobile and capable of a wide range of controlled movements. The hand is a highly mobile and refined grasping and sense organ.

The upper limb is supported by the long bones – the **humerus**, **radius**, and **ulna**. The humerus supports the arm, and the radius and ulna support the forearm (Fig. 14.1). Smaller bones provide additional support and are:

- the **carpal bones** (the wrist bones – the scaphoid, lunate, triquetrum, pisiform, trapezium, trapezoid, capitate, hamate);
- **metacarpals** (palm bones – of which there are five [I to V]);
- the fourteen **phalanges** (two in the thumb, three in each finger).

MUSCLES

The deep fascia of the upper limb provides a supportive investment for the upper limb and, by intermuscular septa and interosseous membranes, divides the various segments of the upper limb into anatomical anterior and posterior compartments. These compartments contain muscles, which mainly act synergistically to carry out specific functions, and nerves and vessels, which supply the contents. The muscles of the anterior compartments are primarily flexors; those of the posterior compartments are extensors.

NERVES

The nerve supply to the upper limb is derived from the brachial plexus (Fig. 14.2). The five major branches of the brachial plexus are the **musculocutaneous**, **median**, **ulnar**, **axillary**, and **radial nerves** (see Chapter 16):

- the musculocutaneous, median, and ulnar nerves supply the anterior flexor compartments of the arm and forearm;
- the posterior extensor compartments of the arm and forearm are supplied by the radial nerve;
- the axillary nerve supplies the deltoid and teres minor muscles, and the skin over the lower part of the deltoid muscle (Fig. 14.3).

In the hand, the thenar (thumb) muscles, the first two lumbricals, the skin of the lateral half of the palm, and the palmar surface of the lateral three and one-half digits are supplied by the median nerve.

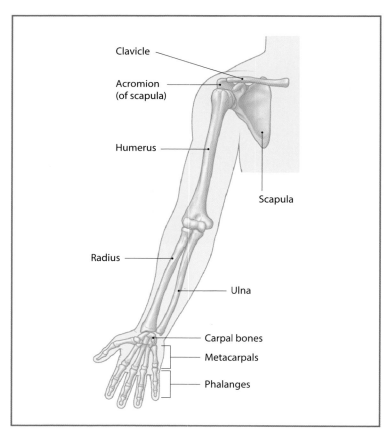

Figure 14.1 Bones of the upper limb

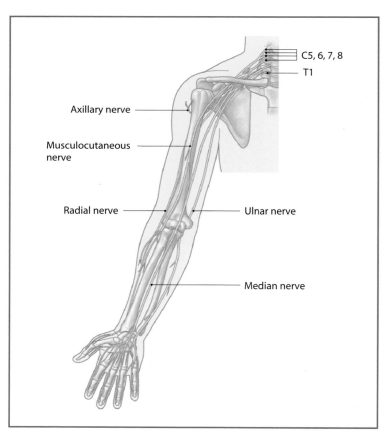

Figure 14.2 Major nerves of the upper limb

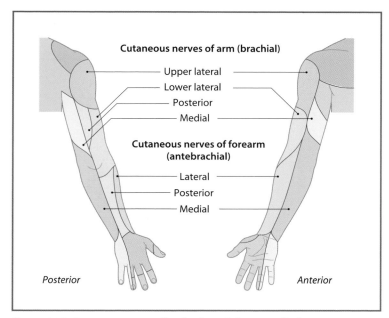

Figure 14.3 Cutaneous nerve distribution of the upper limb

The hypothenar (little finger) muscles, adductor pollicis, third and fourth lumbricals, interossei, palmaris brevis, skin of the medial half of the dorsum and palm of the hand, and of the medial one and one-half digits are supplied by the ulnar nerve.

ARTERIES

The axillary artery supplies blood to the upper limb (Fig. 14.4). It has several branches:

- **superior thoracic artery** (to the upper chest and ribs);
- **thoraco-acromial artery** (to the shoulder and pectoral regions);
- **lateral thoracic artery** (to the breast and lateral chest);
- **subscapular artery** (to the scapular region);
- **posterior circumflex humeral artery** (to upper arm and glenohumeral joint);
- **anterior circumflex humeral artery** (to upper arm and shoulder and glenohumeral joint).

At the lower border of teres major muscle, the axillary artery changes its name to become the **brachial artery**, which continues down the arm, and gives off branches to the anterior and posterior arm and the elbow joint. Just distal to the elbow joint, at the neck of the radius, the brachial artery divides into the **radial** and **ulnar arteries**, which follow the bones after which they are named and supply the lateral (radial) and medial (ulnar) parts of the forearm, respectively.

In the hand, the radial artery terminates by forming the **deep palmar arch**, which gives off a branch for each digit (finger). The ulnar artery contributes primarily to the **superficial palmar arch** superficial to the flexor tendons.

VEINS

The deep veins of the upper limb follow the arteries and flow superiorly toward the axilla. In the axilla, the **axillary vein** travels

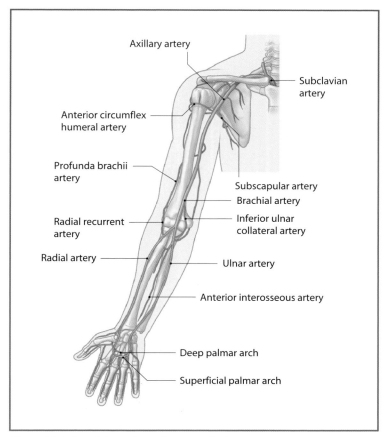

Figure 14.4 Arterial supply to the upper limb

superiorly, becoming the **subclavian vein** at the lateral border of rib I. The subclavian vein continues toward the root of the neck, where it merges with the **internal jugular vein** to form the **brachiocephalic vein**. The right and left brachiocephalic veins merge in the **superior mediastinum** (upper chest) to form the **superior vena cava**, which drains deoxygenated blood into the heart.

Superficial venous drainage of the upper limb originates at the **dorsal venous network** of the hand. The lateral limb of the dorsal venous arch forms the **cephalic vein**, which runs along the upper margin of the upper limb, receiving blood from superficial veins and transporting this blood to the axillary vein, which it joins after passing through the deltopectoral triangle. The medial limb of the dorsal venous network forms the **basilic vein**, which ascends along the medial aspect of the upper limb and empties into the axillary vein within the axilla. Anterior to the elbow, the cephalic vein connects with the basilic vein by way of the median cubital vein.

LYMPHATICS

Lymphatic drainage of the upper limb follows unnamed lymphatic vessels that originate in the hand. Superficial lymphatic drainage follows the superficial veins. Deep lymphatic drainage follows the deep arteries (radial, ulnar, and brachial) and passes superiorly to the axilla. When it reaches the cubital fossa, lymph passes through the **cubital nodes**. From here, lymph vessels run superiorly to the **axillary lymph nodes**. Flow from the axilla is to the **subclavian trunk**, which joins the brachial veins to form the axillary vein.

15 Breast and pectoral region

The breast and pectoral region is on the anterior and superior part of the thorax (chest). In addition to containing muscles and fascia that assist movement of the upper limb, this region also contains the **mammary glands**, which secrete milk (Fig. 15.1). Structural support for the pectoral muscles and the mammary glands is primarily the upper eight ribs along with their attachment to the lateral sternum by way of costal cartilages. The four pectoral muscles listed below all insert either on the clavicle or scapula or on the proximal humerus.

MUSCLES

The upper limb is connected to the chest by the sternoclavicular joint (see Chapter 18), with the pectoral muscles providing muscular attachment to the anterior torso (Fig. 15.2).

The largest muscle (Table 15.1) in the breast and pectoral region is the **pectoralis major** muscle, which is a fan-shaped muscle originating from the anterior chest wall, sternum, and clavicle. Its large **sternocostal head** joins with the smaller **clavicular head** to insert onto the anterior superior humerus (crest of greater tubercle). It adducts, flexes, and medially rotates the arm.

The **pectoralis minor** muscle lies deep to the pectoralis major and covers the second part of the axillary artery and the cords of the brachial plexus. It originates from the chest wall and inserts onto the coracoid process of the scapula, and stabilizes the scapula by pulling it inferiorly and anteriorly. The **subclavius** muscle is small, rounded, and inferior to the clavicle. It joins the inferior surface of the clavicle to rib I and pulls the clavicle inferiorly and anteriorly.

The **serratus anterior** muscle is a thin muscular sheet overlying the lateral part of the thoracic cage and intercostal muscles. It arises from the upper eight ribs and wraps around the rib cage to insert along the entire medial border of the anterior scapula. It becomes the major protractor for the upper limb ('boxer's muscle').

NERVES

Sensory (cutaneous) innervation of the superior pectoral region is by the **supraclavicular nerves** (C3, C4); the inferior pectoral region is supplied by the anterior and lateral pectoral cutaneous branches of the third to sixth **intercostal nerves**.

Motor innervation to the pectoralis major and minor muscles is by the **medial** and **lateral pectoral nerves**, which are branches of the medial and lateral cords of the brachial plexus. The medial pectoral nerve (C7 to T1) arises from the brachial plexus and pierces the pectoralis minor muscle, supplying both it and the overlying pectoralis major muscle. The lateral pectoral nerve (C5, C7) runs medially from the lateral cord of the brachial plexus and innervates the pectoralis major muscle.

The **subclavian nerve** (C5) originates from the superior trunk of the brachial plexus and passes medially to enter the superior posterior part of the subclavius muscle.

The serratus anterior muscle is innervated by the **long thoracic nerve** (C5 to C7). Its three roots arise from the back of the anterior rami.

ARTERIES

Blood supply to the medial part of the pectoral region (Fig. 15.3) is by the **internal thoracic artery**, which branches from the inferior surface of the subclavian artery and runs along the internal surface

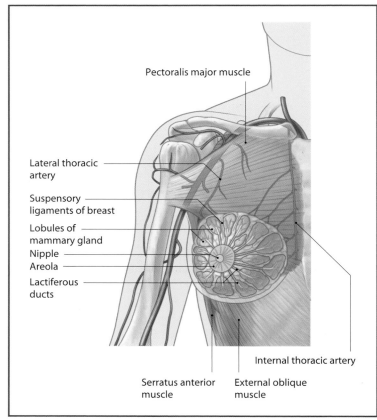

Figure 15.1 Female breast (anterior view)

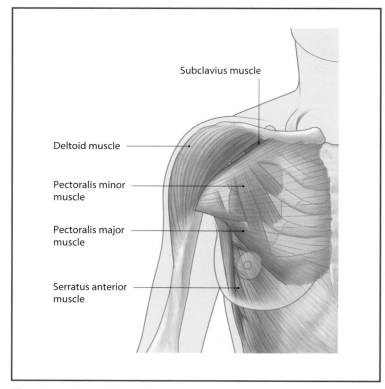

Figure 15.2 Pectoral muscles

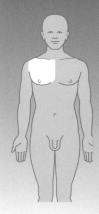

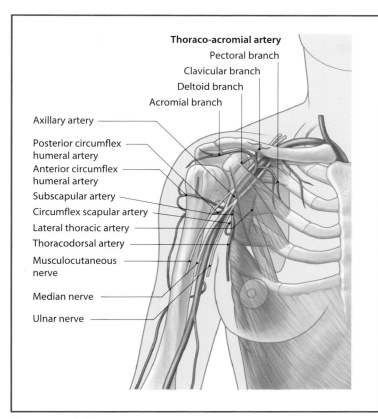

Thoraco-acromial artery
Pectoral branch
Clavicular branch
Deltoid branch
Acromial branch

Axillary artery

Posterior circumflex
humeral artery
Anterior circumflex
humeral artery
Subscapular artery
Circumflex scapular artery
Lateral thoracic artery
Thoracodorsal artery
Musculocutaneous
nerve
Median nerve
Ulnar nerve

Figure 15.3 Axillary artery

of the rib cage toward the anterior abdominal wall muscles, giving off numerous branches. These branches perforate the spaces between the ribs to supply the pectoral muscles and breast.

The lateral part of the pectoral region receives blood from the **thoraco-acromial** and **lateral thoracic** branches of the axillary artery. The thoraco-acromial artery branches four times to form the **acromial**, **deltoid**, **clavicular**, and **pectoral** branches, which are named after the regions they supply.

The lateral thoracic artery branches off the axillary artery just after the thoraco-acromial artery and descends along the lateral border of pectoralis minor muscle to supply it and the serratus anterior muscle. The lateral thoracic artery is also the principal blood supply to the breast.

VEINS

Unnamed vessels empty into the **internal thoracic** and **lateral thoracic veins** and provide superficial venous drainage of the pectoral region. One unique vein from the upper limb, the **cephalic vein**, enters the pectoral region in the deltopectoral triangle and passes deep, just inferior to the clavicle, to enter the axillary vein. The deep venous drainage is along vessels that share the same name as the arteries. The internal thoracic vein empties into the subclavian vein and the lateral thoracic vein drains to the axillary vein.

BREAST

The mammary gland is a modified sweat gland embedded in the superficial fascia of the anterior chest. It overlies the pectoralis muscles. Its superior boundary is usually at the level of rib II, and its inferior boundary is level with rib VI on the anterior chest wall. The lateral aspect of the sternum forms the medial boundary of the breast and the midaxillary line is the lateral boundary. The breast usually contains an extension directed superiorly towards the axilla – the **axillary process** (axillary tail or tail of Spence). This creates a teardrop shape and it is important clinically because it can contain abnormal breast masses.

The breast is in a fascial compartment anterior to the pectoralis muscles and deep to the skin and subcutaneous tissue. Posterior to the breast is the **retromammary space**, which allows movement of the breast on the chest wall. Fascia of the breast form suspensory ligaments oriented in a radial (asterisk-shaped) fashion. These divide the breast into eight to ten lobes, each of which is drained by its own **lactiferous duct**, which in turn drains toward the **areola** (the circular pigmented area on the apex of the breast). Milk is produced during pregnancy and during breastfeeding in the lactiferous lobes, and is then secreted onto the areola via the lactiferous ducts.

The suspensory ligaments (Cooper's ligaments) of the superior breast are usually well developed and support the weight of the breast, while inferiorly, support is provided by a fibrous rim (the inframammary ridge).

The breast is innervated by the intercostal nerves (T2 to T7); the intercostal nerve T4 innervates the nipple.

Blood is supplied to the breast by **anterior intercostal branches** of the **internal thoracic artery**, the **lateral thoracic artery**, and arterial branches of the **thoraco-acromial artery**. The inferior part of the breast also receives a blood supply from the **superior epigastric artery** (on the anterolateral abdominal wall). Venous drainage of the breast is in veins corresponding with the arteries. The **internal thoracic vein** empties into the subclavian vein whereas the **lateral thoracic** and **thoraco-acromial veins** empty into the axillary vein.

Lymphatic drainage of the breast is important clinically because cancer can spread through the lymphatic channels (Fig. 15.4). Lymph drains as follows:

- superiorly to the **supraclavicular** and **inferior deep nodes** (of the neck);
- laterally, to the **axillary lymph nodes**;
- medially, to the **parasternal** and **mediastinal nodes** within the chest; inferiorly, to the skin of the anterior abdominal wall before draining to **lymph nodes along the diaphragm**;
- a small component crosses the midline and enters the **opposite breast**.

■ CLINICAL CORRELATIONS
Breast mass

An abnormal lump (Fig. 15.5) or thickening of the breast tissue is a breast mass. This is more common in women than in men and can occur anywhere within the breast. Two of the more common causes of breast mass in women are fibroadenoma and breast cancer.

Fibroadenoma is a benign tumor that is most common in women under 30 years of age. The tumor is usually a firm, solitary mass that is mobile beneath the skin and sometimes tender on palpation.

Breast cancer usually has unique characteristics, but can be indistinguishable from fibroadenoma on physical examination. Patients may report an asymmetric thickening or palpable mass that is very hard, adherent to underlying tissue, immobile, and sometimes painful. The pain does not usually vary with the menstrual cycle (unlike the pain typically related to fibroadenoma

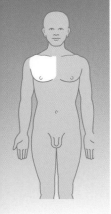
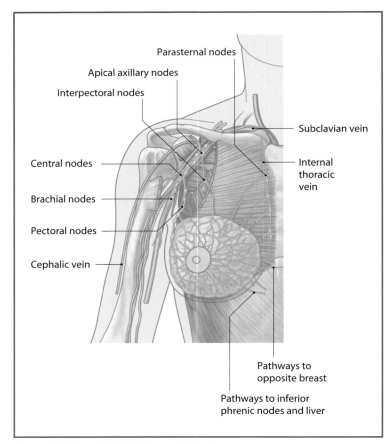

Figure 15.4 Lymphatic drainage of the breast

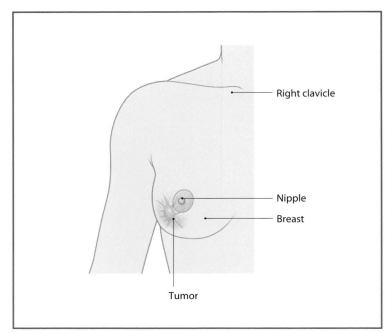

Figure 15.5 Tumor of the right breast

or other benign breast disorders). Additional symptoms and signs of cancer include bloody or watery nipple discharge, inflammatory skin changes, sudden weight loss or gain, and palpable masses in the axilla. Well-known risk factors for breast cancer are: having a close relative with breast cancer, a personal history of ovarian or endometrial cancer, early age of menarche, over 30 years of age at first birth, and late onset of menopause.

Patients with a breast mass may present to their physician with a lump detected on breast self-examination; or the mass might be picked up on routine clinical examination or mammography.

Sometimes, the clinician decides to observe the mass to see if it resolves. A persistent mass is usually scheduled for biopsy. Fine-needle aspiration, core biopsy, or open biopsy in the operating room all provide tissue for microscopic evaluation and a more definite diagnosis. Benign masses are usually scheduled for excisional biopsy (removal of the entire mass). Cancerous masses are diagnosed and, according to tissue type, treated by surgical removal. It is not uncommon for the surgeon to carry out an axillary lymph node removal at the same time because breast cancers typically spread first to the axilla. These nodes are examined histologically and, if cancer is present, this information – combined with the size of the primary tumor – is used to initiate postsurgical treatment with chemotherapy, radiation, or both.

The prognosis for patients with benign tumors is good; for patients with cancer the prognosis depends on its type and size at diagnosis, and the presence or absence of metastasis (distant spread of cancer away from primary location).

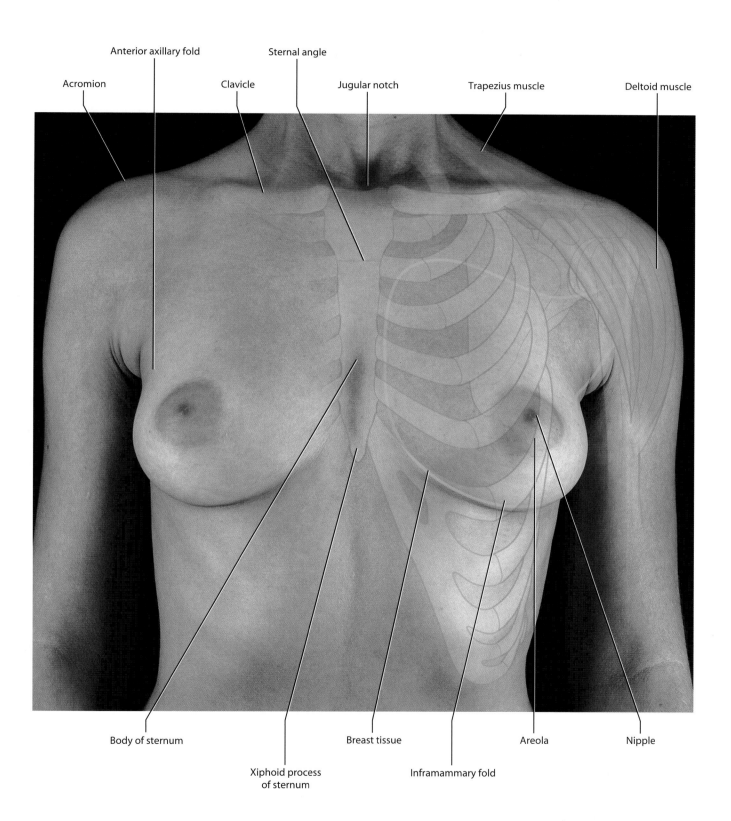

Anterior axillary fold

Sternal angle

Acromion

Clavicle

Jugular notch

Trapezius muscle

Deltoid muscle

Body of sternum

Breast tissue

Areola

Nipple

Xiphoid process
of sternum

Inframammary fold

Figure 15.6 Breast and pectoral region – surface anatomy. Anterior view of the breast and pectoral region of a young woman. There is no breast augmentation

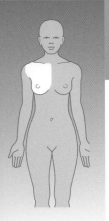

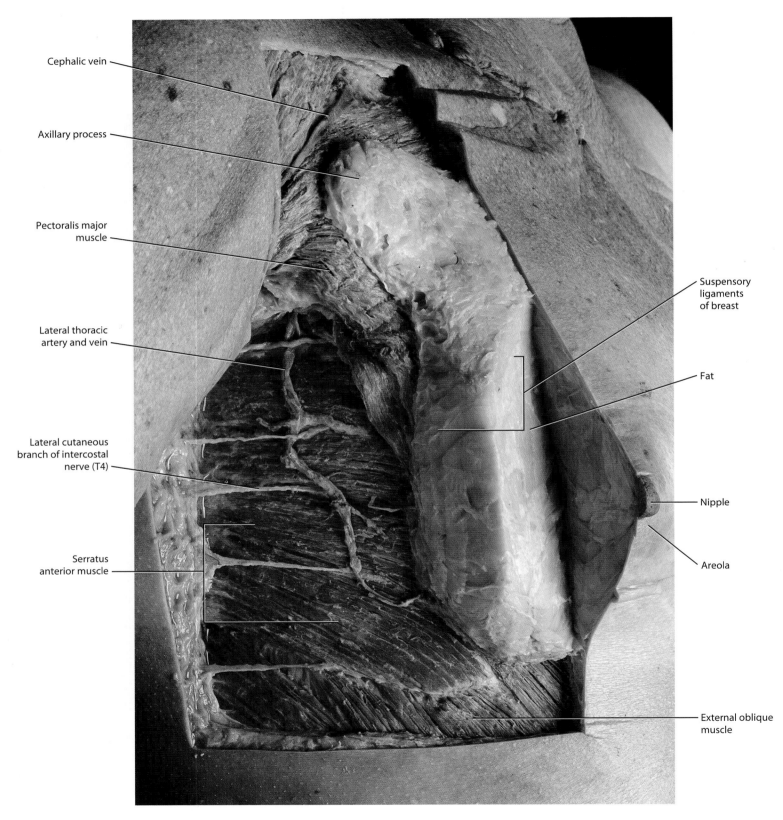

Cephalic vein

Axillary process

Pectoralis major muscle

Lateral thoracic artery and vein

Lateral cutaneous branch of intercostal nerve (T4)

Serratus anterior muscle

Suspensory ligaments of breast

Fat

Nipple

Areola

External oblique muscle

Figure 15.7 Breast – superficial dissection 1. A midsagittal cut of the right breast showing its superficial position on the pectoralis major and serratus anterior muscles. The breast has been dissected using a special layered technique to show the relationships of the nipple, fatty tissue of the breast, and the tail of Spence

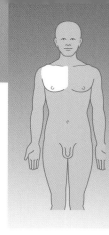

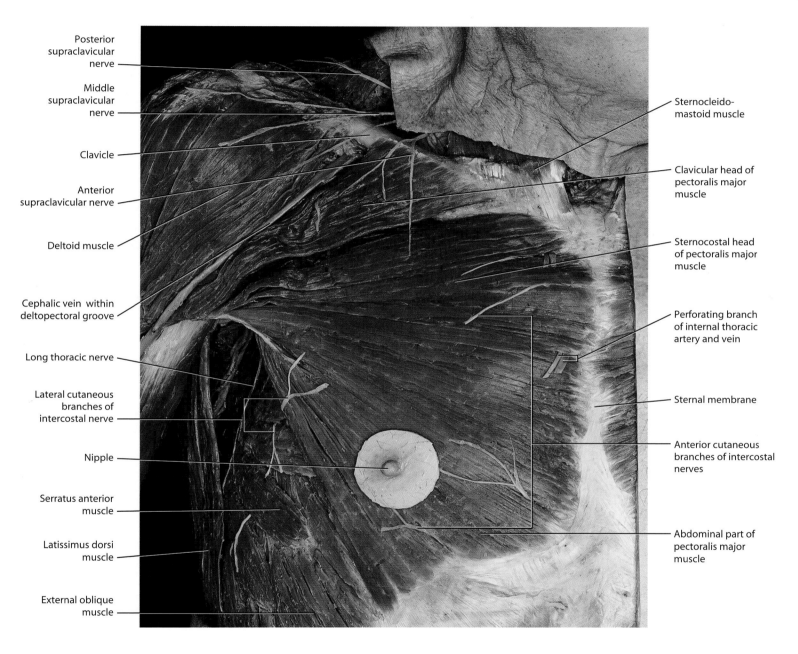

Posterior supraclavicular nerve

Middle supraclavicular nerve

Clavicle

Anterior supraclavicular nerve

Deltoid muscle

Cephalic vein within deltopectoral groove

Long thoracic nerve

Lateral cutaneous branches of intercostal nerve

Nipple

Serratus anterior muscle

Latissimus dorsi muscle

External oblique muscle

Sternocleido-mastoid muscle

Clavicular head of pectoralis major muscle

Sternocostal head of pectoralis major muscle

Perforating branch of internal thoracic artery and vein

Sternal membrane

Anterior cutaneous branches of intercostal nerves

Abdominal part of pectoralis major muscle

Figure 15.8 Pectoral region – superficial dissection 2. Anterior view of the superficial musculature of the right pectoral region. Note the cutaneous nerves over the deltoid and pectoralis major muscles. The nipple and its original location have been preserved as a reference point

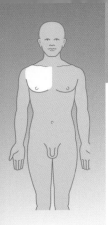

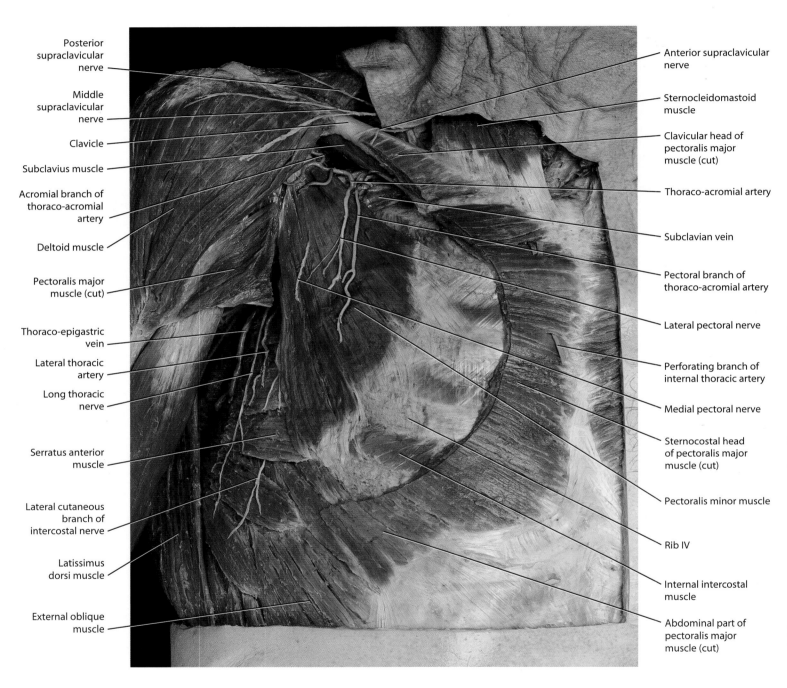

Posterior supraclavicular nerve

Middle supraclavicular nerve

Clavicle

Subclavius muscle

Acromial branch of thoraco-acromial artery

Deltoid muscle

Pectoralis major muscle (cut)

Thoraco-epigastric vein

Lateral thoracic artery

Long thoracic nerve

Serratus anterior muscle

Lateral cutaneous branch of intercostal nerve

Latissimus dorsi muscle

External oblique muscle

Anterior supraclavicular nerve

Sternocleidomastoid muscle

Clavicular head of pectoralis major muscle (cut)

Thoraco-acromial artery

Subclavian vein

Pectoral branch of thoraco-acromial artery

Lateral pectoral nerve

Perforating branch of internal thoracic artery

Medial pectoral nerve

Sternocostal head of pectoralis major muscle (cut)

Pectoralis minor muscle

Rib IV

Internal intercostal muscle

Abdominal part of pectoralis major muscle (cut)

Figure 15.9 Pectoral region – intermediate dissection. Anterior view of an intermediate layer dissection. The pectoralis major muscle has been removed to show the pectoralis minor muscle and some of the interdigitations of the serratus anterior muscle. Note the relationship of pectoralis minor with the medial and lateral pectoral nerves

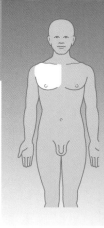

TABLE 15.1 PECTORAL MUSCLES*					
Muscle	Origin	Insertion	Innervation	Action	Blood supply
Pectoralis major	Clavicular head – anterior surface of medial half of clavicle; sternocostal head – anterior sternum, upper six costal cartilages, aponeurosis of external oblique muscle	Lateral lip of intertubercular sulcus of humerus (crest of greater tubercle)	Lateral and medial pectoral nerves: clavicular head (C5, **C6**), sternocostal head (**C7**, **C8**, T1)	Adducts and medially rotates arm; clavicular head flexes arm; sternocostal head extends arm	Pectoral branch of thoraco-acromial artery, perforating branches of internal thoracic artery
Pectoralis minor	Anterior surface of ribs III to V	Medial surface of coracoid process	Medial pectoral nerve (C8, T1)	Stabilizes scapula by pulling it inferiorly and anteriorly	Thoraco-acromial artery, intercostal branches of internal thoracic artery
Subclavius	Junction of rib I and its costal cartilage	Groove on inferior surface of middle third of clavicle	Subclavian nerve (**C5**, C6)	Depresses clavicle down and forward	Clavicular branch of thoraco-acromial artery
Serratus anterior	External surfaces of lateral parts of ribs I to VIII	Anterior surface of medial border of scapula	Long thoracic nerve (C5, **C6**, **C7**)	Abducts and protracts scapula, rotates it so that glenoid cavity faces upwards; also holds scapula firmly against thoracic wall	Lateral thoracic artery

*Main nerve root is indicated in bold

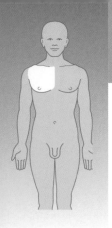

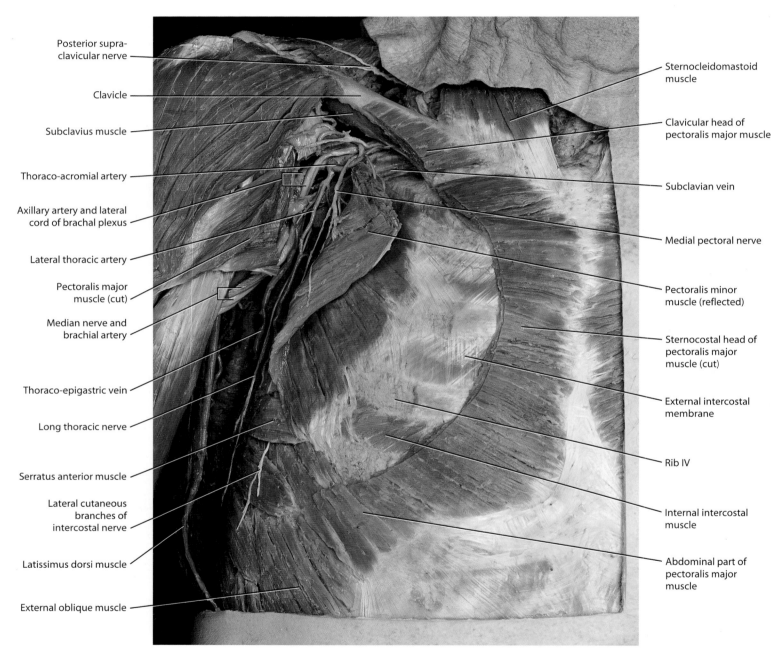

Posterior supra-clavicular nerve

Clavicle

Subclavius muscle

Thoraco-acromial artery

Axillary artery and lateral cord of brachal plexus

Lateral thoracic artery

Pectoralis major muscle (cut)

Median nerve and brachial artery

Thoraco-epigastric vein

Long thoracic nerve

Serratus anterior muscle

Lateral cutaneous branches of intercostal nerve

Latissimus dorsi muscle

External oblique muscle

Sternocleidomastoid muscle

Clavicular head of pectoralis major muscle

Subclavian vein

Medial pectoral nerve

Pectoralis minor muscle (reflected)

Sternocostal head of pectoralis major muscle (cut)

External intercostal membrane

Rib IV

Internal intercostal muscle

Abdominal part of pectoralis major muscle

Figure 15.10 Pectoral region – deep dissection. Anterior view of the deep pectoral layer. The pectoralis major muscle has been partially removed. The pectoralis minor muscle has been reflected medially and inferiorly from its insertion onto the scapula. Note the long thoracic nerve and lateral thoracic artery descending on the serratus anterior muscle

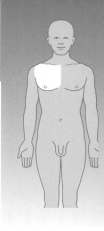

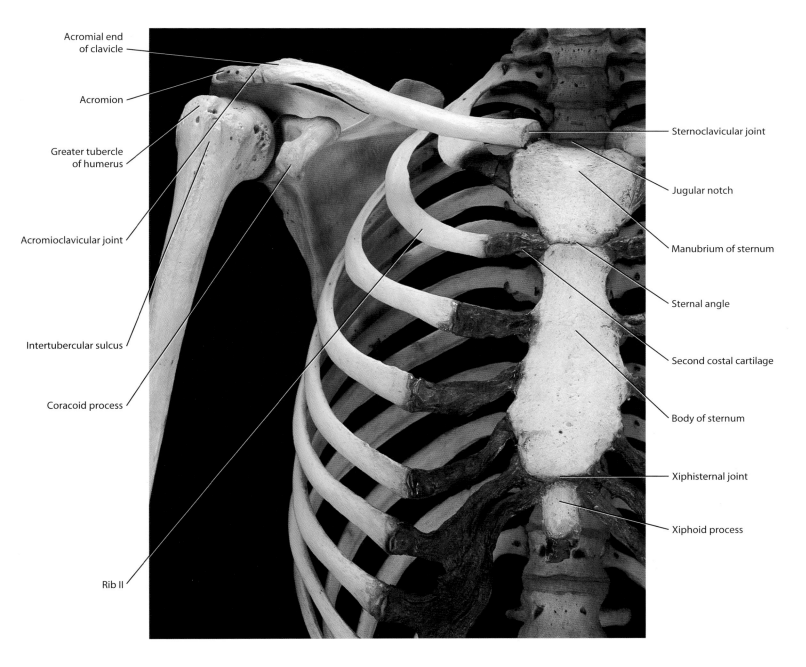

Acromial end
of clavicle

Acromion

Greater tubercle
of humerus

Acromioclavicular joint

Intertubercular sulcus

Coracoid process

Rib II

Sternoclavicular joint

Jugular notch

Manubrium of sternum

Sternal angle

Second costal cartilage

Body of sternum

Xiphisternal joint

Xiphoid process

Figure 15.11 Breast and pectoral region – osteology. Anterior view of the skeletal framework of the right breast and pectoral region

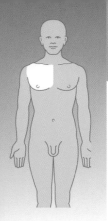

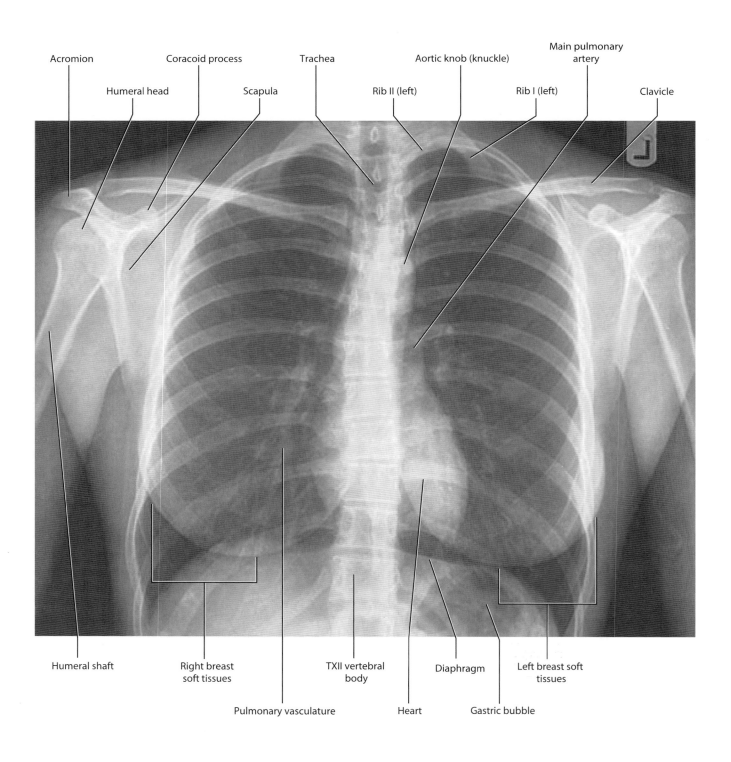

Acromion

Humeral head

Coracoid process

Scapula

Trachea

Rib II (left)

Aortic knob (knuckle)

Main pulmonary artery

Rib I (left)

Clavicle

Humeral shaft

Right breast soft tissues

TXII vertebral body

Diaphragm

Left breast soft tissues

Pulmonary vasculature

Heart

Gastric bubble

Figure 15.12 Breast and pectoral region – plain film radiograph (posteroanterior view). Although the soft tissue of the female breast is clearly visible in this plain film radiograph, the imaging modalities that best identify an abnormal breast mass are ultrasound and mammography. Note that in clinical practice, both anteroposterior and posteroanterior radiographs are viewed as though looking from anterior to posterior, hence the orientation shown here. To obtain a posteroanterior radiograph, the X-rays are projected from behind the patient to a plate that is touching the anterior surface of the patient's chest; structures close to the plate appear very close to actual size, and structures further away appear larger. In anteroposterior views the heart therefore appears much larger (and less distinct) than in this posteroanterior view

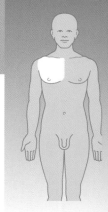

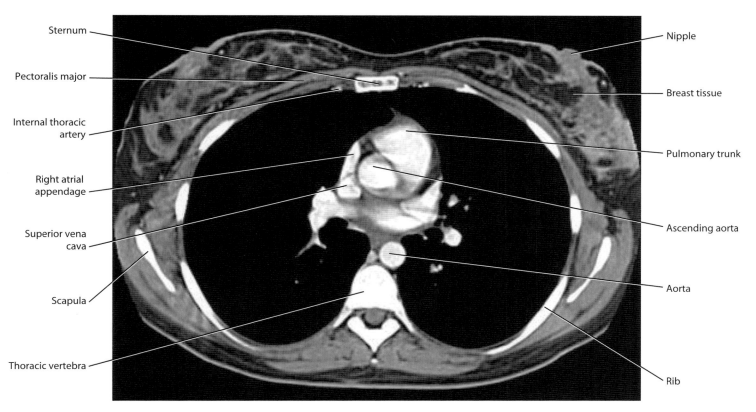

Sternum

Pectoralis major

Internal thoracic artery

Right atrial appendage

Superior vena cava

Scapula

Thoracic vertebra

Nipple

Breast tissue

Pulmonary trunk

Ascending aorta

Aorta

Rib

Figure 15.13 Breast and pectoral region – CT scan (axial view). This scan demonstrates how the breast is located immediately anterior to the pectoralis major muscle

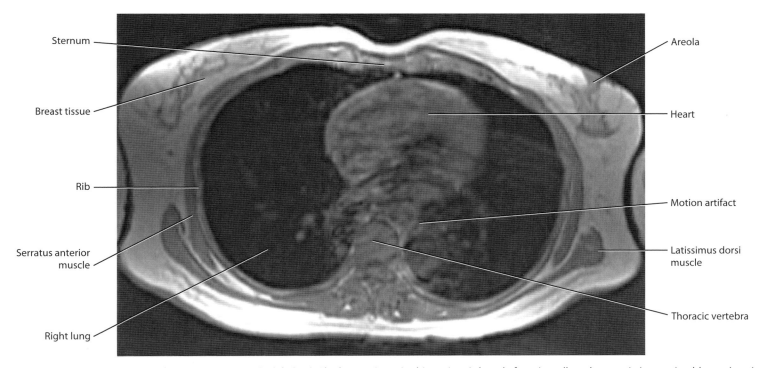

Sternum

Breast tissue

Rib

Serratus anterior muscle

Right lung

Areola

Heart

Motion artifact

Latissimus dorsi muscle

Thoracic vertebra

Figure 15.14 Breast and pectoral region – MRI scan (axial view). The breast tissue in this patient is largely fatty (usually a characteristic seen in older patients). MRI of the chest is generally suboptimal because of cardiac and respiratory motion

171

16   Axilla and brachial plexus

The axilla (armpit) is the concave area on the inferior surface of the junction of the arm with the trunk. It has a base and four walls:

- the base is formed by hairy skin, subcutaneous fat, and axillary fascia;
- the apex is bounded by the posterior border of the clavicle, superior border of the scapula, and rib I;
- the anterior wall (anterior axillary fold) is formed by the pectoralis muscles (major and minor);
- the posterior border (posterior axillary fold) is formed by lateral parts of the latissimus dorsi, teres major, and subscapularis muscles;
- the medial wall is ribs I to IV, and the intercostal and serratus anterior muscles;
- the lateral anterior wall is the intetubercular groove of the humerus.

Structural support to the axilla is provided by the lateral rib cage, clavicle, and scapula.

NERVES

The **brachial plexus** is a branching network of nerves that originates from anterior primary rami of spinal nerves C5 to T1 (Fig. 16.1). It is enclosed with the axillary artery and vein within the axillary sheath, which is a prolongation of the prevertebral layer of cervical fascia that extends inferiorly behind the clavicle and into the axilla. The brachial plexus is composed of nerve roots, trunks, divisions, cords, and branches (Table 16.1).

The nerve roots emerge from the spinal canal through the intervertebral foramina of the lower cervical vertebrae. They are in the deep posterior neck (see Chapter 13) between the anterior

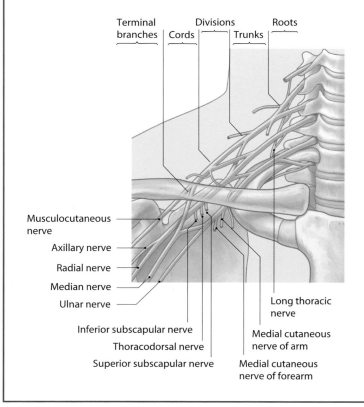

Figure 16.1 Brachial plexus

scalene and middle scalene muscles just superior to rib I. Two nerves come off the spinal roots, the **dorsal scapular nerve** (to the levator scapulae, rhomboid major, and rhomboid minor muscles) and the **long thoracic nerve** (to the serratus anterior muscle).

As they pass laterally, the spinal roots unite to form three trunks (**superior**, **middle**, and **inferior trunks**). The superior trunk is formed by the upper two roots (C5, C6), the middle trunk by C7, and the inferior trunk by C8 and T1. Two nerves leave the superior trunk – the **suprascapular nerve** and **subclavian nerve**.

Behind the clavicle, each trunk divides into **anterior** and **posterior divisions**. Nerves do not usually leave the divisions of the brachial plexus. The anterior division of the superior and middle trunks forms the **lateral cord**, the anterior division of the inferior trunk continues as the **medial cord**, and the posterior divisions of all three trunks form the **posterior cord**. These cords are named according to their relationship to the second part of the axillary artery. Several nerves leave the cords:

- the **lateral pectoral** leaves the lateral cord and becomes the **musculocutaneous nerve**;
- the **medial pectoral nerve, medial cutaneous nerve of arm, medial cutaneous nerve of forearm** and **ulnar nerve** leave the medial cord;
- the **superior subscapular, thoracodorsal, inferior subscapular, radial**, and **axillary nerves** leave the posterior cord.

Five terminal branches (nerves) of the brachial plexus arise from the three cords. Each cord divides into medial and lateral branches:

- the lateral branch of the posterior cord becomes the **axillary nerve** (C5 to C6);
- the medial branch of the posterior cord becomes the **radial nerve** (C5 to T1);
- the lateral branch of the lateral cord becomes the **musculocutaneous nerve** (C5 to C7);
- the medial branch of the lateral cord is joined by the lateral branch of the medial cord to form the **median nerve** (C6 to T1);
- the medial branch of the medial cord becomes the **ulnar nerve** (C7 to T1).

ARTERIES

Branches of the **axillary artery** (Fig. 16.2) supply blood to the structures of the axilla. The axillary artery is a continuation of the subclavian artery, arising at the lateral border of rib I inferior to the roots of the brachial plexus and between the anterior and middle scalene muscles. It continues into the axilla and terminates at the lower border of the teres major muscle, where it becomes the **brachial artery**. The axillary artery is divided into three parts based on its relationship to the pectoralis minor muscle:

- the first part runs between the lateral border of rib I and the superior margin of the pectoralis minor muscle, and has a single branch – the **superior thoracic artery**, which supplies the upper two intercostal spaces and pectoral muscles;
- the second part is posterior to the pectoralis minor muscle and gives rise to two branches: the **thoraco-acromial artery**, which divides into four smaller arteries (the **acromial, deltoid, clavicular**, and **pectoral branches**) to supply the regions after which they are named; and the **lateral thoracic artery**, which provides blood to the lateral chest wall and breast;

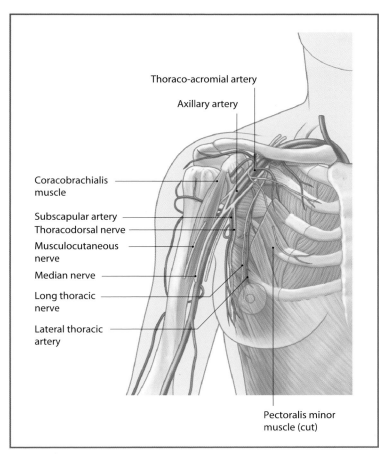

Thoraco-acromial artery

Axillary artery

Coracobrachialis muscle

Subscapular artery

Thoracodorsal nerve

Musculocutaneous nerve

Median nerve

Long thoracic nerve

Lateral thoracic artery

Pectoralis minor muscle (cut)

Figure 16.2 Structures within the axilla

- the third part extends from the inferior border of the pectoralis minor muscle to the lower border of teres major and has three branches: the first is the **subscapular artery**, which divides into the **circumflex scapular** and **thoracodorsal arteries** to supply the scapula and the latissimus dorsi muscle, respectively; the second and third branches are the **posterior** and **anterior circumflex humeral arteries**, which form a ring-like anastomosis around the surgical neck of the humerus to supply blood to the shoulder and surrounding muscles.

VEINS AND LYMPHATICS

The **axillary vein** lies on the medial side of the axillary artery. It begins as the continuation of the brachial companion veins and ends at the lateral border of rib I where it becomes the **subclavian vein**. The axillary vein receives tributaries that correspond to the branches of the axillary artery.

Lymphatic drainage of the axilla is to five lymph node groups named to reflect their relationship to axillary structures:

- **pectoral nodes** deep to the pectoralis major muscle drain the lateral and anterior chest wall, mammary glands, and upper abdominal wall;
- **humeral** (lateral) **nodes** on the lateral wall of the axilla receive lymph from the upper limb;
- **subscapular nodes** on the posterior wall of the axilla drain the back muscles;
- **central nodes** along the axillary vessels receive lymph from the lateral quadrants of the breast;
- **apical nodes** at the apex of the axilla and continuous with the inferior deep nodes (deep neck) drain the other axillary nodes and structures in the deep neck.

■ CLINICAL CORRELATIONS
Injuries to the brachial plexus

The brachial plexus is formed by the union of the anterior rami of spinal nerves C5 to T1. Its branches supply all the structures in the upper limb. The two broad categories of injury are superior and inferior neck injuries, although a penetrating injury to any part of the plexus will cause a specific nerve deficit.

Superior trunk injury can be caused by forceful lateral flexion of the neck away from the affected side concomitant with forceful depression of the affected shoulder. This strains the upper parts of the plexus and results in injury, which depending on severity, may be permanent. Inferior plexus injuries are caused by extreme forceful abduction of the upper limb, which places tension on the lower nerve roots. Plexus injuries can be caused by falling on an outstretched arm, trauma from the poor use of crutches, motor vehicle accidents, sports, radiation, penetrating trauma, and birth injuries.

Superior trunk injuries usually involve the C5 and C6 nerve roots and result in an inability to:

- flex the arm at the elbow;
- abduct the arm;
- supinate the forearm (e.g. turn door knobs).

Patients usually report loss of sensation over the shoulder and lateral forearm and hand, corresponding to the segmental nerve root origin (C5, C6 dermatomes; see Fig. 26.4). On examination, the affected limb is adducted and internally rotated (waiter's tip deformity). The general finding is an inability to use the muscles that flex, abduct, and externally rotate the upper limb (biceps, brachialis, brachioradialis, deltoid, supraspinatus, infraspinatus, and teres minor).

Inferior trunk injuries usually involve C8 and T1 nerve roots and result in paralysis or paresis of the fingers and wrist. This is manifested by an inability to carry out fine motor movements of the hand. Patients also report numbness along the medial arm, forearm, and hand. Examination verifies the complaints, with observed weakness or paralysis of wrist and finger flexors. There may also be some generalized weakness of the flexor and extensor muscles of the entire upper limb. Careful examination may reveal Horner's syndrome with ptosis (drooping eyelid), miosis (small pupil), and anhidrosis (decreased sweating) on the affected side, which occurs when the cervical sympathetic chain is damaged during the initial plexus injury.

A diagnosis of brachial plexus injury can be confirmed by direct electrical stimulation of the muscles using the electromyogram (EMG), myelography (X-ray after dye is injected into the nerve sheath), computed tomography (CT) myelography, or magnetic resonance imaging (MRI). Treatment of brachial plexus injury is based on the mechanism of injury and the final diagnosis. Complete avulsion (separation) of the nerve roots from the spinal cord usually is associated with a poor prognosis; however, with new techniques some function can be restored. Other injuries to the brachial plexus necessitate close observation and consultation with a specialist for possible surgical repair.

MNEMONICS	
Parts of brachial plexus:	**Really Thirsty? Drink Cold Beer** (**R**oots, **T**runks, **D**ivisions, **C**ords, **B**ranches)
Terminal nerves:	**MARMU** (**M**usculocutaneous, **A**xillary, **R**adial, **M**edian, **U**lnar)

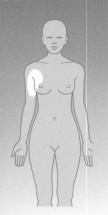

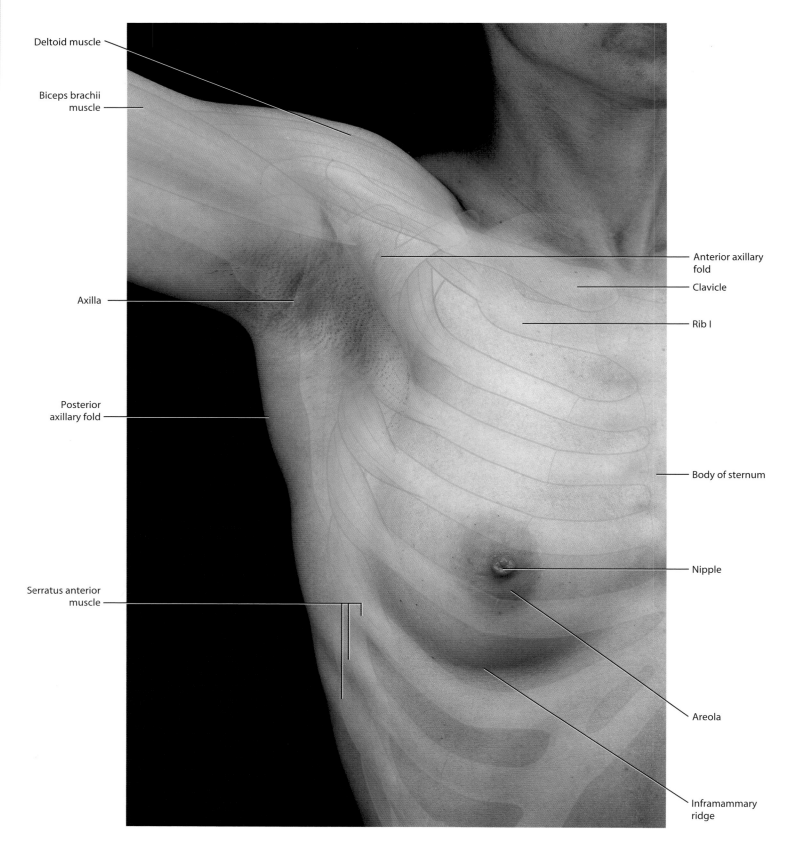

Deltoid muscle

Biceps brachii muscle

Axilla

Posterior axillary fold

Serratus anterior muscle

Anterior axillary fold

Clavicle

Rib I

Body of sternum

Nipple

Areola

Inframammary ridge

Figure 16.3 Axilla and brachial plexus – surface anatomy. Anterior view of the surface features of the right axilla and breast of a young woman. Observe the overall teardrop shape of the breast. The ribs are also visible

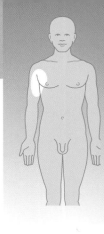

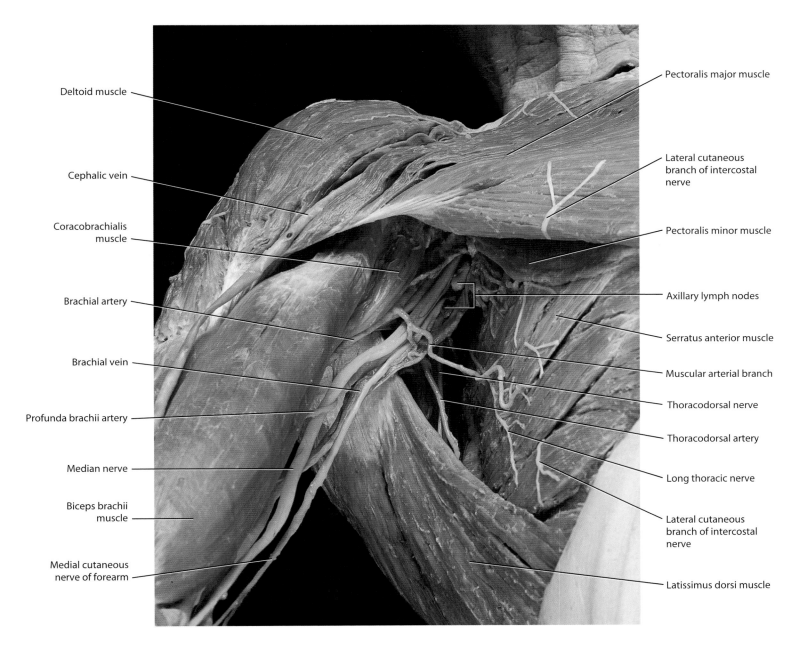

Deltoid muscle

Cephalic vein

Coracobrachialis muscle

Brachial artery

Brachial vein

Profunda brachii artery

Median nerve

Biceps brachii muscle

Medial cutaneous nerve of forearm

Pectoralis major muscle

Lateral cutaneous branch of intercostal nerve

Pectoralis minor muscle

Axillary lymph nodes

Serratus anterior muscle

Muscular arterial branch

Thoracodorsal nerve

Thoracodorsal artery

Long thoracic nerve

Lateral cutaneous branch of intercostal nerve

Latissimus dorsi muscle

Figure 16.4 Axilla – superficial dissection. Inferior view of right axilla showing the anterior wall of the pectoralis major, medial wall of the serratus anterior, and posterior wall of the latissimus dorsi muscles. Many of the lymph nodes of the axilla have been removed to show the nerves and arteries

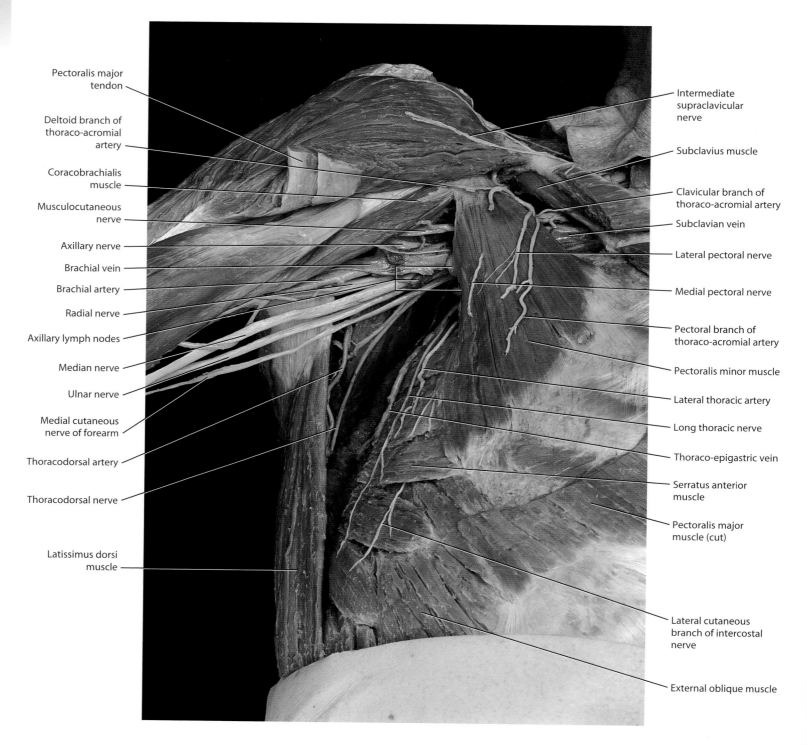

Pectoralis major tendon

Deltoid branch of thoraco-acromial artery

Coracobrachialis muscle

Musculocutaneous nerve

Axillary nerve

Brachial vein

Brachial artery

Radial nerve

Axillary lymph nodes

Median nerve

Ulnar nerve

Medial cutaneous nerve of forearm

Thoracodorsal artery

Thoracodorsal nerve

Latissimus dorsi muscle

Intermediate supraclavicular nerve

Subclavius muscle

Clavicular branch of thoraco-acromial artery

Subclavian vein

Lateral pectoral nerve

Medial pectoral nerve

Pectoral branch of thoraco-acromial artery

Pectoralis minor muscle

Lateral thoracic artery

Long thoracic nerve

Thoraco-epigastric vein

Serratus anterior muscle

Pectoralis major muscle (cut)

Lateral cutaneous branch of intercostal nerve

External oblique muscle

Figure 16.5 Axilla – intermediate dissection. Right axilla with pectoralis major almost completely removed to reveal the neurovasculature of the brachial plexus. The arm is abducted and the clavipectoral fascia removed, together with the axillary sheath, which once enveloped the axillary artery and brachial plexus

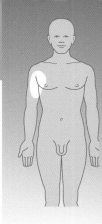

TABLE 16.1   BRANCHES OF THE BRACHIAL PLEXUS

Branches	Origin	Course	Innervation
Dorsal scapular nerve	C5	Pierces middle scalene, descends deep to levator scapulae	Levator scapulae Rhomboid minor Rhomboid major
Long thoracic nerve	C5 to C7	Descends posterior to C8 to T1 roots, descends on external surface of serratus anterior muscle	Serratus anterior
Subclavian nerve	C5, C6	Descends posterior to clavicle, anterior to brachial plexus and subclavian artery	Subclavius Sternoclavicular joint
Suprascapular nerve	C5, C6	Passes laterally through posterior triangle of neck, traverses suprascapular notch under transverse scapular ligament	Supraspinatus Infraspinatus Glenohumeral joint
Lateral pectoral nerve	C5 to C7	Pierces clavipectoral fascia, reaches deep surface of pectoral muscles	Pectoralis major
Medial pectoral nerve	C8, T1	Passes between axillary artery and vein, enters deep surface of pectoralis minor	Pectoralis minor Pectoralis major
Medial cutaneous nerve of arm	C8, T1	Runs along medial side of axillary vein	Skin of medial arm
Medial cutaneous nerve of forearm	C8, T1	Runs between axillary artery and vein	Skin of medial forearm
Upper subscapular nerve	C5, C6	Passes posteriorly and enters subscapularis	Subscapularis
Thoracodorsal nerve	C6 to C8	Arises between superior and inferior subscapular nerves	Latissimus dorsi
Inferior subscapular nerve	C5, C6	Passes inferolaterally, deep to subscapular artery and vein	Subscapularis Teres major
Musculocutaneous nerve	C5 to C7	Pierces coracobrachialis, descends between biceps brachii and brachialis	Coracobrachialis Biceps brachii Brachialis Skin of lateral forearm
Median nerve	C6 to T1	Formed from lateral head joining medial head, descends medially to biceps brachii	Most flexor muscles in forearm Radial half of flexor digitorum profundus Thenar muscles and lumbricals I, II Skin of lateral palm
Ulnar nerve	C7 to T1	Descends medial to brachial artery, runs posteriorly to medial epicondyle of humerus	Flexor carpi ulnaris and ulnar half of flexor digitorum profundus Most intrinsic hand muscles Skin of medial palm
Axillary nerve	C5, C6	Passes through quadrangular space (see Chapter 17), winds around surgical neck of humerus	Teres minor Deltoid Glenohumeral joint Skin of inferior deltoid
Radial nerve	C5 to T1	Descends posterior to axillary artery, enters radial groove with deep brachial artery, passes between long and medial heads of triceps brachii	Triceps brachii Anconeus and brachioradialis Extensor muscles of forearm Skin of posterior arm, forearm, hand

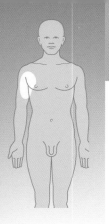

UPPER LIMB

Axilla and brachial plexus

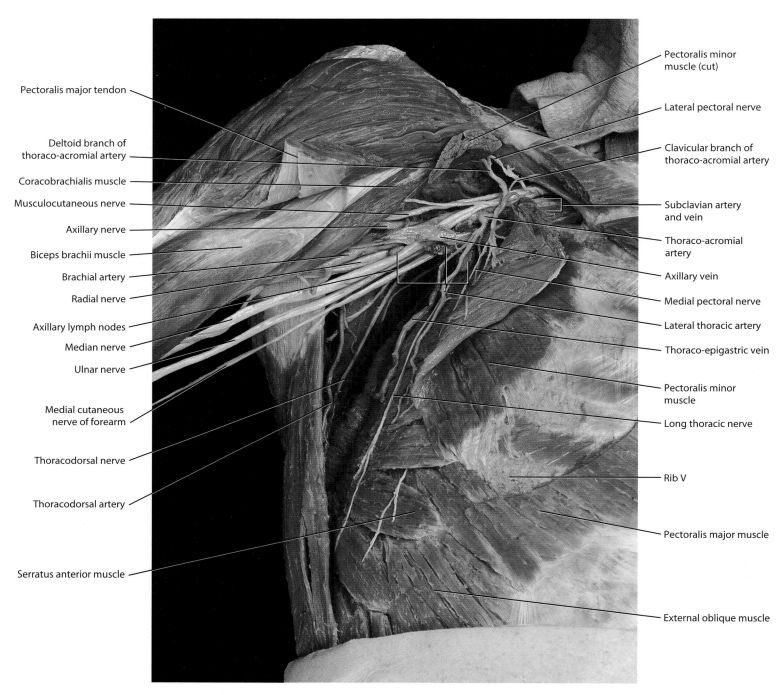

Pectoralis major tendon

Deltoid branch of thoraco-acromial artery

Coracobrachialis muscle

Musculocutaneous nerve

Axillary nerve

Biceps brachii muscle

Brachial artery

Radial nerve

Axillary lymph nodes

Median nerve

Ulnar nerve

Medial cutaneous nerve of forearm

Thoracodorsal nerve

Thoracodorsal artery

Serratus anterior muscle

Pectoralis minor muscle (cut)

Lateral pectoral nerve

Clavicular branch of thoraco-acromial artery

Subclavian artery and vein

Thoraco-acromial artery

Axillary vein

Medial pectoral nerve

Lateral thoracic artery

Thoraco-epigastric vein

Pectoralis minor muscle

Long thoracic nerve

Rib V

Pectoralis major muscle

External oblique muscle

Figure 16.6 Brachial plexus – intermediate dissection 1. Right axilla with the pectoralis major muscle removed and the pectoralis minor muscle cut and reflected medially to show the brachial plexus. The axillary sheath has been removed, showing the relationship of the axillary vein and artery with the brachial plexus. Note the position of the axillary lymph nodes

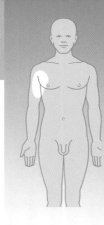

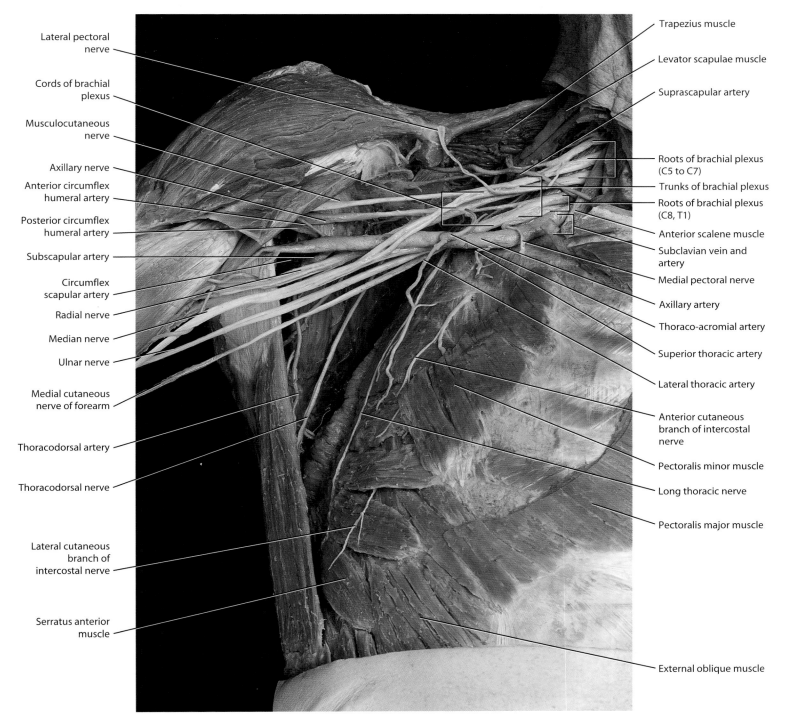

Lateral pectoral nerve

Cords of brachial plexus

Musculocutaneous nerve

Axillary nerve

Anterior circumflex humeral artery

Posterior circumflex humeral artery

Subscapular artery

Circumflex scapular artery

Radial nerve

Median nerve

Ulnar nerve

Medial cutaneous nerve of forearm

Thoracodorsal artery

Thoracodorsal nerve

Lateral cutaneous branch of intercostal nerve

Serratus anterior muscle

Trapezius muscle

Levator scapulae muscle

Suprascapular artery

Roots of brachial plexus (C5 to C7)

Trunks of brachial plexus

Roots of brachial plexus (C8, T1)

Anterior scalene muscle

Subclavian vein and artery

Medial pectoral nerve

Axillary artery

Thoraco-acromial artery

Superior thoracic artery

Lateral thoracic artery

Anterior cutaneous branch of intercostal nerve

Pectoralis minor muscle

Long thoracic nerve

Pectoralis major muscle

External oblique muscle

Figure 16.7 Brachial plexus – deep dissection 1. The pectoralis major and minor muscles along with the clavicle have been removed. The right brachial plexus has been slightly spread out, revealing the branches of the axillary artery. Observe the branching structure of the brachial plexus with respect to the axillary artery

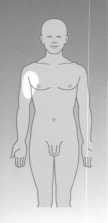

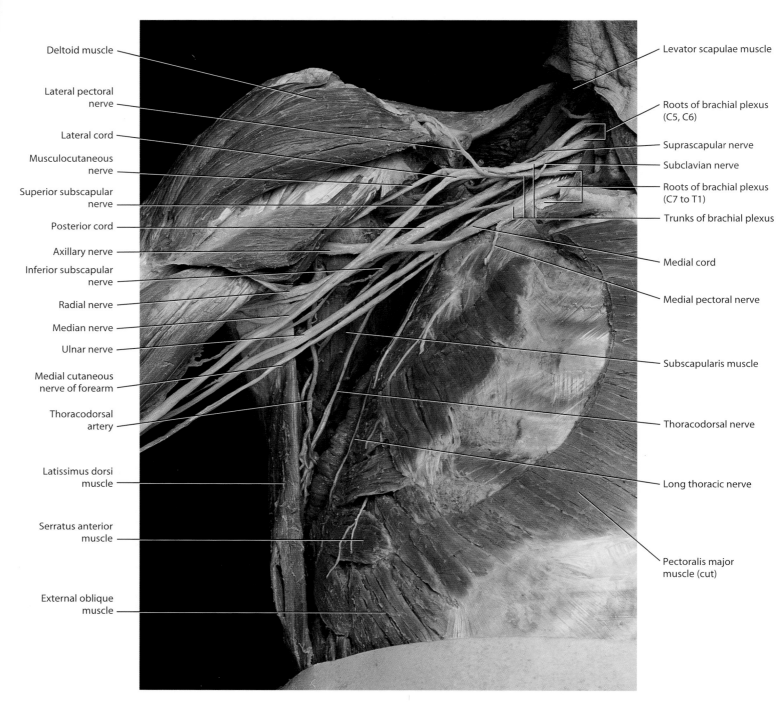

Deltoid muscle

Lateral pectoral nerve

Lateral cord

Musculocutaneous nerve

Superior subscapular nerve

Posterior cord

Axillary nerve

Inferior subscapular nerve

Radial nerve

Median nerve

Ulnar nerve

Medial cutaneous nerve of forearm

Thoracodorsal artery

Latissimus dorsi muscle

Serratus anterior muscle

External oblique muscle

Levator scapulae muscle

Roots of brachial plexus (C5, C6)

Suprascapular nerve

Subclavian nerve

Roots of brachial plexus (C7 to T1)

Trunks of brachial plexus

Medial cord

Medial pectoral nerve

Subscapularis muscle

Thoracodorsal nerve

Long thoracic nerve

Pectoralis major muscle (cut)

Figure 16.8 Brachial plexus – deep dissection 2. The pectoralis major and minor muscles, clavicle and axillary artery have been removed to show the anatomical relationships of the branches of the right brachial plexus – the five roots, three trunks, three cords, and five terminal nerve branches. Note the superior and inferior subscapular nerves

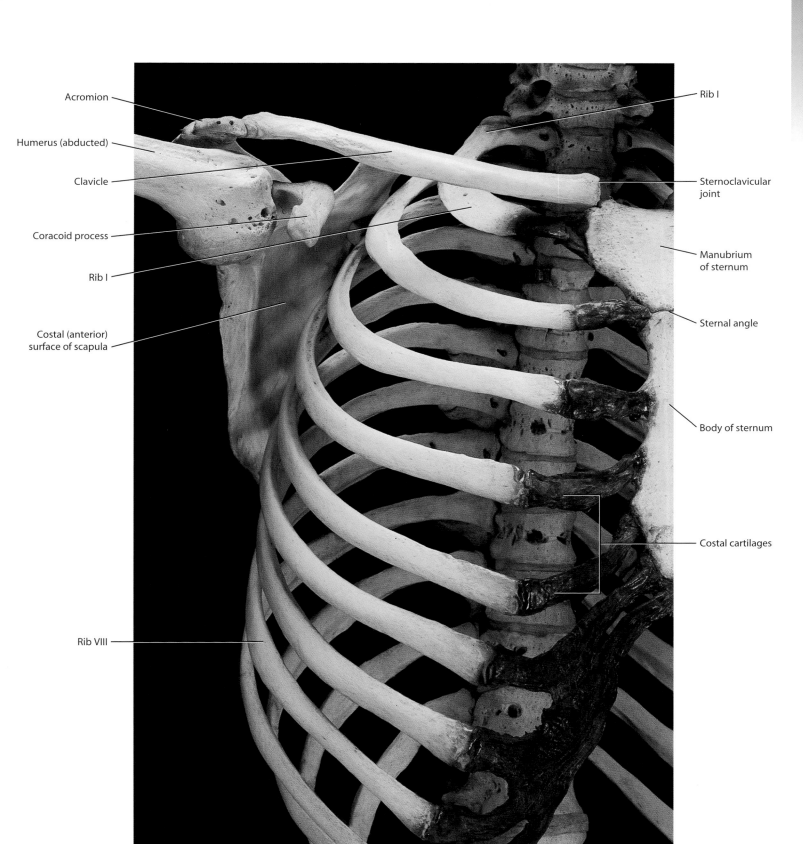

Acromion

Humerus (abducted)

Clavicle

Coracoid process

Rib I

Costal (anterior)
surface of scapula

Rib VIII

Rib I

Sternoclavicular
joint

Manubrium
of sternum

Sternal angle

Body of sternum

Costal cartilages

UPPER LIMB   Axilla and brachial plexus

Figure 16.9 Axilla and brachial plexus – osteology. Anterior view of the bony framework for the apex, lateral, medial, and posterior walls of the axilla. This view of the articulated skeleton replicates the surface anatomy photograph (Figure 16.4)

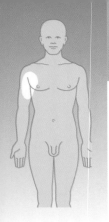

UPPER LIMB

Axilla and brachial plexus

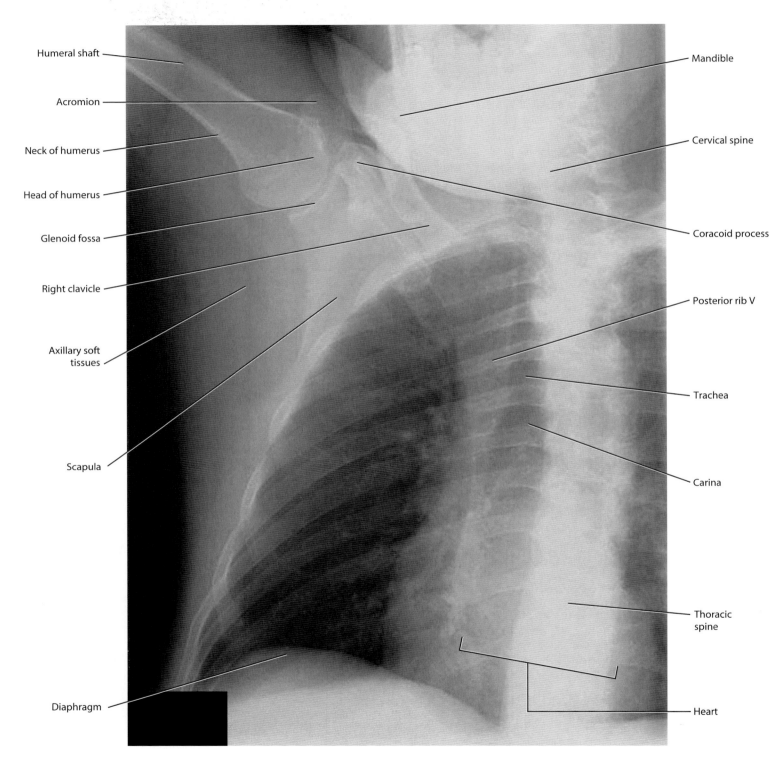

Humeral shaft

Acromion

Neck of humerus

Head of humerus

Glenoid fossa

Right clavicle

Axillary soft
tissues

Scapula

Diaphragm

Mandible

Cervical spine

Coracoid process

Posterior rib V

Trachea

Carina

Thoracic
spine

Heart

182 Figure 16.10 Axilla and brachial plexus – plain film radiograph (left anterior oblique view). Observe how the scapula articulates with the humerus

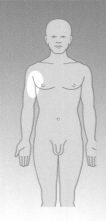

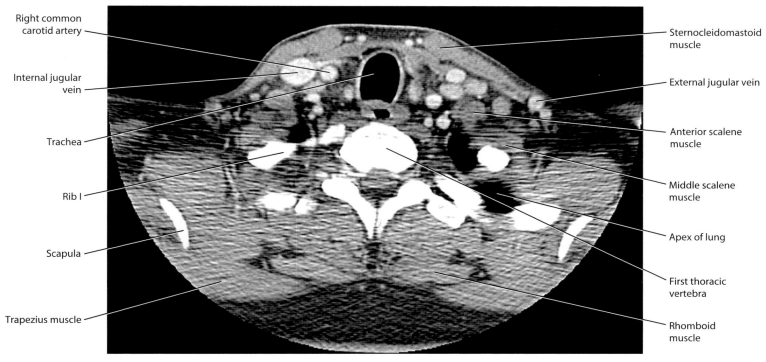

Right common carotid artery

Internal jugular vein

Trachea

Rib I

Scapula

Trapezius muscle

Sternocleidomastoid muscle

External jugular vein

Anterior scalene muscle

Middle scalene muscle

Apex of lung

First thoracic vertebra

Rhomboid muscle

Figure 16.11 Axilla and brachial plexus – CT scan (axial view). Although the brachial plexus is not visible on CT scanning, the anterior and middle scalene muscles, between which they pass, are clearly demonstrated

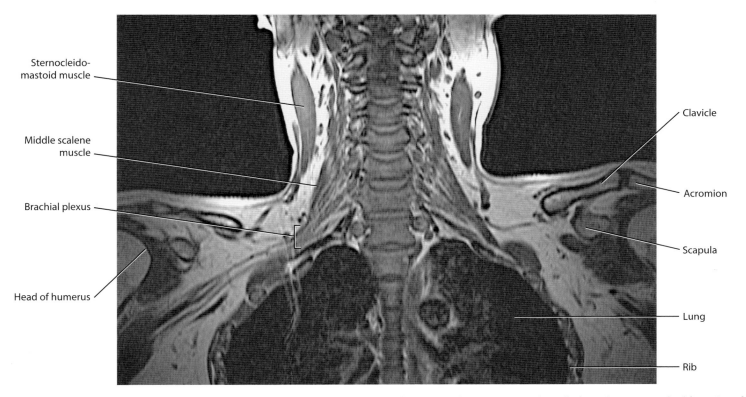

Sternocleido-mastoid muscle

Middle scalene muscle

Brachial plexus

Head of humerus

Clavicle

Acromion

Scapula

Lung

Rib

Figure 16.12 Brachial plexus – MRI scan (coronal view). The nerves of the brachial plexus can be seen passing laterally from the intervertebral foramina of CV to TI

183

17 Scapular region

The scapular region is on the superior posterior surface of the trunk and is defined by the muscles that attach to the **scapula** (shoulder blade). These muscles can be divided into:

- extrinsic muscles, which join the axial to the appendicular skeleton (trapezius, latissimus dorsi, levator scapulae, rhomboid minor, and rhomboid major);
- intrinsic muscles, which join the scapula to the humerus (deltoid, supraspinatus, infraspinatus, teres minor, teres major, and subscapularis).

The principal structural support is from the scapula, a flat triangular bone. The **costal (anterior) surface** of the scapula overlies ribs II to VII, and its three borders are **superior**, **medial** (vertebral), and **lateral** (axillary), The lowest point is the **inferior angle**, and the lateral point is the **lateral angle**. A transverse **spine of scapula** divides the posterior surface of the scapula into a smaller **supraspinous fossa** above and a larger **infraspinous fossa** below. As it continues laterally, this spine forms the **acromion** (the bony high point of the shoulder). The **subscapular fossa** is on the anterior surface of the scapula. At the lateral angle of the scapula the shallow, oval-shaped **glenoid cavity** articulates with the head of the humerus at the glenohumeral joint.

MUSCLES

The muscles of the scapular region (Figs 17.1 and 17.2) join the upper limb to the posterior trunk and facilitate many movements at the shoulder. They can be divided into three groups (Table 17.1).

- The superficial extrinsic muscles join the axial skeleton (chest wall and rib cage) to the appendicular skeleton (bones of the upper limb). The two muscles in this group are the trapezius and latissimus dorsi. The large, triangular **trapezius** muscle slightly overlies the broad **latissimus dorsi** muscle. Together, these muscles originate from the entire length of the thoracic vertebral column (CVII, TI to TXII) and insert laterally onto the clavicle, scapula, and humerus.
- The deep extrinsic muscles (levator scapulae, rhomboid major, and rhomboid minor) elevate and retract the scapula. The strap-like **levator scapulae** muscle is deep to the sternocleidomastoid muscle (see Chapter 13) and trapezius muscles and joins the upper medial border of the scapula to the transverse processes of the upper cervical vertebrae. The rhomboids also originate on the medial border of the scapula, with the **rhomboid minor** being more superior than the **rhomboid major** muscle. These muscles attach to the spinous processes of the upper thoracic vertebrae.
- The deep 'intrinsic' or true scapular muscles are the deltoid, supraspinatus, infraspinatus, teres minor, teres major, and subscapularis muscle. The **deltoid** muscle, which has three parts (clavicular, acromial, and spinal), is superior and forms the roundness of the shoulder over the glenohumeral joint. Inferior to deltoid are four scapular muscles – the **supraspinatus**, **infraspinatus**, **teres minor**, and **subscapularis** – which originate from the scapula and insert laterally on the humerus, forming a protective covering (rotator cuff) over the glenohumeral joint.

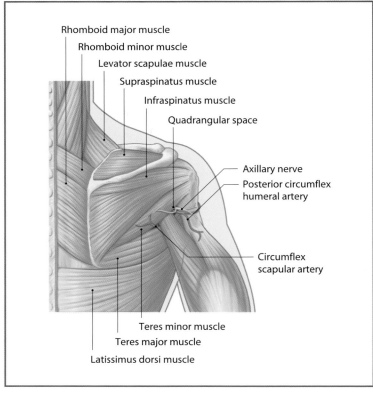

Figure 17.1 Scapular muscles (posterior view)

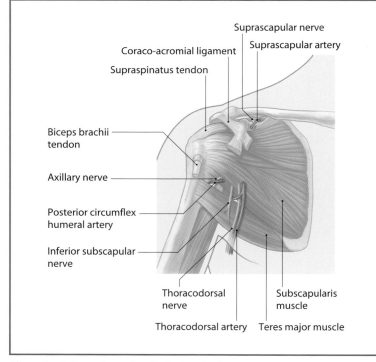

Figure 17.2 Scapular region (anterior view)

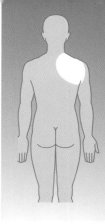

The rotator cuff muscles rotate the humerus to enable actions such as throwing a baseball. In conjunction with the latissimus dorsi muscle, the **teres major** muscle, which is just inferior to the rotator cuff muscles, helps form the posterior axillary fold. The anterior axillary fold is formed by the pectoralis muscles; the axilla lies between these folds.

NERVES

The skin of the scapular region receives sensory information from the medial branches of the **posterior rami of cervical nerves C4 to C8** and **thoracic nerves T1 to T6** (see Chapter 26). The skin over the lateral scapular area overlying the deltoid muscle is innervated by branches of the **superior lateral cutaneous nerve of arm**, which is a branch of the **axillary nerve**. Motor innervation to the muscles of the scapular region is almost entirely by branches of the brachial plexus (see Chapter 16):

- the **dorsal scapular nerve** (levator and rhomboid muscles) is from the anterior ramus of C5;
- the **suprascapular nerve** (supraspinatus and infraspinatus muscles) is from the superior trunk;
- the four other nerves to this region (the **superior** and **inferior subscapular**, **thoracodorsal**, and **axillary**) are branches of the posterior cord and supply the subscapularis, teres major, latissimus dorsi, deltoid, and teres minor muscles. Only the spinal root of accessory nerve [XI], which innervates trapezius, does not originate from the brachial plexus.

ARTERIES

Blood is brought to the scapular region by a network of arteries, which form the scapular anastomosis:

- muscles medial and superior to the scapula receive blood from the **dorsal scapular**, **transverse cervical**, and **suprascapular arteries**, which are branches of the subclavian artery, and also from the **acromial artery**, which is a branch of the axillary artery;
- muscles anterior and lateral to the scapula are supplied by the **subscapular**, **circumflex scapular**, and **posterior circumflex humeral arteries**, which are derived from the axillary artery.

The extensive arterial anastomosis at the scapular region provides a collateral circulation, so if one vessel is blocked or damaged, many others can provide blood to the region. This anastomosis helps preserve the upper limb during injury.

VEINS AND LYMPHATICS

Venous drainage of the scapular region is by veins that correspond to the arteries. Each of these veins drains – directly or indirectly – into the **axillary** or **subclavian veins**. Lymphatic drainage of the scapular region is to the **axillary** and **supraclavicular lymph nodes**.

ANATOMICAL SPACES

Three openings in the scapular region – the triangular space, the quadrangular space, and the triangle of auscultation – contain important neurovascular structures or are of clinical relevance.

The three-sided **triangular space** contains the circumflex scapular artery and is bordered laterally by the long head of the triceps brachii, inferiorly by the teres major, and superiorly by the teres minor muscle.

The **quadrangular space** contains the axillary nerve and posterior circumflex humeral artery and is bordered superiorly by the inferior border of the teres minor, inferiorly by the teres major, and medially by the long head of triceps brachii muscle, and laterally by the shaft of humerus.

The **triangle of auscultation** is a small triangular gap in the musculature, a good place to listen to posterior lungs with a stethoscope when the shoulder is protracted. The triangle is between the horizontal border of latissimus dorsi, the medial border of the scapula, and the inferolateral border of the trapezius.

■ CLINICAL CORRELATIONS
Scapular fracture

Injuries to the scapula are not common because of the triangular structure and its supporting spine. The scapula is also protected by the large number of muscles that cover, surround, and insert onto it. A scapular fracture is a highly significant injury clinically because only high-velocity injuries or great force can fracture the scapula (Fig. 17.3). A patient with a scapular fracture therefore has a high risk of other potentially life-threatening injury (e.g. pneumothorax, hemothorax, pulmonary contusion), so particular attention must be paid to the A, B, C of trauma:

- **A**irway,
- **B**reathing,
- **C**irculation.

In the emergency setting all patients should first be assessed to determine whether their airway is patent (without obstruction). The quality of breathing is then carefully evaluated. After this, the circulatory system of the patient (e.g. pulses, capillary refill) is examined. The entire initial survey of the patient takes a few

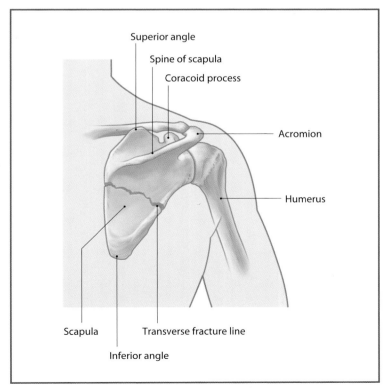

Figure 17.3 Common site of scapular fracture

Superior angle
Spine of scapula
Coracoid process
Acromion
Humerus
Scapula
Transverse fracture line
Inferior angle

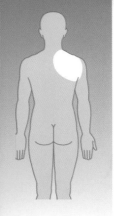
seconds. Once vital functions are confirmed, a full examination, including a complete neurovascular examination, is carried out. Any problem discovered during the initial ABC survey warrants emergency treatment before the next step can be performed.

Most patients with scapular fracture experience extreme upper back pain and cannot lie comfortably; they hold the injured limb in adduction against the chest wall. In addition, because of the high likelihood of associated pulmonary injury, they might have respiratory symptoms (shortness of breath, inability to breathe, pain on deep inspiration). Tenderness on palpation is invariable, as are ecchymoses (bruises) or abrasions. Sometimes crepitance, and

the sensation of a crunching feeling beneath the surface of the skin, is indicative of a pneumothorax. On completion of the trauma survey, and if there are no other life-threatening injuries, the clinician can carefully examine the upper lateral back. Radiographs of the scapula in two views will show the fracture line.

Treatment of most scapular fractures is conservative and consists of immobilization of the affected limb and pain control, and follow-up by an orthopedist. Fractures that damage the nerve and blood supply of the affected limb, open fractures, and fractures involving the glenohumeral joint space should be referred to a specialist for treatment, which in many cases is surgical.

MNEMONICS	
Rotator cuff muscles and their insertion on humerus:	**SITS** (**S**upraspinatus, **I**nfraspinatus, **T**eres major, **S**ubscapularis) (Greater tubercle) (Lesser tubercle)
Transverse scapular ligament:	**Army goes over the 'bridge', Navy goes under the 'bridge'** (Suprascapular **A**rtery over the ligament, suprascapular **N**erve under the ligament)

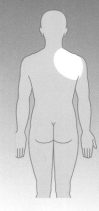

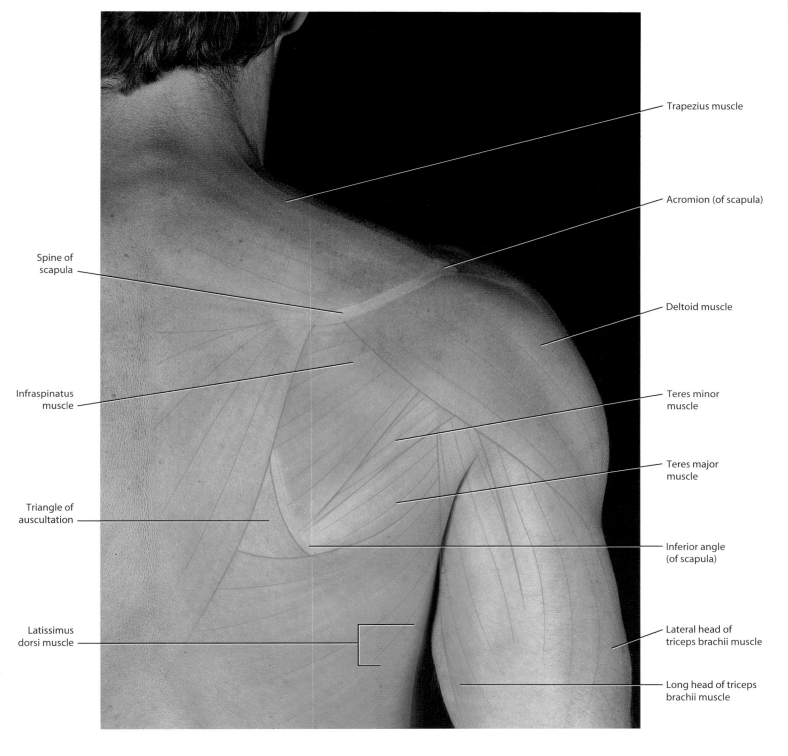

Spine of
scapula

Trapezius muscle

Acromion (of scapula)

Deltoid muscle

Infraspinatus
muscle

Teres minor
muscle

Teres major
muscle

Triangle of
auscultation

Inferior angle
(of scapula)

Latissimus
dorsi muscle

Lateral head of
triceps brachii muscle

Long head of triceps
brachii muscle

Figure 17.4 Scapular region – surface anatomy. Right posterior view of the scapular region of a young male. Observe the muscles that are visible

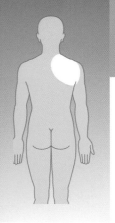

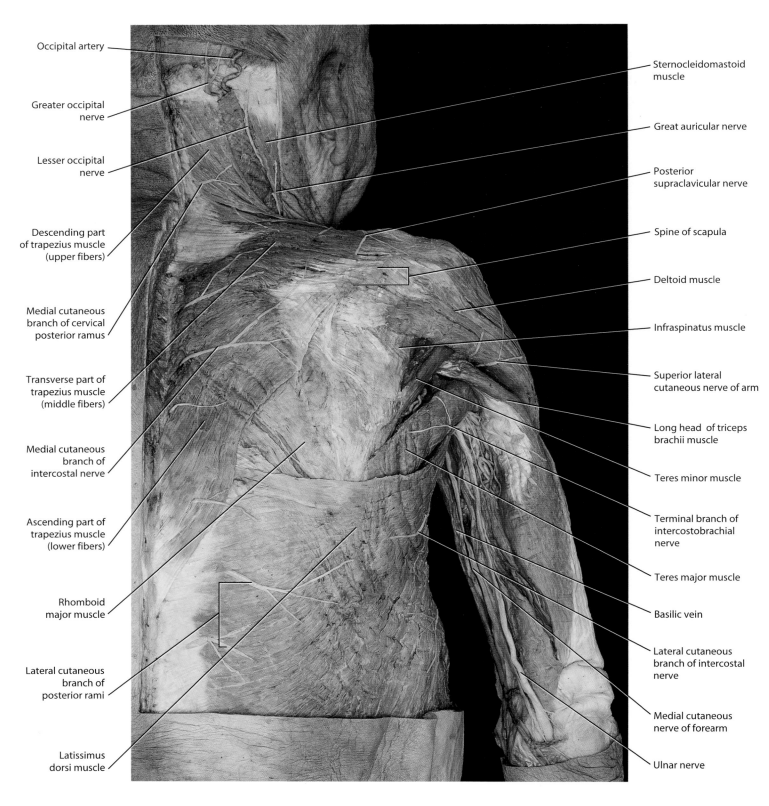

Occipital artery

Greater occipital
nerve

Lesser occipital
nerve

Descending part
of trapezius muscle
(upper fibers)

Medial cutaneous
branch of cervical
posterior ramus

Transverse part of
trapezius muscle
(middle fibers)

Medial cutaneous
branch of
intercostal nerve

Ascending part of
trapezius muscle
(lower fibers)

Rhomboid
major muscle

Lateral cutaneous
branch of
posterior rami

Latissimus
dorsi muscle

Sternocleidomastoid
muscle

Great auricular nerve

Posterior
supraclavicular nerve

Spine of scapula

Deltoid muscle

Infraspinatus muscle

Superior lateral
cutaneous nerve of arm

Long head of triceps
brachii muscle

Teres minor muscle

Terminal branch of
intercostobrachial
nerve

Teres major muscle

Basilic vein

Lateral cutaneous
branch of intercostal
nerve

Medial cutaneous
nerve of forearm

Ulnar nerve

Figure 17.5 Scapular region – superficial dissection. Right posterior shoulder and middle superficial back. The trapezius muscle converges on the spine of the scapula, and the superior margin of the latissimus dorsi muscle overlaps the inferior angle of the scapula and the most inferior part of the teres major muscle

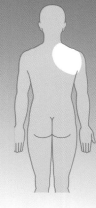

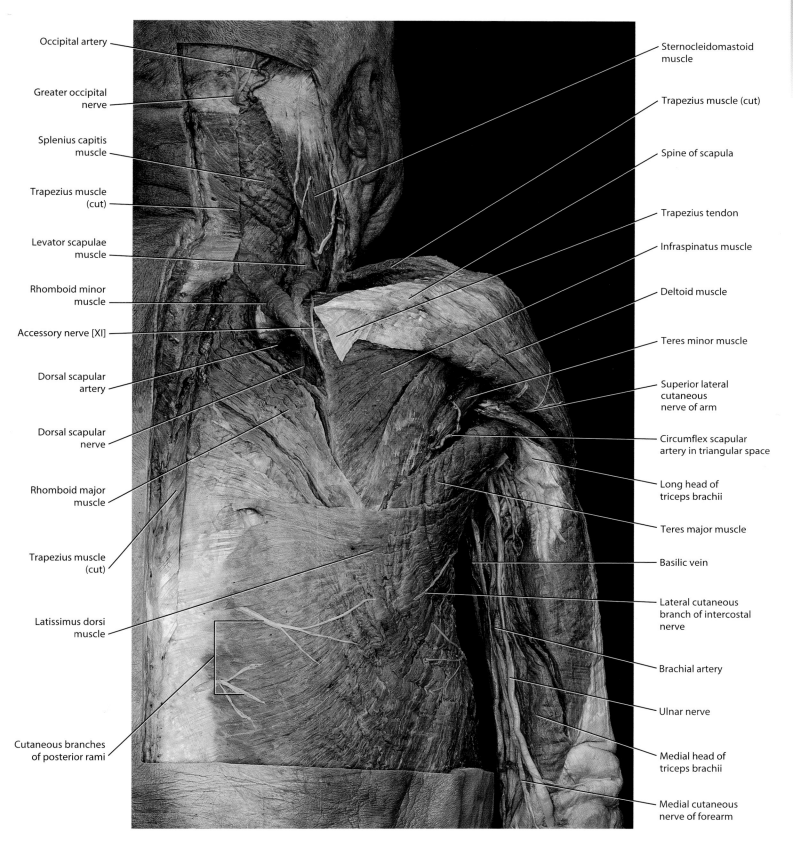

Occipital artery

Greater occipital nerve

Splenius capitis muscle

Trapezius muscle (cut)

Levator scapulae muscle

Rhomboid minor muscle

Accessory nerve [XI]

Dorsal scapular artery

Dorsal scapular nerve

Rhomboid major muscle

Trapezius muscle (cut)

Latissimus dorsi muscle

Cutaneous branches of posterior rami

Sternocleidomastoid muscle

Trapezius muscle (cut)

Spine of scapula

Trapezius tendon

Infraspinatus muscle

Deltoid muscle

Teres minor muscle

Superior lateral cutaneous nerve of arm

Circumflex scapular artery in triangular space

Long head of triceps brachii

Teres major muscle

Basilic vein

Lateral cutaneous branch of intercostal nerve

Brachial artery

Ulnar nerve

Medial head of triceps brachii

Medial cutaneous nerve of forearm

Figure 17.6 Scapular region – intermediate dissection. Right posterior shoulder with the trapezius cut and removed to show the muscles deep to it in the scapular region. The underlying levator scapulae and rhomboid muscles are seen converging on the medial border of the scapula

189

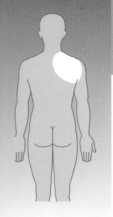

UPPER LIMB

Scapular region

		TABLE 17.1 SCAPULAR MUSCLES*			
Muscle	**Origin**	**Insertion**	**Innervation**	**Action**	**Blood supply**
Superficial extrinsic muscles Trapezius	Medial third of superior nuchal line, external occipital protuberance, ligamentum nuchae, spinous processes of CVII to TXII	Lateral third of posterior clavicle, medial acromion, superior edge of spine of scapula	Spinal root of accessory nerve [XI] and C3, C4	Elevates scapula (descending part), retracts scapula (transverse part), depresses scapula (ascending part); rotates scapula (descending & ascending parts acting together)	Transverse cervical artery, dorsal scapular artery
Latissimus dorsi	Spinous processes of TVII to TXII, thoracolumbar fascia, iliac crest, lower three to four ribs	Floor of intertubercular sulcus of humerus	Thoracodorsal nerve (**C6**, **C7**, C8)	Extends, adducts and medially rotates arm, draws shoulder downward and backward	Thoracodorsal artery
Deep extrinsic muscles Levator scapulae	Posterior tubercles of transverse processes CI to CIV	Medial border of scapula above base of spine of scapula	Dorsal scapular nerve (C5) and C3, C4	Elevates the scapula medially, inferiorly rotates glenoid cavity	Dorsal scapular artery, transverse cervical artery
Rhomboid minor	Ligamentum nuchae, spinous processes of CVII, TI	Medial border of scapula at base of spine of scapula	Dorsal scapular nerve (C4, **C5**)	Retracts and stabilizes the scapula	Dorsal scapular artery
Rhomboid major	Spinous processes of TII–TV	Medial border of scapula below base of spine of scapula	Dorsal scapular nerve (C4, **C5**)	Retracts and rotates scapula to depress the glenoid cavity	Dorsal scapular artery
Intrinsic muscles Deltoid	Lateral third of anterior clavicle, lateral acromion, inferior edge of spine of scapula	Deltoid tuberosity of humerus	Anterior and posterior branches of axillary nerve (**C5**, C6)	Clavicular part – flexes and medially rotates arm; acromial part – abducts arm; spinal part – extends and laterally rotates arm	Posterior circumflex humeral artery, deltoid branch of thoraco-acromial artery
Supraspinatus	Supraspinous fossa of scapula	Superior facet of greater tubercle of humerus	Suprascapular nerve (C4, **C5**, C6)	Initiates arm abduction, acts with rotator cuff muscles	Suprascapular artery
Infraspinatus	Infraspinous fossa of scapula	Middle facet of greater tubercle of humerus	Suprascapular nerve (**C5**, C6)	Lateral rotation of arm, (with teres minor)	Suprascapular artery
Teres minor	Upper two-thirds of posterior surface of lateral border of scapula	Inferior facet of greater tubercle of humerus	Posterior branch of axillary nerve (**C5**, C6)	Lateral rotation of arm, adduction	Circumflex scapular artery
Teres major	Posterior surface of inferior angle of scapula	Medial lip of intertubercular sulcus	Inferior subscapular nerve (**C6**, C7)	Adducts and medially rotates arm	Circumflex scapular artery
Subscapularis	Subscapular fossa	Lesser tubercle of humerus	Superior and inferior subscapular nerves (C5, **C6**, C7)	Medially rotates arm and adducts it	Subscapular artery, lateral thoracic artery

*Main nerve root is indicated in bold

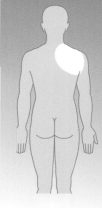

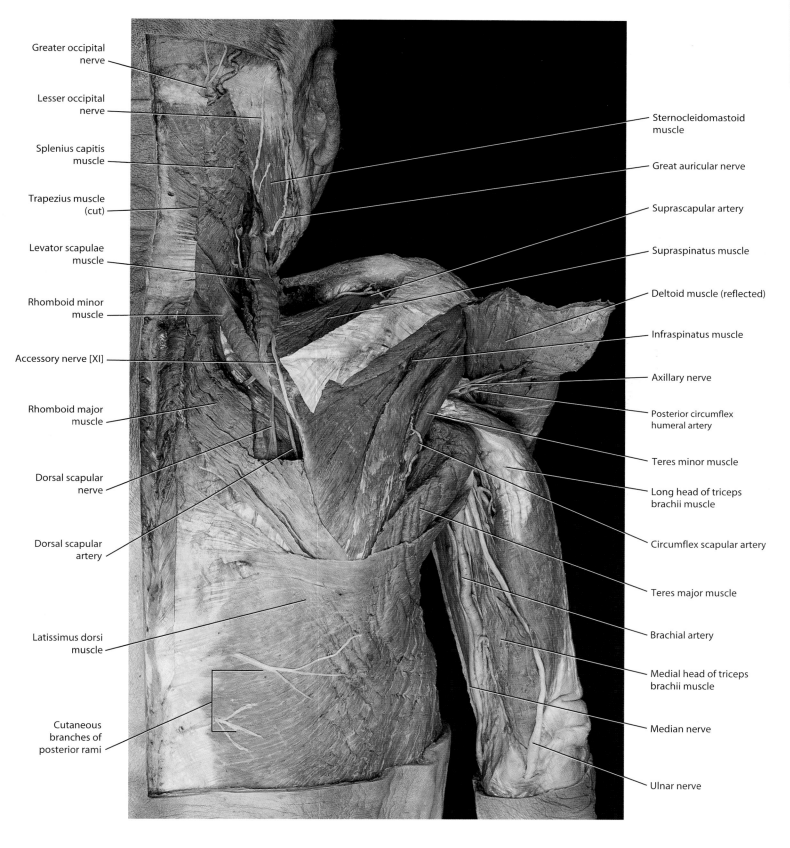

Greater occipital nerve

Lesser occipital nerve

Splenius capitis muscle

Trapezius muscle (cut)

Levator scapulae muscle

Rhomboid minor muscle

Accessory nerve [XI]

Rhomboid major muscle

Dorsal scapular nerve

Dorsal scapular artery

Latissimus dorsi muscle

Cutaneous branches of posterior rami

Sternocleidomastoid muscle

Great auricular nerve

Suprascapular artery

Supraspinatus muscle

Deltoid muscle (reflected)

Infraspinatus muscle

Axillary nerve

Posterior circumflex humeral artery

Teres minor muscle

Long head of triceps brachii muscle

Circumflex scapular artery

Teres major muscle

Brachial artery

Medial head of triceps brachii muscle

Median nerve

Ulnar nerve

Figure 17.7 Scapular region – deep dissection 1. Right posterior shoulder with the trapezius muscle removed and the posterior deltoid muscle cut and reflected laterally to show the muscles immediately attached to the scapula (supraspinatus, infraspinatus). Note the window in the rhomboid major muscle showing the dorsal scapular artery and nerve. The axillary nerve, with the posterior circumflex humeral artery is visible under the relected deltoid

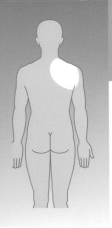

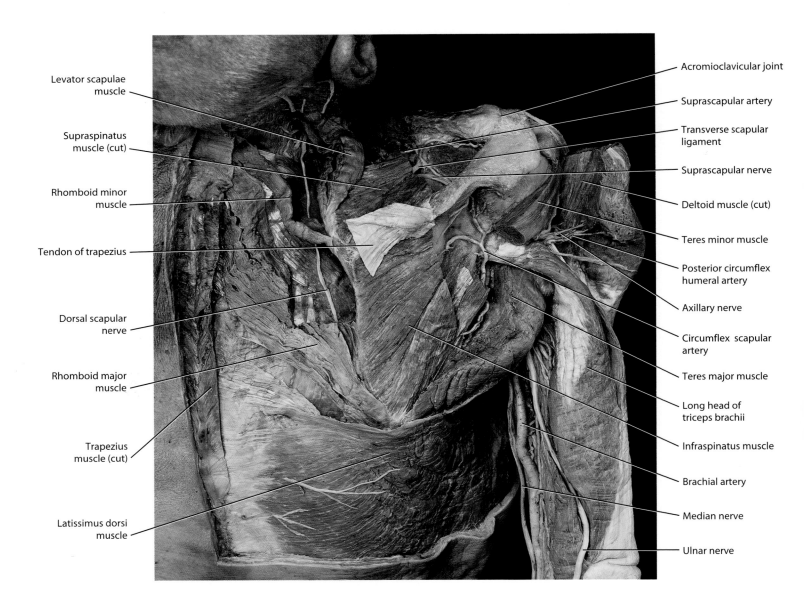

Levator scapulae muscle

Supraspinatus muscle (cut)

Rhomboid minor muscle

Tendon of trapezius

Dorsal scapular nerve

Rhomboid major muscle

Trapezius muscle (cut)

Latissimus dorsi muscle

Acromioclavicular joint

Suprascapular artery

Transverse scapular ligament

Suprascapular nerve

Deltoid muscle (cut)

Teres minor muscle

Posterior circumflex humeral artery

Axillary nerve

Circumflex scapular artery

Teres major muscle

Long head of triceps brachii

Infraspinatus muscle

Brachial artery

Median nerve

Ulnar nerve

Figure 17.8 Scapular region – deep dissection 2. Right shoulder with the trapezius muscle removed and posterior half of the deltoid muscle reflected laterally. Note that the central parts of the supraspinatus and infraspinatus and teres minor muscles have been removed to show the anastomosis between the suprascapular artery and the circumflex scapular branch of the subscapular artery. Part of the rhomboid major muscle has been removed to show the dorsal scapular nerve

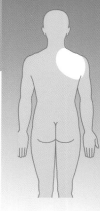

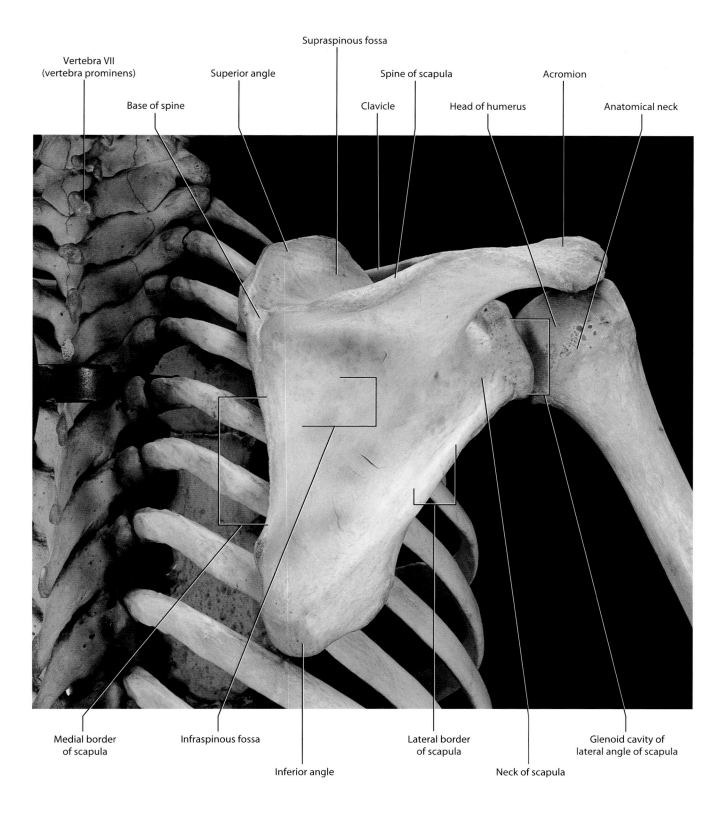

Vertebra VII
(vertebra prominens)

Base of spine

Superior angle

Supraspinous fossa

Spine of scapula

Clavicle

Head of humerus

Acromion

Anatomical neck

Medial border
of scapula

Infraspinous fossa

Inferior angle

Lateral border
of scapula

Neck of scapula

Glenoid cavity of
lateral angle of scapula

Figure 17.9 Scapular region – osteology. Posterior view of the articulated right scapula showing its position on the upper posterior rib cage, along with the proximal humerus

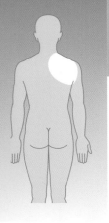

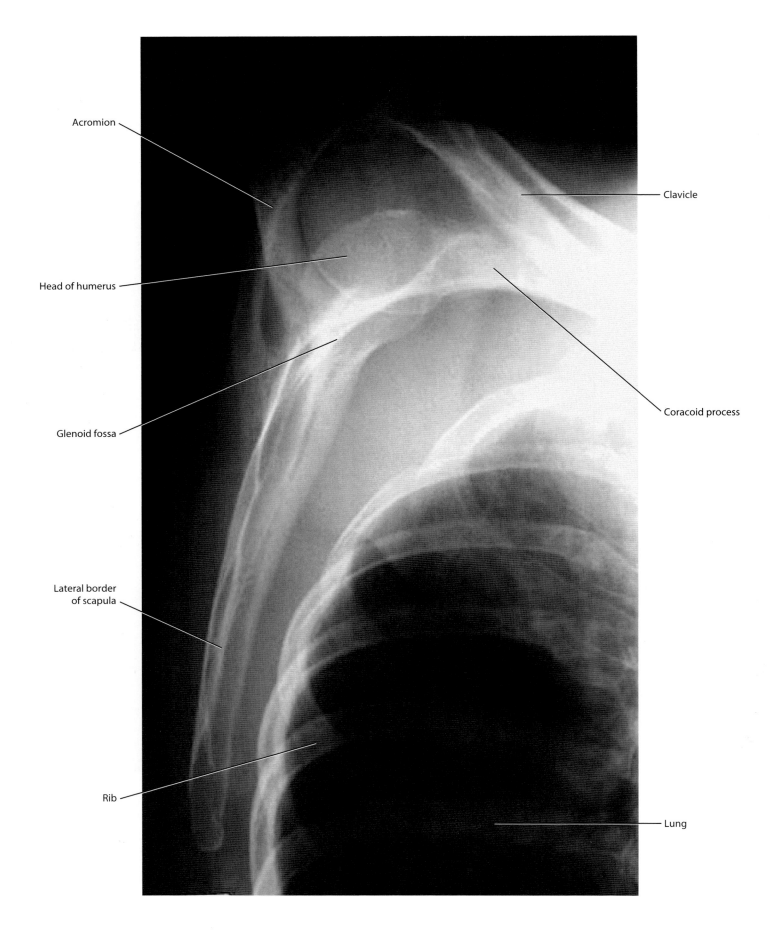

Acromion

Clavicle

Head of humerus

Coracoid process

Glenoid fossa

Lateral border
of scapula

Rib

Lung

Figure 17.10 Scapular region – plain film radiograph (lateral or 'Y' view). The humeral head sits centrally in the glenoid fossa with respect to the coracoid process (anterior) and acromion process (posterior). When there is displacement of the head of humerus towards the coracoid or acromion process, this suggests anterior or posterior dislocation, respectively.

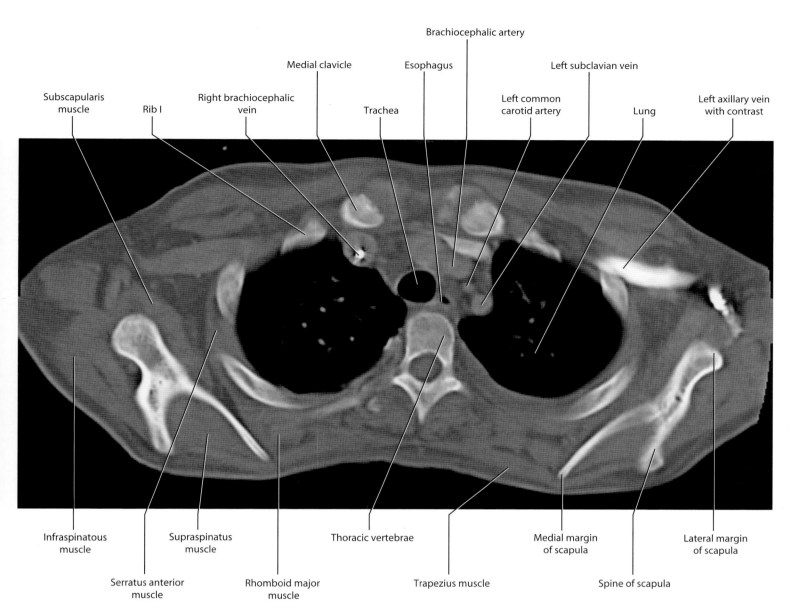

Figure 17.11 Scapular region – CT scan (axial view). The scapula is completely surrounded by muscles. This provides extensive protection to the scapula and also enables its mobility in supplementing the movements of the upper limb

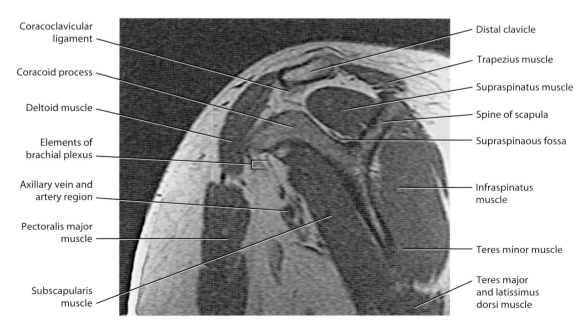

Figure 17.12 Scapular region – MRI scan (coronal oblique view). In the view here, note how the appearance of the scapula is similar to that in the 'Y' view plain film radiograph

195

Shoulder complex

The shoulder joint complex is composed of three joints – the sternoclavicular, acromioclavicular, and glenohumeral joints (Table 18.1). As a group, these attach the upper limb to the scapula and sternum (Figs 18.1 and 18.2). The mobility provided by three joints working together gives the shoulder complex a wide range of movement. The extensive mobility in the shoulder joint complex also results from the flexible support provided by numerous muscles, ligaments, and tendons. The bones articulating as part of the shoulder joint complex are the humerus, scapula, clavicle, and sternum.

STERNOCLAVICULAR JOINT

The sternoclavicular joint is a saddle synovial joint that joins the medial end of the clavicle to the manubrium of the sternum. It is the only point of osseous attachment of the upper limb to the torso. The glenohumeral and acromioclavicular joints join the upper limb to the scapula and clavicle.

Like the acromioclavicular joint (see below), the sternoclavicular joint has a thick fibrous capsule and an articular disc within the joint space. **Anterior** and **posterior sternoclavicular ligaments** reinforce the joint capsule. The **costoclavicular ligament** is a very strong ligament providing support to the posterior side of the joint as it joins the inferior surface of the medial clavicle to rib I. An additional **interclavicular ligament** bridges the space between the clavicles and prevents excessive inferior movement of the clavicle at the sternoclavicular joint.

Innervation of the sternoclavicular joint is provided by branches of the anterior supraclavicular nerves (C3 to C4) and by the subclavian nerve (C5, C6). Blood is supplied by the **internal**

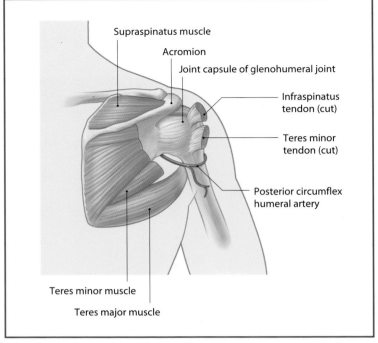

Figure 18.2 Glenohumeral joint (posterior view)

thoracic artery and venous drainage is to the suprascapular veins. Lymphatic drainage is to the supraclavicular, mediastinal, and axillary lymph nodes.

ACROMIOCLAVICULAR JOINT

The acromioclavicular joint connects the acromion of the scapula to the lateral end of the clavicle. It is a plane synovial joint with an articular disc within the joint space. The articular disc increases flexibility. The exterior surface of the joint is completely surrounded by the fibrous joint capsule. Superiorly the capsule is reinforced by the **superior acromioclavicular ligament**, and inferiorly by the **inferior acromioclavicular ligament**. The **coracoclavicular ligament**, which contains two parts (the lateral **trapezoid ligament** and the medial **conoid ligament**), provides the acromioclavicular joint with considerable stability without actually inserting onto the joint.

Innervation to the acromioclavicular joint is from the **supraclavicular** (C3 to C4), **suprascapular**, **lateral pectoral**, and axillary nerves, which are all components of the brachial plexus (see Chapter 16).

The primary blood supply to the acromioclavicular joint is from the **suprascapular artery** (from the thyrocervical trunk) and the **thoraco-acromial artery** (from the axillary artery). Venous drainage follows vessels named after the corresponding arteries and is towards the axillary vein. Lymphatic drainage is to the axillary lymph nodes.

GLENOHUMERAL JOINT

The glenohumeral joint (commonly referred to as the shoulder joint) is a ball-and-socket synovial joint formed by the articulation of the **head of humerus** with the **glenoid cavity** of the scapula.

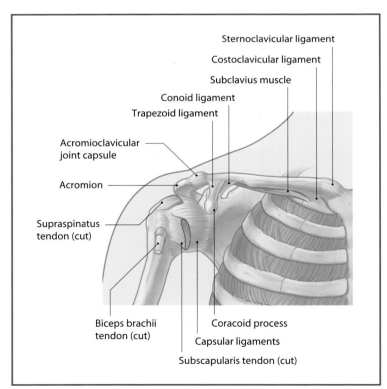

Figure 18.1 Glenohumeral joint (anterior view)

The shallow glenoid cavity is made more bowl-like by a fibrocartilaginous rim – the **glenoid labrum**. The glenohumeral joint is surrounded by a loose fibrous tissue joint capsule. The **glenohumeral ligaments** (superior, middle, and inferior) are three thickened areas forming a 'Z'-shaped line on the internal surface of the anterior wall of the joint capsule and prevent extreme lateral rotation of the humerus.

Laterally, the band-like **coracohumeral ligament** originates from the coracoid process of the scapula and inserts onto the superior part of the joint capsule and anatomical neck of the humerus next to the greater tubercle. The joint capsule is thickened by the **transverse humeral ligament** and is protected superiorly by the arching of the **coraco-acromial ligament**.

The head of the humerus is held in the glenoid cavity by four scapular muscles commonly referred to as the **rotator cuff** muscles – the supraspinatus, infraspinatus, teres minor, and subscapularis muscles.

The **suprascapular**, **axillary**, and **subscapular nerves** innervate the glenohumeral joint, and branch to form small nerve branches to the joint as they pass en route to the muscles they innervate.

Blood is supplied by the **anterior** and **posterior circumflex humeral arteries** (from the axillary artery) and the **suprascapular artery** (from the thyrocervical trunk) (Fig. 18.3).

Venous drainage is by the **anterior** and **posterior circumflex humeral veins** and the **suprascapular vein**, which together empty towards the axillary vein. Lymphatic drainage is to the **axillary lymph nodes**.

■ CLINICAL CORRELATIONS
Rotator cuff tears

The rotator cuff is a bowl- or 'cuff'-shaped structure that acts with the glenoid labrum to hold the head of the humerus to the glenoid cavity of the scapula at the glenohumeral joint. Four muscles – supraspinatus, infraspinatus, teres minor, and subscapularis – contribute to the rotator cuff, which is the tendon–ligament complex by which these muscles insert onto the humerus.

The rotator cuff can be injured by:

- fast repetitive movements of the upper limb, such as throwing a ball (baseball) or swinging a racket (tennis);
- traumatic movements that pull the humerus away from the glenoid cavity, for example reaching upward and grabbing hold of a stationary object during a fall to the ground or reaching down to catch and prevent a heavy object from hitting the floor.

These actions can pull the head of humerus partially 'out of socket', resulting in a strain (partial tear) or complete tearing of part of the rotator cuff (Fig. 18.4). The supporting tissues of the rotator cuff may also be injured, for example the bursae (connective tissue sacs containing small amounts of fluid) that decrease friction as muscles and tendons slide over other tissues. The tendon sheaths may also become inflamed, usually from overuse. A rotator cuff injury causes pain at and around the shoulder. In overuse injuries, patients may seek medical attention after a week and complain of pain when carrying out activities such as combing the hair or reaching up to open a cupboard.

Patients with traumatic injuries usually present to the hospital immediately. On examination, there may be swelling, ecchymosis (bruising), and tenderness over the involved shoulder. Its range of movement is reduced, as demonstrated by limited abduction of the arm beyond the horizontal plane because of pain. Specific movements are evaluated by the physician to determine the stability or laxity of the glenohumeral joint. The rotator cuff muscles are also tested individually to determine the site of injury. Radiographically, the modality that best demonstrates rotator cuff injury is magnetic resonance imaging (MRI).

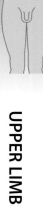
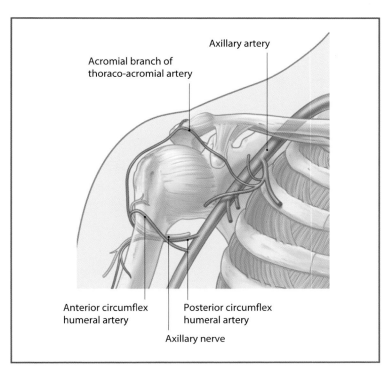

Figure 18.3 Nerves and vessels around the glenohumeral joint (anterior view)

Axillary artery

Acromial branch of thoraco-acromial artery

Anterior circumflex humeral artery

Posterior circumflex humeral artery

Axillary nerve

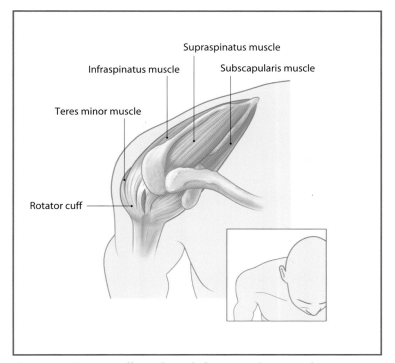

Figure 18.4 Rotator cuff tear through the supraspinatus tendon

Supraspinatus muscle

Infraspinatus muscle

Subscapularis muscle

Teres minor muscle

Rotator cuff

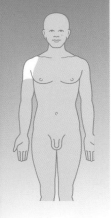

Treatment depends on the diagnosis, which may be bursitis, tendonitis (inflammation of the tendon), strain, or tear. The hallmark of treatment is to rest the shoulder and upper limb. Less severe problems, such as bursitis and tendonitis, are usually treated with rest, anti-inflammatory medications, and sometimes physical therapy. More severe injuries, such as a complete tear of the rotator cuff, should be referred to the orthopedist for possible surgical repair.

Acromioclavicular joint injuries

The acromioclavicular joint is superior to the glenohumeral joint and can be palpated as a bony prominence along the superior lateral margin of the shoulder region. It is one of two ligamentous articulations joining the clavicle to the scapula (acromioclavicular and sternoclavicular). Injuries in which a strong downward force is applied to the lateral shoulder can damage or separate the acromioclavicular joint (Fig. 18.5).

Patients complain of pain, swelling, and deformity at the lateral upper shoulder, which usually occur immediately after injury. They may also report an uneasy, painful sensation of instability at the acromioclavicular joint when the upper limb moves, and usually hold the injured limb very still.

On examination, there is deformity secondary to upward displacement and protrusion of the lateral clavicle, and the injured joint is also tender to palpation, Radiographs are usually obtained to determine the severity of the injury.

- Low-grade injuries to the acromioclavicular joint involve only minor strains (small tears) of the acromioclavicular joint capsule and there is no abnormality on radiography.
- Mid-grade injuries cause instability of the joint and radiography demonstrates some elevation of the lateral clavicle compared to the acromion of the scapula (subluxation). This discrepancy is usually less than the thickness of the clavicle.
- High-grade injuries cause dislocation of the acromioclavicular joint and tearing of the coracoclavicular ligament. Radiography

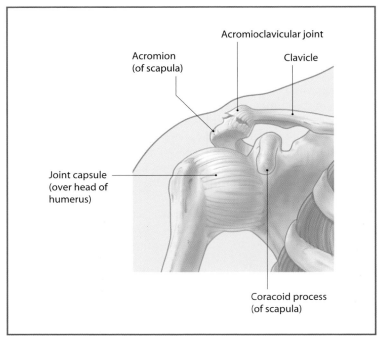

Figure 18.5 Partial disruption of the acromioclavicular joint due to falling on the top of the shoulder

demonstrates disparity greater than the thickness of the clavicle between the clavicle and acromion.

Treatment of most acromioclavicular joint injuries is nonsurgical, and includes medication for pain relief, the application of ice (cool packs), and immobilization with an arm sling. Return to normal activities is encouraged as comfort permits. More serious injuries may require surgical stabilization of the joint and repair of the torn acromioclavicular and coracoclavicular ligaments.

MNEMONIC

Rotator cuff muscles and their insertion on humerus: **SITS**
(**S**upraspinatus, **I**nfraspinatus, **T**eres major, **S**ubscapularis)
(Greater tubercle)   (Lesser tubercle)

TABLE 18.1 JOINTS OF THE SHOULDER COMPLEX

Joints	Type	Articular surface	Ligaments	Movement
Sternoclavicular	Saddle-type synovial joint	Concave facet of manubrium of sternum and concave facet of clavicle	Anterior sternoclavicular Posterior sternoclavicular Costoclavicular Interclavicular	Elevation ≅ 45° Depression ≅ 15° Protraction ≅ 15° Retraction ≅ 15° Transverse rotation ≅ 30°
Acromioclavicular	Plane-type synovial joint	Concave facet of acromion and convex facet of clavicle	Superior acromioclavicular Inferior acromioclavicular Coracoclavicular (medial – conoid, lateral – trapezoid)	Maintains clavicle/scapula relationship (no measurable movements)
Glenohumeral	Ball and socket-type synovial joint	Glenoid cavity of scapula and hemispheric head of humerus	Joint capsule Glenohumeral Coracohumeral Transverse humeral Coraco-acromial	Flexion ≅ 90° Extension ≅ 50° Abduction: 60–90° – 60° in internal rotation – 90° in external rotation External rotation ≅ 90° Internal rotation ≅ 90°

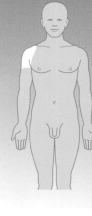

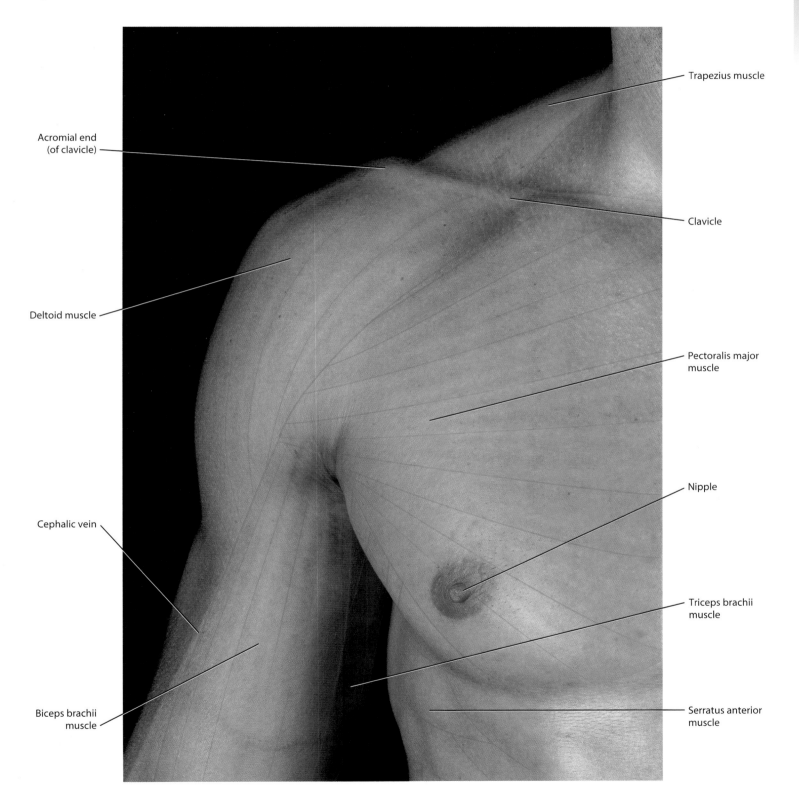

Trapezius muscle

Acromial end (of clavicle)

Clavicle

Deltoid muscle

Pectoralis major muscle

Nipple

Cephalic vein

Triceps brachii muscle

Biceps brachii muscle

Serratus anterior muscle

Figure 18.6 Shoulder complex – surface anatomy 1. Anterior view of the right shoulder of a young man

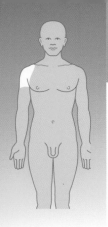

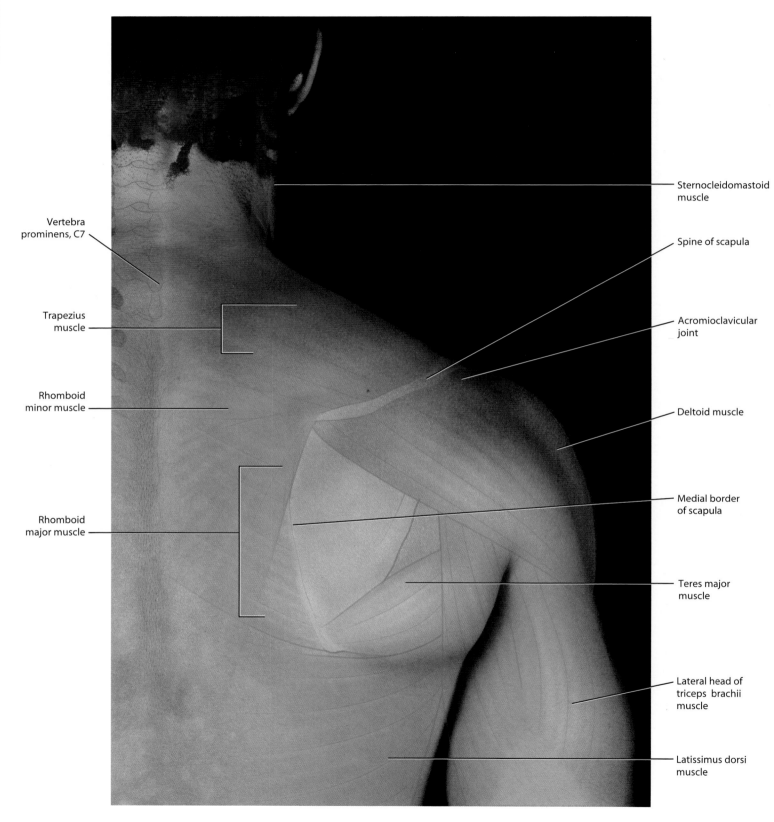

Sternocleidomastoid
muscle

Vertebra
prominens, C7

Spine of scapula

Trapezius
muscle

Acromioclavicular
joint

Rhomboid
minor muscle

Deltoid muscle

Rhomboid
major muscle

Medial border
of scapula

Teres major
muscle

Lateral head of
triceps brachii
muscle

Latissimus dorsi
muscle

Figure 18.7 Shoulder complex – surface anatomy 2. Posterior view of the right shoulder of a young man

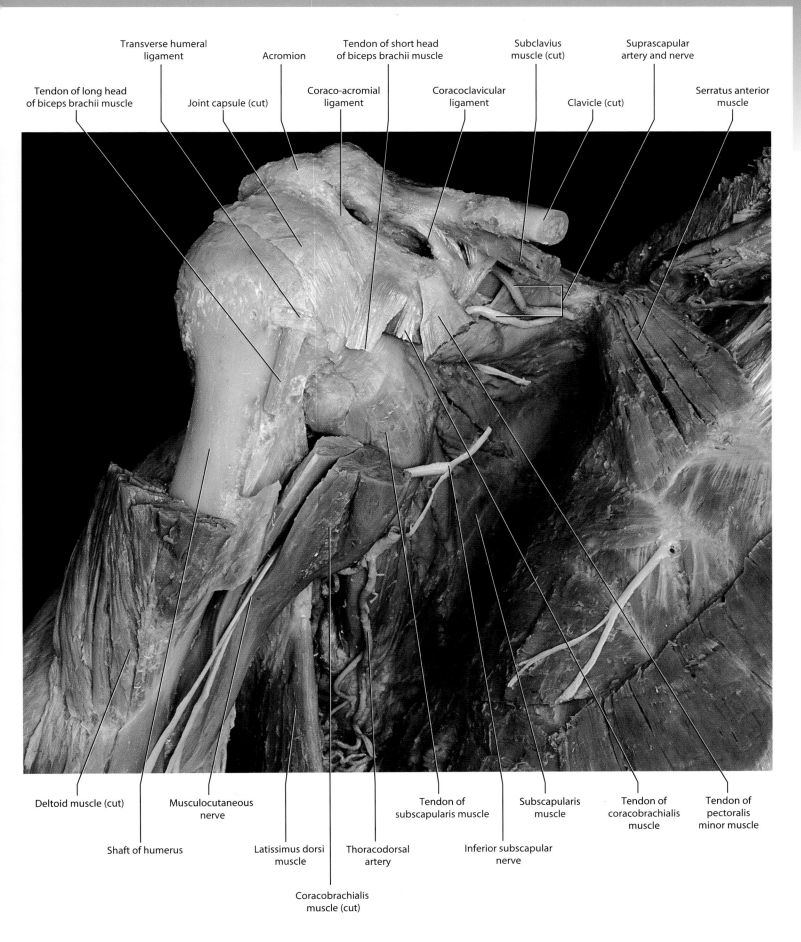

Transverse humeral ligament

Acromion

Tendon of short head of biceps brachii muscle

Subclavius muscle (cut)

Suprascapular artery and nerve

Tendon of long head of biceps brachii muscle

Joint capsule (cut)

Coraco-acromial ligament

Coracoclavicular ligament

Clavicle (cut)

Serratus anterior muscle

Deltoid muscle (cut)

Musculocutaneous nerve

Tendon of subscapularis muscle

Subscapularis muscle

Tendon of coracobrachialis muscle

Tendon of pectoralis minor muscle

Shaft of humerus

Latissimus dorsi muscle

Thoracodorsal artery

Inferior subscapular nerve

Coracobrachialis muscle (cut)

Figure 18.8 Shoulder complex – superficial dissection 1. Anterior view of a superficial dissection of the right shoulder joints (glenohumeral and acromioclavicular). The clavicle has been cut so that the joint could be mobilized laterally showing the muscles on the anterior surface of the scapula that insert onto the glenohumeral joint. The joint capsule is reinforced superiorly by the coraco-acromial ligament and anteriorly by the tendon of the subscapular muscle

201

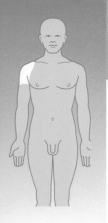

UPPER LIMB

Shoulder complex

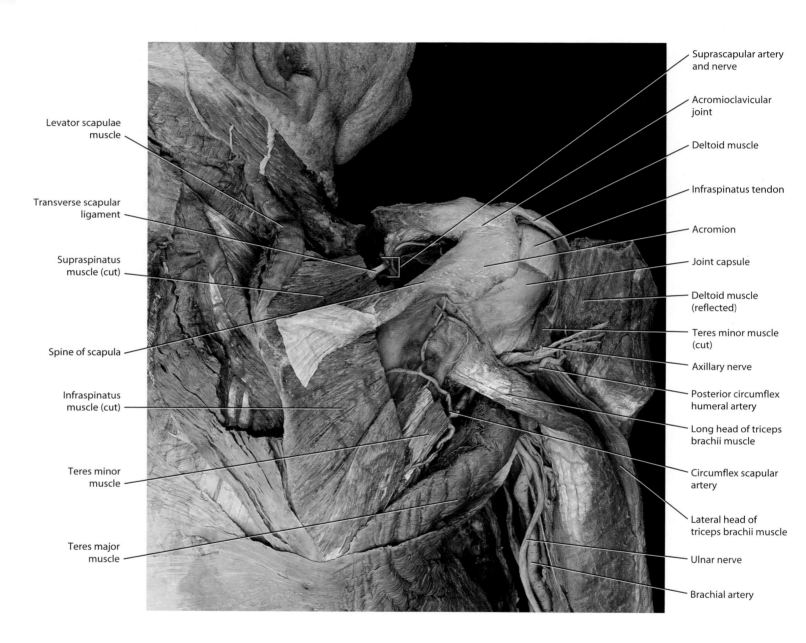

Levator scapulae muscle

Transverse scapular ligament

Supraspinatus muscle (cut)

Spine of scapula

Infraspinatus muscle (cut)

Teres minor muscle

Teres major muscle

Suprascapular artery and nerve

Acromioclavicular joint

Deltoid muscle

Infraspinatus tendon

Acromion

Joint capsule

Deltoid muscle (reflected)

Teres minor muscle (cut)

Axillary nerve

Posterior circumflex humeral artery

Long head of triceps brachii muscle

Circumflex scapular artery

Lateral head of triceps brachii muscle

Ulnar nerve

Brachial artery

Figure 18.9 Shoulder complex – superficial dissection 2. Posterior view of a superficial dissection of the right glenohumeral joint. The posterior glenohumeral joint capsule is reinforced by the deltoid muscle and the tendons of the infraspinatus and teres minor muscles. Observe how the muscles of the joint are related to the acromion process of the scapula

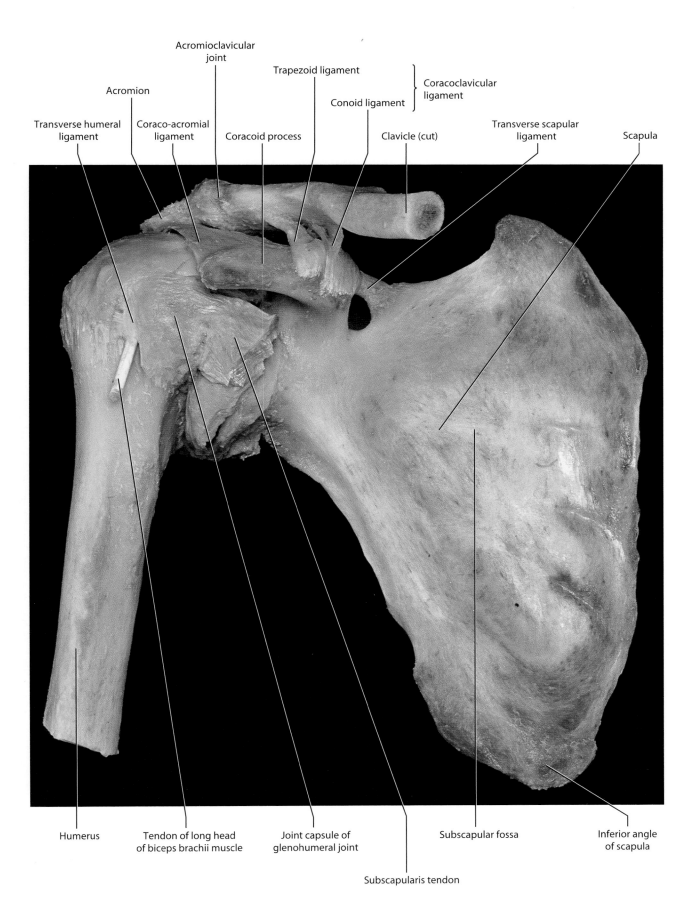

Acromioclavicular joint

Acromion

Trapezoid ligament

Conoid ligament

Coracoclavicular ligament

Transverse humeral ligament

Coraco-acromial ligament

Coracoid process

Clavicle (cut)

Transverse scapular ligament

Scapula

Humerus

Tendon of long head of biceps brachii muscle

Joint capsule of glenohumeral joint

Subscapular fossa

Inferior angle of scapula

Subscapularis tendon

Figure 18.10 Shoulder complex – deep dissection 1. Anterior view of a deep dissection of the right glenohumeral joint showing the capsule of the glenohumeral joint and the two parts of the coracoclavicular ligament (conoid and trapezoid ligaments), which support this region

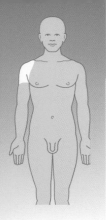

UPPER LIMB

Shoulder complex

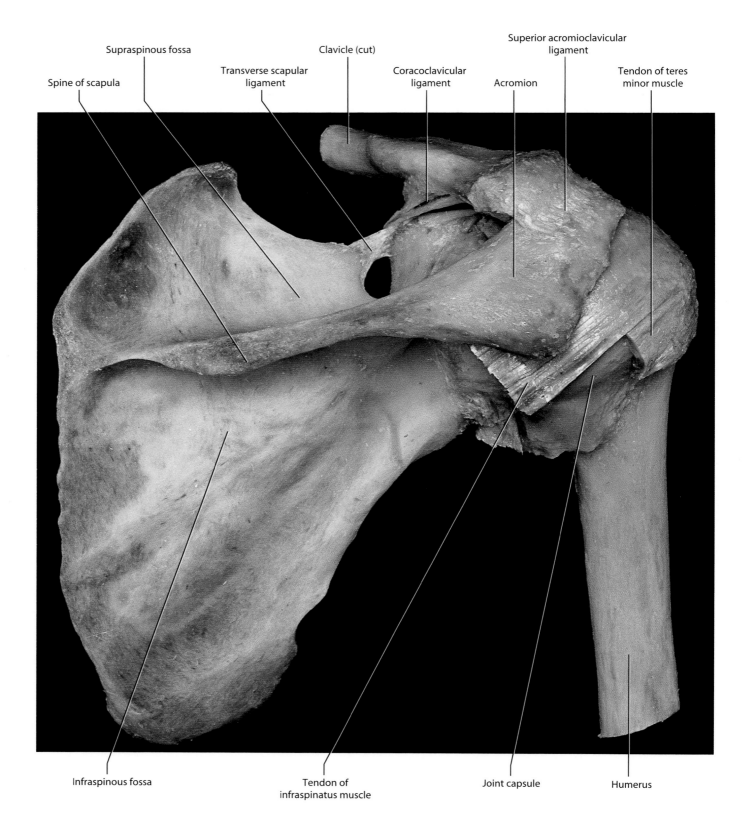

Supraspinous fossa

Spine of scapula

Transverse scapular ligament

Clavicle (cut)

Coracoclavicular ligament

Acromion

Superior acromioclavicular ligament

Tendon of teres minor muscle

Infraspinous fossa

Tendon of infraspinatus muscle

Joint capsule

Humerus

Figure 18.11 Shoulder complex – deep dissection 2. Posterior view of a deep dissection of the right glenohumeral joint. The scapula is still attached to the lateral clavicle and upper humerus by the supporting ligaments and joint sheaths. The spine of the scapula is visible

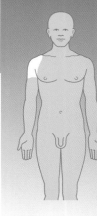

Spine of scapula

Tendon of long head of biceps
brachii muscle

Joint capsule (cut)

Infraspinatus muscle

Glenoid labrum

Acromion

Tendon of
infraspinatus muscle

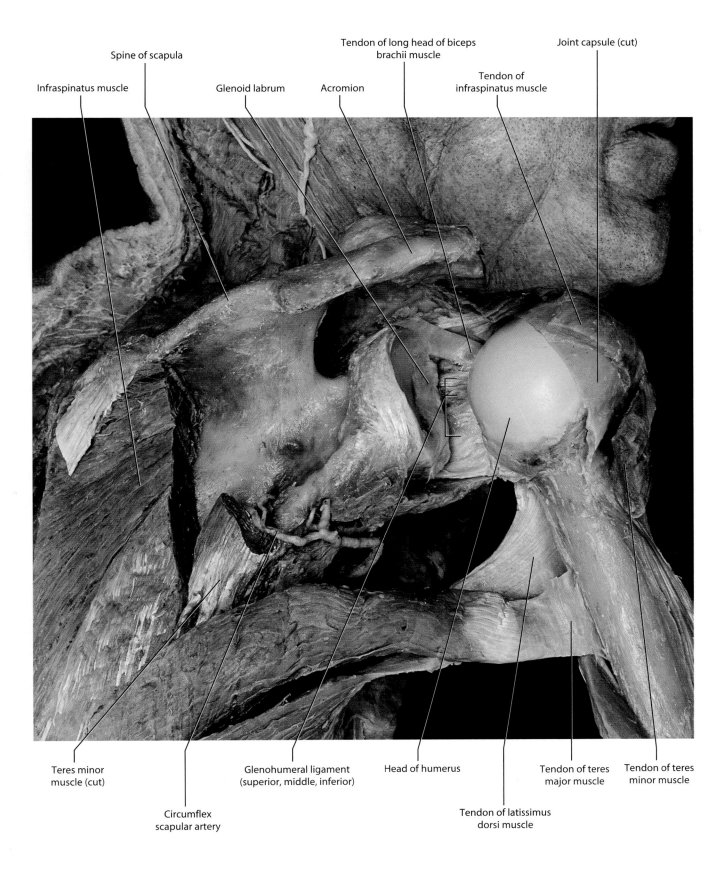

Teres minor
muscle (cut)

Glenohumeral ligament
(superior, middle, inferior)

Head of humerus

Tendon of teres
major muscle

Tendon of teres
minor muscle

Circumflex
scapular artery

Tendon of latissimus
dorsi muscle

Figure 18.12 Shoulder complex – deep dissection 3. Posterolateral view of the right glenohumeral joint. The posterior wall of the capsule has been cut and the arm is medially rotated to show the glenohumeral ligaments that reinforce the inside of the anterior capsule wall

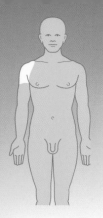

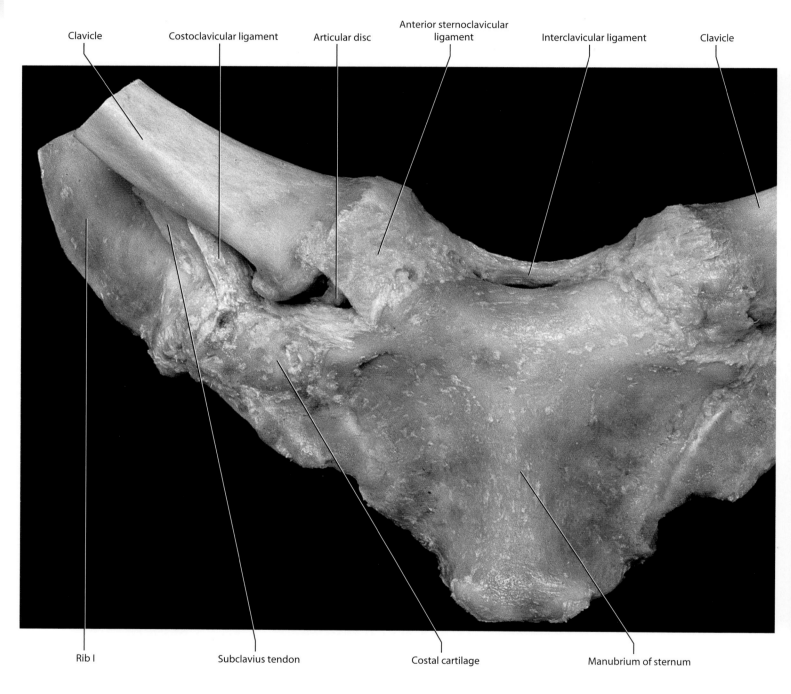

Clavicle Costoclavicular ligament Articular disc Anterior sternoclavicular ligament Interclavicular ligament Clavicle

Rib I Subclavius tendon Costal cartilage Manubrium of sternum

Figure 18.13 Sternoclavicular joint – isolated. Anterior view of the manubrium of sternum showing the uppermost part of the sternum and the medial ends of the clavicles as they join the sternum at the sternoclavicular joint. The first rib is also visible, contributing to this joint. Part of the anterior sternoclavicular ligament has been removed to show the anterior part of the articular disc

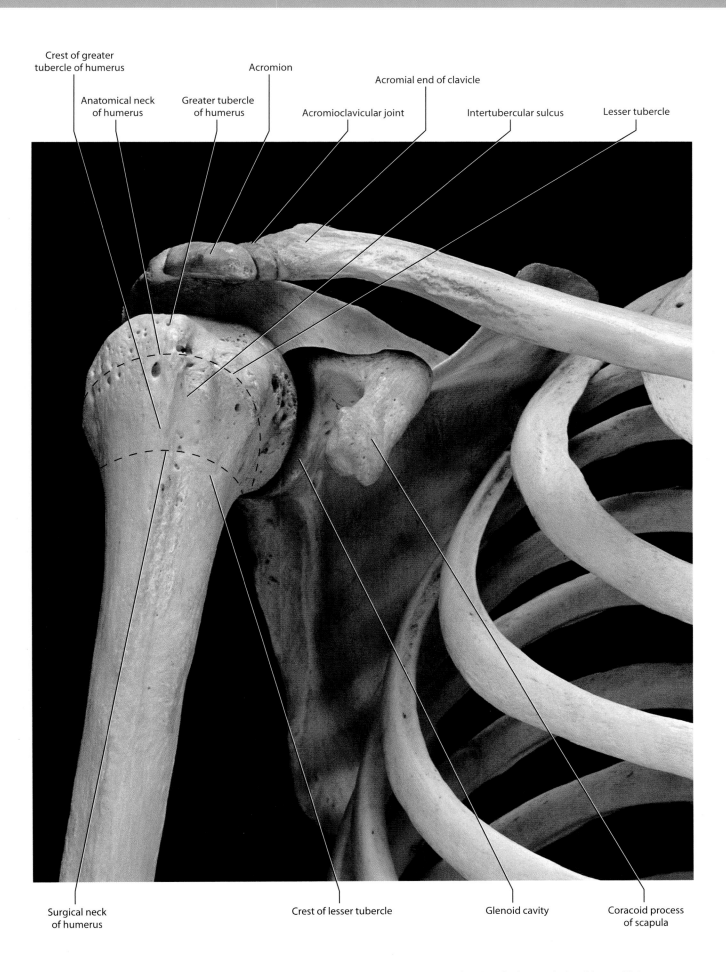

Crest of greater
tubercle of humerus

Anatomical neck
of humerus

Greater tubercle
of humerus

Acromion

Acromioclavicular joint

Acromial end of clavicle

Intertubercular sulcus

Lesser tubercle

Surgical neck
of humerus

Crest of lesser tubercle

Glenoid cavity

Coracoid process
of scapula

Figure 18.14 Shoulder complex – osteology. Anterior articulated view of the right shoulder joints showing the bony relationships and joints

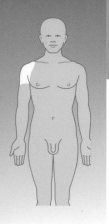

UPPER LIMB

Shoulder complex

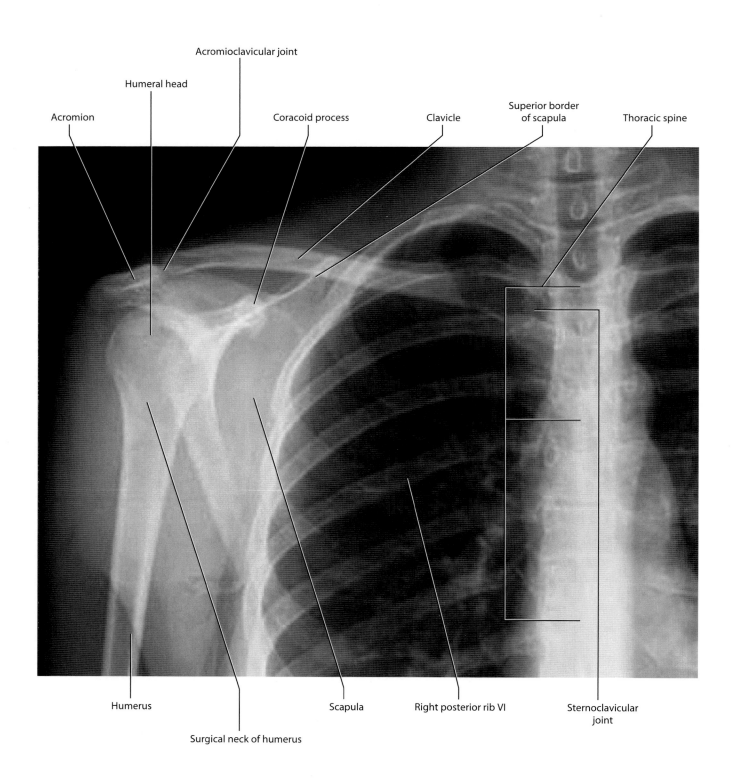

Acromioclavicular joint

Humeral head

Acromion

Coracoid process

Clavicle

Superior border of scapula

Thoracic spine

Humerus

Surgical neck of humerus

Scapula

Right posterior rib VI

Sternoclavicular joint

Figure 18.15 Shoulder complex – plain film radiograph (anteroposterior view). From this view it is clear how the acromioclavicular joint can prevent the humerus from dislocating superiorly. Also note the two-part articulation between the scapula and humerus through the glenohumeral joint, and the scapula and clavicle through the acromioclavicular joint

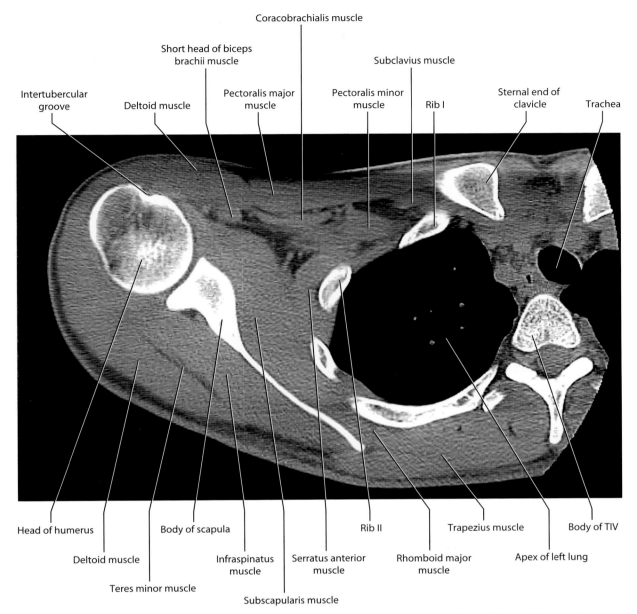

Coracobrachialis muscle

Short head of biceps brachii muscle

Subclavius muscle

Intertubercular groove

Deltoid muscle

Pectoralis major muscle

Pectoralis minor muscle

Rib I

Sternal end of clavicle

Trachea

Head of humerus

Deltoid muscle

Body of scapula

Infraspinatus muscle

Rib II

Serratus anterior muscle

Trapezius muscle

Body of TIV

Rhomboid major muscle

Apex of left lung

Teres minor muscle

Subscapularis muscle

Figure 18.16 Shoulder complex – CT scan (axial view). Note how the head of humerus articulates with the glenoid fossa of the scapula

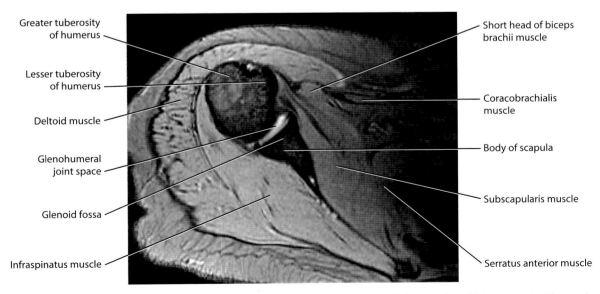

Greater tuberosity of humerus

Lesser tuberosity of humerus

Deltoid muscle

Glenohumeral joint space

Glenoid fossa

Infraspinatus muscle

Short head of biceps brachii muscle

Coracobrachialis muscle

Body of scapula

Subscapularis muscle

Serratus anterior muscle

Figure 18.17 Shoulder complex – MRI scan (axial view). This view shows the glenohumeral joint and the muscles which support it. Observe how the deltoid muscle protects the lateral portion of the joint. MRI is valuable in imaging the integrity of muscles and tendons of the shoulder. If rotator cuff tears are present they are easily visualized

The arm is the part of the upper limb that extends from the shoulder to the elbow. The upper part of the arm receives tendons from the shoulder and scapular region whereas the lower part sends tendons to the forearm. This unique arrangement enables the arm to take part in:

- flexion, extension, abduction, adduction, and circumduction at the glenohumeral joint;
- flexion and extension at the elbow joint.

The arm is supported by the **humerus** (arm bone), the upper end of which (the **head** of humerus) is ball-shaped to enable articulation with the glenoid cavity of the scapula. The **anatomical neck** separates the head from the proximal part of the shaft of the humerus and has two prominences:

- the anteriorly facing **lesser tubercle**;
- the laterally placed **greater tubercle**.

These tubercles are separated by the **intertubercular sulcus**, which receives the tendon of the long head of the biceps brachii muscle. The region where the tubercles join the shaft of humerus is the **surgical neck** of the humerus and is a common fracture site. The long slender shaft of humerus provides attachment areas for the arm muscles. Near its distal end, the humerus is expanded medially and laterally by the **medial** and **lateral supracondylar ridges** and the subjacent **medial** and **lateral epicondyles**. The distal end of the humerus has articular surfaces:

- the **trochlea** articulates with the ulna;
- the **capitulum** articulates with the radius;
- the **olecranon fossa** on the posterior surface accommodates the olecranon of the ulna at the elbow joint during extension.

MUSCLES

The deep fascia that surrounds the arm gives rise to the **medial** and **lateral intermuscular septa of arm**. These fascial walls divide the arm into the **anterior** (flexor) and **posterior** (extensor) **compartments**:

- the medial intermuscular septum of arm extends from the medial lip of the intertubercular sulcus at the superior humerus to the inferiorly located medial epicondyle;
- the lateral intermuscular septum of arm extends from the lateral lip of the intertubercular sulcus at the superior humerus to the inferiorly placed lateral epicondyle.

Superiorly, the compartmentalization of the arm is completed by the blending of the medial and lateral intermuscular septa with the deep fascia of the coracobrachialis and deltoid muscles, respectively. The posterior compartment of arm contains the **triceps brachii** muscle, which has three heads originating superiorly from the humerus and scapula and joining inferiorly to insert onto the olecranon process of the ulna (Figs 19.1 and 19.2). This arrangement makes the triceps brachii a strong extensor of the forearm at the elbow joint. The radial nerve (from the brachial

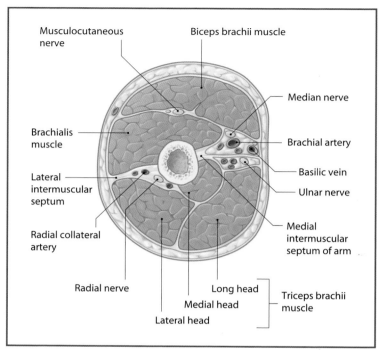

Figure 19.1 Cross-section through the mid right arm (viewed from distal to proximal)

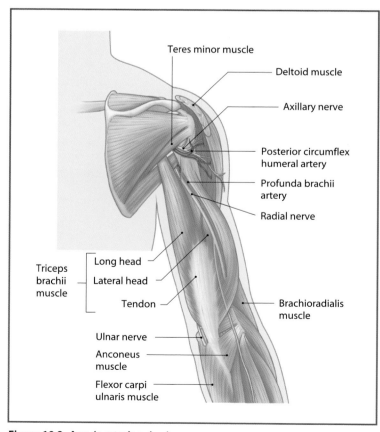

Figure 19.2 Arm (posterior view)

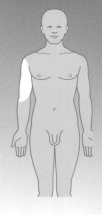

plexus) provides innervation and the profunda brachii (deep brachial artery branching off the brachial artery) supplies blood. The ulnar nerve passes through the inferior part of the posterior compartment of the arm on its way to the hand.

The flexor compartment of the arm contains the **biceps brachii** muscle, which has two heads of origin, and the **coracobrachialis** and **brachialis** muscles (Fig. 19.3). These three muscles have points of origin on the humerus and scapula and insert inferiorly onto the radius and **bicipital aponeurosis** (a thickening of the dense fascia of the forearm). This arrangement enables the anterior arm muscles to help flex the arm at the glenohumeral joint and to flex the forearm at the elbow joint. Innervation to the anterior arm muscles is by the musculocutaneous nerve (from the brachial plexus) and blood is supplied by the brachial artery (Table 19.1).

NERVES

The anterior and posterior compartments of the arm are innervated by the musculocutaneous and radial nerves. In addition, two major nerves from the brachial plexus (the median and ulnar nerves) pass through the arm to innervate structures in the forearm and hand.

The **musculocutaneous nerve** (C5 to C7 from the lateral cord of the brachial plexus) pierces the coracobrachialis muscle and descends between the biceps brachii and brachialis muscles to the lateral arm. It supplies the three flexor muscles of the arm, sends an articular branch to the elbow joint, and terminates as the **lateral cutaneous nerve of forearm**, which conveys sensation to the lateral forearm.

The **radial nerve** (C5 to T1 from the posterior cord of the brachial plexus) passes posteriorly with the profunda brachii artery and winds around the shaft of the humerus in the **radial groove** inferior to the long and lateral heads of the triceps brachii muscle. It innervates the triceps brachii and elbow joint and branches to form the **posterior cutaneous nerve of arm**, which innervates the skin of the posterior arm, and the **posterior cutaneous nerve of forearm**, which innervates the skin of the posterior forearm. On reaching the distal part of the posterior forearm the radial nerve turns anteriorly toward the cubital fossa, between the brachioradialis and brachialis muscles (see Chapter 20). The radial nerve terminates by dividing into **superficial** and **deep branches** at the level of the lateral epicondyle of the humerus. The superficial branch conveys sensation to the distal lateral forearm and hand; the deep branch innervates the muscles of the posterior forearm and skin on the dorsum of the hand.

The **median nerve** (C6 to T1 from the medial and lateral cords of the brachial plexus) is lateral to the brachial artery in the anterior compartment of the upper arm but passes medially as it descends, crossing the elbow joint medial to the brachial artery to enter the forearm.

The **ulnar nerve** (C8 to T1 from the medial cord of the brachial plexus) is in the anterior compartment of the arm medial to the brachial artery in the upper arm. It pierces the medial intermuscular septum to enter the posterior compartment of the arm at the level of the insertion of the coracobrachialis muscle in the mid-arm. It descends in the medial posterior compartment toward the elbow, where it is just deep to the skin at a point on the posterior elbow between the medial epicondyle of the humerus and the olecranon of the ulna.

ARTERIES

The **brachial artery** and its branches supply blood to the arm. This blood vessel is a continuation of the axillary artery at the lower border of the teres major muscle. It descends medial to the humerus within the anterior compartment of arm and branches to form the deep **profunda brachii artery** and the **superior** and **inferior** ulnar collateral arteries. On reaching the cubital fossa, the brachial artery is lateral to the median nerve. It ends at the level of the neck of the radius by dividing into the **radial** and **ulnar arteries**.

VEINS AND LYMPHATICS

The **cephalic** and **basilic veins** are the main superficial veins of the arm. They are formed from the lateral and medial ends of the dorsal venous network of hand (see Chapter 24).

- The cephalic vein ascends lateral to the biceps brachii muscle (on its anterior surface), then enters the deltopectoral groove formed by the adjacent deltoid and pectoralis muscles, from where it pierces the fascia in the deltopectoral triangle to enter the **axillary vein**.
- The basilic vein ascends medial to the biceps brachii muscle (on its medial surface) and accompanies the brachial artery to the axilla, where it joins the **brachial vein**, which becomes the axillary vein at the inferior border of the teres major muscle.

Deep venous drainage of the arm is through veins that share the names of the corresponding arteries and empty into the brachial

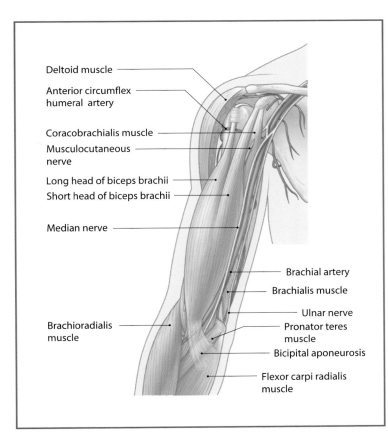

Deltoid muscle

Anterior circumflex humeral artery

Coracobrachialis muscle

Musculocutaneous nerve

Long head of biceps brachii

Short head of biceps brachii

Median nerve

Brachioradialis muscle

Brachial artery

Brachialis muscle

Ulnar nerve

Pronator teres muscle

Bicipital aponeurosis

Flexor carpi radialis muscle

Figure 19.3 Arm (anterior view)

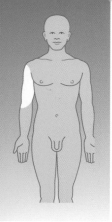
vein. Lymphatic drainage of the arm is to the **cubital** and **axillary lymph nodes**.

■ CLINICAL CORRELATIONS
Glenohumeral joint dislocation

The glenohumeral joint is the ball-and-socket joint that gives the shoulder its wide range of movement. It is one of the most commonly dislocated major joints, partly because of its flexibility and orientation. Dislocation of the head of humerus from the glenoid cavity can be anterior, posterior, inferior, or superior. Anterior dislocations are most common. In younger people, glenohumeral dislocation usually occurs during athletic injuries in which abnormal force is applied to the shoulder while the arm is extended, abducted, and externally rotated (similar to the position adopted to wave to a friend). In older people, glenohumeral dislocation can occur from a fall onto an outstretched arm.

Anterior glenohumeral dislocation causes severe pain and patients usually hold the dislocated arm in external rotation and slight abduction. Many try to support the injured shoulder using the uninjured limb. On examination, there will also be abnormal prominence of the acromion of the scapula. The gentle sloping of the shoulder lateral to the acromion is deficient and appears 'dented'. Anteriorly, the shoulder will protrude abnormally. The neurovasculature of the affected limb must be examined because there may be nerve or arterial injury. The most commonly injured nerve is the axillary nerve. Careful examination of sensation around the shoulder and muscle strength of the deltoid is essential because it is innervated by the axillary nerve.

Radiographs in two viewing angles (anteroposterior and lateral) should be obtained before attempting to reduce the dislocated joint. Findings on radiography usually show the head of humerus anterior and inferior to the glenoid cavity of the scapula. The radiograph must be carefully examined for an associated fracture of the humerus or scapula, which is not uncommon.

Treatment aims to replace the head of humerus into the glenoid cavity. Adequate muscle relaxation and pain control are helpful before reduction because there are many supporting muscles around the shoulder. The examiner then carries out a specific maneuver to reduce the dislocation. Post-reduction radiographs are required to reveal any residual fracture and ensure proper replacement of the joint. A repeat neurovascular examination is also necessary. The limb is immobilized using a simple arm sling or other immobilization method.

Glenohumeral dislocation treated by nonoperative reduction may be associated with a concomitant rotator cuff injury or persistent instability of the joint, and close follow-up is indicated to monitor healing and initiate any further treatment. Only severe or refractory cases of glenohumeral joint dislocation are managed operatively.

Humeral fracture

Fractures of the humerus (Fig. 19.4) tend to be caused by a high-energy impact to the upper limb; motor vehicle accidents are one of the more common causes. Because of its size, fractures can occur at any point along the humerus.

The extreme pain associated with such injuries means that patients cannot use the injured limb and usually seek immediate medical attention. Sometimes, impingement of one of the nerves of the brachial plexus causes a neurologic deficit, which the patient reports as a region of numbness. Patients with a nerve injury do not usually complain of paralysis because of the extreme pain, which results in them holding the injured arm very still.

Vascular injuries can also go unnoticed during the initial examination if a thorough neurovascular examination is not carried out. It is very important for the clinician to examine the patient carefully and to search for additional injuries, such as a fractured clavicle or scapula.

Radiographs reveal the site of the fracture. In proximal humeral fractures, the radiograph should be checked for bone fragments in the glenohumeral joint. Likewise, distal fractures necessitate examination of the elbow joint.

Fractures of the shaft of the humerus are unstable and must be stabilized to prevent neurovascular damage. In children, stabilization can usually be achieved using a 'hanging' arm cast. Surgery is almost always necessary in adults.

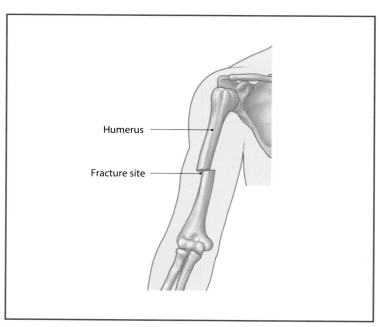

Figure 19.4 Fracture of the humerus

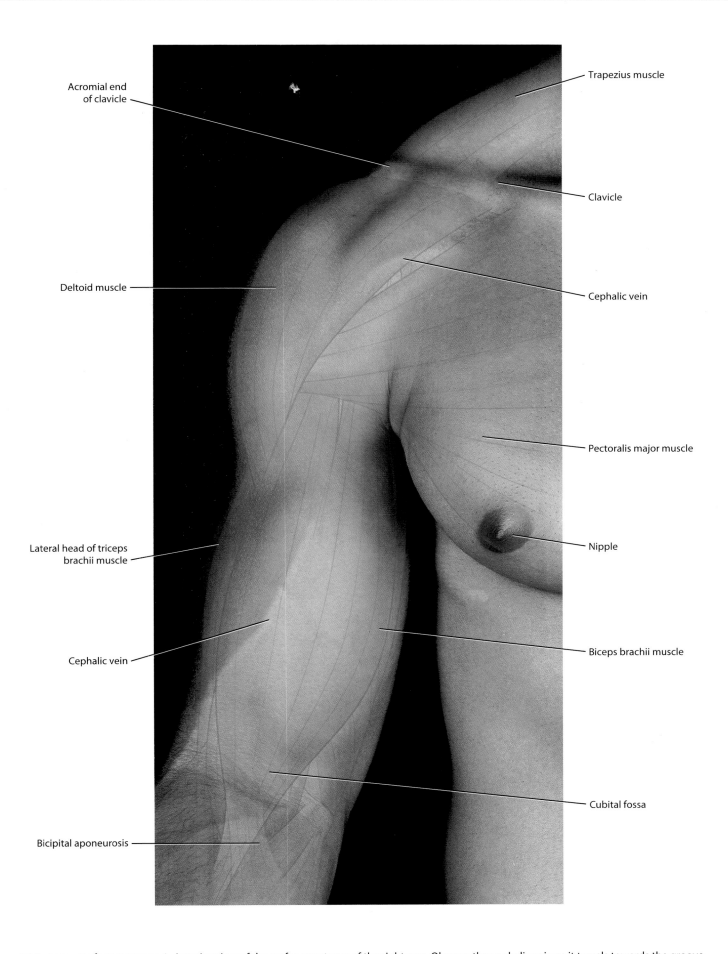

Acromial end
of clavicle

Deltoid muscle

Lateral head of triceps
brachii muscle

Cephalic vein

Bicipital aponeurosis

Trapezius muscle

Clavicle

Cephalic vein

Pectoralis major muscle

Nipple

Biceps brachii muscle

Cubital fossa

Figure 19.5 Arm – surface anatomy 1. Anterior view of the surface anatomy of the right arm. Observe the cephalic vein as it travels towards the groove between the deltoid and pectoralis muscles

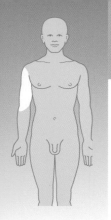

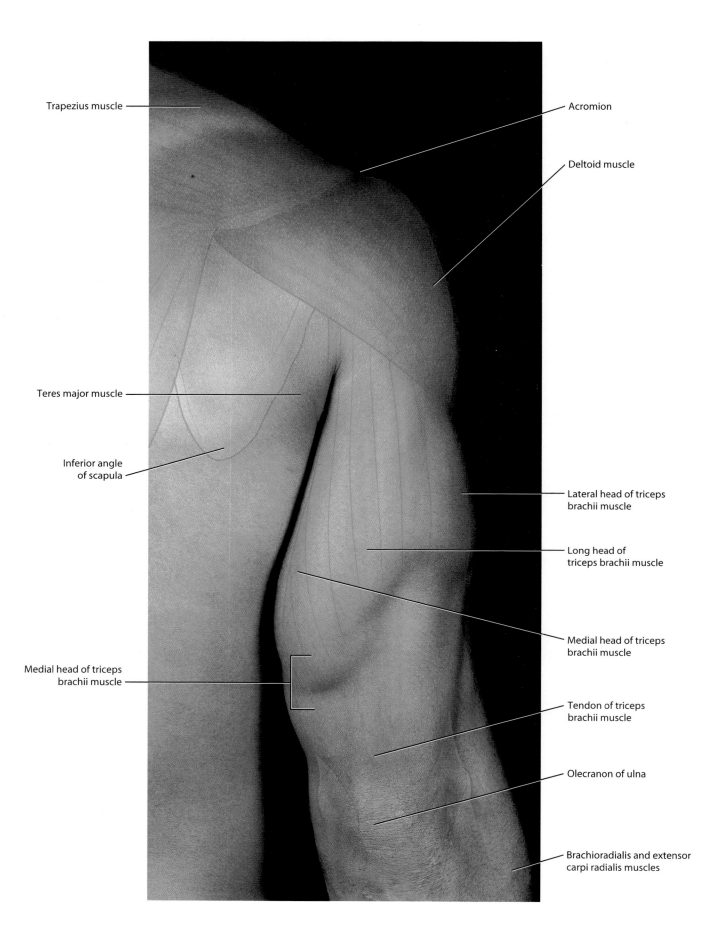

Trapezius muscle

Acromion

Deltoid muscle

Teres major muscle

Inferior angle
of scapula

Lateral head of triceps
brachii muscle

Long head of
triceps brachii muscle

Medial head of triceps
brachii muscle

Medial head of triceps
brachii muscle

Tendon of triceps
brachii muscle

Olecranon of ulna

Brachioradialis and extensor
carpi radialis muscles

Figure 19.6 Arm – surface anatomy 2. Posterior view of the surface anatomy of the right arm. Observe the three heads of the triceps brachii muscle

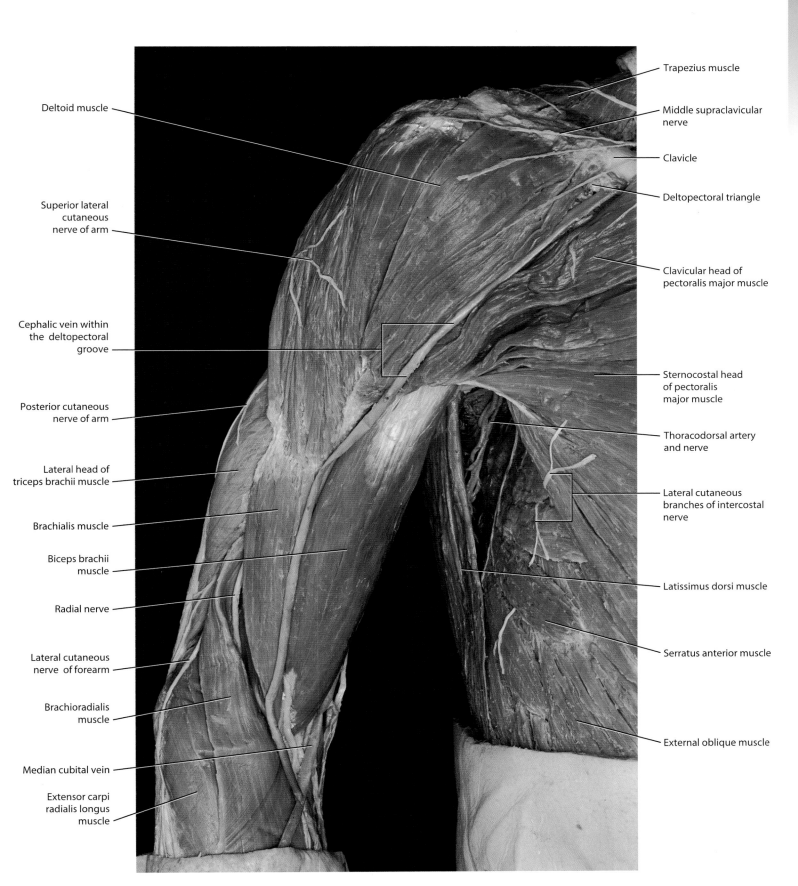

Deltoid muscle

Superior lateral
cutaneous
nerve of arm

Cephalic vein within
the deltopectoral
groove

Posterior cutaneous
nerve of arm

Lateral head of
triceps brachii muscle

Brachialis muscle

Biceps brachii
muscle

Radial nerve

Lateral cutaneous
nerve of forearm

Brachioradialis
muscle

Median cubital vein

Extensor carpi
radialis longus
muscle

Trapezius muscle

Middle supraclavicular
nerve

Clavicle

Deltopectoral triangle

Clavicular head of
pectoralis major muscle

Sternocostal head
of pectoralis
major muscle

Thoracodorsal artery
and nerve

Lateral cutaneous
branches of intercostal
nerve

Latissimus dorsi muscle

Serratus anterior muscle

External oblique muscle

Figure 19.7 Arm – superficial dissection 1. Right anterior arm showing the cephalic vein between the brachialis and biceps brachii muscles. Note the radial nerve between brachialis and brachioradialis. Observe the cephalic vein as it ascends the arm and enters the groove between the deltoid and pectoralis muscles and deltopectoral triangle

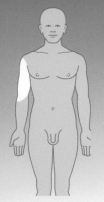

TABLE 19.1 ARM MUSCLES*					
Muscle	**Origin**	**Insertion**	**Innervation**	**Action**	**Blood supply**
Biceps brachii	Long head – supraglenoid tubercle of humerus; Short head: tip of coracoid process of scapula	Radial tuberosity, fascia of forearm via bicipital aponeurosis	Musculocutaneous nerve (C5, **C6**)	Flexes and supinates forearm Flexes arm when forearm is fixed	Muscular branches of brachial artery
Coracobrachialis	Tip of coracoid process of scapula	Middle third of medial surface of humerus	Musculocutaneous nerve (C5, **C6**, C7)	Flexes and adducts arm	Muscular branches of brachial artery
Brachialis	Distal half of anterior surface of humerus	Coronoid process and tuberosity of ulna	Musculocutaneous nerve (C5, **C6**)	Flexes forearm	Radial recurrent artery, muscular branches of brachial artery
Triceps brachii	Long head – infraglenoid tubercle of scapula; Lateral head – upper half of posterior humerus; Medial head – distal two-thirds of medial and posterior humerus	Posterior surface of olecranon process of ulna	Radial nerve (C6, **C7**, C8)	Extends forearm, long head stabilizes head of abducted humerus	Branch of profunda brachii artery

*Main nerve root is indicated in bold

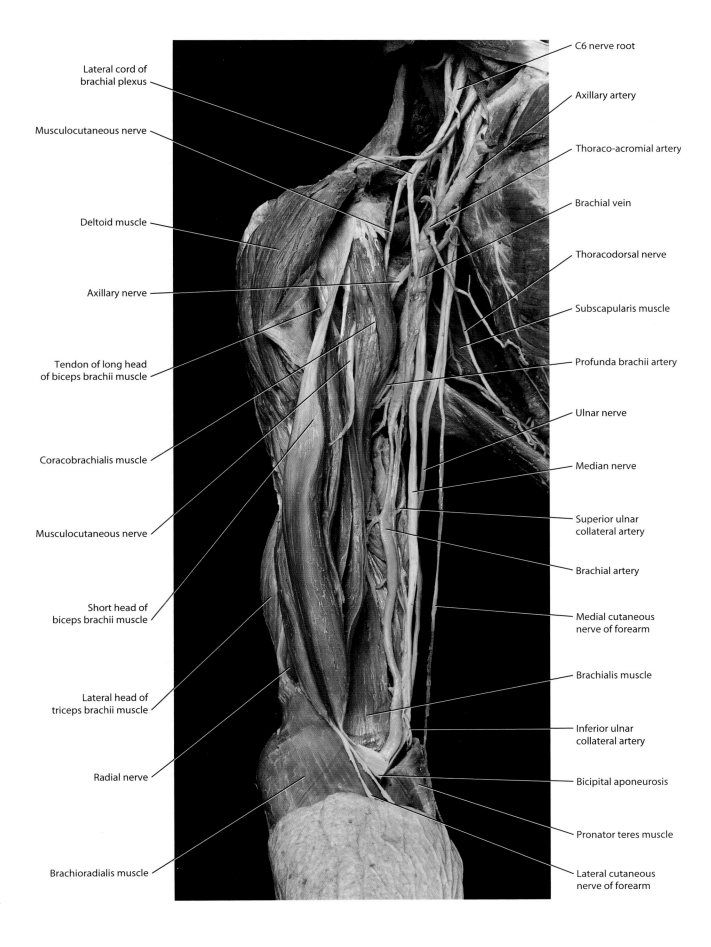

Lateral cord of brachial plexus

Musculocutaneous nerve

Deltoid muscle

Axillary nerve

Tendon of long head of biceps brachii muscle

Coracobrachialis muscle

Musculocutaneous nerve

Short head of biceps brachii muscle

Lateral head of triceps brachii muscle

Radial nerve

Brachioradialis muscle

C6 nerve root

Axillary artery

Thoraco-acromial artery

Brachial vein

Thoracodorsal nerve

Subscapularis muscle

Profunda brachii artery

Ulnar nerve

Median nerve

Superior ulnar collateral artery

Brachial artery

Medial cutaneous nerve of forearm

Brachialis muscle

Inferior ulnar collateral artery

Bicipital aponeurosis

Pronator teres muscle

Lateral cutaneous nerve of forearm

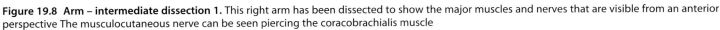

Figure 19.8 Arm – intermediate dissection 1. This right arm has been dissected to show the major muscles and nerves that are visible from an anterior perspective The musculocutaneous nerve can be seen piercing the coracobrachialis muscle

217

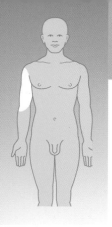

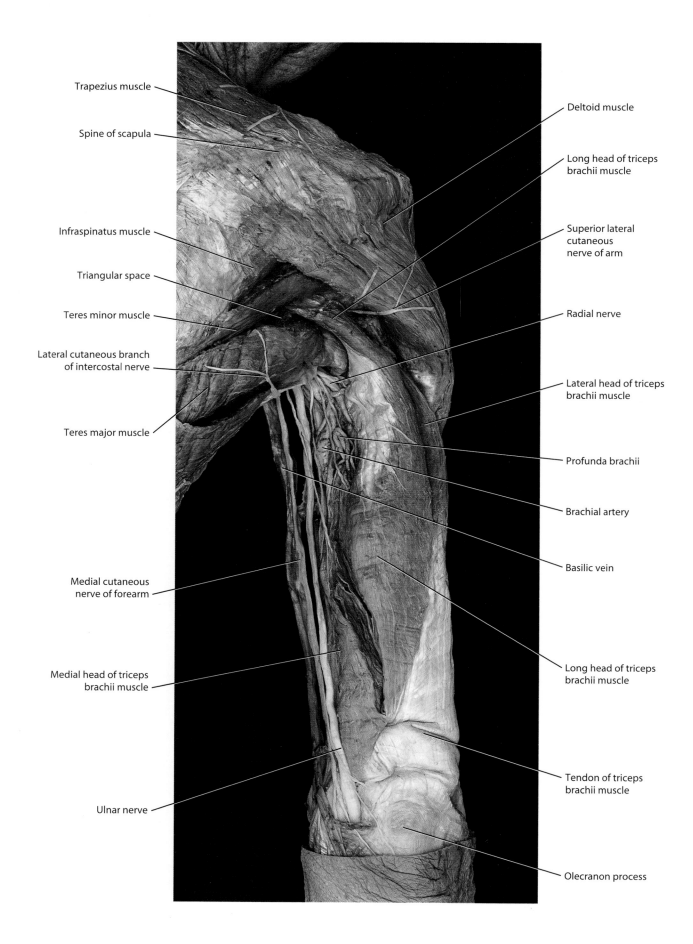

Trapezius muscle

Spine of scapula

Infraspinatus muscle

Triangular space

Teres minor muscle

Lateral cutaneous branch
of intercostal nerve

Teres major muscle

Medial cutaneous
nerve of forearm

Medial head of triceps
brachii muscle

Ulnar nerve

Deltoid muscle

Long head of triceps
brachii muscle

Superior lateral
cutaneous
nerve of arm

Radial nerve

Lateral head of triceps
brachii muscle

Profunda brachii

Brachial artery

Basilic vein

Long head of triceps
brachii muscle

Tendon of triceps
brachii muscle

Olecranon process

Figure 19.9 Arm – superficial dissection 2. A dissection of the right posterior arm that shows the interrelationships of the triceps brachii muscle with the neurovasculature. Observe the three heads of the triceps brachii muscle

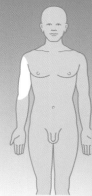

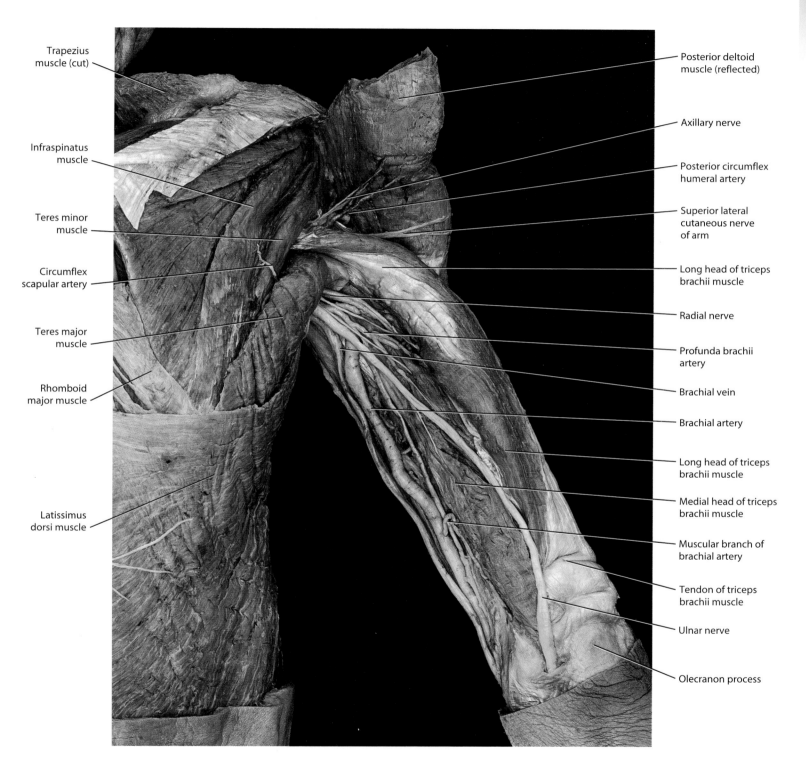

Trapezius muscle (cut)

Infraspinatus muscle

Teres minor muscle

Circumflex scapular artery

Teres major muscle

Rhomboid major muscle

Latissimus dorsi muscle

Posterior deltoid muscle (reflected)

Axillary nerve

Posterior circumflex humeral artery

Superior lateral cutaneous nerve of arm

Long head of triceps brachii muscle

Radial nerve

Profunda brachii artery

Brachial vein

Brachial artery

Long head of triceps brachii muscle

Medial head of triceps brachii muscle

Muscular branch of brachial artery

Tendon of triceps brachii muscle

Ulnar nerve

Olecranon process

Figure 19.10 Arm – intermediate dissection 2. Right posterior arm with a view of the entire medial head of triceps brachii. The posterior deltoid muscle is reflected laterally to show the emerging contents of the quadrangular space

219

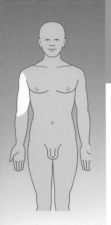

UPPER LIMB

Arm

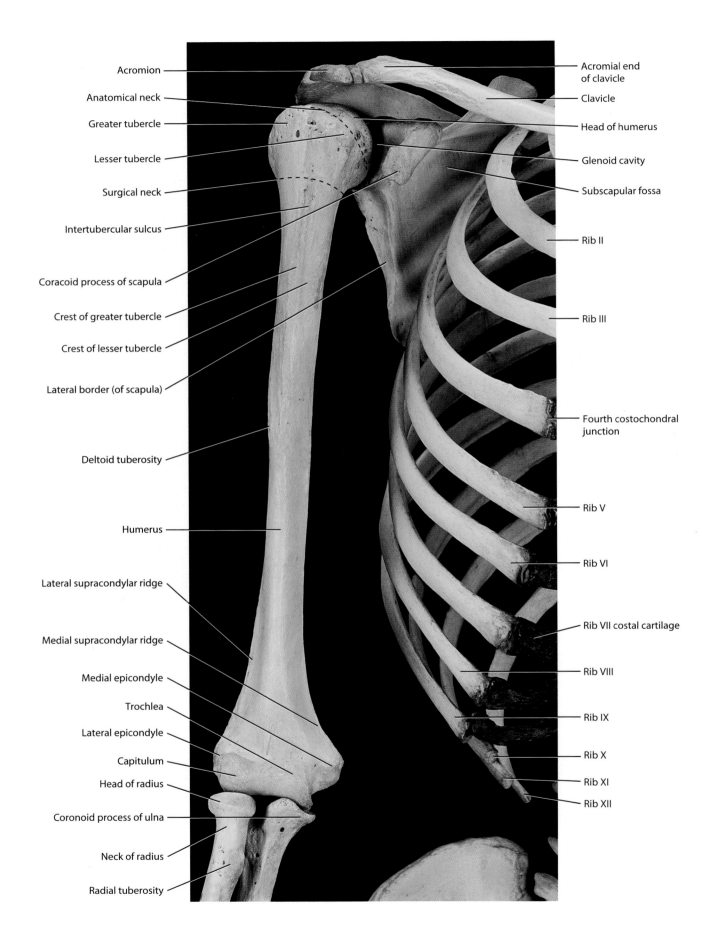

Acromion

Anatomical neck

Greater tubercle

Lesser tubercle

Surgical neck

Intertubercular sulcus

Coracoid process of scapula

Crest of greater tubercle

Crest of lesser tubercle

Lateral border (of scapula)

Deltoid tuberosity

Humerus

Lateral supracondylar ridge

Medial supracondylar ridge

Medial epicondyle

Trochlea

Lateral epicondyle

Capitulum

Head of radius

Coronoid process of ulna

Neck of radius

Radial tuberosity

Acromial end
of clavicle

Clavicle

Head of humerus

Glenoid cavity

Subscapular fossa

Rib II

Rib III

Fourth costochondral
junction

Rib V

Rib VI

Rib VII costal cartilage

Rib VIII

Rib IX

Rib X

Rib XI

Rib XII

Figure 19.11 Arm – osteology 1. Anterior view of the articulated right humerus

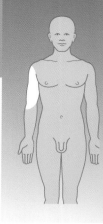

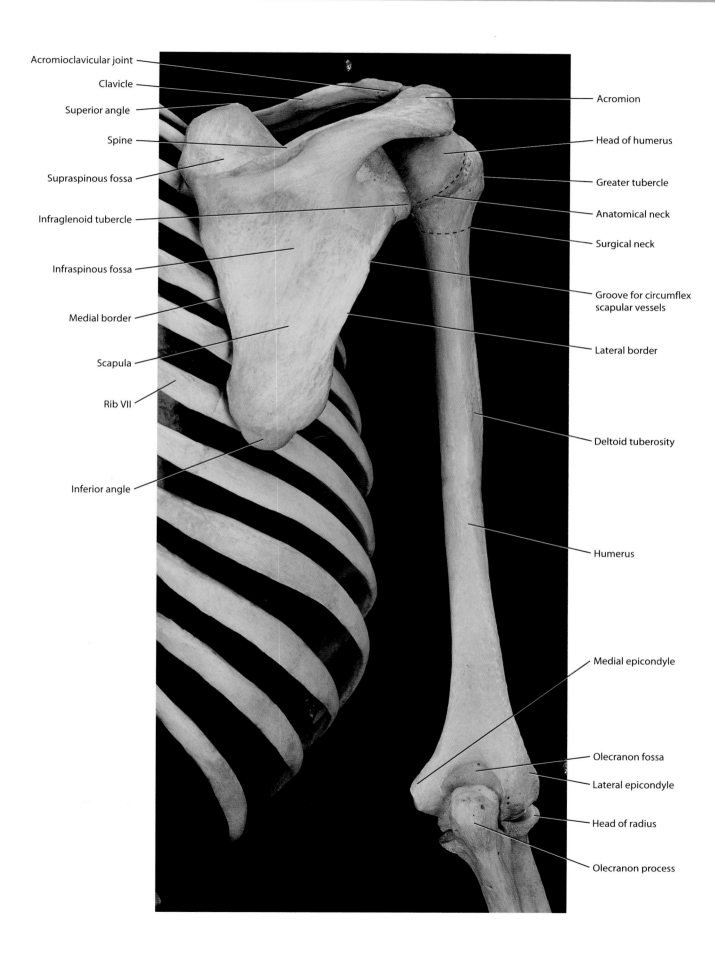

Acromioclavicular joint

Clavicle

Superior angle

Spine

Supraspinous fossa

Infraglenoid tubercle

Infraspinous fossa

Medial border

Scapula

Rib VII

Inferior angle

Acromion

Head of humerus

Greater tubercle

Anatomical neck

Surgical neck

Groove for circumflex scapular vessels

Lateral border

Deltoid tuberosity

Humerus

Medial epicondyle

Olecranon fossa

Lateral epicondyle

Head of radius

Olecranon process

Figure 19.12 Arm – osteology 2. Posterior view of the articulated right humerus

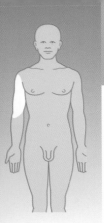

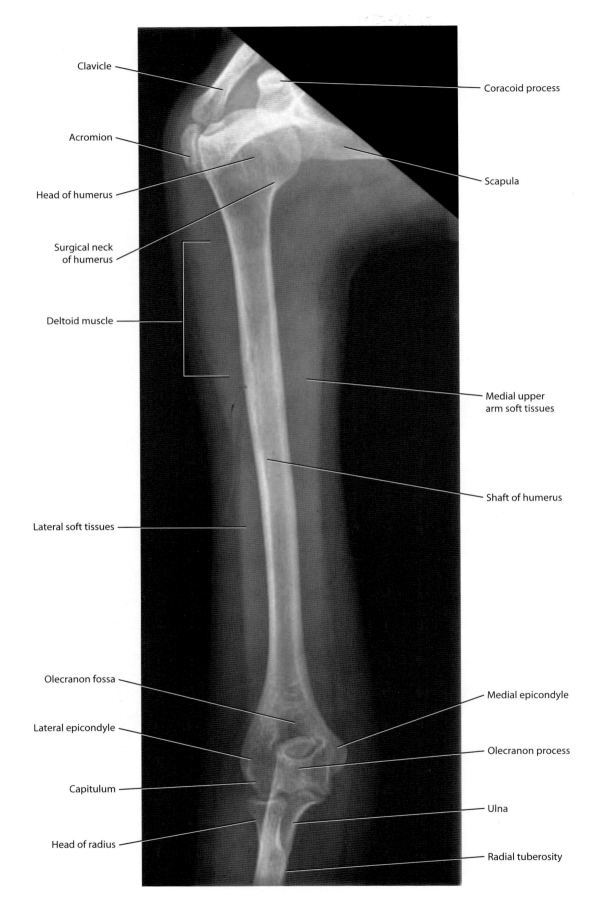

Clavicle

Coracoid process

Acromion

Scapula

Head of humerus

Surgical neck
of humerus

Deltoid muscle

Medial upper
arm soft tissues

Shaft of humerus

Lateral soft tissues

Olecranon fossa

Medial epicondyle

Lateral epicondyle

Olecranon process

Capitulum

Ulna

Head of radius

Radial tuberosity

Figure 19.13 Arm – plain film radiograph (anteroposterior view). The muscles of the arm are visible as a light gray region surrounding the bone. The skin and subcutaneous tissue are then seen as a second slightly darker gray zone more superficial to the muscles. A view like this, showing the joints above and below a long bone, should be assessed for injury in trauma patients

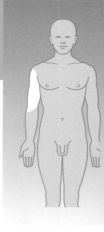

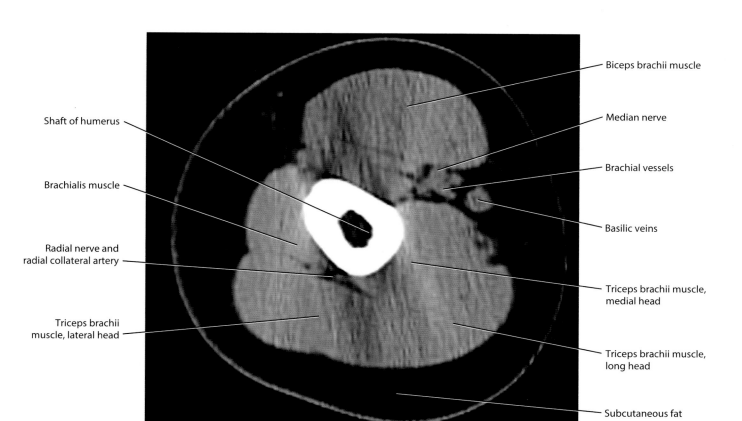

Biceps brachii muscle

Median nerve

Brachial vessels

Basilic veins

Triceps brachii muscle, medial head

Triceps brachii muscle, long head

Subcutaneous fat

Shaft of humerus

Brachialis muscle

Radial nerve and radial collateral artery

Triceps brachii muscle, lateral head

Figure 19.14 Arm – CT scan (axial view, from distal to proximal). Note that the muscle mass of the triceps brachii is much larger than that of the biceps brachii

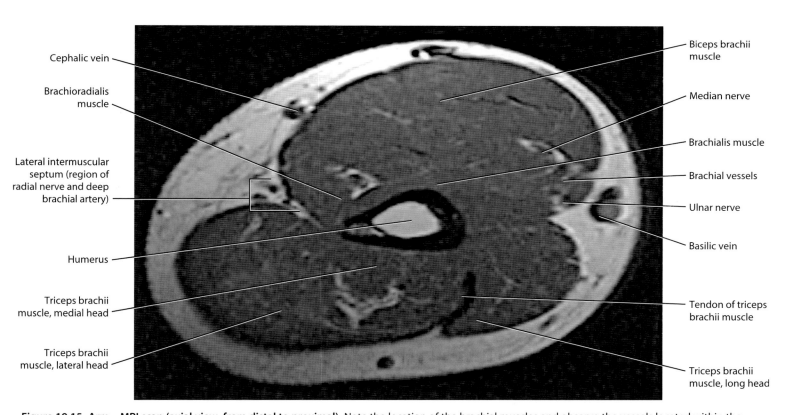

Cephalic vein

Brachioradialis muscle

Lateral intermuscular septum (region of radial nerve and deep brachial artery)

Humerus

Triceps brachii muscle, medial head

Triceps brachii muscle, lateral head

Biceps brachii muscle

Median nerve

Brachialis muscle

Brachial vessels

Ulnar nerve

Basilic vein

Tendon of triceps brachii muscle

Triceps brachii muscle, long head

Figure 19.15 Arm – MRI scan (axial view, from distal to proximal). Note the location of the brachial muscles and observe the vessels located within the subcutaneous tissues

20 Cubital fossa and elbow joint

CUBITAL FOSSA

The cubital fossa is a triangular area on the anterior surface of the elbow joint formed by the borders of the arm and forearm muscles:

- the apex points inferiorly toward the hand;
- the medial side is formed by the pronator teres muscle;
- the lateral border is the brachioradialis muscle;
- the superior border is an imaginary line joining the medial and lateral epicondyles of the humerus;
- the floor is formed by the supinator and brachialis muscles;
- the roof is the deep fascia of the forearm reinforced by the bicipital aponeurosis.

The superficial fascia of the cubital fossa contains a variable arrangement of superficial veins as well as the **medial** and **lateral cutaneous nerves of the forearm** (see Chapter 16). The **cephalic vein** is lateral, the **basilic vein** medial, and the **median cubital vein** joins the two. The median vein of forearm ends in the median cubital vein. The contents of the cubital fossa from lateral to medial are the **tendon of biceps brachii**, the **brachial artery**, and the **median nerve** (Fig. 20.1).

THE ELBOW JOINT

The elbow is a synovial joint at the junction of the arm and forearm. It joins the distal humerus to the proximal radius and ulna, and is primarily mobile in only one axis, which allows active flexion up to about 135° to 145°. The elbow joint comprises three distinct articulations all contained within a single joint capsule:

- the **humero-ulnar joint** between the trochlea of the humerus and the trochlear notch of the ulna (a hinge joint);
- the **humeroradial joint** between the capitulum of the humerus and the head of the radius (a ball and socket joint);
- the **proximal radio-ulnar joint** between the head of the radius and the radial notch of the ulna.

The humero-ulnar and humeroradial joints act as a single hinge joint during extension and flexion of the forearm; the proximal radio-ulnar joint allows rotation of the head of the radius during pronation and supination of the forearm. These three articulations are enclosed within the joint capsule of the elbow. This is thickened laterally to form the **radial collateral** and **ulnar collateral ligaments**, which stabilize the elbow joint and prevent lateral flexion (Fig. 20.2):

- the radial collateral ligament is fanlike and joins the lateral epicondyle of the humerus to the anular ligament of the radius;
- the ulnar collateral ligament is triangular, extending from the medial epicondyle of the humerus to the coronoid process and olecranon of the ulna.

Distally, the joint capsule forms the **anular ligament of radius**, which is a strong band of connective tissue lined by hyaline cartilage that forms a ring-like shape around the head of the radius. This unique shape allows the head of the radius to rotate while the ulna remains stationary, an action needed during pronation and

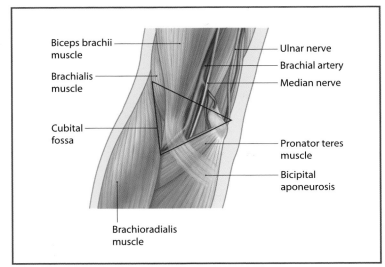

Figure 20.1 Cubital fossa (outlined) and neighboring structures

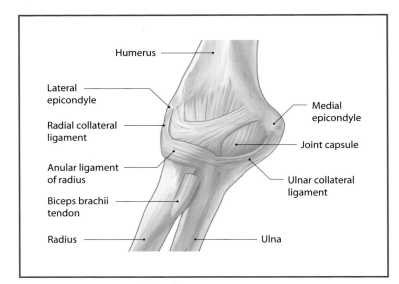

Figure 20.2 Ligaments of the elbow

supination of the forearm. The distal radio-ulnar joint is not part of the elbow joint complex but moves in conjunction with the proximal radio-ulnar joint and facilitates pronation and supination of the forearm and hand (Table 20.1).

The elbow joint is supported by the joint capsule, the radial collateral and ulnar collateral ligaments, the muscles that cross the joint (biceps brachii, brachialis, brachioradialis, triceps brachii, and anconeus), and by the articular surfaces between the humerus and ulna. The **interosseous membrane** that connects the radius and ulna adds stability to the elbow joint complex. Its fibers are directed medially and inferiorly to facilitate the transmission of forces from the hand to the radius, then to the ulna, and finally to the humerus through the elbow joint complex.

Sensory innervation of the elbow is anteriorly from the musculocutaneous, median, radial, ulnar, and posterior interosseous nerves, and posteriorly from the ulnar nerve.

The elbow joint receives its blood supply from anastomoses between the **collateral arteries of the brachial** and **profunda brachii arteries** and the **recurrent branches of the radial** and **ulnar arteries** (Fig. 20.3), and also from small, unnamed branches of the radial and ulnar arteries. Vessels supplying blood to the elbow joint are the:

- ulnar artery;
- radial artery;
- superior ulnar collateral artery (from the brachial artery);
- inferior ulnar collateral artery (from the brachial artery);
- radial collateral artery (from profunda brachii artery);
- middle collateral artery (from profunda brachii artery);
- radial recurrent artery (from the radial artery);
- anterior ulnar recurrent artery (from the ulnar artery – this vessel anastomoses with the inferior ulnar recurrent artery);
- posterior ulnar recurrent artery (from the ulnar artery – this vessel anastomoses with the superior ulnar collateral artery).

Superficial venous drainage of the skin and subcutaneous tissues around the elbow joint is to the cephalic and basilic veins. The deep veins run alongside the arteries (radial and ulnar) and are usually paired. Near the elbow they coalesce to form the brachial veins, which continue into the arm. Lymphatic drainage of the elbow is to the **cubital nodes** at the anterior elbow and vessels that empty into the axillary lymph nodes.

■ CLINICAL CORRELATIONS
Dislocation of the elbow

Dislocation of the elbow (Fig. 20.4) usually results in a fracture to either the humerus or ulna. It can result from falling forcefully onto the outstretched twisted arm, and although uncommon, it is important clinically because immediate reduction is required to prevent neurovascular damage.

A dislocated elbow causes extreme pain and inability to move the forearm at the elbow. Deficiencies in sensation or cyanosis of the distal forearm and arm may occur, depending on the severity of the injury. Medical attention is usually sought quickly.

On examination the patient has an obvious deformity at the elbow. The dislocation must be reduced immediately by an expert to prevent further damage. Careful vascular examination is necessary to ensure that blood is reaching the hand and digits, and palpation of the brachial and radial pulses and examination of capillary refill of the digits are vital to confirm adequate blood flow. Neurological examination of the distal forearm and hand is carried out to assess for nerve damage and includes testing sensation in the injured limb. Radiographs may show joint damage. If joint stability is not maintained after reduction, surgical treatment may be necessary.

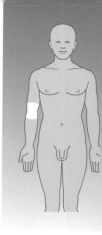

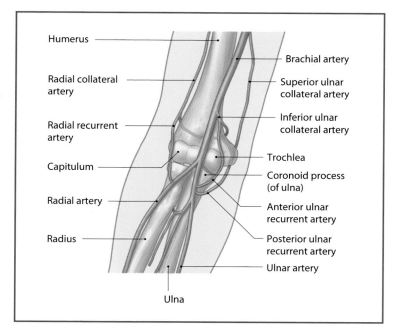

Figure 20.3 The elbow and its arteries

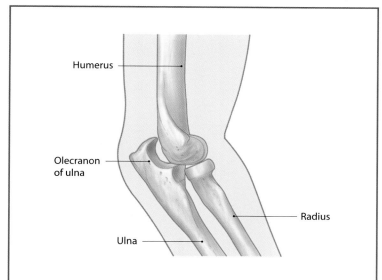

Figure 20.4 Posterior dislocation of the right elbow

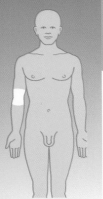

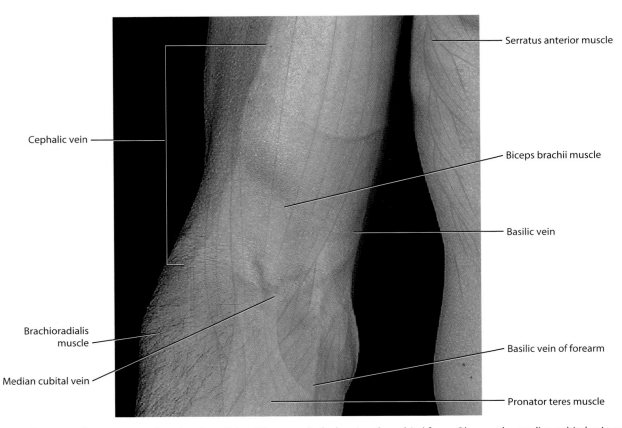

Cephalic vein

Brachioradialis muscle

Median cubital vein

Serratus anterior muscle

Biceps brachii muscle

Basilic vein

Basilic vein of forearm

Pronator teres muscle

Figure 20.5 Cubital fossa – surface anatomy. Anterior view of the right upper limb showing the cubital fossa. Observe the median cubital vein connecting the cephalic with the basilic vein as it crosses the fossa

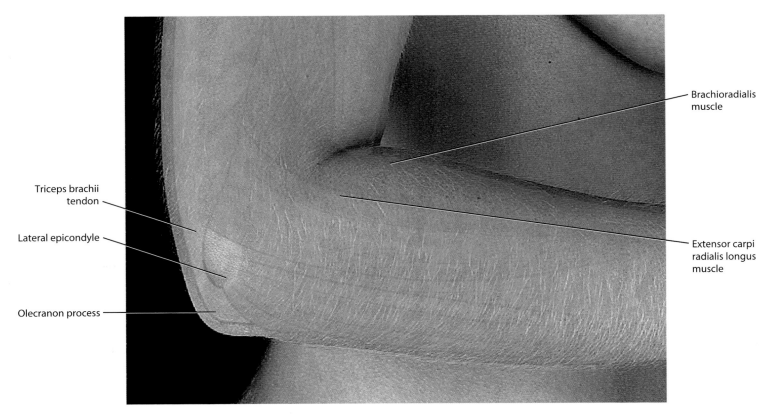

Triceps brachii tendon

Lateral epicondyle

Olecranon process

Brachioradialis muscle

Extensor carpi radialis longus muscle

Figure 20.6 Elbow joint – surface anatomy. Lateral view of the right elbow

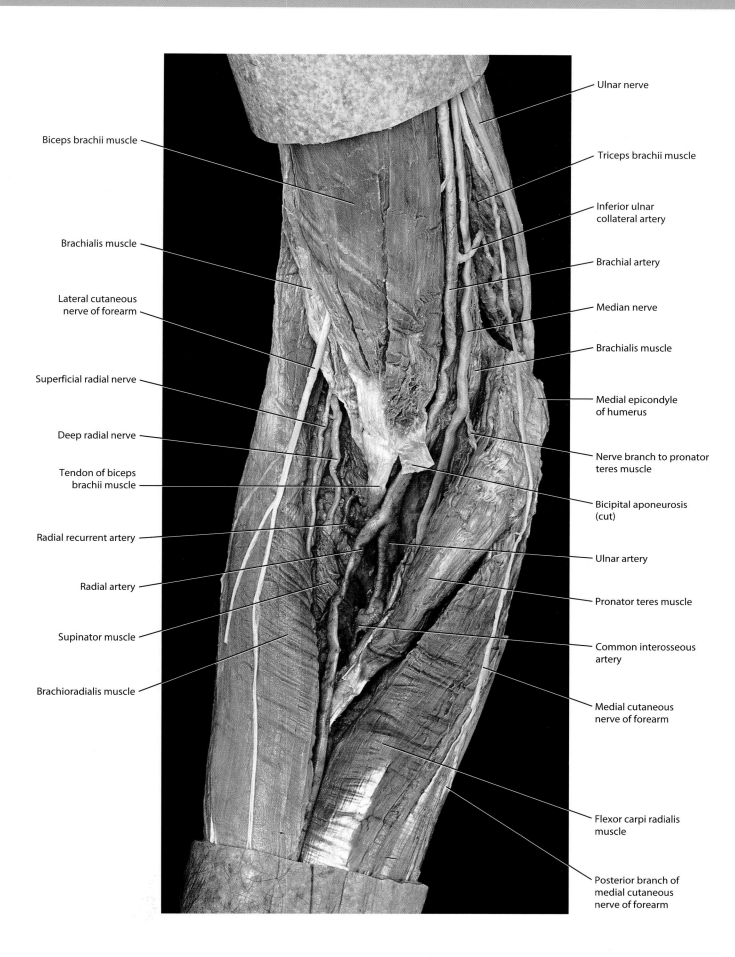

Biceps brachii muscle

Brachialis muscle

Lateral cutaneous
nerve of forearm

Superficial radial nerve

Deep radial nerve

Tendon of biceps
brachii muscle

Radial recurrent artery

Radial artery

Supinator muscle

Brachioradialis muscle

Ulnar nerve

Triceps brachii muscle

Inferior ulnar
collateral artery

Brachial artery

Median nerve

Brachialis muscle

Medial epicondyle
of humerus

Nerve branch to pronator
teres muscle

Bicipital aponeurosis
(cut)

Ulnar artery

Pronator teres muscle

Common interosseous
artery

Medial cutaneous
nerve of forearm

Flexor carpi radialis
muscle

Posterior branch of
medial cutaneous
nerve of forearm

UPPER LIMB   Cubital fossa and elbow joint

Figure 20.7 Cubital fossa – superficial dissection. Anterior view of the right cubital fossa. The bicipital aponeurosis has been cut to show the median nerve, and the pronator teres and brachioradialis muscles have been pulled slightly apart to show the contents of the cubital fossa

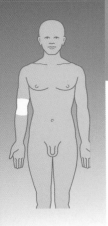

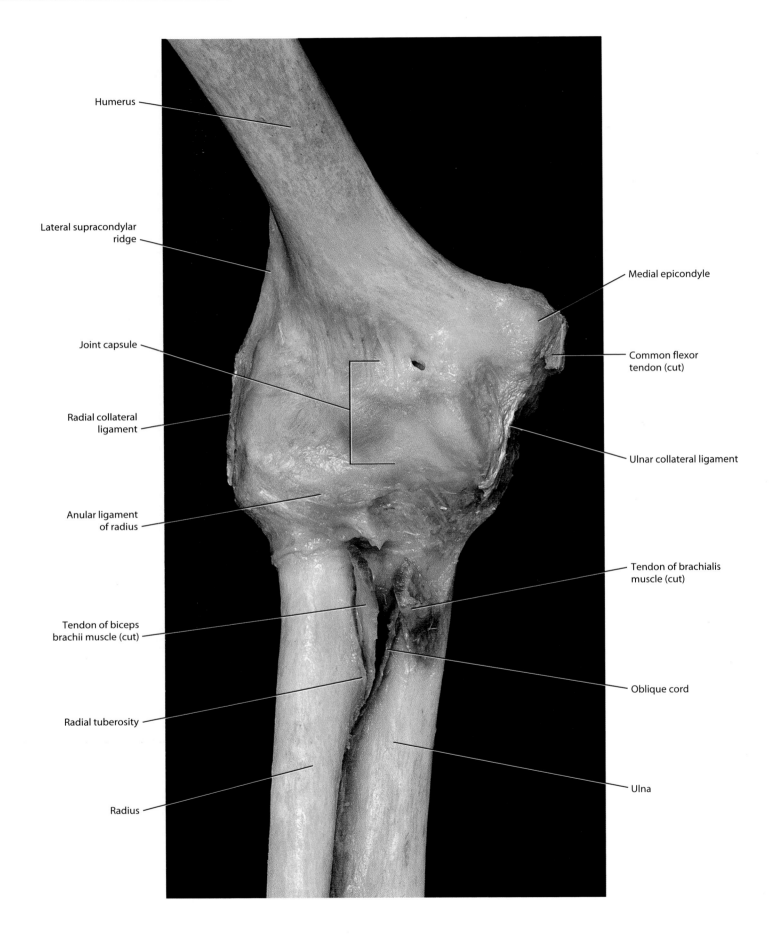

Humerus

Lateral supracondylar ridge

Joint capsule

Radial collateral ligament

Anular ligament of radius

Tendon of biceps brachii muscle (cut)

Radial tuberosity

Radius

Medial epicondyle

Common flexor tendon (cut)

Ulnar collateral ligament

Tendon of brachialis muscle (cut)

Oblique cord

Ulna

Figure 20.8 Elbow joint – dissection 1. Anterior view of the right elbow joint. The joint capsule is relatively thin anteriorly but has collateral thickenings along both sides. All muscles and neurovasculature have been removed to show the ligaments. Observe the anular ligament which holds the head of the radius within the joint

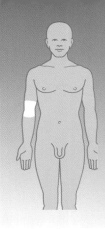

TABLE 20.1 JOINTS OF THE ELBOW AND FOREARM

Joint	Type	Articular surfaces	Ligaments	Movement
Elbow ROM = 10–0–150°	Hinge-type synovial joint	Humero-ulnar – trochlea of humerus with trochlear notch of ulna; humeroradial – capitulum of humerus with head of radius	Ulnar collateral with anterior, posterior, and transverse bands Radial collateral	Flexion/extension (active) range of movement approximately 160°
Proximal (superior) radio-ulnar	Pivot-type synovial joint	Radial notch of ulna with head of radius	Anular ligament of radius – forms collar Quadrate – reinforces inferior joint capsule Oblique cord – flat fascial band	Pronation approx. 70° Supination approx. 85°
Distal (inferior) radio-ulnar	Pivot-type synovial joint	Ulnar notch of radius with head of ulna and articular disk	Anterior radio-ulnar Posterior radio-ulnar Interosseous membrane – fibers running obliquely downwards and medially	Pronation approx. 70° Supination approx. 85° (works with superior radio-ulnar joint)

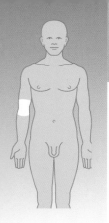

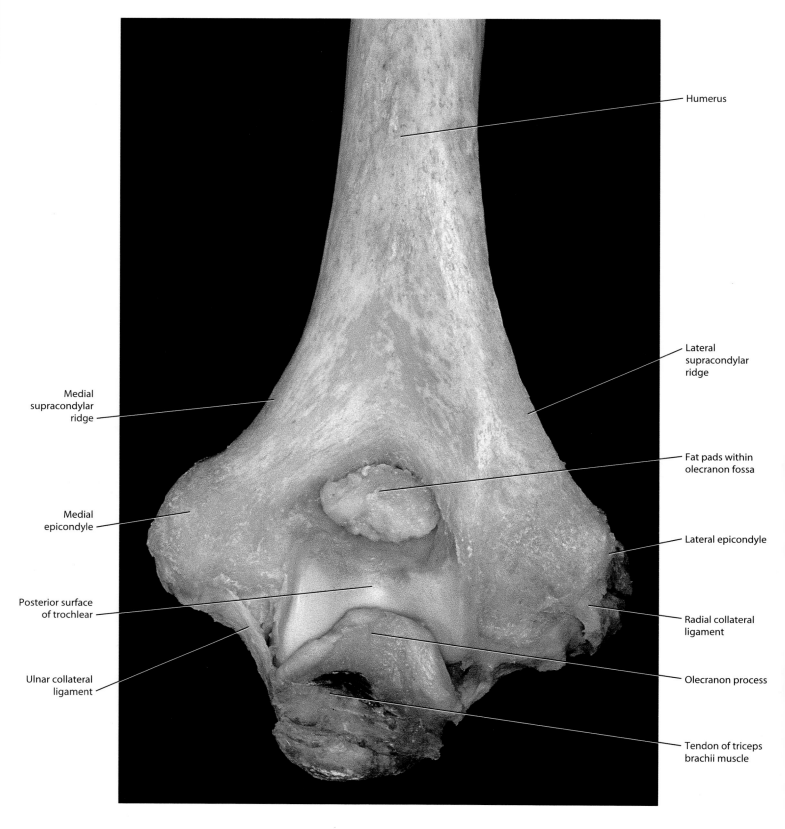

Medial
supracondylar
ridge

Medial
epicondyle

Posterior surface
of trochlear

Ulnar collateral
ligament

Humerus

Lateral
supracondylar
ridge

Fat pads within
olecranon fossa

Lateral epicondyle

Radial collateral
ligament

Olecranon process

Tendon of triceps
brachii muscle

Figure 20.9 Elbow joint – dissection 2. Posterior view of the right elbow joint. The joint capsule has been removed revealing the fat pads above the smooth surface of the trochlea of the humerus. Observe how the olecranon process of the ulna would slide across the trochlea of the humerus during flexion and extension of the elbow joint

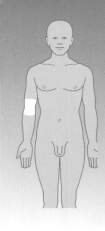

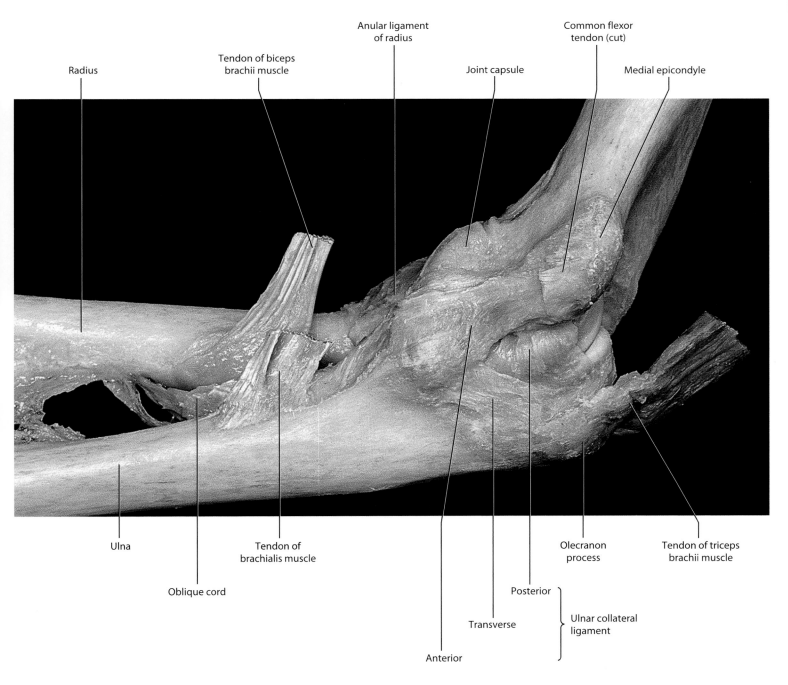

Radius

Tendon of biceps
brachii muscle

Anular ligament
of radius

Joint capsule

Common flexor
tendon (cut)

Medial epicondyle

Ulna

Oblique cord

Tendon of
brachialis muscle

Anterior

Transverse

Posterior

Olecranon
process

Ulnar collateral
ligament

Tendon of triceps
brachii muscle

Figure 20.10 Elbow joint – dissection 3. Medial view of the right elbow joint with the major tendons and ligaments visible. All three parts of the ulnar collateral ligament are shown

231

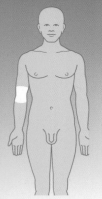

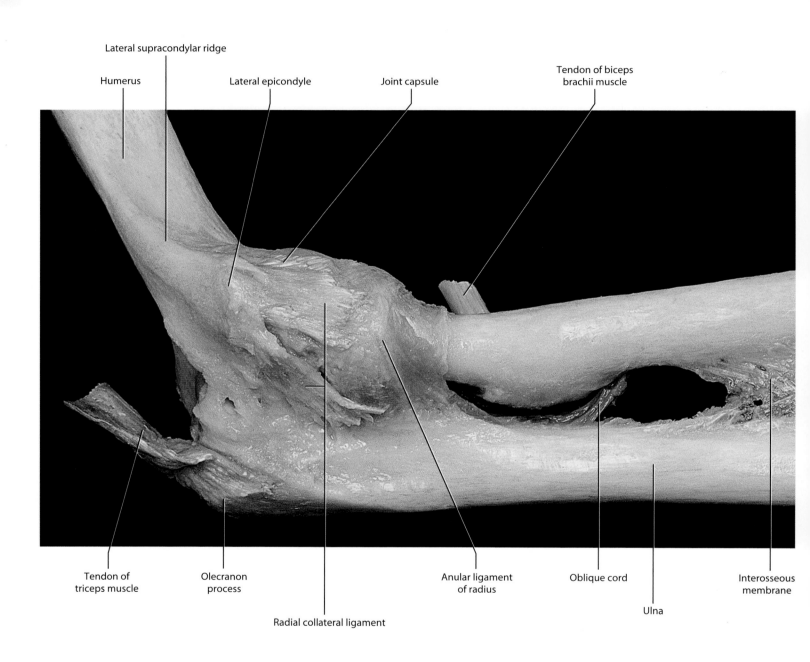

Lateral supracondylar ridge

Humerus

Lateral epicondyle

Joint capsule

Tendon of biceps brachii muscle

Tendon of triceps muscle

Olecranon process

Radial collateral ligament

Anular ligament of radius

Oblique cord

Ulna

Interosseous membrane

Figure 20.11 Elbow joint – dissection 4. Lateral view of the right elbow joint with the major tendons and ligaments visible. The radial collateral ligament lies distally over part of the anular ligament of radius

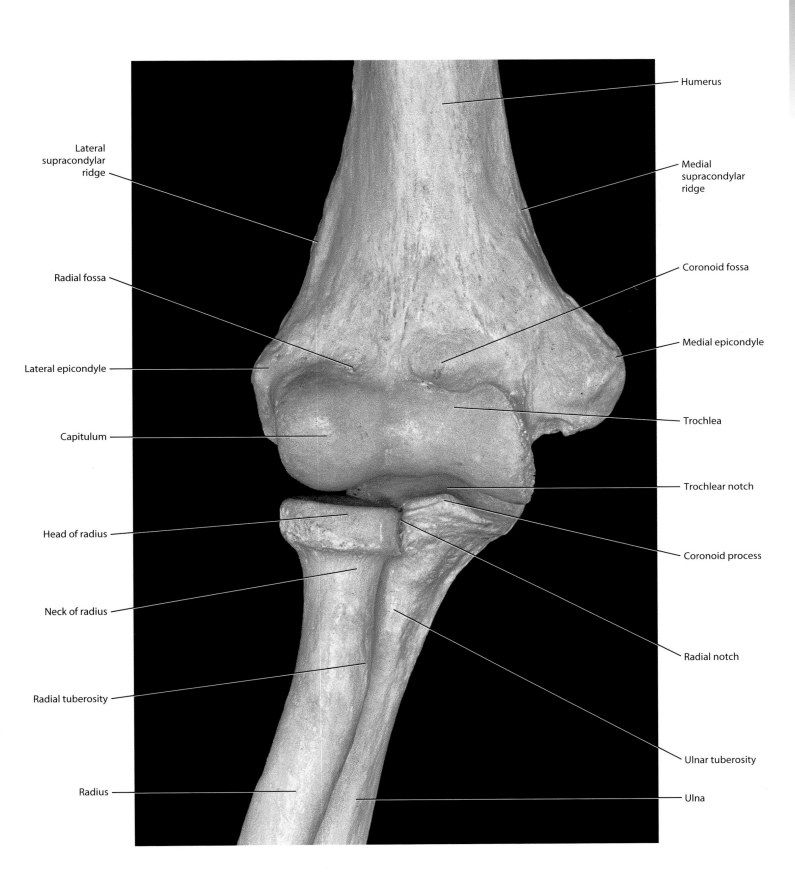

Humerus

Lateral supracondylar ridge

Medial supracondylar ridge

Radial fossa

Coronoid fossa

Lateral epicondyle

Medial epicondyle

Capitulum

Trochlea

Head of radius

Trochlear notch

Neck of radius

Coronoid process

Radial tuberosity

Radial notch

Ulnar tuberosity

Radius

Ulna

UPPER LIMB Cubital fossa and elbow joint

Figure 20.12 Elbow joint – osteology 1. Anterior view of the articulated bones of the right elbow joint. Note the large trochlear notch and the slight indentation of the radial notch of the ulna

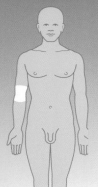

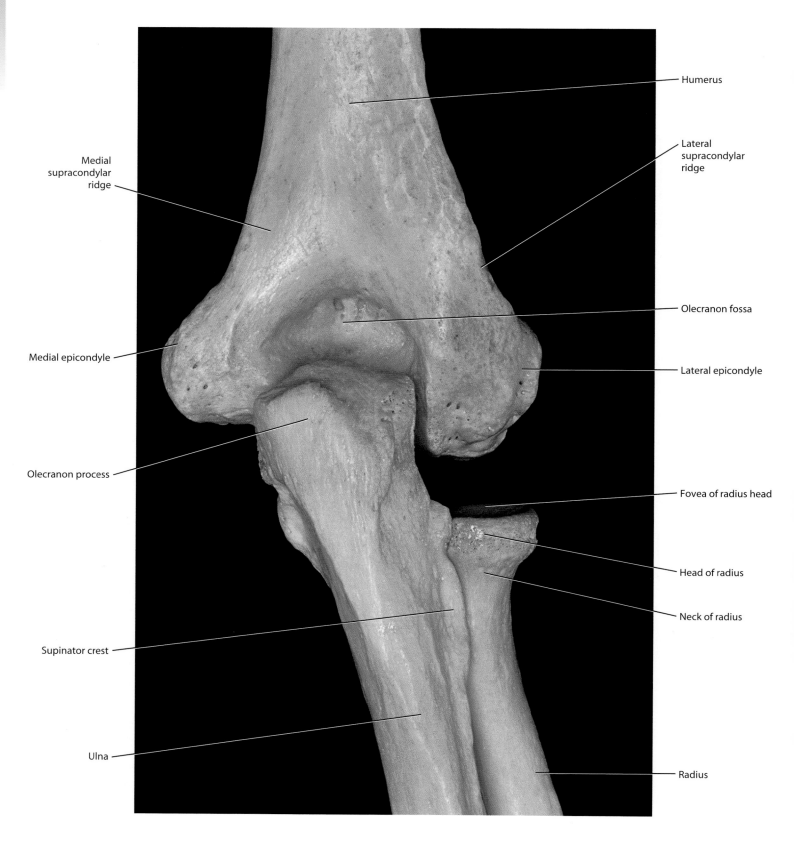

Medial
supracondylar
ridge

Medial epicondyle

Olecranon process

Supinator crest

Ulna

Humerus

Lateral
supracondylar
ridge

Olecranon fossa

Lateral epicondyle

Fovea of radius head

Head of radius

Neck of radius

Radius

Figure 20.13 Elbow joint – osteology 2. Posterior view of the bones of the right elbow joint. The ulna and radius are slightly displaced inferiorly to show the olecranon fossa

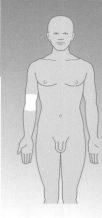

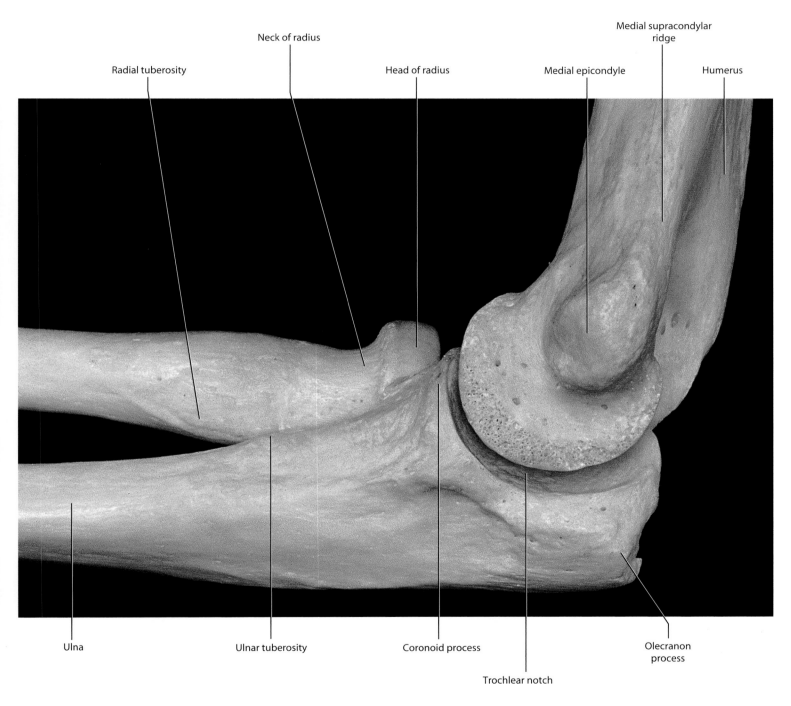

Radial tuberosity

Neck of radius

Head of radius

Medial epicondyle

Medial supracondylar ridge

Humerus

Ulna

Ulnar tuberosity

Coronoid process

Trochlear notch

Olecranon process

Figure 20.14 Elbow joint – osteology 3. Medial view of the right elbow in 90° flexion. The trochlea of the humerus within the trochlear notch of the ulna comprises the humero-ulnar joint

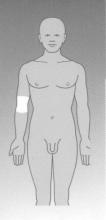

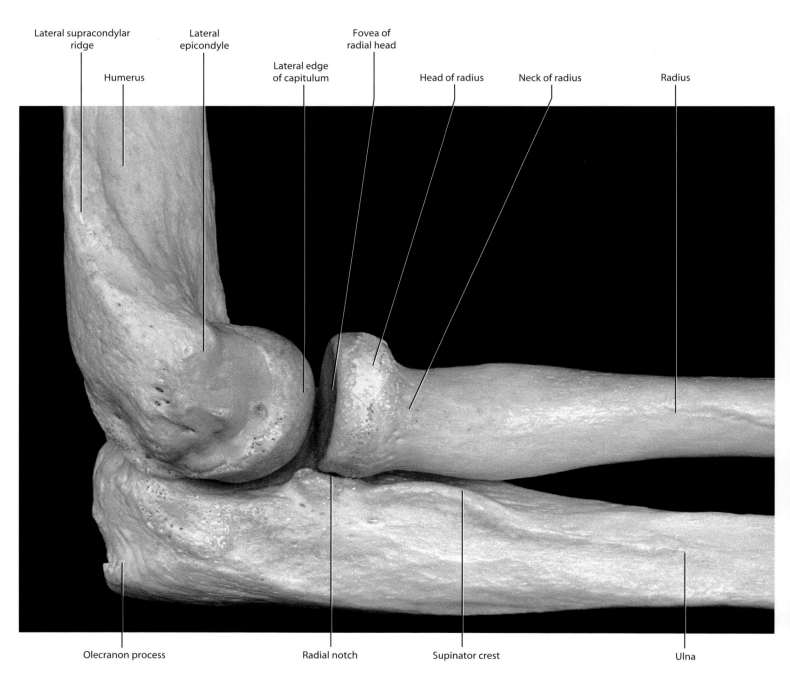

Lateral supracondylar ridge

Lateral epicondyle

Fovea of radial head

Humerus

Lateral edge of capitulum

Head of radius

Neck of radius

Radius

Olecranon process

Radial notch

Supinator crest

Ulna

Figure 20.15 Elbow joint – osteology 4. Lateral view of the articulated right elbow bones in 90º flexion. The capitulum of the humerus with the head of the radius comprises the humeroradial joint

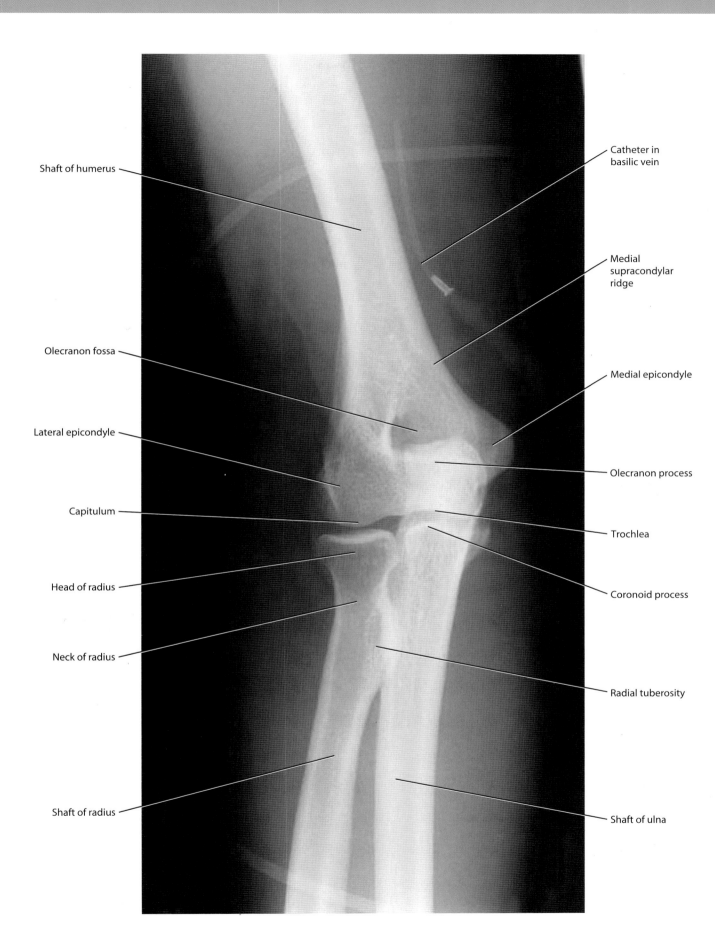

Shaft of humerus

Olecranon fossa

Lateral epicondyle

Capitulum

Head of radius

Neck of radius

Shaft of radius

Catheter in basilic vein

Medial supracondylar ridge

Medial epicondyle

Olecranon process

Trochlea

Coronoid process

Radial tuberosity

Shaft of ulna

Figure 20.16 Elbow joint – plain film radiograph (anteroposterior view). There is an intravenous catheter in the basilic vein. Note that the head of the radius does not make direct contact with the humerus, instead weight is transferred from the forearm to the arm via the humeroulnar articulation

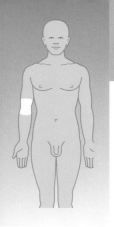

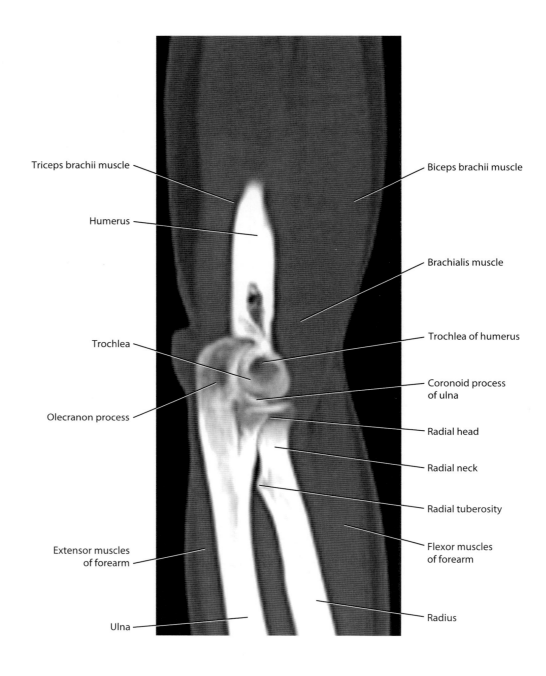

Triceps brachii muscle

Humerus

Trochlea

Olecranon process

Extensor muscles of forearm

Ulna

Biceps brachii muscle

Brachialis muscle

Trochlea of humerus

Coronoid process of ulna

Radial head

Radial neck

Radial tuberosity

Flexor muscles of forearm

Radius

Figure 20.17 **Elbow joint – CT scan (sagittal view).** Note how the olecranon process of the ulna wraps around the trochlea of the humerus

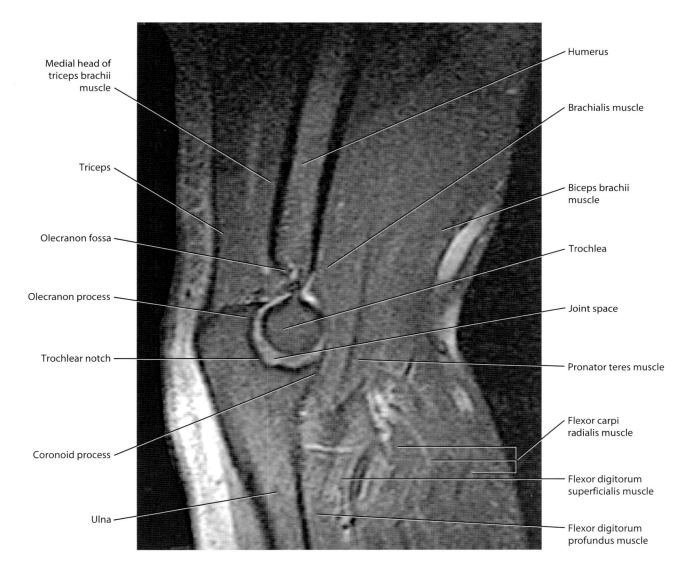

Medial head of
triceps brachii
muscle

Triceps

Olecranon fossa

Olecranon process

Trochlear notch

Coronoid process

Ulna

Humerus

Brachialis muscle

Biceps brachii
muscle

Trochlea

Joint space

Pronator teres muscle

Flexor carpi
radialis muscle

Flexor digitorum
superficialis muscle

Flexor digitorum
profundus muscle

Figure 20.18 Elbow joint – MRI scan (sagittal view). Note that the external surface of the ulna is not covered by muscle, unlike the humerus which is well protected by muscles. The triceps muscle attaches to the olecranon process of the ulna and is the primary extensor of the forearm at the elbow joint

The forearm is the part of the upper limb between the elbow and wrist. It is divided into **anterior** and **posterior compartments of forearm** by the **interosseous membrane**, which joins the radius and ulna. The anterior forearm contains several muscles that flex the wrist and digits (fingers). The forearm is supported by the radius and ulna.

The superior part of the **ulna** bears the coronoid process and olecranon, which articulate with the humerus at the elbow joint. Distally, the ulna is narrow; its small head articulates with the radius through the distal radio-ulnar joint and indirectly with carpal (wrist) bones via an interarticular disk.

The **radius** is shorter than the ulna and is lateral in the forearm. Its distal end is large and articulates directly with the carpal bones at the radiocarpal joint. Proximally, the anular ligament of radius binds the head of the radius to the ulna and allows the rotation of the forearm necessary for pronation and supination. The arrangement of the radius and ulna is unique in that weight is transferred from the wrist to the radius and then to the humerus via the ulna.

MUSCLES

The muscles of the anterior forearm (Figs 21.1 and 21.2) can be divided into a superficial group of five muscles and a deep group of three muscles. The superficial group comprises, from lateral to medial:

- pronator teres
- flexor carpi radialis
- palmaris longus
- flexor carpi ulnaris
- flexor digitorum superficialis.

The superficial muscles have a similar origin at the common flexor tendon, which originates from the front of the medial epicondyle of the humerus. The **flexor digitorum** muscle is unique in that it has three heads of origin (Table 21.1) and sends four tendons to the middle phalanx of each of the index, middle, ring, and little fingers. The **flexor digitorum superficialis** and other superficial muscles flex the hand and fingers.

The deep muscles of the anterior forearm are:

- flexor digitorum profundus
- flexor pollicis longus
- pronator quadratus.

The **flexor digitorum profundus** muscle arises from the upper three-quarters of the medial and anterior surface of the ulna and interosseous membrane (Fig. 21.3). The insertion is onto the base of the distal phalanx of the medial four digits by four tendons.

The **flexor pollicis longus** muscle arises from the upper two-thirds of the anterior surface of the radius and inserts into the distal phalanx of the thumb. The flexor digitorum profundus and flexor pollicis longus muscles flex the digits and assist in flexion of the hand.

The **pronator quadratus** muscle takes origin from the distal anterior surface of the ulna and inserts onto the medial and anterior surfaces of the distal radius. With this unique layout it acts to pronate the forearm.

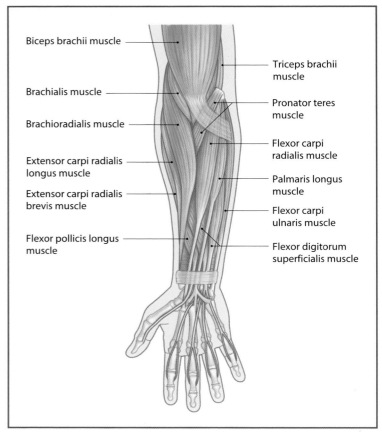

Figure 21.1 Superficial muscles of right anterior forearm

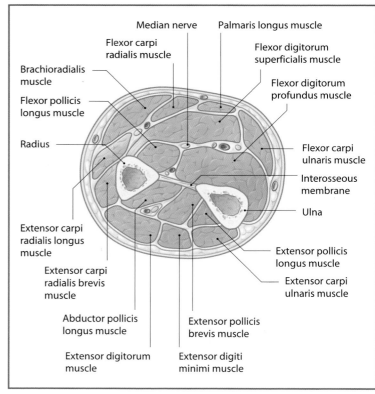

Figure 21.2 Cross-section through the right forearm (viewed from distal to proximal)

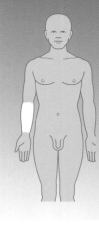

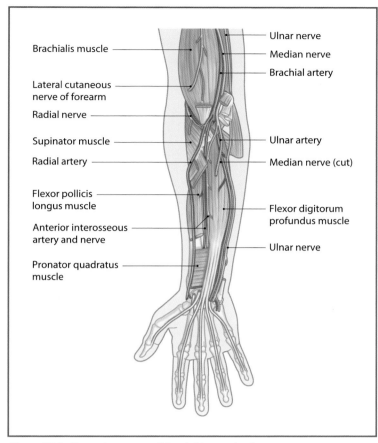

Figure 21.3 Deep structures of the right anterior forearm

Labels on figure:
Brachialis muscle
Lateral cutaneous nerve of forearm
Radial nerve
Supinator muscle
Radial artery
Flexor pollicis longus muscle
Anterior interosseous artery and nerve
Pronator quadratus muscle
Ulnar nerve
Median nerve
Brachial artery
Ulnar artery
Median nerve (cut)
Flexor digitorum profundus muscle
Ulnar nerve

NERVES

The **median nerve** (C6 to T1) is the main nerve to the anterior forearm, innervating six and a half of the eight muscles. It originates from the brachial plexus, descends in the arm, and passes into the cubital fossa where it supplies pronator teres, flexor carpi radialis, and palmaris longus muscles. In the cubital fossa the median nerve pierces the pronator teres muscle, and on leaving this muscle it branches to give off the **anterior interosseous nerve**, which supplies the three deep muscles – the radial half of flexor digorum profundus, flexor pollicis longus, and pronator quadratus. The **ulnar nerve** supplies the flexor carpi ulnaris muscle and the ulnar half of the flexor digitorum profundus muscle.

The median nerve descends in the forearm deep to the flexor digitorum superficialis muscle, to emerge at the radial side of the flexor digitorum superficialis tendons just superior to the wrist. Here, it branches to form a **palmar cutaneous branch**, which supplies the skin over the radial side of the palm. The median nerve continues deep and traverses the carpal tunnel of the wrist anterior to the tendons of the flexor digitorum superficialis muscle. On leaving the carpal tunnel, the median nerve supplies muscles and skin of the medial part of the hand (see Chapter 24).

The **ulnar nerve** (C7 to T1) is also a branch of the brachial plexus and enters the anterior forearm by passing between the heads of the flexor carpi ulnaris muscle. It runs alongside the ulnar artery between the flexor carpi ulnaris and flexor digitorum profundus muscles, and branches to supply these muscles. The ulnar nerve is superficial at the wrist and provides sensation to the skin on the medial side of the hand.

ARTERIES

Blood is supplied to the anterior forearm by the two terminal branches of the brachial artery – the radial and ulnar arteries – which divide at the level of the neck of the radius. The **radial artery** is smaller than the ulnar artery and runs inferiorly into the forearm deep to the brachioradialis muscle and lateral to the flexor carpi radialis tendon. The **ulnar artery** gives off the **common interosseous artery** to supply the deep muscles of the anterior and posterior forearm, and descends in the anterior forearm medial to the tendons of the flexor digitorum superficialis muscle. Both the ulnar and radial arteries continue into the hand to form two anastomotic connections – the **superficial** and **deep palmar arches**.

VEINS AND LYMPHATICS

The cephalic and basilic veins drain the superficial soft tissue of the anterior forearm. The **cephalic vein** arises from the veins of the **dorsal venous network of hand**. From the lateral forearm the cephalic vein ascends to the arm and is observed over the biceps brachii muscle (see Chapter 19). The **basilic vein** arises from the medial side of the dorsal venous network of hand, ascends in the medial anterior forearm and crosses the cubital fossa (see Chapter 20) to enter the medial arm. Both the cephalic and basilic veins are usually bridged at the cubital fossa by the median cubital vein.

The deep veins of the anterior forearm follow the ulnar and radial arteries as venae comitantes. For example, the radial artery has two venae comitantes, which drain blood from the deep structures of the hand and lateral anterior forearm.

Superficial lymphatic drainage of the anterior forearm is by lymphatic vessels that drain the hand and ascend with the superficial veins to empty into the cubital nodes at the medial elbow. Deep lymphatic vessels follow the deep veins of the anterior forearm and empty into the lymph nodes at the axilla.

■ CLINICAL CORRELATIONS
Colles' fracture

A Colles' fracture (Fig. 21.4) occurs when the distal radius and ulna break and the resultant fragments are displaced posteriorly, for example as may occur on falling onto an outstretched hand. The transverse fracture through the radius may extend into the wrist joints. Symptoms include pain, swelling, and instability of the distal forearm and wrist.

On examination, the neurovascular function of the injured limb must be evaluated and the motor and sensory function of the median nerve and the radial arterial pulse checked. Further examination of the fractured forearm will reveal deformity and point tenderness along the fractured (broken) bones. Radiographs will show fracture lines through the radial metaphysis and/or

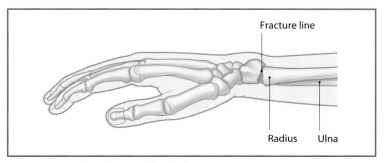

Figure 21.4 Colles' fracture of right forearm

Labels on figure:
Fracture line
Radius
Ulna

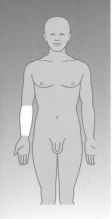
extension of the fracture into the radiocarpal or radio-ulnar joints (see Chapter 23) with posterior displacement of the distal wrist hand bones in relation to the proximal forearm.

Closed reduction (re-orienting the broken bones without surgery) of a closed fracture can be attempted. Radiographs must be evaluated after reduction to check the position of the bones. If satisfactory, a cast or splint is applied. Immediate referral to the orthopedic surgeon is indicated if the Colles' fracture is complicated by an open wound along the fracture site or by neurovascular damage. Open reduction and internal fixation is classically carried out for all open fractures. Neurovascular injuries are treated surgically based on the site and type of injury.

Golfer's elbow (medial epicondylitis)

Golfer's elbow is an inflammatory condition involving the medial epicondyle of the humerus through its origin for attachment of the flexor carpi radialis muscle and other forearm flexors by the common flexor tendon. It is thought to occur in people who participate in activities that involve repetitive wrist flexion, which

over time causes inflammation and microinjury to the origin of the flexor carpi radialis muscle or surrounding flexor muscles. In addition, there may be bursitis and synovitis. A constellation of these conditions may occur, causing pain on flexion of the wrist joint. Patients usually complain of a gradual development of pain over the medial epicondylar region of the humerus.

On examination, there is tenderness over the medial epicondyle of the humerus and pain on forced pronation. Radiographs are usually normal. Treatment includes resting the limb, elevating the joint to decrease swelling, and pain medications as needed. Referral to an orthopedic surgeon for possible surgery is indicated if there is persistent pain after a prescribed rest and rehabilitation period.

MNEMONIC	
Flexor carpi superficialis and profundus insertions:	**Superficialis splits in two, to permit profundus to pass through**

TABLE 21.1 ANTERIOR FOREARM MUSCLES					
Muscle	Origin	Insertion	Innervation	Action	Blood supply
Superficial Pronator teres	Medial epicondyle of humerus and coranoid process of ulna	Middle of lateral surface of radius	Median nerve (C6, C7)	Pronates forearm, assists in flexion	Anterior ulnar recurrent artery
Flexor carpi radialis	Medial epicondyle of humerus	Base of metacarpals II and III	Median nerve (C6, C7)	Flexes hand, assists in abduction	Radial artery
Palmaris longus	Medial epicondyle of humerus	Distal half of flexor retinaculum and palmar aponeurosis	Median nerve (C7, C8)	Flexes hand and tenses palmar fascia	Posterior ulnar recurrent artery
Flexor carpi ulnaris	Humeral head – medial epicondyle of humerus; ulnar head – olecranon and posterior border of ulna	Pisiform bone, hook of hamate, base of metacarpal V	Ulnar nerve (C7, C8)	Flexes hand, assists in adduction	Posterior ulnar recurrent artery
Flexor digitorum superficialis	Humeral head – medial epicondyle; ulnar head – coronoid process; radial head – anterior border of radius	Bodies of middle phalanges of index, middle, ring and little fingers	Median nerve (C7 to T1)	Flexes middle and proximal phalanges of index, middle, ring and little fingers; assists in hand flexion	Ulnar and radial arteries
Deep Flexor digitorum profundus	Medial and anterior surface of proximal three-quarters of ulna, and interosseous membrane	Anterior base of distal phalanges of index, middle, ring and little fingers	Medial part – ulnar nerve (C8, T1); lateral part – median nerve (C8, T1)	Flexes distal phalanges of index, middle, ring and little fingers; assists in hand flexion	Anterior interosseous artery and muscular branches of ulnar artery
Flexor pollicis longus	Anterior surface of radius, and interosseous membrane	Palmar base of distal phalanx of thumb	Anterior interosseous branch of median nerve (C8, T1)	Flexes phalanges of thumb	Anterior interosseous artery
Pronator quadratus	Distal fourth of anterior ulna	Distal fourth of anterior radius	Anterior interosseous branch of median nerve (C8, T1)	Pronates forearm	Anterior interosseous artery

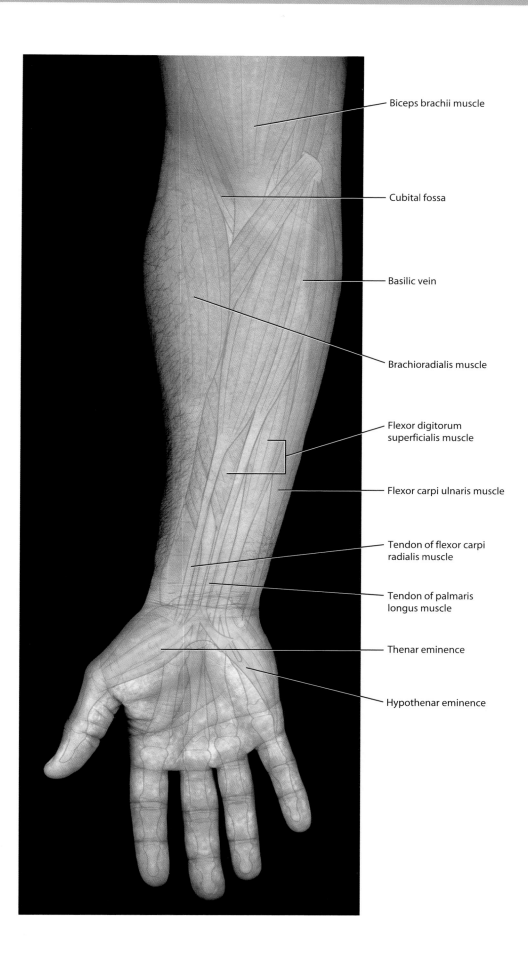

Biceps brachii muscle

Cubital fossa

Basilic vein

Brachioradialis muscle

Flexor digitorum superficialis muscle

Flexor carpi ulnaris muscle

Tendon of flexor carpi radialis muscle

Tendon of palmaris longus muscle

Thenar eminence

Hypothenar eminence

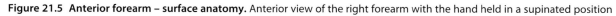

Figure 21.5 Anterior forearm – surface anatomy. Anterior view of the right forearm with the hand held in a supinated position

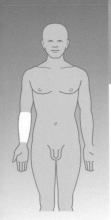

UPPER LIMB

Anterior forearm

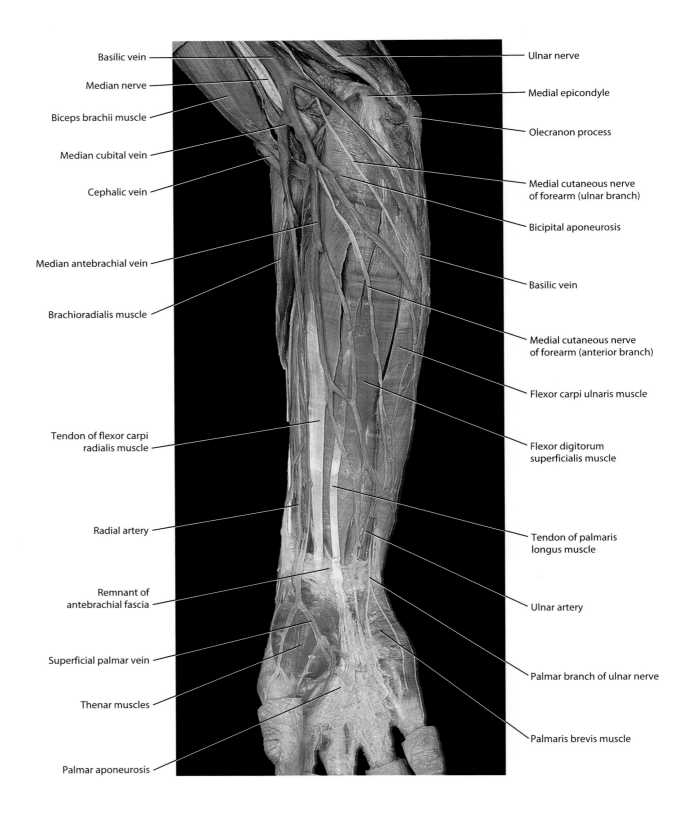

Basilic vein

Median nerve

Biceps brachii muscle

Median cubital vein

Cephalic vein

Median antebrachial vein

Brachioradialis muscle

Tendon of flexor carpi radialis muscle

Radial artery

Remnant of antebrachial fascia

Superficial palmar vein

Thenar muscles

Palmar aponeurosis

Ulnar nerve

Medial epicondyle

Olecranon process

Medial cutaneous nerve of forearm (ulnar branch)

Bicipital aponeurosis

Basilic vein

Medial cutaneous nerve of forearm (anterior branch)

Flexor carpi ulnaris muscle

Flexor digitorum superficialis muscle

Tendon of palmaris longus muscle

Ulnar artery

Palmar branch of ulnar nerve

Palmaris brevis muscle

Figure 21.6 Anterior forearm – superficial dissection 1. A dissection of the right anterior forearm. Observe the tributaries of the superficial veins, forming the larger basilic vein

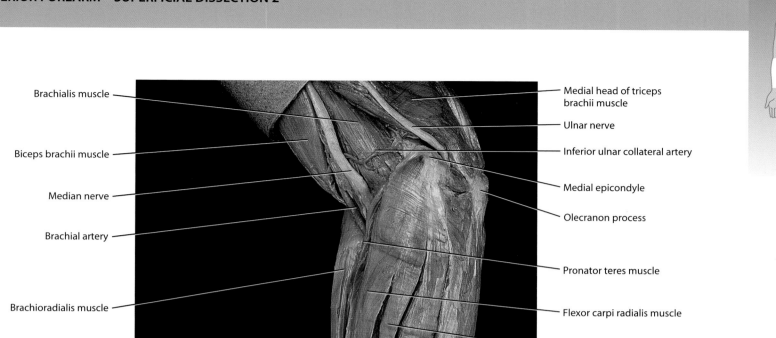
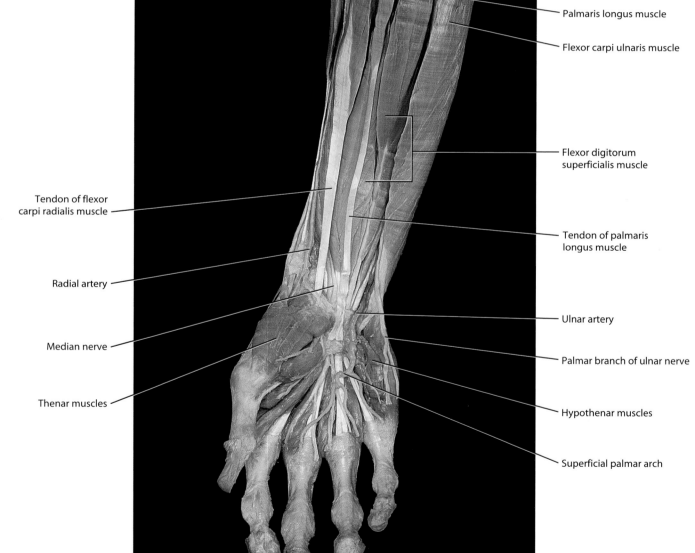

Brachialis muscle

Biceps brachii muscle

Median nerve

Brachial artery

Brachioradialis muscle

Tendon of flexor
carpi radialis muscle

Radial artery

Median nerve

Thenar muscles

Medial head of triceps
brachii muscle

Ulnar nerve

Inferior ulnar collateral artery

Medial epicondyle

Olecranon process

Pronator teres muscle

Flexor carpi radialis muscle

Palmaris longus muscle

Flexor carpi ulnaris muscle

Flexor digitorum
superficialis muscle

Tendon of palmaris
longus muscle

Ulnar artery

Palmar branch of ulnar nerve

Hypothenar muscles

Superficial palmar arch

Figure 21.7 Anterior forearm – superficial dissection 2. A dissection of the right anterior forearm with the superficial veins removed to show the musculature

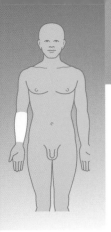

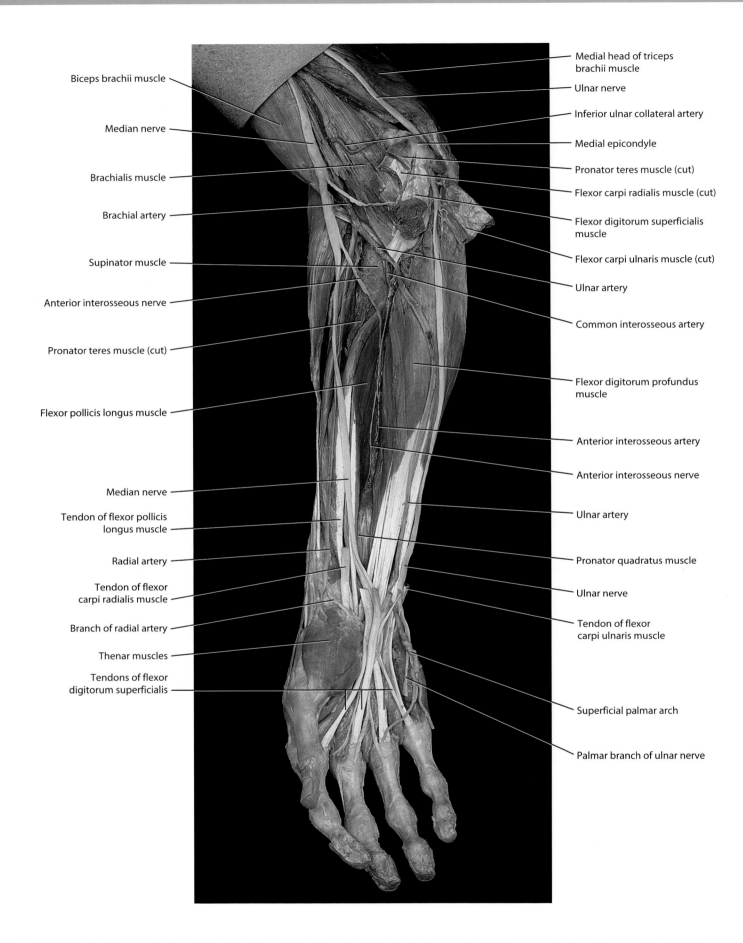

Biceps brachii muscle

Median nerve

Brachialis muscle

Brachial artery

Supinator muscle

Anterior interosseous nerve

Pronator teres muscle (cut)

Flexor pollicis longus muscle

Median nerve

Tendon of flexor pollicis longus muscle

Radial artery

Tendon of flexor carpi radialis muscle

Branch of radial artery

Thenar muscles

Tendons of flexor digitorum superficialis

Medial head of triceps brachii muscle

Ulnar nerve

Inferior ulnar collateral artery

Medial epicondyle

Pronator teres muscle (cut)

Flexor carpi radialis muscle (cut)

Flexor digitorum superficialis muscle

Flexor carpi ulnaris muscle (cut)

Ulnar artery

Common interosseous artery

Flexor digitorum profundus muscle

Anterior interosseous artery

Anterior interosseous nerve

Ulnar artery

Pronator quadratus muscle

Ulnar nerve

Tendon of flexor carpi ulnaris muscle

Superficial palmar arch

Palmar branch of ulnar nerve

Figure 21.8 Anterior forearm – intermediate dissection. A dissection of a right anterior forearm in which the pronator teres, flexor carpi radialis, flexor digitorum superficialis, and flexor carpi ulnaris muscles have been removed. The flexor pollicis longus muscle has been reflected to show the anterior interosseous artery and nerve traveling on the interosseous membrane

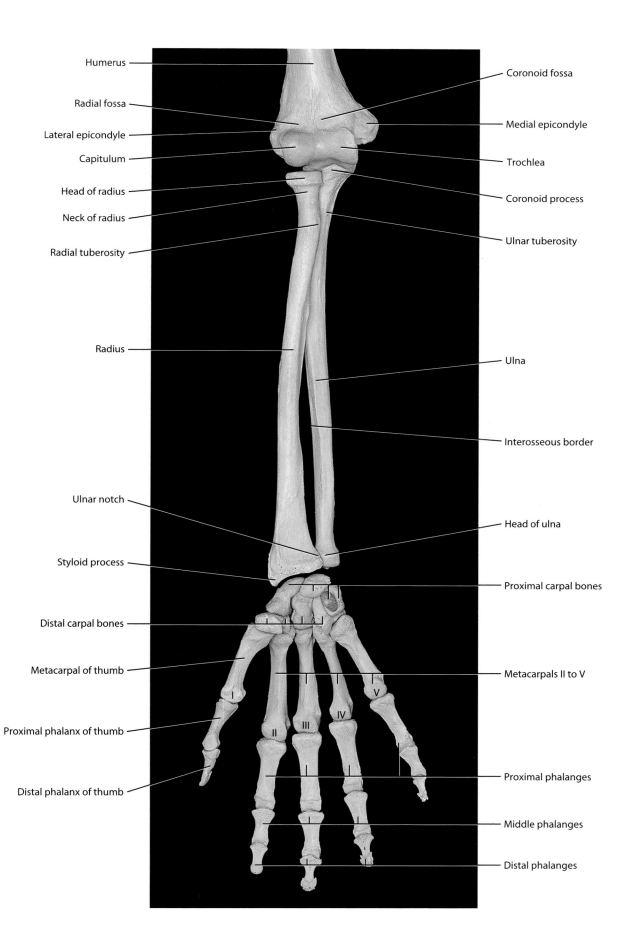

Humerus

Radial fossa

Lateral epicondyle

Capitulum

Head of radius

Neck of radius

Radial tuberosity

Radius

Ulnar notch

Styloid process

Distal carpal bones

Metacarpal of thumb

Proximal phalanx of thumb

Distal phalanx of thumb

Coronoid fossa

Medial epicondyle

Trochlea

Coronoid process

Ulnar tuberosity

Ulna

Interosseous border

Head of ulna

Proximal carpal bones

Metacarpals II to V

Proximal phalanges

Middle phalanges

Distal phalanges

Figure 21.9 The anterior forearm – osteology. Anterior view of the articulated bones of the right anterior forearm, wrist, and hand

247

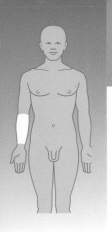

UPPER LIMB

Anterior forearm

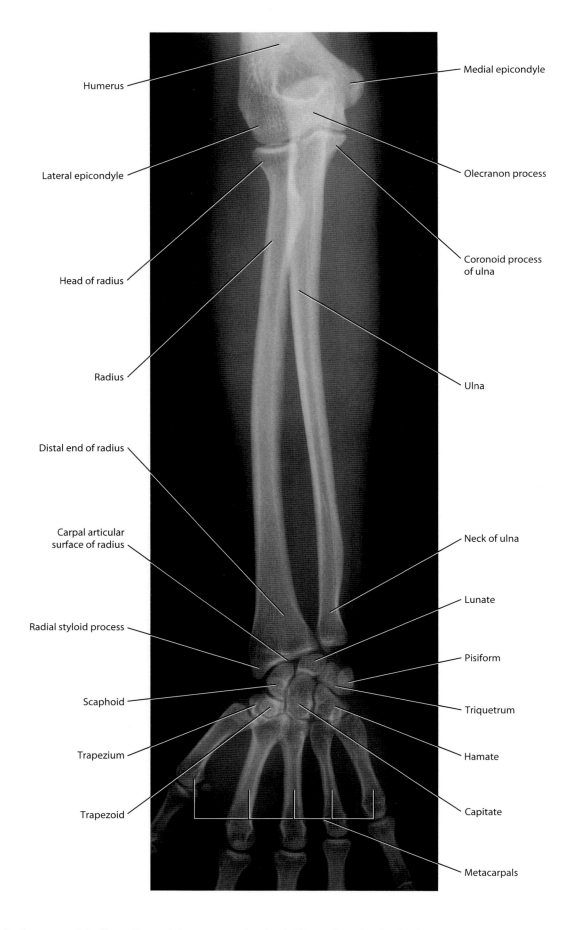

Humerus

Lateral epicondyle

Head of radius

Radius

Distal end of radius

Carpal articular
surface of radius

Radial styloid process

Scaphoid

Trapezium

Trapezoid

Medial epicondyle

Olecranon process

Coronoid process
of ulna

Ulna

Neck of ulna

Lunate

Pisiform

Triquetrum

Hamate

Capitate

Metacarpals

Figure 21.10 Anterior forearm – plain film radiograph (anteroposterior view). Observe how the distal radius articulates primarily with the carpal bones and the proximal ulna makes primary articulation with the humerus. This causes the unique transfer of weight from the carpal bones to the radius, then from the radius to the ulna and finally from the ulna to the humerus

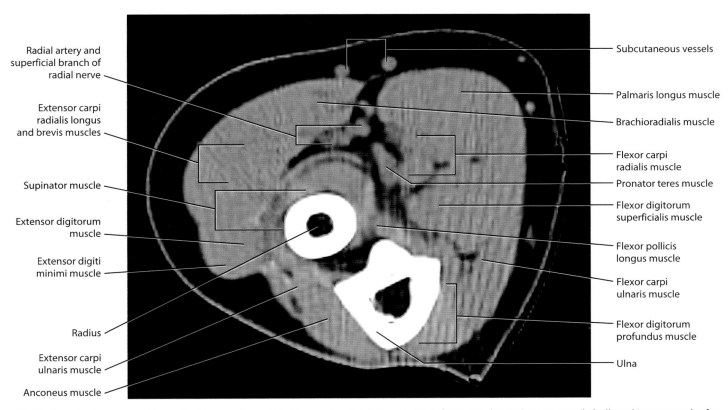

Radial artery and superficial branch of radial nerve

Extensor carpi radialis longus and brevis muscles

Supinator muscle

Extensor digitorum muscle

Extensor digiti minimi muscle

Radius

Extensor carpi ulnaris muscle

Anconeus muscle

Subcutaneous vessels

Palmaris longus muscle

Brachioradialis muscle

Flexor carpi radialis muscle

Pronator teres muscle

Flexor digitorum superficialis muscle

Flexor pollicis longus muscle

Flexor carpi ulnaris muscle

Flexor digitorum profundus muscle

Ulna

Figure 21.11 Anterior forearm – CT scan (axial view, from distal to proximal). Intermuscular definition is dependent on muscle bulk and intermuscular fat planes. Definition of muscles is suboptimal in this scan because the patient was very slim and had low body fat content

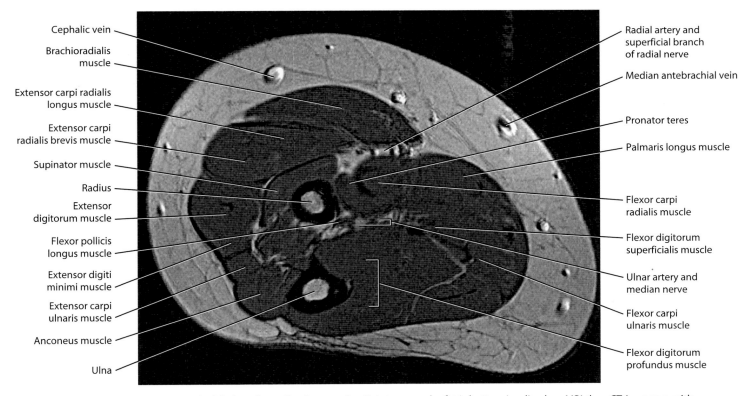

Cephalic vein

Brachioradialis muscle

Extensor carpi radialis longus muscle

Extensor carpi radialis brevis muscle

Supinator muscle

Radius

Extensor digitorum muscle

Flexor pollicis longus muscle

Extensor digiti minimi muscle

Extensor carpi ulnaris muscle

Anconeus muscle

Ulna

Radial artery and superficial branch of radial nerve

Median antebrachial vein

Pronator teres

Palmaris longus muscle

Flexor carpi radialis muscle

Flexor digitorum superficialis muscle

Ulnar artery and median nerve

Flexor carpi ulnaris muscle

Flexor digitorum profundus muscle

Figure 21.12 Anterior forearm – MRI scan (axial view, from distal to proximal). Intermuscular fat is better visualized on MRI than CT (compare with Fig. 21.11). Observe the location of the median nerve

249

The posterior forearm is between the elbow and wrist joints, contains 12 muscles divided into superficial and deep groups (Figs 22.1 and 22.2), and is supported by the radius and ulna (see Chapter 21). The main function of the forearm muscles (except brachioradialis and supinator) is extension of the wrist and fingers. Brachioradialis and supinator flex and laterally rotate (supinate) the forearm and hand, respectively.

MUSCLES

The superficial muscles of the posterior forearm, from lateral to medial, are:

- brachioradialis
- extensor carpi radialis longus
- extensor carpi radialis brevis
- extensor digitorum
- extensor digiti minimi
- extensor carpi ulnaris
- anconeus.

These superficial muscles have a similar superior attachment to the humerus, mostly through the common extensor tendon attached to the lateral epicondyle (extensor carpi radialis brevis, extensor digitorum, extensor digiti minimi and extensor carpi ulnaris muscles). The **brachioradialis** and **extensor carpi radialis longus** muscles originate from the lateral supracondylar ridge and the

anconeus muscle from the posterior surface of the lateral epicondyle. From this common area, the muscle bellies of the superficial muscles run parallel to the axis of the forearm toward the wrist and hand. The primary action of these superficial muscles is to extend or abduct the wrist. Unique to the superficial muscle group, because they perform elbow functions, are the brachioradialis and anconeus muscles.

The **brachioradialis** inserts on the distal radius, and is a fast flexor and stabilizer of the forearm and hand.

The **anconeus** muscle is a small muscle on the lateral elbow that extends from the lateral epicondyle of the humerus to the lateral olecranon process of the ulna. It assists the triceps brachii muscle in extending the forearm.

The deep group of muscles of the posterior forearm from lateral to medial, are:

- supinator
- abductor pollicis longus (pollex means thumb)
- extensor pollicis brevis
- extensor pollicis longus
- extensor indicis.

These deep muscles originate from the shafts of the radius and ulna, and from the interosseous membrane, and their slender tendons insert onto the metacarpals and phalanges (wrist and hand bones). They all extend the thumb and index finger, except

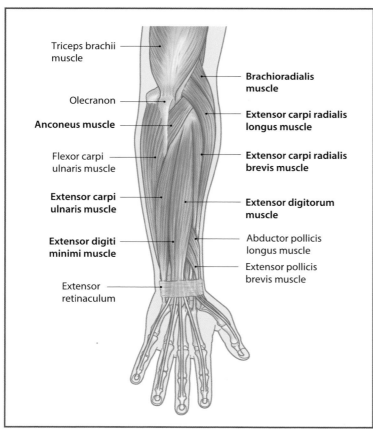

Figure 22.1 Superficial muscles (bold) of right posterior forearm

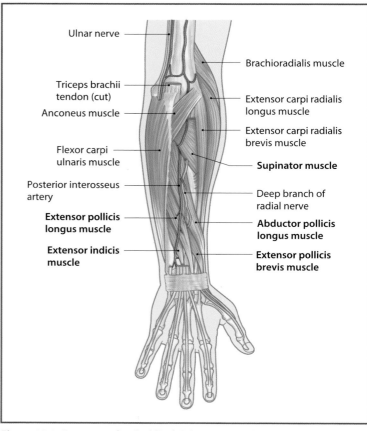

Figure 22.2 Deep muscles (bold) of right posterior forearm

supinator, which originates from the lateral epicondyle of the humerus and wraps medially onto the proximal third of the shaft of the radius. This unique path enables the supinator to supinate the forearm by rotating the radius and palm of the hand laterally (Table 22.1).

NERVES

The **radial nerve** (spinal nerves C5 to T1) innervates all of the structures of the posterior forearm. It starts as a branch of the brachial plexus (see Chapter 16), descends into the cubital fossa and then enters the anterior forearm between the brachialis and brachioradialis muscles (see Chapter 21). The radial nerve innervates the brachioradialis, extensor carpi radialis longus, and anconeus muscles before dividing into superficial and deep branches.

The **deep branch** of the radial nerve innervates the extensor carpi radialis brevis muscle and then enters the supinator muscle. On leaving the supinator muscle, it enters the posterior forearm and becomes the **posterior interosseous nerve**, which innervates the other muscles of the posterior forearm (Table 22.1). The **superficial branch** of the radial nerve conveys sensation of the skin of the distal lateral forearm, hand, and joints of the hand; it does not innervate any muscles.

ARTERIES

The **posterior interosseous artery**, a branch of the ulnar artery, supplies blood to most of the posterior forearm muscles. Its course in the posterior forearm lies along the interosseous membrane with the posterior interosseous nerve. The posterior interosseous artery terminates at the wrist where it anastomoses with the dorsal terminal branch of the anterior interosseous artery (see Chapter 21) and contributes to the dorsal carpal arch.

The **radial artery** and **recurrent radial artery** supply blood to the brachioradialis, extensor carpi radialis longus, and extensor carpi radialis brevis muscles; the anconeus receives blood from the profunda brachii artery (see Chapter 19).

VEINS AND LYMPHATICS

Venous drainage of the superficial posterior forearm is along unnamed vessels that empty into the **cephalic** and **basilic veins** (see Chapter 21). Deep venous drainage is by **venae comitantes**, which follow the posterior interosseous and radial arteries. Superficial lymphatic vessels follow the course of the superficial veins and empty into the **cubital nodes**. Deep lymphatic vessels follow the course of the posterior interosseous artery and drain to the **axillary lymph nodes**.

■ CLINICAL CORRELATIONS
Tennis elbow (lateral epicondylitis)

Tennis elbow is an inflammatory condition involving the common extensor tendon of the lateral elbow. Repetitive supination and pronation movements of the forearm cause microinjury and inflammation along the origin for attachment of the extensor carpi radialis brevis and other muscles that insert into the common extensor tendon. The inflammation around the lateral epicondyle (lateral epicondylitis) can be compounded by bursitis or synovitis at the elbow joint. Tennis elbow generally causes a dull, aching sensation on the lateral aspect of the elbow, which usually develops over a period of several months. On examination, there is tenderness over the lateral epicondyle. The pain specific to this condition can be elicited by asking the patient to extend the middle fingers of the outstretched arm against resistance; pain on active dorsiflexion of the wrist also suggests the diagnosis. Radiographs do not usually show fracture but may help in diagnosing rare coexistent conditions. The treatment of lateral epicondylitis is directed at preventing further injury – the RICE regimen is recommended:

- **R**est
- **I**ce or cool packs
- **C**ompression (e.g. Ace bandages – elasticated bandages)
- **E**levation of the affected region to decrease swelling.

Smith's fracture (reverse Colles' fracture)

A Smith's fracture can occur on falling onto the dorsum of a flexed wrist, or by direct trauma to the distal posterior forearm. Transverse fracture of the distal radius with palmar (anterior) displacement of the hand and wrist is observed. Patients complain of pain, swelling, and instability of the distal forearm and wrist.

The injured limb must be examined for any injury to the median nerve or arteries to the hand (radial and ulnar). Usually there is a visible deformity and point tenderness on the bones at the fracture site. Radiographs show fracture lines through the distal radial metaphysis with angulation of the hand and wrist towards the palm.

Closed reduction is attempted if there is minimal angulation of the distal hand and wrist and there are no findings on examination suggesting neurovascular injury. If postreduction radiographs are satisfactory and no neurovascular changes have occurred, a splint or cast is applied. In the presence of open or complex fractures, immediate orthopedic referral for open reduction and internal fixation (surgery with possible plate or screw placement) is recommended.

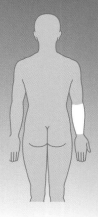

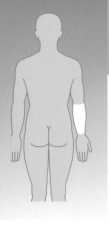

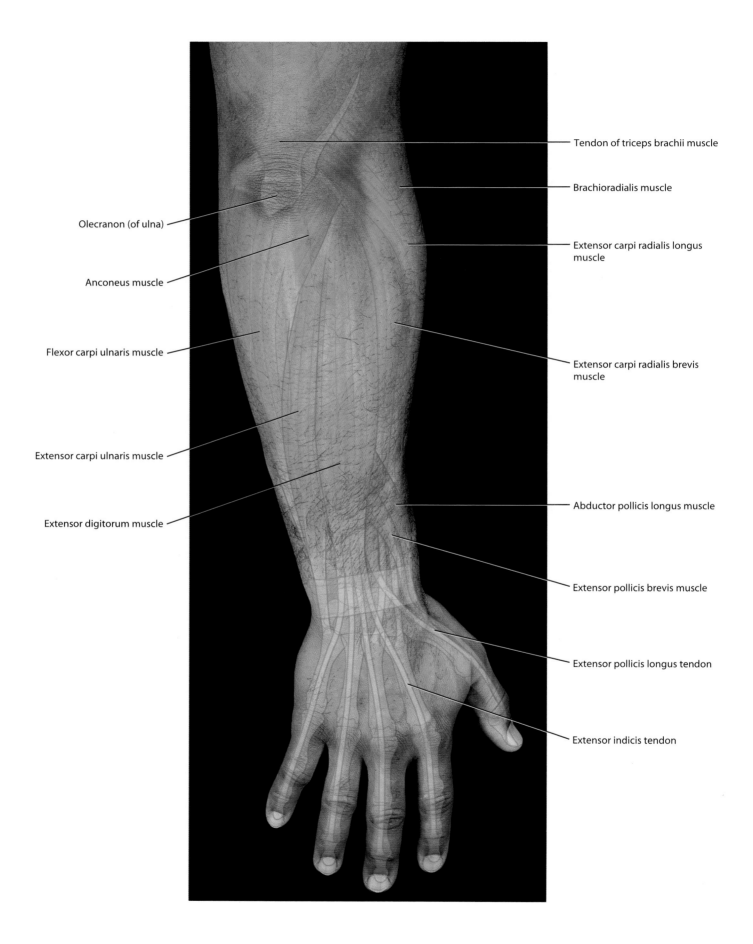

Tendon of triceps brachii muscle

Brachioradialis muscle

Extensor carpi radialis longus muscle

Extensor carpi radialis brevis muscle

Abductor pollicis longus muscle

Extensor pollicis brevis muscle

Extensor pollicis longus tendon

Extensor indicis tendon

Olecranon (of ulna)

Anconeus muscle

Flexor carpi ulnaris muscle

Extensor carpi ulnaris muscle

Extensor digitorum muscle

Figure 22.3 Posterior forearm – surface anatomy. Posterior view of the right forearm

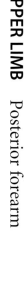

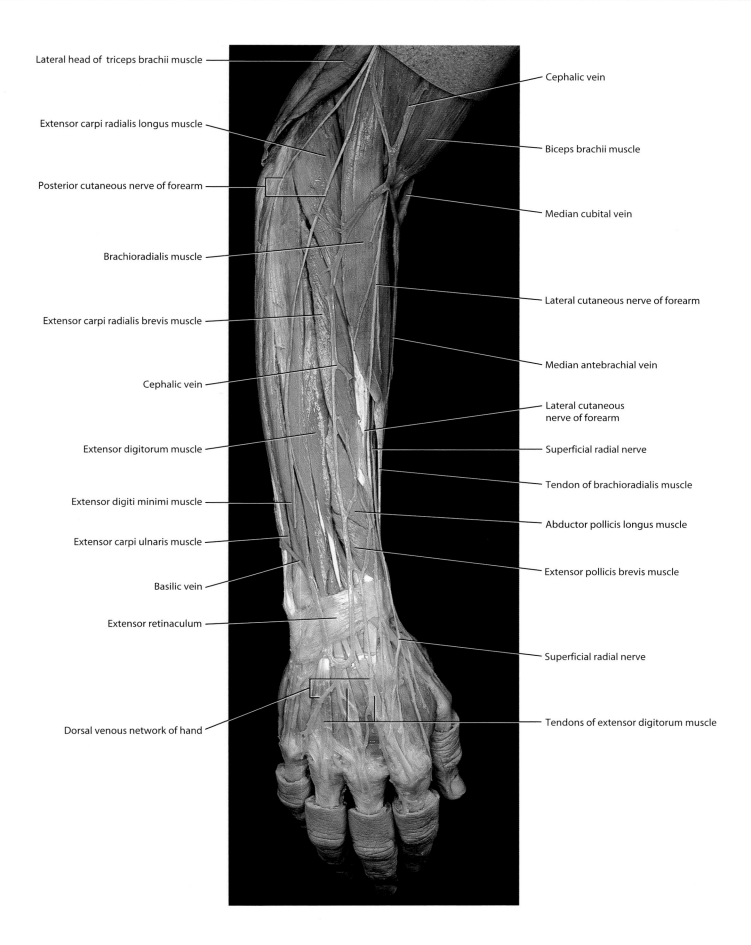

Lateral head of triceps brachii muscle

Extensor carpi radialis longus muscle

Posterior cutaneous nerve of forearm

Brachioradialis muscle

Extensor carpi radialis brevis muscle

Cephalic vein

Extensor digitorum muscle

Extensor digiti minimi muscle

Extensor carpi ulnaris muscle

Basilic vein

Extensor retinaculum

Dorsal venous network of hand

Cephalic vein

Biceps brachii muscle

Median cubital vein

Lateral cutaneous nerve of forearm

Median antebrachial vein

Lateral cutaneous nerve of forearm

Superficial radial nerve

Tendon of brachioradialis muscle

Abductor pollicis longus muscle

Extensor pollicis brevis muscle

Superficial radial nerve

Tendons of extensor digitorum muscle

Figure 22.4 Posterior forearm – superficial dissection. Posterior view of a dissected right forearm. Observe the branching structure of the superficial veins and the cutaneous nerves

253

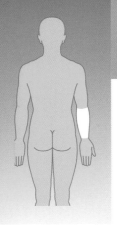

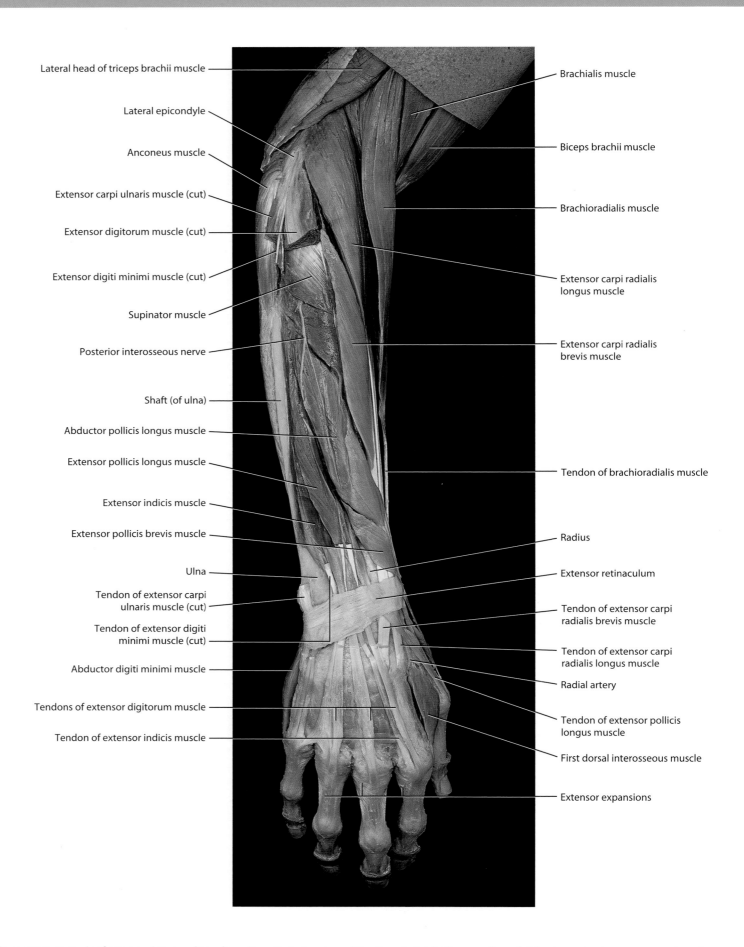

Lateral head of triceps brachii muscle

Lateral epicondyle

Anconeus muscle

Extensor carpi ulnaris muscle (cut)

Extensor digitorum muscle (cut)

Extensor digiti minimi muscle (cut)

Supinator muscle

Posterior interosseous nerve

Shaft (of ulna)

Abductor pollicis longus muscle

Extensor pollicis longus muscle

Extensor indicis muscle

Extensor pollicis brevis muscle

Ulna

Tendon of extensor carpi ulnaris muscle (cut)

Tendon of extensor digiti minimi muscle (cut)

Abductor digiti minimi muscle

Tendons of extensor digitorum muscle

Tendon of extensor indicis muscle

Brachialis muscle

Biceps brachii muscle

Brachioradialis muscle

Extensor carpi radialis longus muscle

Extensor carpi radialis brevis muscle

Tendon of brachioradialis muscle

Radius

Extensor retinaculum

Tendon of extensor carpi radialis brevis muscle

Tendon of extensor carpi radialis longus muscle

Radial artery

Tendon of extensor pollicis longus muscle

First dorsal interosseous muscle

Extensor expansions

Figure 22.5 Posterior forearm – intermediate dissection. Posterior view of the dissected right forearm. Superficial veins and cutaneous nerves have been removed. The extensor carpi ulnaris and extensor digitorum muscles have been cut and removed to show the five posterior muscles and their relationship to the posterior interosseous nerve

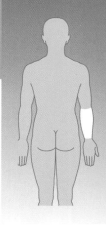

TABLE 22.1 POSTERIOR FOREARM MUSCLES					
Muscle	Origin	Insertion	Innervation	Action	Blood supply
Superficial group Brachioradialis	Proximal two-thirds of lateral supracondylar ridge of humerus	Lateral side of base of styloid process of radius	Radial nerve (C5 to C7)	Flexes forearm	Radial recurrent artery
Extensor carpi radialis longus	Distal one-third of lateral supracondylar ridge of humerus	Dorsal base of metacarpal II	Radial nerve (C6, C7)	Extends wrist and abducts hand	Radial and radial recurrent arteries
Extensor carpi radialis brevis	Lateral epicondyle of humerus (common extensor tendon)	Dorsal base of metacarpal III	Deep branch of radial nerve (C7, C8)	Extends wrist and abducts hand	Radial and radial recurrent arteries
Extensor digitorum	Lateral epicondyle of humerus (common extensor tendon)	Lateral and dorsal surfaces of phalanges of index, middle, ring and little fingers	Posterior interosseous nerve (C7, C8)	Extends index, middle, ring and little fingers; assists in wrist extension	Posterior interosseous artery
Extensor digiti minimi	Lateral epicondyle of humerus (common extensor tendon)	Dorsal base of proximal phalanx of little finger	Posterior interosseous nerve (C7, C8)	Extends little finger	Posterior interosseous artery
Extensor carpi ulnaris	Lateral epicondyle of humerus and posterior border of ulna (common extensor tendon)	Dorsal base of metacarpal V	Posterior interosseous nerve (C7, C8)	Extends wrist and adducts hand	Posterior interosseous artery
Anconeus	Posterior surface of lateral epicondyle of humerus	Lateral surface of olecranon and posterior proximal ulna	Radial nerve (C7 to T1)	Assists triceps brachii in extending forearm	Deep brachial artery
Deep group Supinator	Lateral epicondyle of humerus, supinator crest	Lateral, posterior, and anterior surfaces of proximal third of radius	Deep radial nerve (C5, C6)	Supinates forearm	Radial recurrent and posterior interosseous arteries
Abductor pollicis longus	Posterior surface of ulna, radius, and interosseous membrane	Base of metacarpal I	Posterior interosseous nerve (C7, C8)	Abducts and extends thumb	Posterior interosseous artery
Extensor pollicis brevis	Posterior surface of radius and interosseous membrane	Base of proximal phalanx of thumb	Posterior interosseous nerve (C7, C8)	Extends proximal phalanx of thumb	Posterior interosseous artery
Extensor pollicis longus	Posterior surface of middle third of ulna and interosseous membrane	Base of distal phalanx of thumb	Posterior interosseous nerve (C7, C8)	Extends distal phalanx of thumb	Posterior interosseous artery
Extensor indicis	Posterior surface of ulna and interosseous membrane	Dorsal base of proximal phalanx of second digit	Posterior interosseous nerve (C7, C8)	Extends proximal phalanx of index finger	Posterior interosseous artery

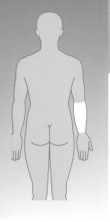

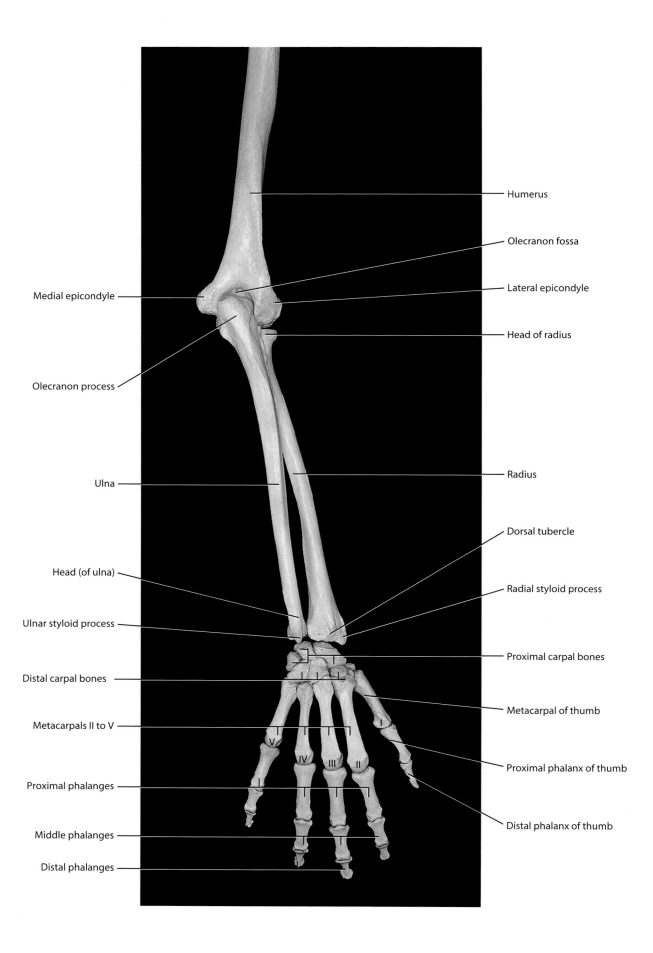

Humerus

Olecranon fossa

Medial epicondyle

Lateral epicondyle

Head of radius

Olecranon process

Ulna

Radius

Dorsal tubercle

Head (of ulna)

Radial styloid process

Ulnar styloid process

Distal carpal bones

Proximal carpal bones

Metacarpal of thumb

Metacarpals II to V

I

V

IV

III

II

Proximal phalanx of thumb

Proximal phalanges

Middle phalanges

Distal phalanx of thumb

Distal phalanges

Figure 22.6 Posterior forearm – osteology. Posterior view of the articulated bones of the right forearm, wrist, and hand

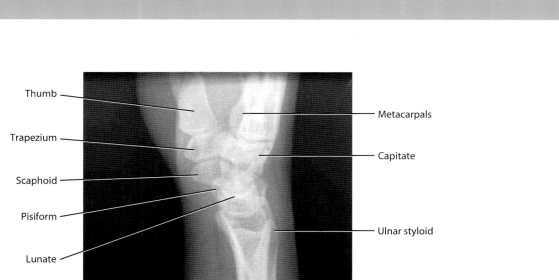

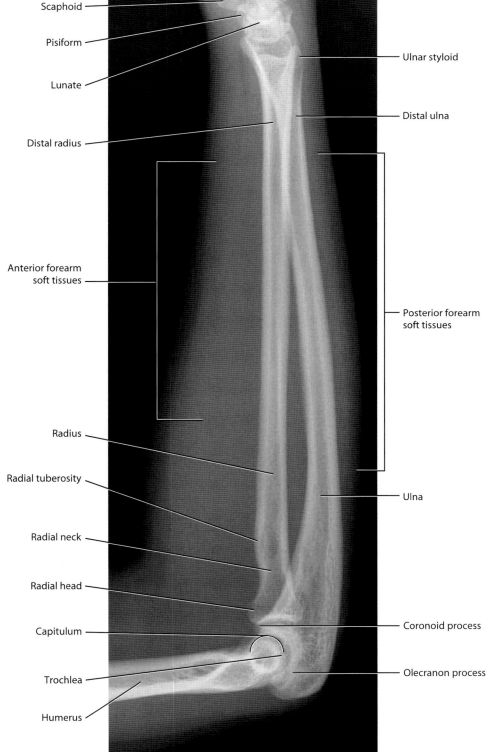

Thumb

Trapezium

Scaphoid

Pisiform

Lunate

Distal radius

Anterior forearm soft tissues

Radius

Radial tuberosity

Radial neck

Radial head

Capitulum

Trochlea

Humerus

Metacarpals

Capitate

Ulnar styloid

Distal ulna

Posterior forearm soft tissues

Ulna

Coronoid process

Olecranon process

Figure 22.7 Posterior forearm – plain film radiograph (lateral view). Note that the bulk of the soft tissue of the forearm is anterior

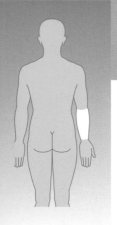

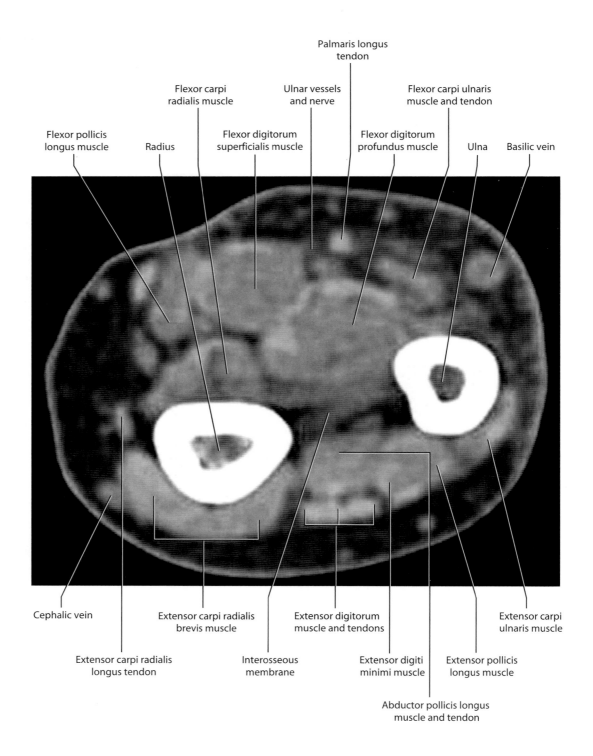

Palmaris longus
tendon

Flexor carpi
radialis muscle

Ulnar vessels
and nerve

Flexor carpi ulnaris
muscle and tendon

Flexor pollicis
longus muscle

Radius

Flexor digitorum
superficialis muscle

Flexor digitorum
profundus muscle

Ulna

Basilic vein

Cephalic vein

Extensor carpi radialis
brevis muscle

Extensor digitorum
muscle and tendons

Extensor carpi
ulnaris muscle

Extensor carpi radialis
longus tendon

Interosseous
membrane

Extensor digiti
minimi muscle

Extensor pollicis
longus muscle

Abductor pollicis longus
muscle and tendon

Figure 22.8 Posterior forearm – CT scan (axial view, from distal to proximal). The bulk of the posterior forearm muscles is usually less than that of the anterior forearm because the hand requires more strength to perform grasping maneuvers than it does to 'ungrasp' an object. The interosseous membrane separates the two compartments and also aids in the transfer of weight from the radius to the ulna during weight bearing activities

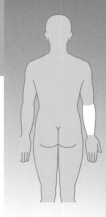

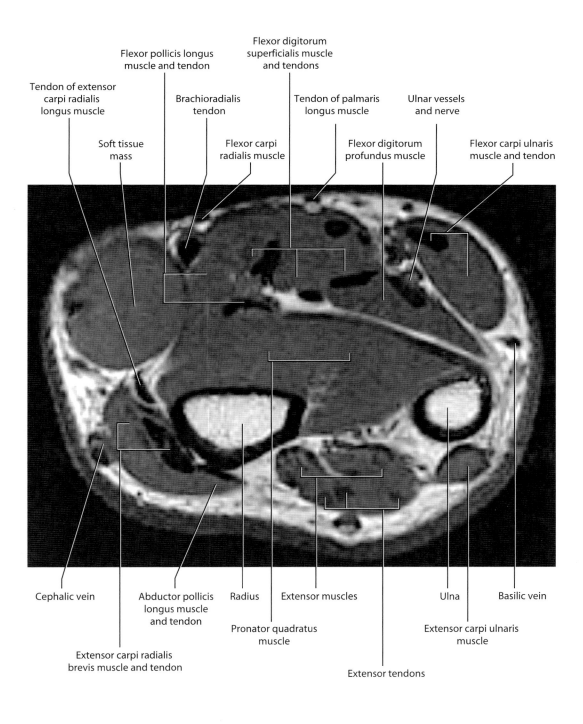

Figure 22.9 Posterior forearm – MRI scan (axial view, from distal to proximal). The extensor carpi radialis brevis and extensor carpi ulnaris muscles are easily seen in this scan of the distal forearm. An abnormal soft tissue mass is seen in the lateral subcutaneous fat

23 Wrist and hand joints

The joints of the wrists and hands are an array of small interconnections at the distal upper limb that enable complex movements such as writing and sewing. The wrist contains eight bones arranged in two rows (proximal and distal) while the hand and its five digits contains 19 bones (Figs 23.1 and 23.2).

WRIST

The eight carpal bones of the wrist are oriented in two rows and collectively connect the forearm to the hand. From lateral to medial, the first (proximal) row of bones in the wrist (**carpal bones**) comprise the scaphoid, lunate, triquetrum, and pisiform bones. The second (distal) row from lateral to medial comprise the trapezium, trapezoid, capitate, and hamate bones. The carpal bones form three primary articulations:

- wrist joint (**radiocarpal joint**) between the forearm and wrist;
- **midcarpal joints** between the proximal and distal rows of carpal bones;
- **carpometacarpal joints** between the distal row of carpal bones and the hand.

The carpal bones are contained within a single joint capsule, which encloses the entire group. The joint capsule has many thickenings, which are named as ligaments (e.g. **palmar radiocarpal** and **ulnocarpal** and **dorsal radiocarpal** and **ulnocarpal ligaments**, and **ulnar** and **radial collateral ligaments of wrist joint**). In addition, **interosseous intercarpal ligaments** bind the proximal row of carpals with the distal row, and **palmar** and **dorsal intercarpal ligaments** connect the individual carpal bones within a row.

The scaphoid, lunate, and triquetrum bones within the joint capsule of the wrist form an arch, which fits into a concave depression on the surface of the distal radius. These bones articulate with the radius at the radiocarpal joint. The arch is bridged by the **flexor retinaculum** to form the **carpal tunnel**, through which pass the tendons of the flexor digitorum superficialis, flexor digitorum profundus, and flexor pollicis longus muscles, and the median nerve.

On the dorsum of the wrist is the **extensor retinaculum**, which encloses the tendons on the dorsum of the hand to prevent bowstringing during extension of the wrist and hand.

Innervation to the carpal bones and joints is from the **anterior interosseous nerve** (a branch of the median nerve), the **posterior interosseous nerve** (a branch of the radial nerve), and the **dorsal** and **deep branches of the ulnar nerve**. The blood supply is from the **dorsal** and **palmar carpal arches**, which are formed from branches of the radial and ulnar arteries. Venous drainage is to the **radial** and **ulnar veins** through venae comitantes. Lymphatic drainage is to the **cubital** and **axillary lymph nodes**; there are no lymph node groups at the wrist.

HAND

The hand contains 19 bones divided into two groups, five metacarpals (which form the palm) and 14 phalanges (which form the fingers and thumb).

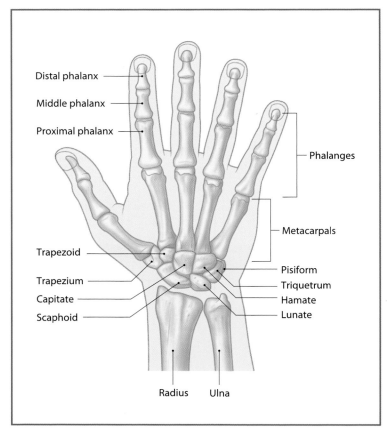

Figure 23.1 Bones of the wrist and hand, posterior (dorsal) view

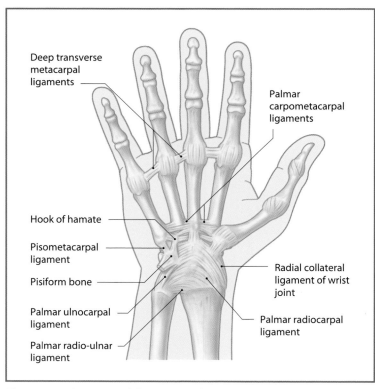

Figure 23.2 Ligaments of the wrist and hand, anterior (palmar) view

The **metacarpals** are slim bones with their **heads** distal and their **bases** proximal. The bases articulate with the carpal bones (Table 23.1) through carpometacarpal (CMC) joints:

- the CMC joint of the thumb is between the base of metacarpal I and the trapezium;
- metacarpal II articulates primarily with the trapezoid, and secondarily with the trapezium and capitate;
- metacarpal III articulates with the capitate;
- metacarpal IV articulates with the capitate and hamate;
- metacarpal V is medial in the hand and articulates with the hamate.

The four metacarpals of the fingers are supported by strong intermetacarpal ligaments and are united by dorsal, palmar, and interosseous ligaments. This adds strength to the distal palm and creates a natural concave curvature to the palm to increase stability when handling objects.

The head of each metacarpal articulates with the proximal phalanx of each digit through the metacarpophalangeal (MCP) joints (knuckle joints). These joints join the head of each metacarpal with the corresponding proximal phalanx of each digit. All MCP joints have an anterior **palmar ligament** (volar plate) to reinforce the joint capsule anteriorly. The palmar ligaments of the four fingers are united transversely by **deep transverse metacarpal ligaments** and **collateral ligaments**.

The **interphalangeal joints of hand**, created by the union of the phalanges, are all synovial joints, and the joint capsules show considerable laxity. These loose ligamentous attachments onto each finger permit the wide range of movements of the digits.

All of the joints of the wrist and hand are supplied by the anterior interosseous branch of the median nerve, the posterior interosseous branch of the radial nerve, and the dorsal and deep branches of the ulnar nerve. Blood is supplied by the **superficial** and **deep palmar arches**, and by the digital arteries that originate from these arches. Venous drainage is along small unnamed digital and deep veins that drain to the radial and ulnar veins. Lymphatic drainage follows the venous drainage and empties to the cubital lymph nodes and axillary lymph nodes.

■ CLINICAL CORRELATIONS
Carpal tunnel syndrome

Carpal tunnel syndrome is caused by injury to the median nerve as it passes along the palmar surface of the carpal bones from the anterior forearm to the hand. The median nerve and the tendons of the flexor digitorum superficialis, flexor digitorum profundus, and flexor pollicis longus muscles run through the carpal tunnel. Overuse of these muscles, injury, or inflammatory diseases (e.g. rheumatoid arthritis) can lead to swelling within the narrow carpal tunnel, exerting pressure on the median nerve (Fig. 23.3).

Symptoms usually result from carrying out some type of repetitive action involving the wrist and hand for a long period of time, and include pain in the thumb, index, and middle fingers, vague pain in the hand, and numbness and paresthesias ('pins and needles' sensation) throughout the hand. The symptoms usually reflect the distribution of the median nerve in the hand and resolve with rest.

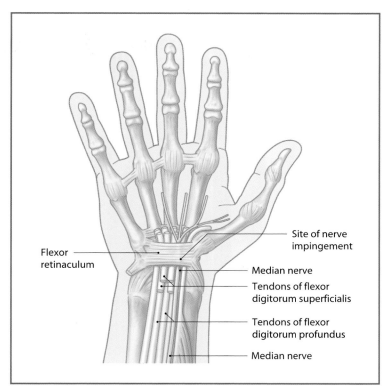

Flexor retinaculum

Site of nerve impingement

Median nerve

Tendons of flexor digitorum superficialis

Tendons of flexor digitorum profundus

Median nerve

Figure 23.3 Carpal tunnel syndrome

On examination an adequate blood supply to the hand should be verified by checking the peripheral pulses and capillary refill within the pads of the fingers. The nerves to the hand are then examined, first checking sensation to the hand, then muscle strength. A sensitive test for carpal tunnel syndrome is Phalen's maneuver. With the forearms in a vertical position, the patient is asked to flex the wrists maximally and to hold them in this position for 1 minute. The result is positive and indicative of probable carpal tunnel syndrome if the patient reports paresthesias in the hand along the distribution of the median nerve.

Specialized nerve conduction studies are sometimes used to determine the extent of median nerve injury.

Initial treatment is to avoid actions that might have led to the condition and rest of the involved upper limb. Splints and oral anti-inflammatory medications are commonly used. After a course of nonoperative treatment, the patient might be referred to the surgeon for definitive management. A carpal tunnel release is a procedure in which the transverse carpal ligament (the ligament that bridges the gap between the carpal bones to create the carpal tunnel) is incised surgically.

MNEMONICS			
Carpal bones:	**Simply Learn The Parts That The Carpus Has**		
	(Proximal row, lateral to medial:	**S**caphoid, **L**unate, **T**riquetrum, **P**isiform)	
	(Distal row, lateral to medial:	**T**rapezium, **T**rapezoid, **C**apitate, **H**amate)	
	Trapezi**UM** at the Th**UM**b		

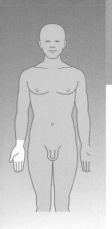

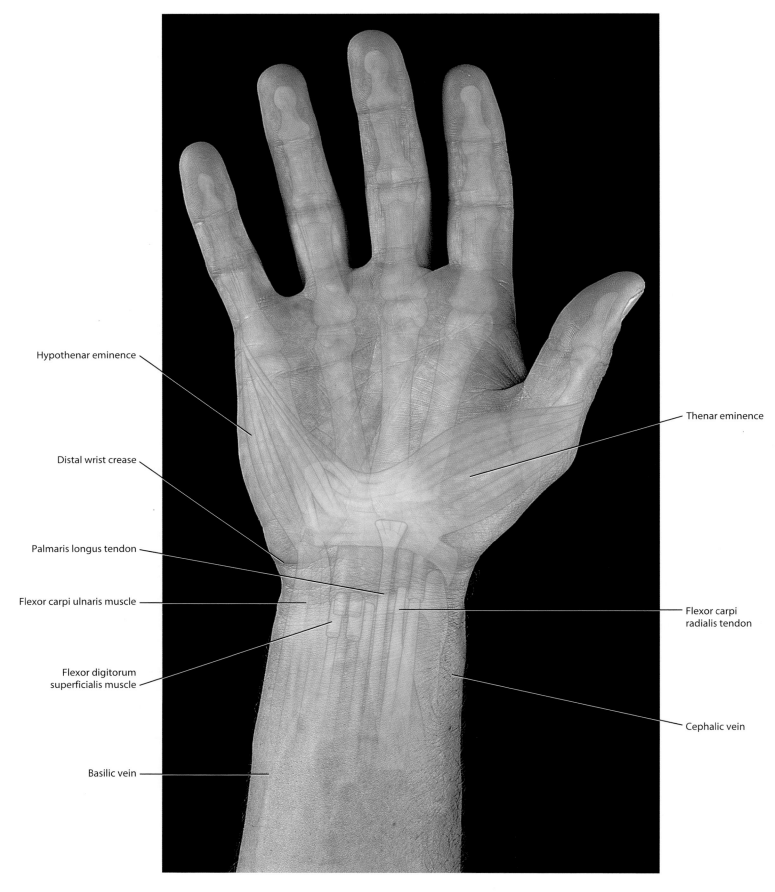

Hypothenar eminence

Distal wrist crease

Palmaris longus tendon

Flexor carpi ulnaris muscle

Flexor digitorum
superficialis muscle

Basilic vein

Thenar eminence

Flexor carpi
radialis tendon

Cephalic vein

Figure 23.4 Wrist and hand joints – anterior surface anatomy. Anterior view of the right wrist and hand showing the features of the palmar (anterior) surface. Markings of tendons, muscles, veins, and creases are visible

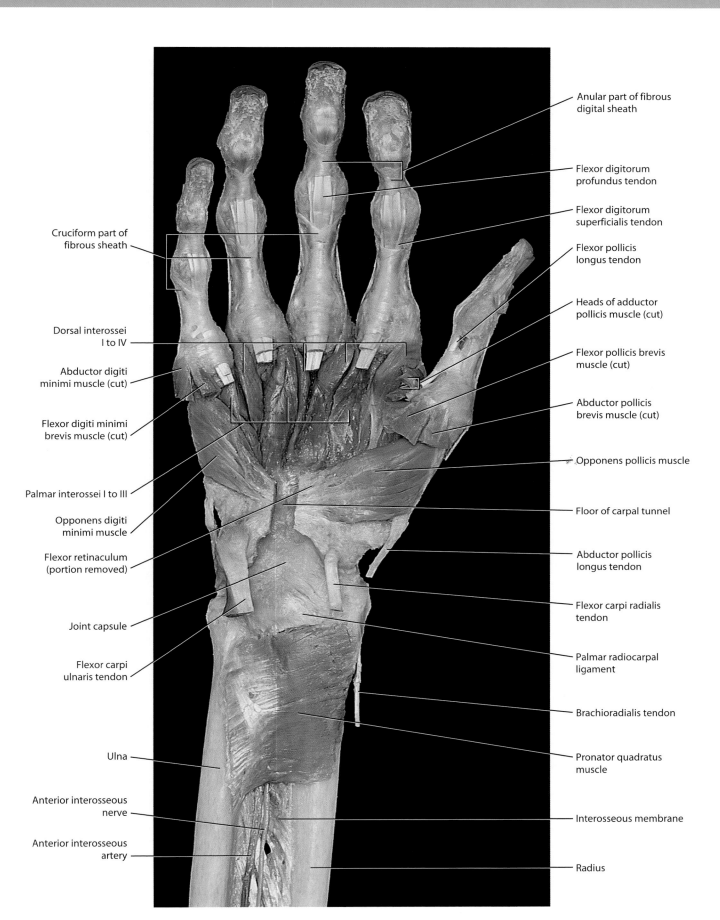

Anular part of fibrous digital sheath

Flexor digitorum profundus tendon

Flexor digitorum superficialis tendon

Flexor pollicis longus tendon

Heads of adductor pollicis muscle (cut)

Flexor pollicis brevis muscle (cut)

Abductor pollicis brevis muscle (cut)

Opponens pollicis muscle

Floor of carpal tunnel

Abductor pollicis longus tendon

Flexor carpi radialis tendon

Palmar radiocarpal ligament

Brachioradialis tendon

Pronator quadratus muscle

Interosseous membrane

Radius

Cruciform part of fibrous sheath

Dorsal interossei I to IV

Abductor digiti minimi muscle (cut)

Flexor digiti minimi brevis muscle (cut)

Palmar interossei I to III

Opponens digiti minimi muscle

Flexor retinaculum (portion removed)

Joint capsule

Flexor carpi ulnaris tendon

Ulna

Anterior interosseous nerve

Anterior interosseous artery

Figure 23.5 Wrist and hand joints – anterior superficial dissection. Anterior (palmar) view of the dissected right hand. Observe that the tendons of the flexor digitorum superficialis and flexor digitorum profundus muscles have been cut and removed. Also observe the cut ligament, exposing the floor of the carpal tunnel. Note the position of the seven interossei muscles and the joint capsule

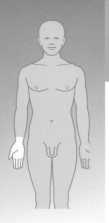

Wrist and hand joints

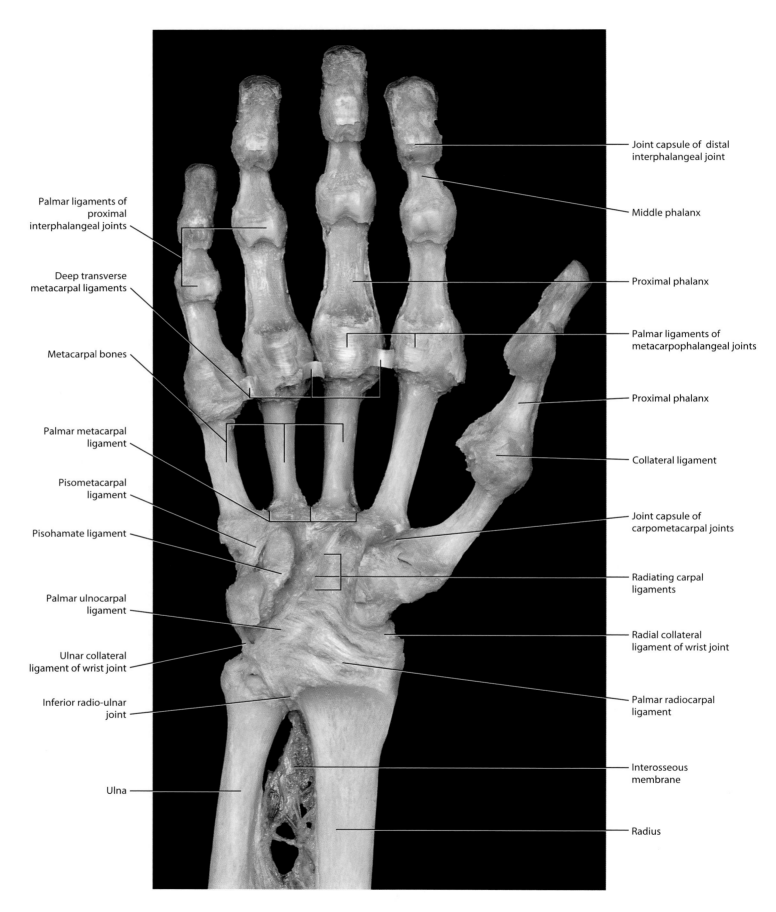

Palmar ligaments of proximal interphalangeal joints

Deep transverse metacarpal ligaments

Metacarpal bones

Palmar metacarpal ligament

Pisometacarpal ligament

Pisohamate ligament

Palmar ulnocarpal ligament

Ulnar collateral ligament of wrist joint

Inferior radio-ulnar joint

Ulna

Joint capsule of distal interphalangeal joint

Middle phalanx

Proximal phalanx

Palmar ligaments of metacarpophalangeal joints

Proximal phalanx

Collateral ligament

Joint capsule of carpometacarpal joints

Radiating carpal ligaments

Radial collateral ligament of wrist joint

Palmar radiocarpal ligament

Interosseous membrane

Radius

Figure 23.6 Wrist and hand joints – anterior deep dissection. Anterior (palmar) view of a deep dissection of the right wrist and hand with all the muscles, their tendons, and and other soft tissues removed to show the ligaments of the wrist and hand. Note the various carpal ligaments reinforcing the joint capsule

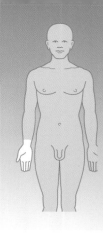

TABLE 23.1 JOINTS OF THE WRIST AND HAND

Joint	Type	Articular surfaces	Ligaments	Movements
Wrist complex Radiocarpal	Condyloid-type synovial joint	Radius and articular disk proximally. Scaphoid, lunate, and triquetrum distally	Palmar and dorsal ligaments strengthen the capsule. Radial collateral to lateral scaphoid. Ulnar collateral to pisiform and triquetrum	Flexion (50°) Extension (35°) Ulnar deviation (30°) Radial deviation (7°) Circumduction
Midcarpal	Plane-type synovial joint	Scaphoid, lunate and triquetrum proximally. Trapezium, trapezoid, capitate and hamate distally	Interosseous intercarpal between proximal and distal rows. Intercarpals among the carpal bones	Extension (50°) Flexion (35°) Ulnar deviation (15°) Radial deviation (8°)
Hand complex Carpometacarpal (CMC)	Plane-type synovial joint; CMCI is saddle joint	MCI → trapezium MCII → trapezium, trapezoid, and capitate MCIII → capitate MCIV → capitate and hamate MCV → hamate	Each metacarpal receives palmar and dorsal ligaments. Intermetacarpal ligaments between metacarpals	CMCI → flexion–extension also, abduction–adduction CMCII, III → immovable CMCIV, V → slight gliding
Metacarpophalangeal (MCP)	Condyloid-type synovial joint	Heads of metacarpals articulate with bases of proximal phalanges	Palmar ligaments between phalanges and metacarpals. Deep transverse metacarpal ligaments bind metacarpal heads. Collateral ligaments unite metacarpal heads to bases of phalanges	MCP II–V: – flexion–extension – abduction–adduction – circumduction – MCPI – flexion–extension – abduction–adduction – opposition
Interphalangeal: – proximal (PIP) – distal (DIP)	Hinge-type synovial joint	Heads of phalanges with bases of more distally located phalanges	Collateral ligaments along sides. Palmar ligaments (plates) anteriorly	Flexion–extension (increases ulnarly)

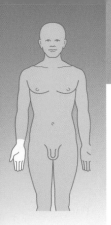

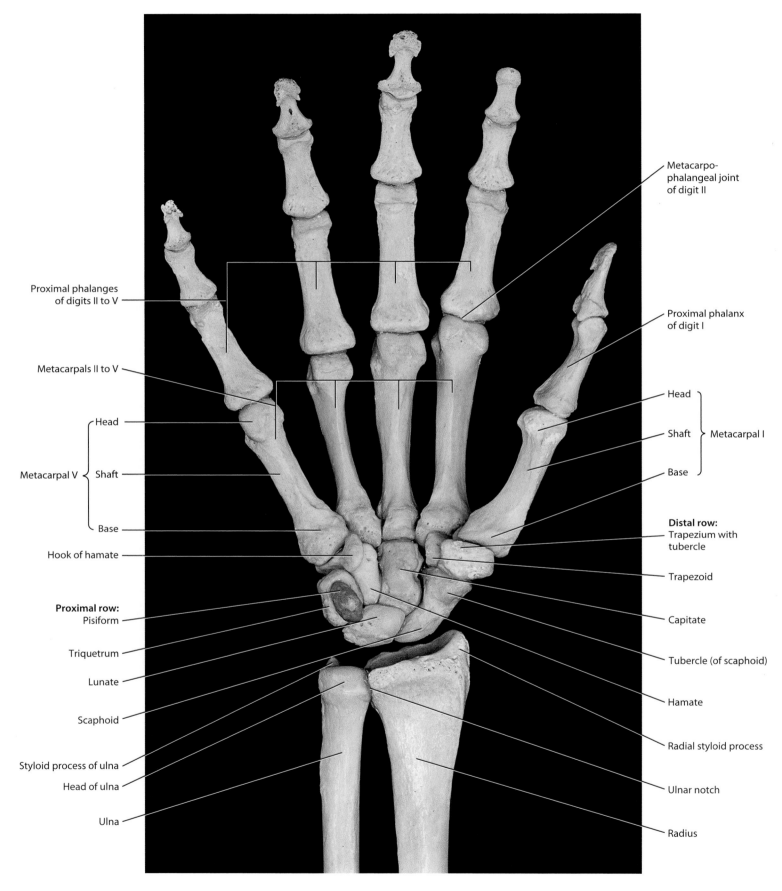

Metacarpo-phalangeal joint of digit II

Proximal phalanges of digits II to V

Proximal phalanx of digit I

Metacarpals II to V

Head

Head

Shaft

Shaft ⎬ Metacarpal I

Metacarpal V ⎨ Shaft

Base

Base

Distal row:
Trapezium with tubercle

Hook of hamate

Trapezoid

Proximal row:
Pisiform

Capitate

Triquetrum

Tubercle (of scaphoid)

Lunate

Scaphoid

Hamate

Styloid process of ulna

Head of ulna

Radial styloid process

Ulna

Ulnar notch

Radius

Figure 23.7 Wrist and hand joints – anterior osteology. Anterior (palmar) view of the articulated bones of the right wrist and hand. The ulna and radius have been separated slightly to show the concave socket of the wrist joint.

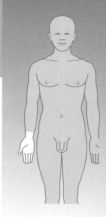

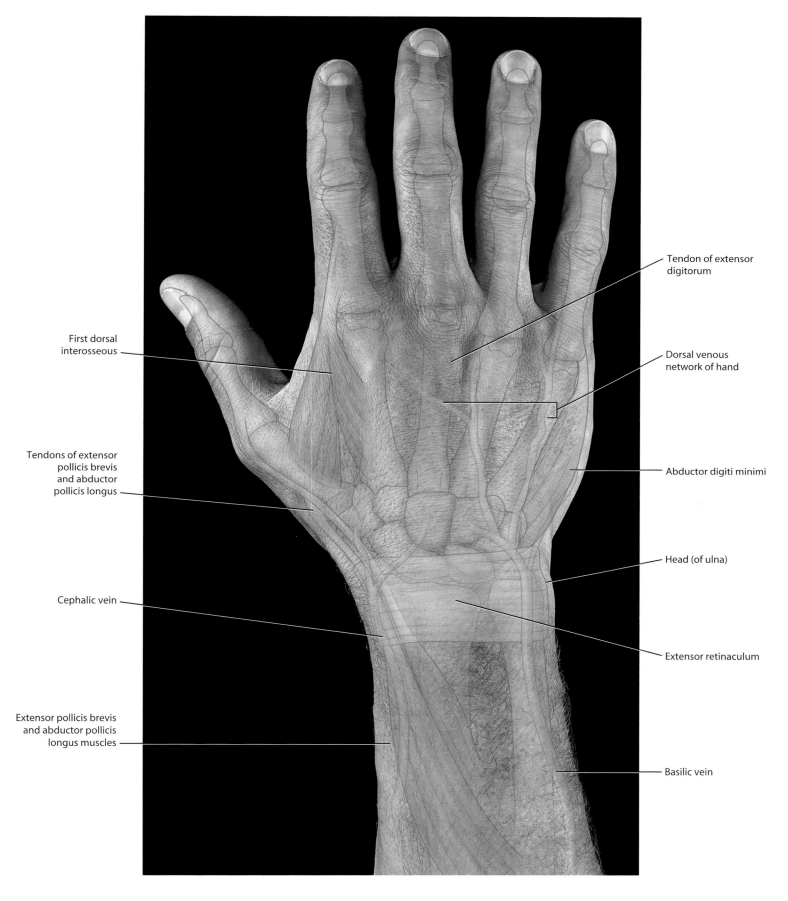

First dorsal
interosseous

Tendons of extensor
pollicis brevis
and abductor
pollicis longus

Cephalic vein

Extensor pollicis brevis
and abductor pollicis
longus muscles

Tendon of extensor
digitorum

Dorsal venous
network of hand

Abductor digiti minimi

Head (of ulna)

Extensor retinaculum

Basilic vein

Figure 23.8 Wrist and hand joints – posterior surface anatomy. Posterior view of the right wrist and hand showing the features of the dorsal (posterior) surface

267

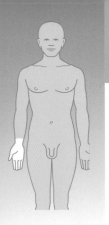

UPPER LIMB

Wrist and hand joints

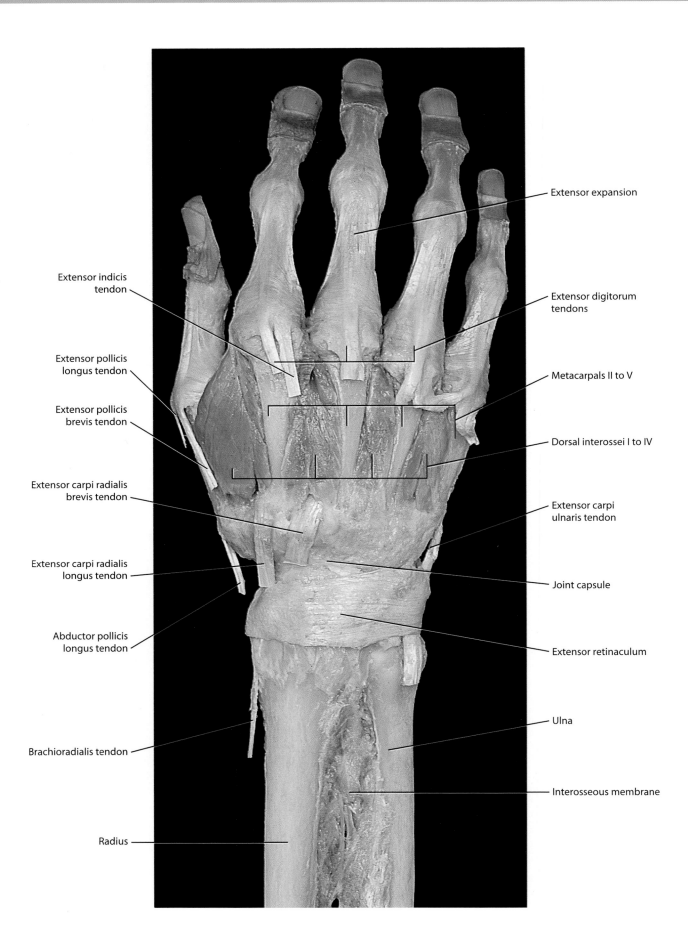

Extensor indicis tendon

Extensor pollicis longus tendon

Extensor pollicis brevis tendon

Extensor carpi radialis brevis tendon

Extensor carpi radialis longus tendon

Abductor pollicis longus tendon

Brachioradialis tendon

Radius

Extensor expansion

Extensor digitorum tendons

Metacarpals II to V

Dorsal interossei I to IV

Extensor carpi ulnaris tendon

Joint capsule

Extensor retinaculum

Ulna

Interosseous membrane

Figure 23.9 Wrist and hand joints – posterior intermediate dissection. Posterior (dorsal) view of the right wrist and hand with the extensor retinaculum intact. The tendons of the extensor digitorum and extensor indicis muscles have been removed to demonstrate the interossei muscles and the metacarpals

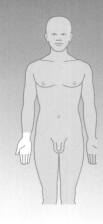

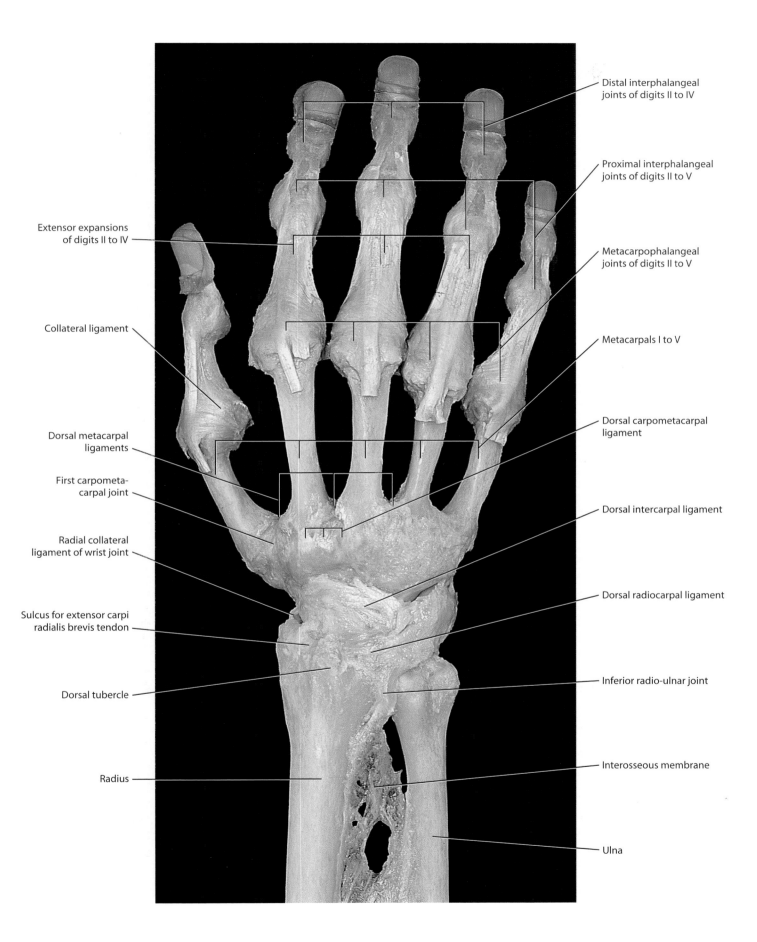

Distal interphalangeal joints of digits II to IV

Proximal interphalangeal joints of digits II to V

Metacarpophalangeal joints of digits II to V

Metacarpals I to V

Dorsal carpometacarpal ligament

Dorsal intercarpal ligament

Dorsal radiocarpal ligament

Inferior radio-ulnar joint

Interosseous membrane

Ulna

Extensor expansions of digits II to IV

Collateral ligament

Dorsal metacarpal ligaments

First carpometa-carpal joint

Radial collateral ligament of wrist joint

Sulcus for extensor carpi radialis brevis tendon

Dorsal tubercle

Radius

Figure 23.10 Wrist and hand joints – posterior deep dissection. Posterior (dorsal) view of the wrist and hand ligaments showing the joint capsules. The dorsal surface of the wrist joint is reinforced by the dorsal intercarpal ligament

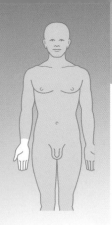

UPPER LIMB

Wrist and hand joints

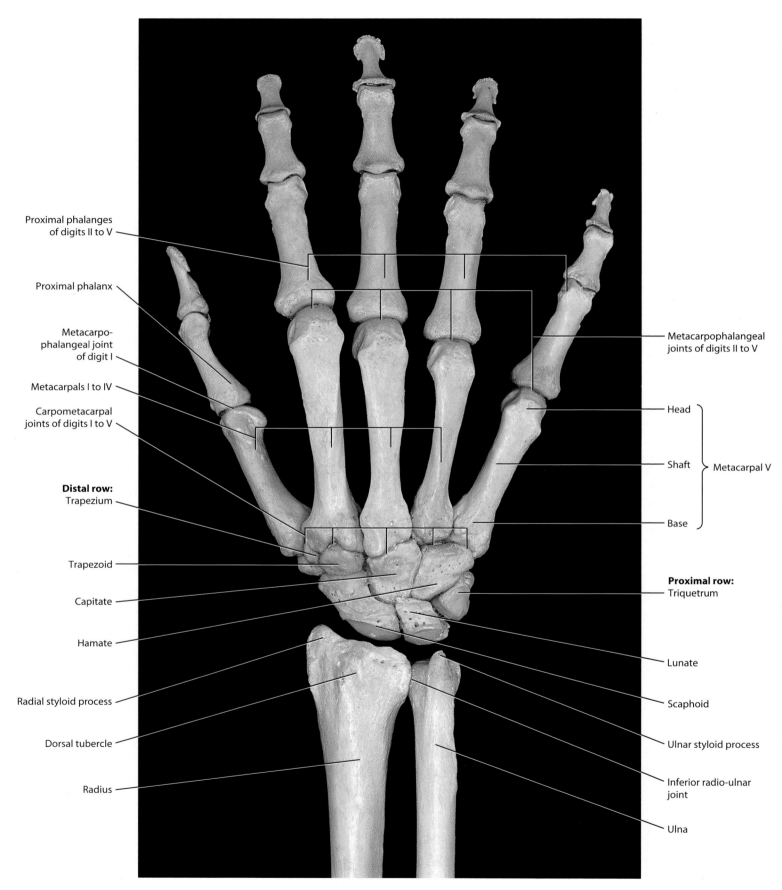

Proximal phalanges of digits II to V

Proximal phalanx

Metacarpo-phalangeal joint of digit I

Metacarpals I to IV

Carpometacarpal joints of digits I to V

Distal row:
Trapezium

Trapezoid

Capitate

Hamate

Radial styloid process

Dorsal tubercle

Radius

Metacarpophalangeal joints of digits II to V

Head

Shaft   } Metacarpal V

Base

Proximal row:
Triquetrum

Lunate

Scaphoid

Ulnar styloid process

Inferior radio-ulnar joint

Ulna

Figure 23.11 Wrist and hand joints – posterior osteology. Posterior (dorsal) view of the articulated right wrist and hand bones. Note the midcarpal joint between the proximal and distal rows of carpal bones

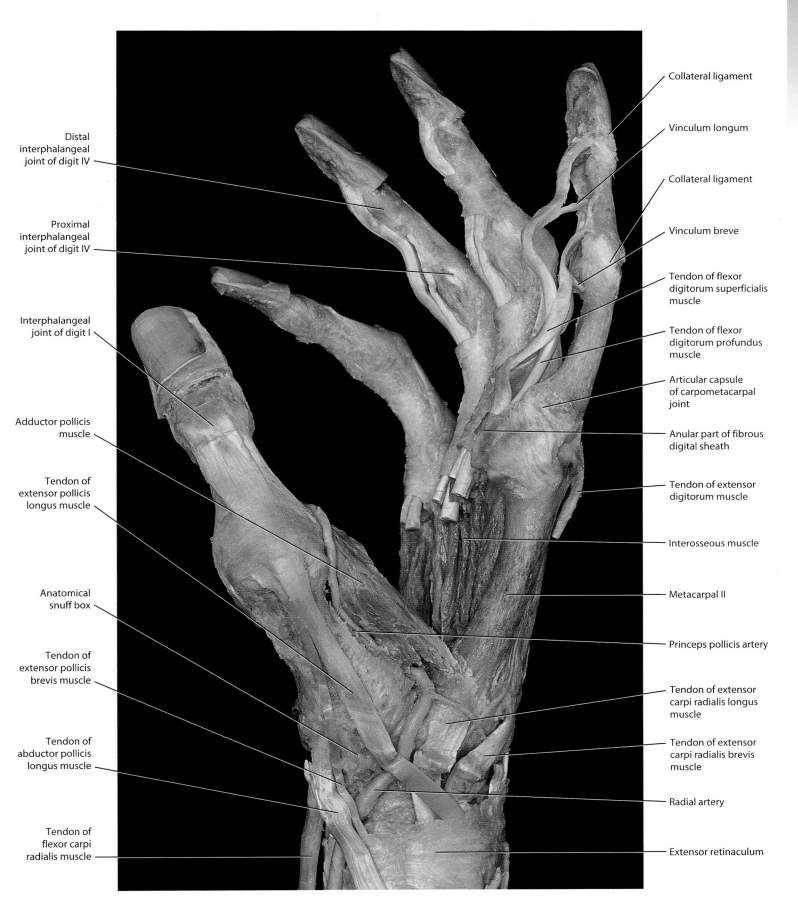

Distal
interphalangeal
joint of digit IV

Proximal
interphalangeal
joint of digit IV

Interphalangeal
joint of digit I

Adductor pollicis
muscle

Tendon of
extensor pollicis
longus muscle

Anatomical
snuff box

Tendon of
extensor pollicis
brevis muscle

Tendon of
abductor pollicis
longus muscle

Tendon of
flexor carpi
radialis muscle

Collateral ligament

Vinculum longum

Collateral ligament

Vinculum breve

Tendon of flexor
digitorum superficialis
muscle

Tendon of flexor
digitorum profundus
muscle

Articular capsule
of carpometacarpal
joint

Anular part of fibrous
digital sheath

Tendon of extensor
digitorum muscle

Interosseous muscle

Metacarpal II

Princeps pollicis artery

Tendon of extensor
carpi radialis longus
muscle

Tendon of extensor
carpi radialis brevis
muscle

Radial artery

Extensor retinaculum

UPPER LIMB   Wrist and hand joints

Figure 23.12 Wrist and hand joints – intermediate dissection. Lateral view of the right hand illustrating two relationships: the lateral finger with vincula and
the collateral ligaments; and the thumb tendons bordering the anatomical snuffbox at the base of the thumb. The tendons of the flexor digitorum superficialis
and flexor digitorum profundus muscles are visible as they insert onto the middle and distal phalanges, respectively

271

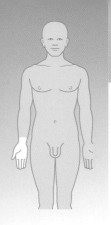

UPPER LIMB

Wrist and hand joints

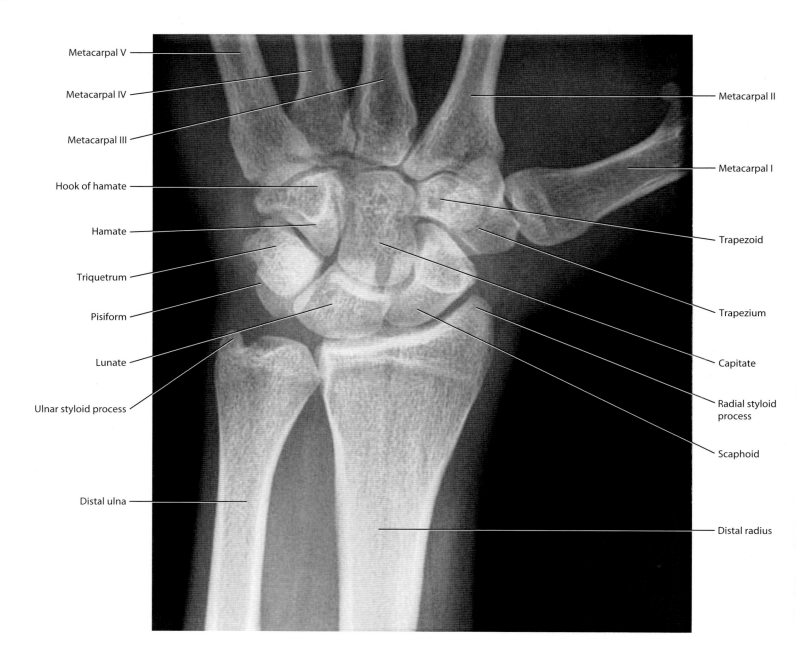

Metacarpal V

Metacarpal IV

Metacarpal III

Hook of hamate

Hamate

Triquetrum

Pisiform

Lunate

Ulnar styloid process

Distal ulna

Metacarpal II

Metacarpal I

Trapezoid

Trapezium

Capitate

Radial styloid process

Scaphoid

Distal radius

Figure 23.13 Wrist joints - plain film radiograph (anteroposterior view). The carpal bones are arranged in two rows: proximal (scaphoid, lunate, triquetrum, and pisiform) and distal (trapezium, trapezoid, capitate, and hamate). Observe how the scaphoid articulates with the distal radius in this normal radiograph. The most frequently fractured carpal bone is the scaphoid

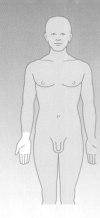

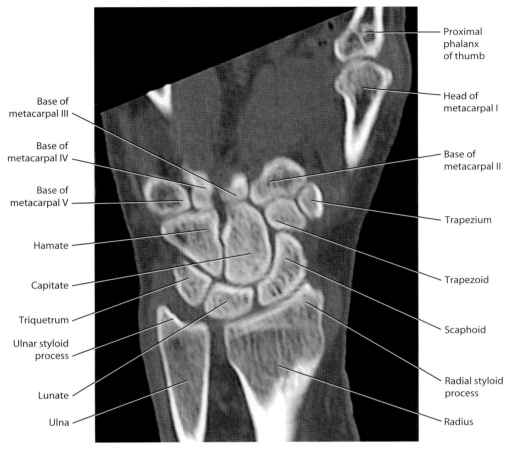

Proximal
phalanx
of thumb

Head of
metacarpal I

Base of
metacarpal II

Trapezium

Trapezoid

Scaphoid

Radial styloid
process

Radius

Base of
metacarpal III

Base of
metacarpal IV

Base of
metacarpal V

Hamate

Capitate

Triquetrum

Ulnar styloid
process

Lunate

Ulna

Figure 23.14 Wrist joints – CT scan (coronal view). The carpals are arranged in a unique fashion to facilitate smooth transfer of weight from the hand to the forearm as well as to enable a wide range of motion. Note that the pisiform is not visible because it is anterior to the plane of the scan

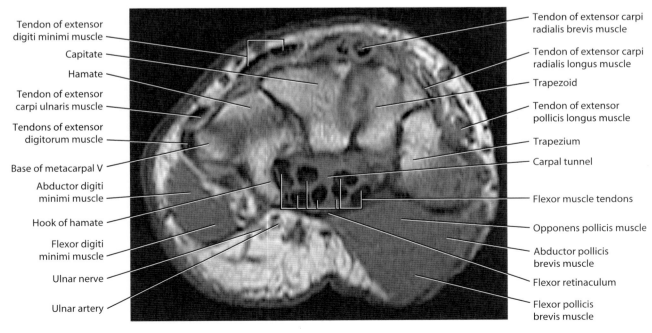

Tendon of extensor
digiti minimi muscle

Capitate

Hamate

Tendon of extensor
carpi ulnaris muscle

Tendons of extensor
digitorum muscle

Base of metacarpal V

Abductor digiti
minimi muscle

Hook of hamate

Flexor digiti
minimi muscle

Ulnar nerve

Ulnar artery

Tendon of extensor carpi
radialis brevis muscle

Tendon of extensor carpi
radialis longus muscle

Trapezoid

Tendon of extensor
pollicis longus muscle

Trapezium

Carpal tunnel

Flexor muscle tendons

Opponens pollicis muscle

Abductor pollicis
brevis muscle

Flexor retinaculum

Flexor pollicis
brevis muscle

Figure 23.15 Wrist joints – MRI scan (axial view, from distal to proximal). This scan is at the level of the distal row of carpal bones (trapezium, trapezoid, capitate, and hamate). Observe the flexor muscle tendons, which more distally will pass through the carpal tunnel

24 Hand muscles

The hand is the most distal part of the upper limb. It can carry out complex movements because of the unique arrangement of four digits with the opposing thumb. The digits (fingers) are numbered with the thumb as digit I and the little finger as digit V. The digits can also be referred to as the thumb, index finger, middle finger, ring finger, and little finger. There are 19 bones in the hand: five metacarpals and 14 phalanges. The wrist contains eight bones (carpal bones) and is described in Chapter 23.

DORSUM OF THE HAND

The skin on the dorsal (posterior) surface of the hand is thin and contains visible superficial veins comprising the **dorsal venous network of hand**. The medial end of the dorsal venous network coalesces to form the **basilic vein**, and the veins on the lateral end form the **cephalic vein**. Deep to the veins are the long extensor tendons from the forearm, which are bound down as they cross the wrist by the extensor retinaculum. The dorsum (dorsal surface) of the hand contains only four dorsal interossei muscles between the metacarpal bones (Table 24.1).

Cutaneous innervation to the dorsum of the hand is from the **radial**, **median**, and **ulnar nerves** (Fig. 24.1). The blood is supplied by branches of the **radial artery**. At the distal lateral wrist the radial artery gives off the **princeps pollicis artery** (to the thumb) and the **dorsalis indices artery** to the index finger. From this point, the radial artery continues as the **dorsal carpal arch**, giving rise to the **dorsal metacarpal arteries**, which in turn become the **dorsal digital arteries** to each finger.

PALMAR SURFACE OF THE HAND

The skin on the palmar (anterior) surface of the hand is thick and hairless and displays numerous longitudinal and transverse flexion creases. The palm is unique in that its ridged surface combined with the many intrinsic muscles of the hand enables it to participate in grasping, lifting, and fine movements.

The deep fascia of the palm is a continuation of the antebrachial fascia of the forearm. In the middle of the palm the fascia becomes thickened as the **palmar aponeurosis**, which provides distal attachment for the palmaris longus muscle from the anterior forearm, and protects and contains the tendons and muscles of the hand. Two septa arising from the internal (deep) surface of the palmar aponeurosis, one medial and one lateral, divide the hand into three compartments – medial, central, and lateral. The flexor retinaculum proximal to the palmar aponeurosis is a strong transverse band of fascia that confines the flexor tendons of the forearm as they pass through the hand towards the fingers.

MUSCLES OF THE HAND

The intrinsic muscles of the hand are divided into three groups named after the three major (medial, central, and lateral) compartments of the hand described below. **Intrinsic hand muscles** originate and have insertion points on the hand whereas **extrinsic hand muscles** (e.g. flexor digitorum longus) originate outside the hand.

The **medial** or **hypothenar compartment** contains three intrinsic muscles – abductor digiti minimi, flexor digiti minimi brevis, and opponens digiti minimi (Fig. 24.3), which take their general proximal origin from the carpal bones and extend distally towards the little finger. These muscles are innervated by the deep branch of the ulnar nerve and, as a group, flex, abduct, and oppose the little finger. The hypothenar muscle group creates the small bulge (**hypothenar eminence**) on the medial palm.

The **central compartment** of the hand contains three short intrinsic muscle groups – lumbricals (I to IV), three palmar interossei, and four dorsal interossei. These small muscles are oriented so that digit III (the middle finger) delineates the central axis of the hand.

- The **lumbrical muscles** are four small hand muscles that originate proximally on the tendons of the flexor digitorum profundus and insert onto the lateral surface of the extensor expansion. They assist flexion of the MCP joint and extension of the interphalangeal joints.

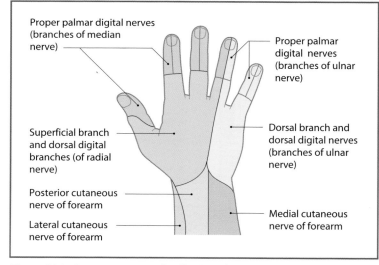

Figure 24.1 Cutaneous nerve distribution of the posterior (dorsal) surface of the hand

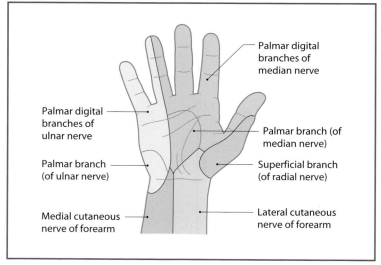

Figure 24.2 Cutaneous nerve distribution of the anterior (palmar) surface of the hand

- The three **palmar interossei** muscles adduct the fingers toward the central axis created by the middle finger. Each arises from the metacarpal shaft of the digit it abducts and inserts onto the fascial extensor expansion on the first, third, and fourth fingers.
- The four **dorsal interossei** muscles abduct the fingers away from the central axis. Each arises by two heads from the adjacent sides of the metacarpal bones and inserts onto the extensor expansion of the first, second, and third fingers.

The lateral or **thenar compartment** of the hand contains abductor pollicis brevis, flexor pollicis brevis, opponens pollicis, and adductor pollicis muscles. These muscles flex, abduct, and oppose the thumb. The first three muscles form the **thenar eminence**. The adductor pollicis muscle contains two points of origin (heads) and inserts onto the proximal phalanx of the thumb. The adductor pollicis muscle adducts the thumb.

NERVES

Innervation to the intrinsic hand muscles is from **muscular branches** of the median and ulnar nerves.

The **median nerve** enters the hand through the carpal tunnel and supplies the three thenar muscles via the recurrent branch and then the lateral two lumbricals. The median nerve also innervates the skin over part of the proximal hand, palm, and medial three and a half digits (Figs 24.1 and 24.2).

Before entering the hand, the **ulnar nerve** gives off two branches – the **dorsal** and the **palmar branches**. These cutaneous branches leave the ulnar nerve proximal to the wrist and enter the hand to supply the skin over the medial part of the dorsal and palmar hand and lateral one and a half digits. The ulnar nerve crosses the palmar surface of the wrist superficial to the flexor retinaculum, and divides into **superficial** and **deep branches**:

- the superficial branch supplies the palmaris brevis muscle before dividing into smaller common palmar digital nerves, which pass to the medial one and a half fingers (medial half of the ring finger plus the little finger);
- the deep branch innervates the hypothenar muscles, the two medial lumbrical muscles, the interosseous muscles (dorsal and palmar), and adductor pollicis.

The **radial nerve** crosses the dorsal wrist into the hand and conveys sensation to the skin over most of the medial dorsum of the hand. It does not innervate any hand muscles.

ARTERIES

Blood supply to the hand is from the radial and ulnar arteries (Fig. 24.4).

The **radial artery** at the lateral anterior wrist in the distal forearm branches to form a **superficial palmar branch**, which enters the hand to form the lateral half of the **superficial palmar arch**. From the lateral wrist the radial artery runs posteriorly to the dorsum of the hand, then turns anteriorly to enter the deep palmar hand between the thumb and index finger. Several digital branches leave the radial artery while it is still on the dorsum of the hand:

- the **princeps pollicis artery**, which supplies the thumb;
- the **radialis indicis artery**, which supplies the index finger;
- digital arteries 1 and 2.

The radial artery is the primary contributor to the **deep palmar arch**, which is where it terminates.

The **ulnar artery** crosses the wrist medially, superficial to the flexor retinaculum. It then branches to form a **deep palmar branch**, which is a secondary contributor to the deep palmar arch. The ulnar artery then travels deeper into the hand and ends as a major contributor to the superficial palmar arch as it meets the superficial palmar branch from the radial artery. The blood supply to the digits

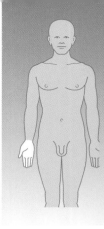

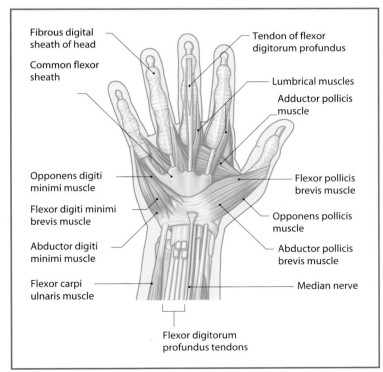

Figure 24.3 Muscles of the anterior (palmar) hand – intermediate layer

Labels:
- Fibrous digital sheath of head
- Common flexor sheath
- Opponens digiti minimi muscle
- Flexor digiti minimi brevis muscle
- Abductor digiti minimi muscle
- Flexor carpi ulnaris muscle
- Flexor digitorum profundus tendons
- Tendon of flexor digitorum profundus
- Lumbrical muscles
- Adductor pollicis muscle
- Flexor pollicis brevis muscle
- Opponens pollicis muscle
- Abductor pollicis brevis muscle
- Median nerve

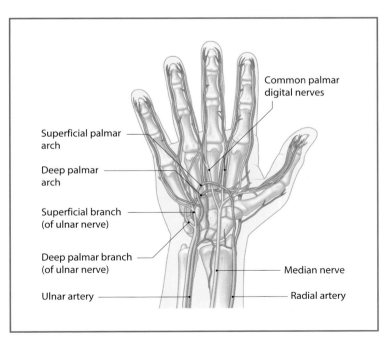

Figure 24.4 Arteries and nerves of the anterior (palmar) aspect of the hand

Labels:
- Superficial palmar arch
- Deep palmar arch
- Superficial branch (of ulnar nerve)
- Deep palmar branch (of ulnar nerve)
- Ulnar artery
- Common palmar digital nerves
- Median nerve
- Radial artery

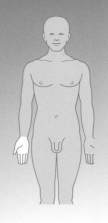

is from individual digital arteries, which are branches of the superficial and deep palmar arches.

VEINS AND LYMPHATICS

Deep venous drainage of the hand follows the digital arteries and arterial arches through venae comitantes. These accompanying veins empty into larger vessels, which follow the course of the radial and ulnar arteries into the forearm. Superficial venous drainage of the dorsum of the hand flows into the **dorsal venous network of hand**. The medial end of this network coalesces to form the **basilic vein** whereas the lateral end becomes the **cephalic vein**.

Lymphatic drainage of the hand follows the superficial and deep venous systems and flows towards the **cubital nodes** at the anterior elbow.

■ CLINICAL CORRELATIONS
Hand fracture

Fractures of the hand bones are common. They may result when the hand is injured when falling to the ground or a finger is injured by a blow from a heavy object. Symptoms include swelling and bruising over the injured part of the hand, and pain, which is worse when the hand is held in a dependent position (below the level of the heart). Patients usually seek early medical attention because of the severity of the pain when trying to carry out normal activities with the injured hand.

On examination, the injured hand is swollen and edematous, usually with ecchymoses (bruises). Point tenderness can be elicited over the broken (fractured) bone, and there is usually some deformity at the fracture site. Careful examination of the radial pulse and capillary refill is important to rule out vascular injury, which is rare. Neurologic examination of the injured hand involving light touch and pinprick testing is valuable in determining whether there has been any nerve injury. Because hand fractures are relatively common with hand trauma, radiographic evaluation usually comprises a minimum of two views of the injured area.

In general, transverse fractures are stable whereas oblique, spiral, or comminuted fractures are unstable. In the emergency setting, a patient with a stable closed hand fracture is usually managed with a splint to immobilize the fracture and then followed up by a physician with expertise in hand fracture treatment. Open fractures (an open wound with visible bone fragments) should be evaluated by an orthopedic surgeon immediately. Unstable closed fractures also need orthopedic evaluation. In some cases, unstable closed fractures are repaired with K-wire fixation (holes drilled into the fracture fragments and wire threaded through the holes to bind the site and create stability).

MNEMONICS		
Interosseus muscles and their function:	**PAD**	(**P**almar muscles, **AD**duct)
	DAB	(**D**orsal muscles, **AB**duct)
Intrinsic muscles of the hand (medial to lateral):	**All For One And One For All**	
	(**A**bductor digiti minimi, **F**lexor digiti minimi, **O**pponens digiti minimi, **A**dductor pollicis, **O**pponens pollicis, **F**lexor pollicis brevis, **A**bductor pollicis brevis)	

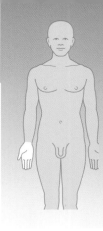

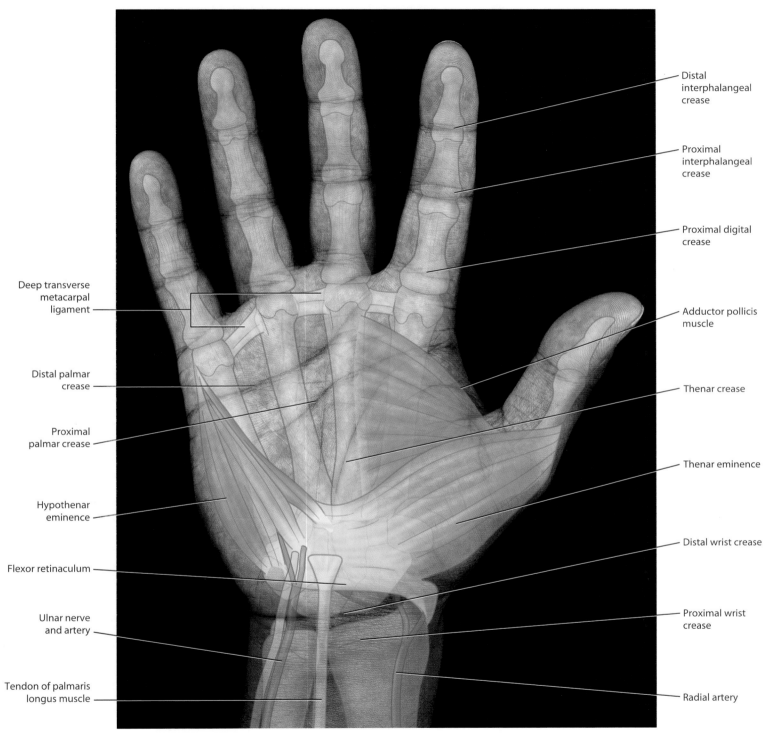

Distal
interphalangeal
crease

Proximal
interphalangeal
crease

Proximal digital
crease

Adductor pollicis
muscle

Thenar crease

Thenar eminence

Distal wrist crease

Proximal wrist
crease

Radial artery

Deep transverse
metacarpal
ligament

Distal palmar
crease

Proximal
palmar crease

Hypothenar
eminence

Flexor retinaculum

Ulnar nerve
and artery

Tendon of palmaris
longus muscle

Figure 24.5 Hand muscles – anterior surface anatomy. Anterior (palmar) surface of the right hand showing muscles, tendons, vessels, and creases

277

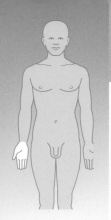

Hand muscles

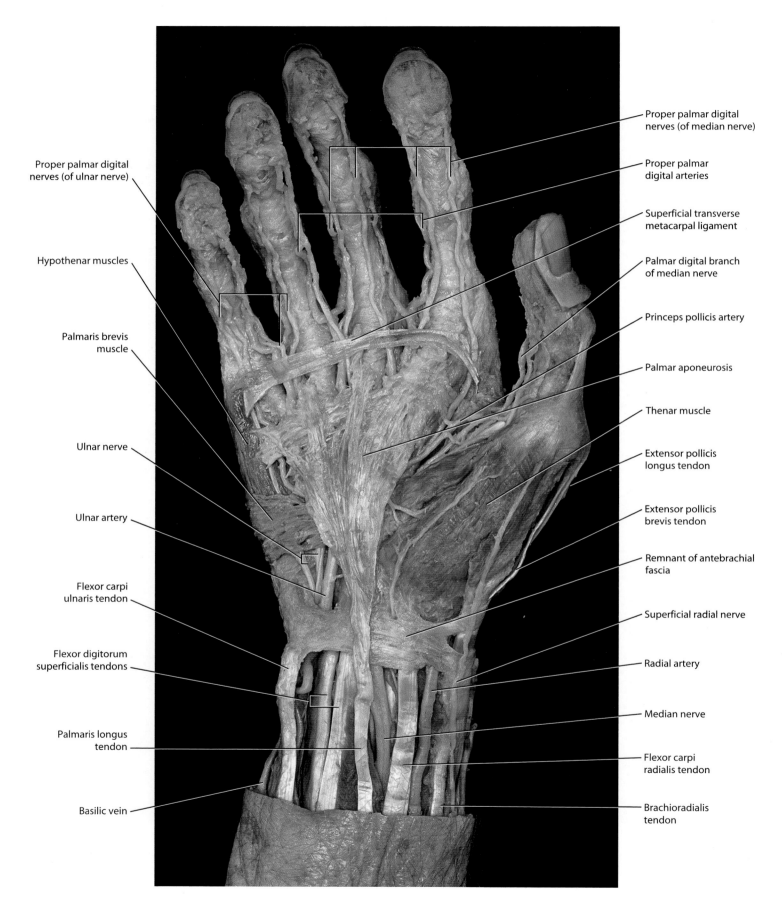

Proper palmar digital
nerves (of ulnar nerve)

Hypothenar muscles

Palmaris brevis
muscle

Ulnar nerve

Ulnar artery

Flexor carpi
ulnaris tendon

Flexor digitorum
superficialis tendons

Palmaris longus
tendon

Basilic vein

Proper palmar digital
nerves (of median nerve)

Proper palmar
digital arteries

Superficial transverse
metacarpal ligament

Palmar digital branch
of median nerve

Princeps pollicis artery

Palmar aponeurosis

Thenar muscle

Extensor pollicis
longus tendon

Extensor pollicis
brevis tendon

Remnant of antebrachial
fascia

Superficial radial nerve

Radial artery

Median nerve

Flexor carpi
radialis tendon

Brachioradialis
tendon

Figure 24.6 Hand muscles – anterior superficial dissection. Anterior (palmar) view of a superficial dissection of the anterior (palmar) surface of the right hand.
Observe the superficial transverse metacarpal ligament, the palmar aponeurosis and the palmaris brevis muscle.

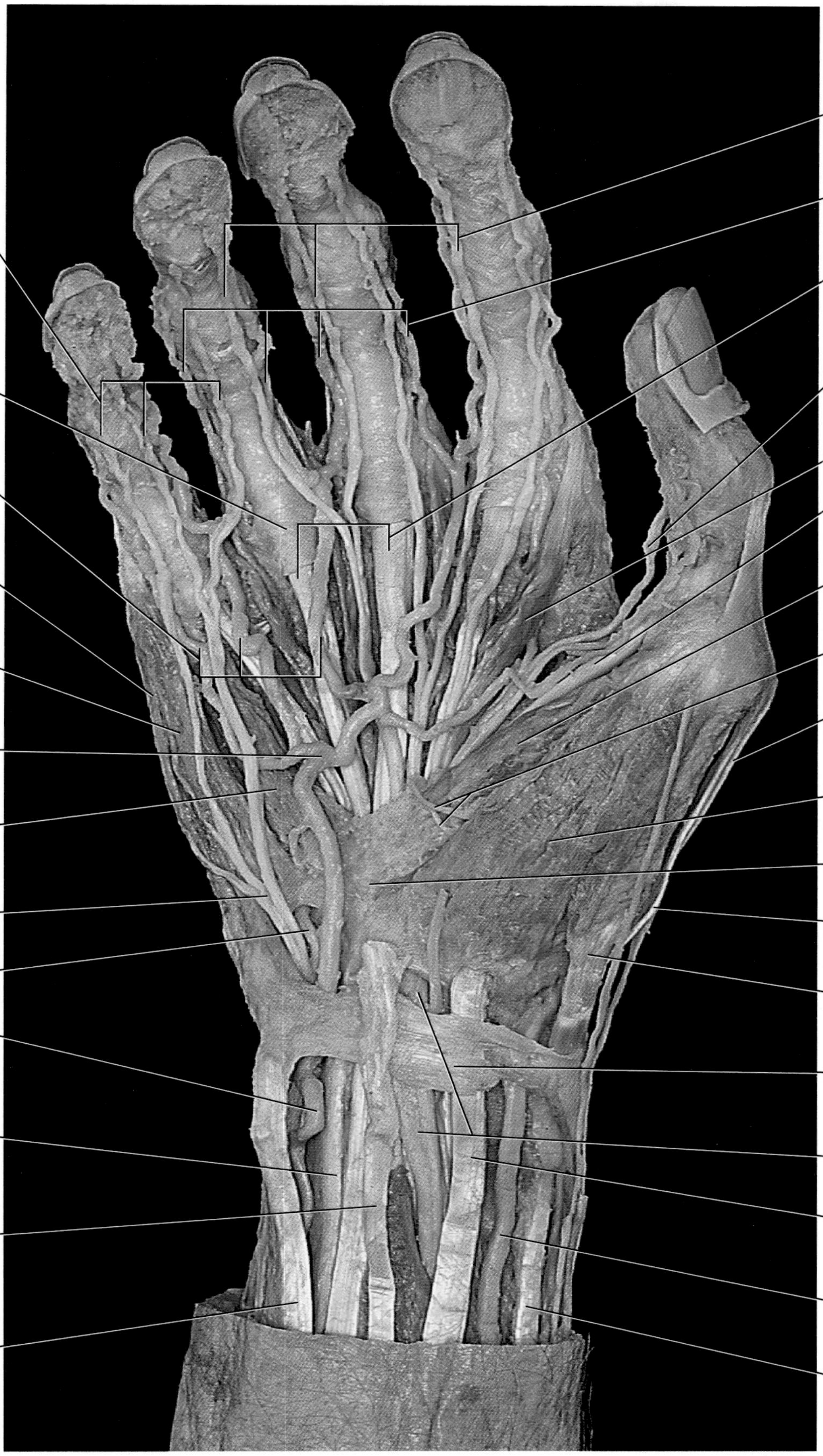

Proper palmar digital nerves (of ulnar nerve)

Fibrous digital sheath

Common palmar digital arteries

Abductor digiti minimi muscle

Flexor digiti minimi brevis muscle

Superficial palmar arch

Opponens digiti minimi muscle

Superficial ulnar nerve

Deep ulnar nerve

Ulnar artery

Flexor digitorum superficialis tendon

Palmaris longus tendon

Flexor carpi ulnaris tendon

Proper palmar digital nerves (of median nerve)

Proper palmar digital arteries

Flexor digitorum superficialis tendon

Palmar digital branch of median nerve

Lumbrical muscle I

Flexor pollicis longus tendon

Flexor pollicis brevis muscle

Recurrent median nerve

Extensor pollicis longus tendon

Abductor pollicis brevis muscle

Flexor retinaculum

Extensor pollicis brevis tendon

Abductor pollicis longus tendon

Remnant of antebrachial fascia

Median nerve

Flexor carpi radialis tendon

Radial artery

Brachioradialis tendon

Figure 24.7 Hand muscles – anterior intermediate dissection 1. Superficial dissection of the anterior (palmar) surface of the right hand. The palmar aponeurosis has been removed. The superficial palmar arterial arch of the ulnar artery is visible anterior to the tendons of the flexor digitorum superficialis and flexor digitorum profundus muscles and gives rise to the common palmar digital arteries to the fingers

279

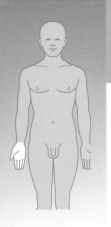

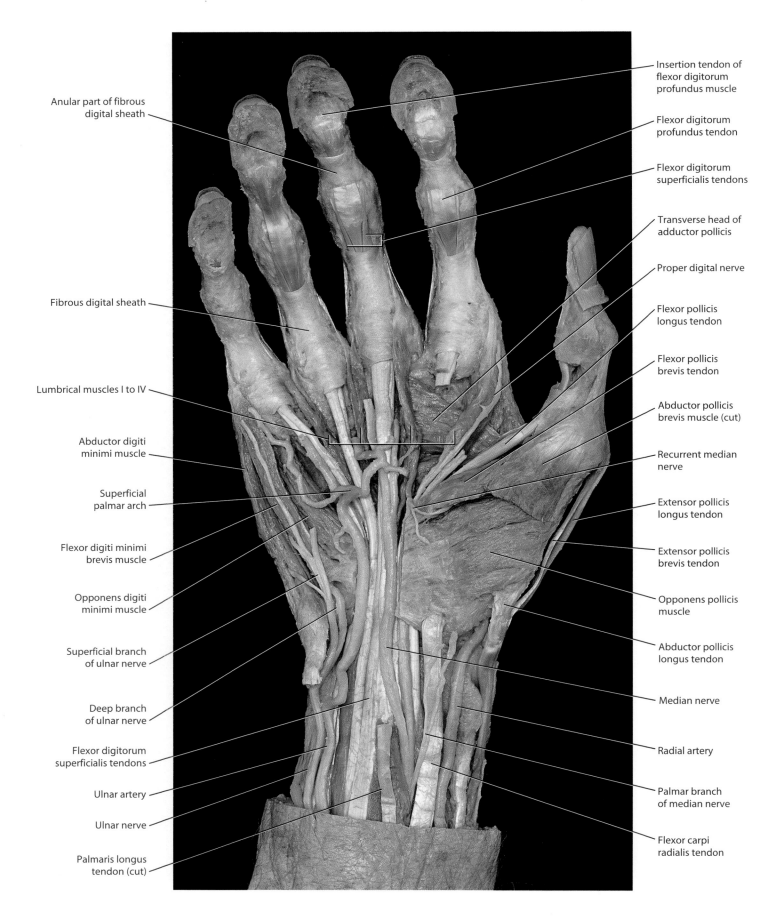

Anular part of fibrous digital sheath

Fibrous digital sheath

Lumbrical muscles I to IV

Abductor digiti minimi muscle

Superficial palmar arch

Flexor digiti minimi brevis muscle

Opponens digiti minimi muscle

Superficial branch of ulnar nerve

Deep branch of ulnar nerve

Flexor digitorum superficialis tendons

Ulnar artery

Ulnar nerve

Palmaris longus tendon (cut)

Insertion tendon of flexor digitorum profundus muscle

Flexor digitorum profundus tendon

Flexor digitorum superficialis tendons

Transverse head of adductor pollicis

Proper digital nerve

Flexor pollicis longus tendon

Flexor pollicis brevis tendon

Abductor pollicis brevis muscle (cut)

Recurrent median nerve

Extensor pollicis longus tendon

Extensor pollicis brevis tendon

Opponens pollicis muscle

Abductor pollicis longus tendon

Median nerve

Radial artery

Palmar branch of median nerve

Flexor carpi radialis tendon

Figure 24.8 Hand muscles – anterior intermediate dissection 2. Anterior (palmar) view of the dissected right hand. The flexor retinaculum has been removed to show the constituents of the carpal tunnel. Flexor tendons of the index finger have been removed to show the transverse head of the adductor pollicis muscle. All four lumbricals are present along with the flexor digitorum profundus tendon

280

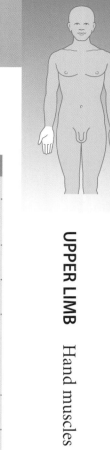

TABLE 24.1 INTRINSIC HAND MUSCLES

Muscle	Origin	Insertion	Innervation	Action	Blood supply
Abductor pollicis brevis	Flexor retinaculum, scaphoid and trapezium bones	Lateral side of proximal phalanx of thumb	Recurrent branch of median nerve (C8, T1)	Abducts and assists opposition of the thumb	Superficial palmar branch of radial artery
Flexor pollicis brevis	Flexor retinaculum and trapezium bone	Lateral side of proximal phalanx of thumb	Recurrent branch of median nerve (C8, T1)	Flexes proximal phalanx of thumb	Superficial palmar branch of radial artery
Opponens pollicis	Flexor retinaculum and trapezium bone	Lateral side of metacarpal I	Recurrent branch of median nerve (C8, T1)	Draws metacarpal I forward and medially	Superficial palmar branch of radial artery
Adductor pollicis	Oblique head – bases of metacarpals II and III; capitate and trapezoid bones; transverse head – anterior surface of metacarpal III	Medial side of base of proximal phalanx of thumb	Deep branch of ulnar nerve (C8, T1)	Adducts and flexes thumb	Deep palmar arch
Palmaris brevis	Palmar aponeurosis	Skin on ulnar border of palm	Superficial palmar branch of ulnar nerve (C8)	Deepens the hollow of the hand	Superficial palmar arch
Abductor digiti minimi	Pisiform bone, tendon of flexor carpi ulnaris	Medial side of base of proximal phalanx of little finger	Deep branch of ulnar nerve (C8, T1)	Abducts the little finger	Deep palmar branch of ulnar artery
Flexor digiti minimi brevis	Flexor retinaculum and hook of hamate bone	Medial side of base of proximal phalanx of little finger	Deep branch of ulnar nerve (C8, T1)	Flexes proximal phalanx of the little finger	Deep palmar branch of ulnar artery
Opponens digiti minimi	Flexor retinaculum and hook of hamate bone	Medial border of metacarpal V	Deep branch of ulnar nerve (C8, T1)	Draws metacarpal V forward to face thumb	Deep palmar branch of ulnar artery
Lumbricals I and II	Lateral two tendons of flexor digitorum profundus	Lateral sides of extensor expansion of index and middle fingers	Median nerve (C8, T1)	Extends index and middle fingers at the interphalangeal joints and flexes metacarpophalangeal joints 1 and 2	Superficial and deep palmar arches
Lumbricals III and IV	Medial three tendons of flexor digitorum profundus	Lateral sides of extensor expansion of digits 4 and ring finger	Deep branch of ulnar nerve (C8, T1)	Extends ring and little fingers at the interphalangeal joints and flexes metacarpophalangeal joints 3 and 4	Superficial and deep palmar arches
Dorsal interossei I to IV	Adjacent sides of two metacarpal bones	I to lateral side of proximal phalanx (PP) of index finger II to lateral side of PP of middle finger III to medial side of PP of middle finger IV to medial side of PP of ring finger	Deep branch of ulnar nerve (C8, T1)	Abducts the index and ring fingers from the middle finger	Deep palmar arch
Palmar interossei I to III	Palmar surfaces of metacarpals II, IV and V	I to medial side of PP of index finger II to lateral side of PP of ring finger III to lateral side of PP of little finger	Deep branch of ulnar nerve (C8, T1)	Adducts the index, ring, and little finger towards the middle finger	Deep palmar arch

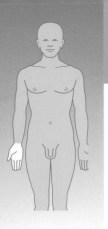

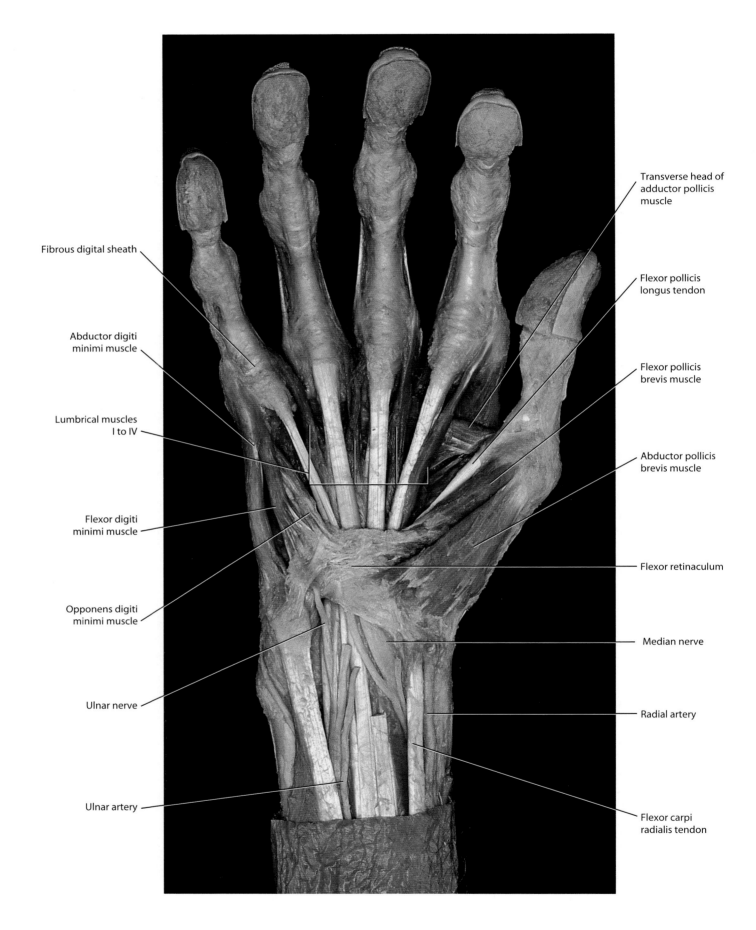

Fibrous digital sheath

Abductor digiti
minimi muscle

Lumbrical muscles
I to IV

Flexor digiti
minimi muscle

Opponens digiti
minimi muscle

Ulnar nerve

Ulnar artery

Transverse head of
adductor pollicis
muscle

Flexor pollicis
longus tendon

Flexor pollicis
brevis muscle

Abductor pollicis
brevis muscle

Flexor retinaculum

Median nerve

Radial artery

Flexor carpi
radialis tendon

Figure 24.9 Hand muscles – anterior deep dissection 1. Anterior (palmar) view of the dissected right hand. The flexor retinaculum is intact, but the arteries and nerves have been removed to clearly show the hypothenar and thenar muscles. Observe the lumbrical muscles as they relate to the flexor digitorum superficialis tendons

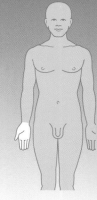

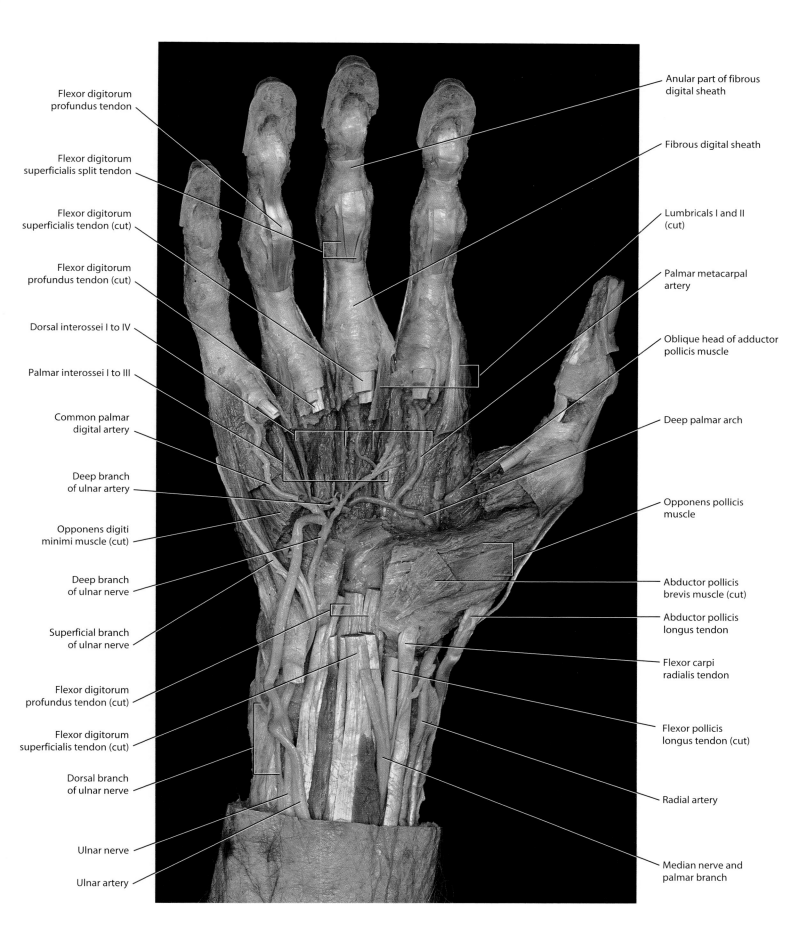

Flexor digitorum profundus tendon

Flexor digitorum superficialis split tendon

Flexor digitorum superficialis tendon (cut)

Flexor digitorum profundus tendon (cut)

Dorsal interossei I to IV

Palmar interossei I to III

Common palmar digital artery

Deep branch of ulnar artery

Opponens digiti minimi muscle (cut)

Deep branch of ulnar nerve

Superficial branch of ulnar nerve

Flexor digitorum profundus tendon (cut)

Flexor digitorum superficialis tendon (cut)

Dorsal branch of ulnar nerve

Ulnar nerve

Ulnar artery

Anular part of fibrous digital sheath

Fibrous digital sheath

Lumbricals I and II (cut)

Palmar metacarpal artery

Oblique head of adductor pollicis muscle

Deep palmar arch

Opponens pollicis muscle

Abductor pollicis brevis muscle (cut)

Abductor pollicis longus tendon

Flexor carpi radialis tendon

Flexor pollicis longus tendon (cut)

Radial artery

Median nerve and palmar branch

Figure 24.10 Hand muscles – anterior deep dissection 2. Anterior (palmar) view of a deep dissection of the right hand. Flexor tendons and lumbricals are removed to reveal the seven dorsal and palmar interossei muscles and the deep palmar arch from the radial artery

UPPER LIMB

Hand muscles

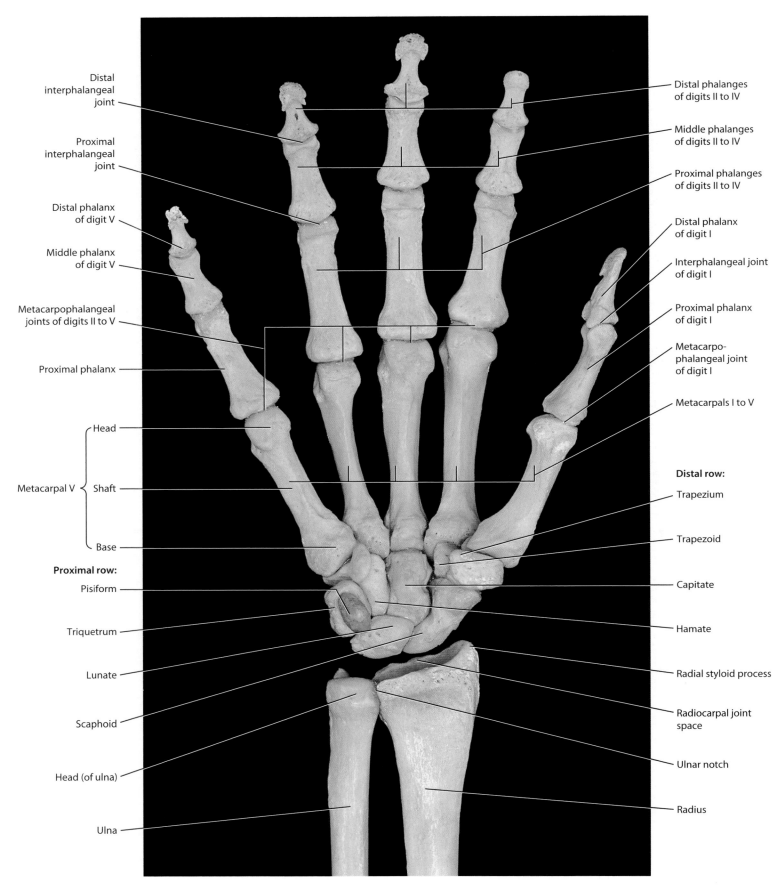

Distal interphalangeal joint

Proximal interphalangeal joint

Distal phalanx of digit V

Middle phalanx of digit V

Metacarpophalangeal joints of digits II to V

Proximal phalanx

Head

Metacarpal V — Shaft

Base

Proximal row:

Pisiform

Triquetrum

Lunate

Scaphoid

Head (of ulna)

Ulna

Distal phalanges of digits II to IV

Middle phalanges of digits II to IV

Proximal phalanges of digits II to IV

Distal phalanx of digit I

Interphalangeal joint of digit I

Proximal phalanx of digit I

Metacarpo-phalangeal joint of digit I

Metacarpals I to V

Distal row:

Trapezium

Trapezoid

Capitate

Hamate

Radial styloid process

Radiocarpal joint space

Ulnar notch

Radius

Figure 24.11 Hand muscles – anterior osteology 1. Anterior (palmar) view of the articulated bones of the right hand. All bones and joints are numbered I to V from the thumb

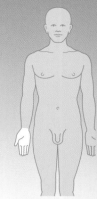

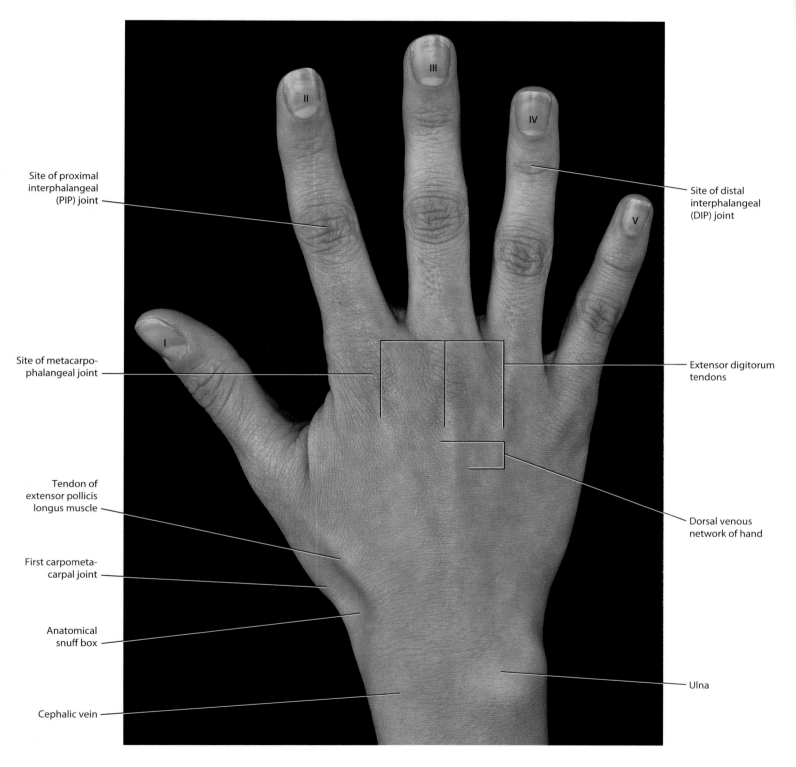

Site of proximal interphalangeal (PIP) joint

Site of distal interphalangeal (DIP) joint

Site of metacarpo-phalangeal joint

Extensor digitorum tendons

Tendon of extensor pollicis longus muscle

Dorsal venous network of hand

First carpometa-carpal joint

Anatomical snuff box

Ulna

Cephalic vein

Figure 24.12 Hand muscles – posterior surface anatomy. Posterior (dorsal) view of the right hand showing joint sites and tendons (see also Fig. 23.8)

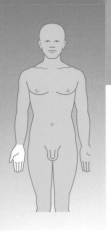

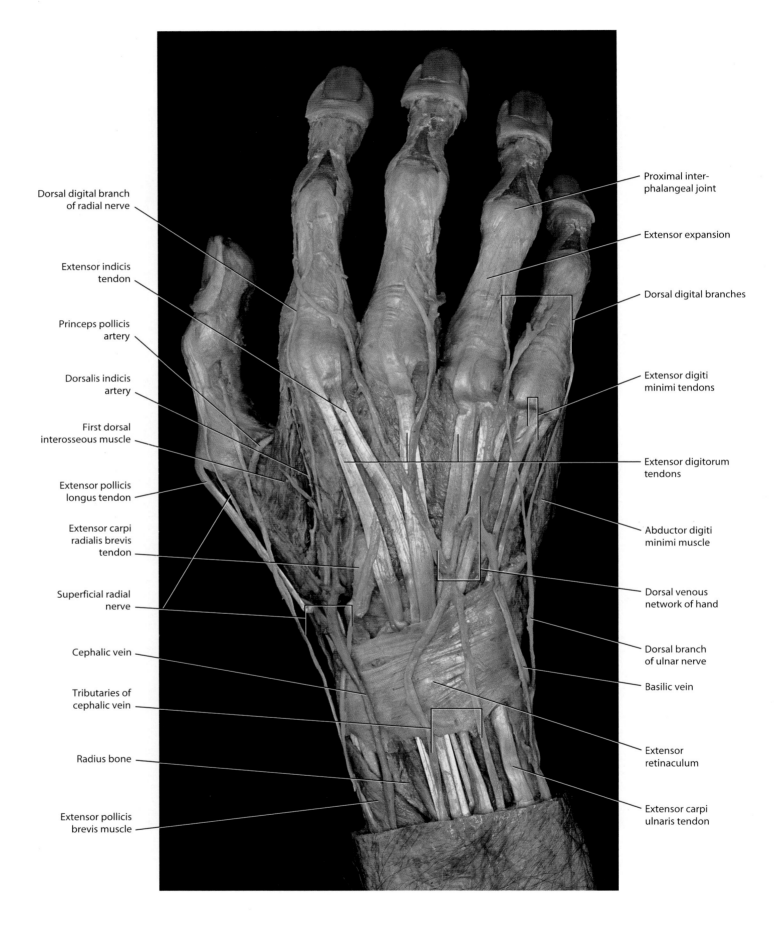

Dorsal digital branch
of radial nerve

Extensor indicis
tendon

Princeps pollicis
artery

Dorsalis indicis
artery

First dorsal
interosseous muscle

Extensor pollicis
longus tendon

Extensor carpi
radialis brevis
tendon

Superficial radial
nerve

Cephalic vein

Tributaries of
cephalic vein

Radius bone

Extensor pollicis
brevis muscle

Proximal inter-
phalangeal joint

Extensor expansion

Dorsal digital branches

Extensor digiti
minimi tendons

Extensor digitorum
tendons

Abductor digiti
minimi muscle

Dorsal venous
network of hand

Dorsal branch
of ulnar nerve

Basilic vein

Extensor
retinaculum

Extensor carpi
ulnaris tendon

Figure 24.13 Hand muscles – posterior superficial dissection. Posterior (dorsal) view of the dissected right hand. Observe the veins that contribute to the formation of the dorsal venous network. The cephalic vein originates from the radial side and the basilic vein from the ulnar side

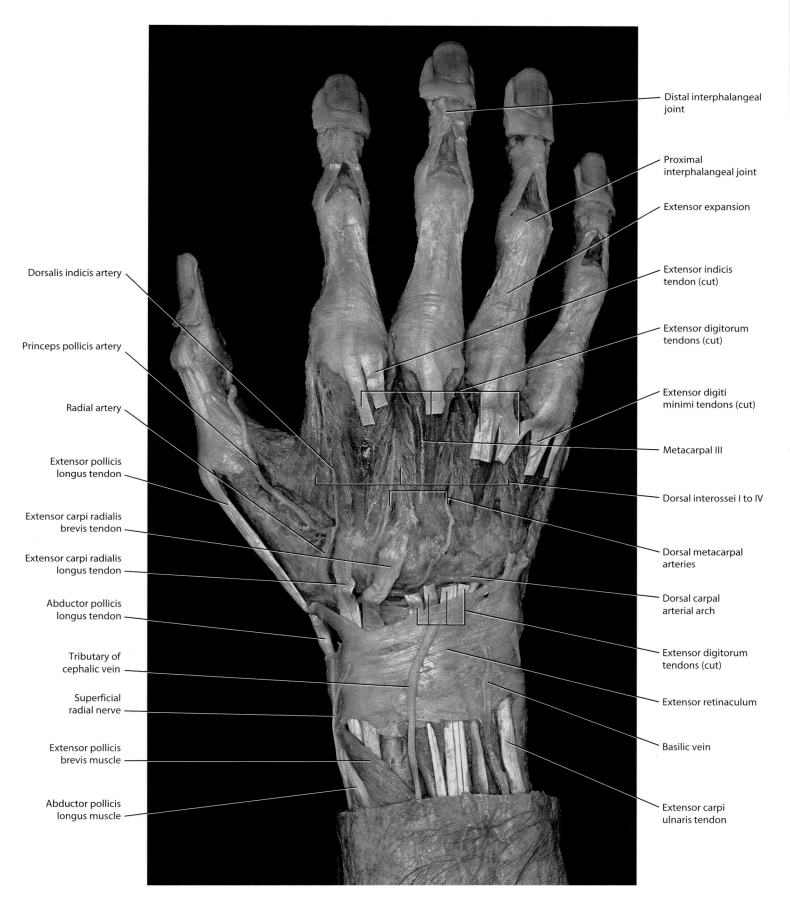

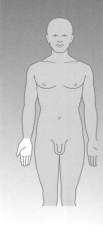

Distal interphalangeal joint

Proximal interphalangeal joint

Extensor expansion

Extensor indicis tendon (cut)

Extensor digitorum tendons (cut)

Extensor digiti minimi tendons (cut)

Metacarpal III

Dorsal interossei I to IV

Dorsal metacarpal arteries

Dorsal carpal arterial arch

Extensor digitorum tendons (cut)

Extensor retinaculum

Basilic vein

Extensor carpi ulnaris tendon

Dorsalis indicis artery

Princeps pollicis artery

Radial artery

Extensor pollicis longus tendon

Extensor carpi radialis brevis tendon

Extensor carpi radialis longus tendon

Abductor pollicis longus tendon

Tributary of cephalic vein

Superficial radial nerve

Extensor pollicis brevis muscle

Abductor pollicis longus muscle

Figure 24.14 Hand – posterior intermediate dissection. Posterior (dorsal) view of the dissected right hand. The tendons of the extensor digitorum have been cut and the extensor muscles have been removed over the metacarpal area to view all four dorsal interossei muscles

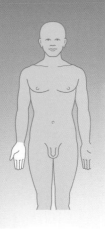

UPPER LIMB

Hand muscles

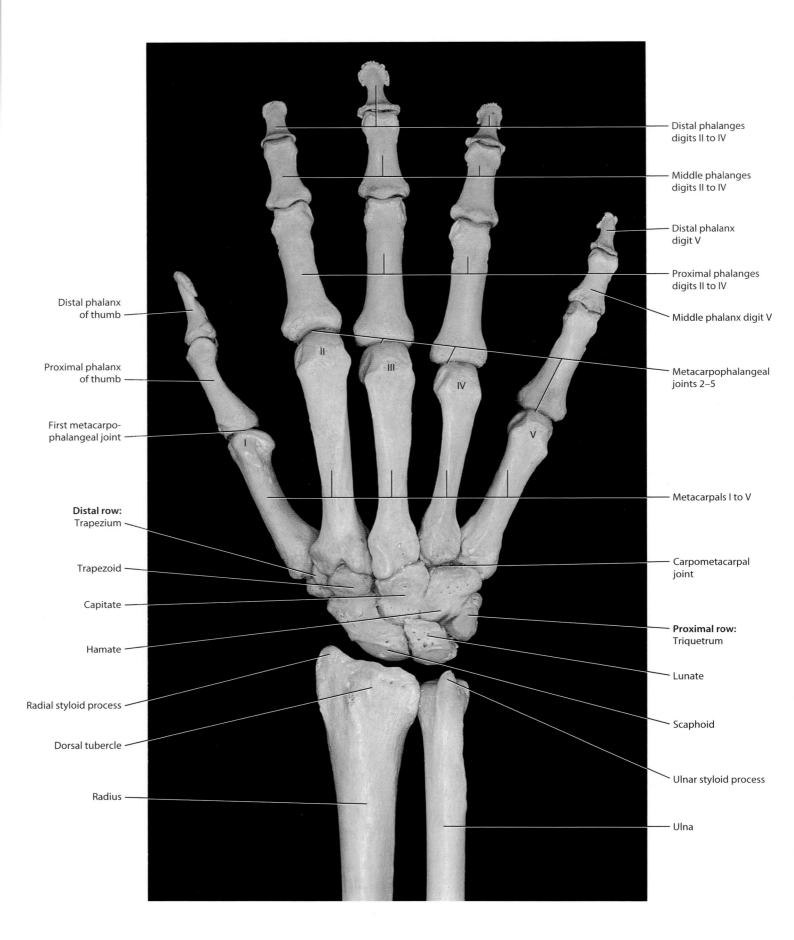

Distal phalanges
digits II to IV

Middle phalanges
digits II to IV

Distal phalanx
digit V

Proximal phalanges
digits II to IV

Middle phalanx digit V

Metacarpophalangeal
joints 2–5

Metacarpals I to V

Carpometacarpal
joint

Proximal row:
Triquetrum

Lunate

Scaphoid

Ulnar styloid process

Ulna

Distal phalanx
of thumb

Proximal phalanx
of thumb

First metacarpo-
phalangeal joint

Distal row:
Trapezium

Trapezoid

Capitate

Hamate

Radial styloid process

Dorsal tubercle

Radius

288   **Figure 24.15 Hand – posterior osteology.** Posterior (dorsal) view of the articulated bone of the right hand. The pisiform is not visible in this view

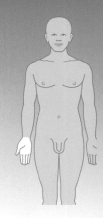

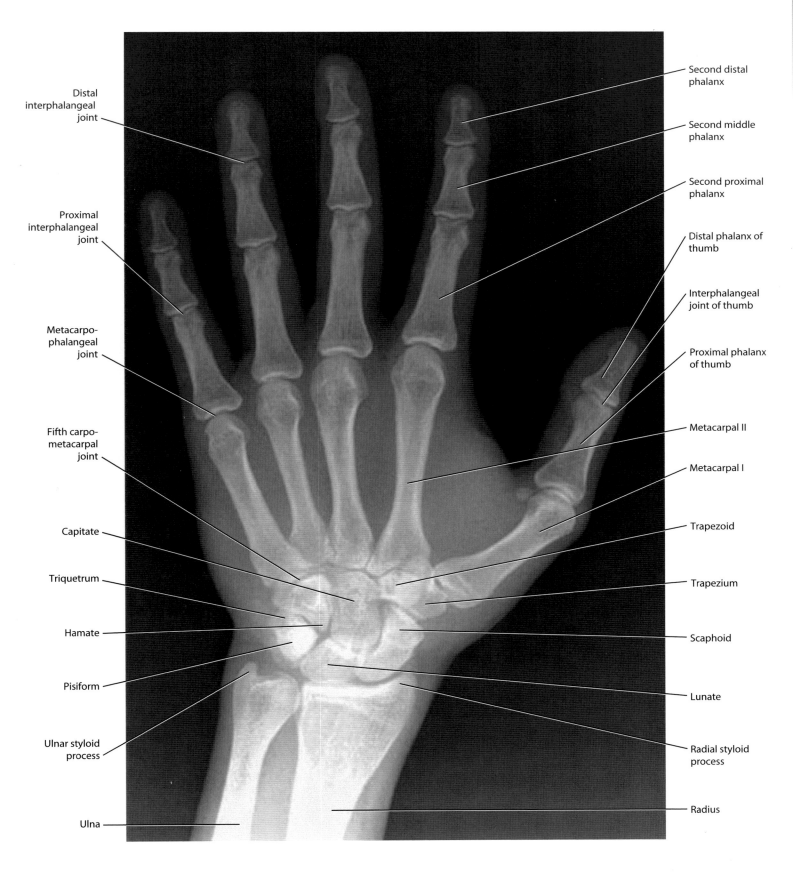

Distal interphalangeal joint

Proximal interphalangeal joint

Metacarpo-phalangeal joint

Fifth carpo-metacarpal joint

Capitate

Triquetrum

Hamate

Pisiform

Ulnar styloid process

Ulna

Second distal phalanx

Second middle phalanx

Second proximal phalanx

Distal phalanx of thumb

Interphalangeal joint of thumb

Proximal phalanx of thumb

Metacarpal II

Metacarpal I

Trapezoid

Trapezium

Scaphoid

Lunate

Radial styloid process

Radius

Figure 24.16 Hand – plain film radiograph (anteroposterior view). This radiograph shows the junction of the carpal bones with the metacarpal bones. In addition, the phalanges (fingers) are seen articulating with the metacarpals at the metacarpophalangeal joints

289

Hand muscles

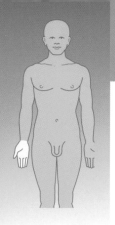

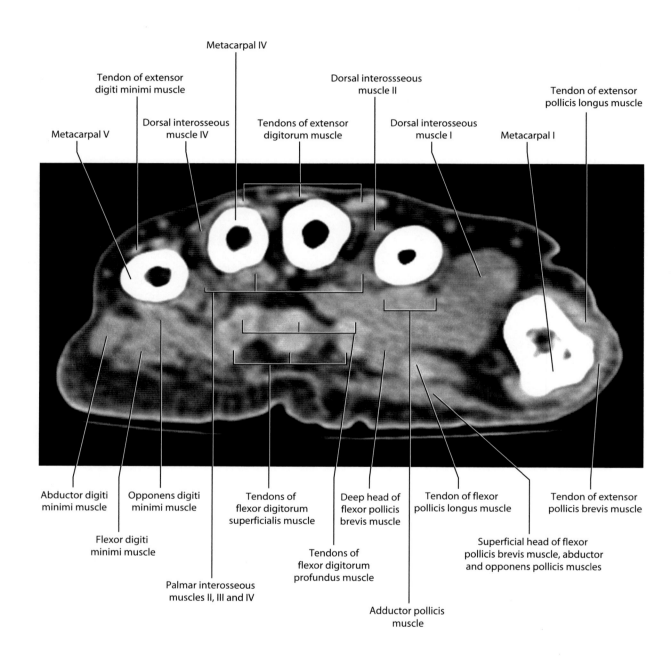

Metacarpal IV

Tendon of extensor
digiti minimi muscle

Dorsal interossseous
muscle II

Tendon of extensor
pollicis longus muscle

Metacarpal V

Dorsal interosseous
muscle IV

Tendons of extensor
digitorum muscle

Dorsal interosseous
muscle I

Metacarpal I

Abductor digiti
minimi muscle

Opponens digiti
minimi muscle

Tendons of
flexor digitorum
superficialis muscle

Deep head of
flexor pollicis
brevis muscle

Tendon of flexor
pollicis longus muscle

Tendon of extensor
pollicis brevis muscle

Flexor digiti
minimi muscle

Tendons of
flexor digitorum
profundus muscle

Superficial head of flexor
pollicis brevis muscle, abductor
and opponens pollicis muscles

Palmar interosseous
muscles II, III and IV

Adductor pollicis
muscle

Figure 24.17 Hand muscles – CT scan (axial view, from distal to proximal). In this scan at mid-metacarpal level observe the flexor and extensor tendons which have high attenuation (visibility)

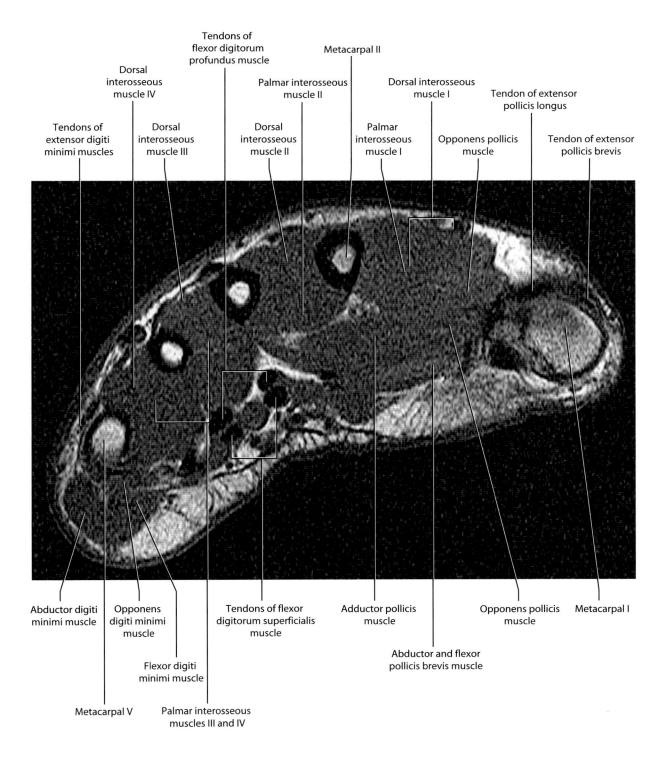

Tendons of
flexor digitorum
profundus muscle

Metacarpal II

Dorsal
interosseous
muscle IV

Palmar interosseous
muscle II

Dorsal interosseous
muscle I

Tendon of extensor
pollicis longus

Tendons of
extensor digiti
minimi muscles

Dorsal
interosseous
muscle III

Dorsal
interosseous
muscle II

Palmar
interosseous
muscle I

Opponens pollicis
muscle

Tendon of extensor
pollicis brevis

Abductor digiti
minimi muscle

Opponens
digiti minimi
muscle

Tendons of flexor
digitorum superficialis
muscle

Adductor pollicis
muscle

Opponens pollicis
muscle

Metacarpal I

Flexor digiti
minimi muscle

Abductor and flexor
pollicis brevis muscle

Metacarpal V

Palmar interosseous
muscles III and IV

Figure 24.18 Hand muscles – MRI scan (axial view, from distal to proximal). In this scan at mid-metacarpal level the tendons are black. The space between the thumb (metacarpal I) and index finger (metacarpal II) is larger than the other interdigital spaces, which together with the muscles between the finger and thumb, provides a great amount of mobility between them

The thorax, abdomen, and pelvis – together with the back – are collectively referred to as the 'trunk'. These areas are described here together because of their close interrelationships.

The **thorax** is the part of the trunk above the diaphragm. It contains and protects the principal organs of respiration (lungs) and circulation (heart), and part of the gastrointestinal tract (esophagus) (Fig. 25.1).

The thorax communicates with the neck at the **superior thoracic aperture** (thoracic inlet) and is enclosed by the diaphragm at the **inferior thoracic aperture** (thoracic outlet). Its walls are:

• posteriorly, the 12 thoracic vertebrae;
• anteriorly, the sternum;
• laterally, the 12 pairs of ribs and their costal cartilages.

The superior thoracic aperture is kidney-shaped, slopes downward and forward, and is bounded posteriorly by vertebra TI, anteriorly by the superior border of the manubrium of sternum, and laterally by rib I and its costal cartilage. It is a passageway for the trachea and esophagus, and the large vessels and nerves of the head, neck, and upper limbs. The cervical pleura (external lining of the lung) and apex of each lung are at its lateral margins.

Inferiorly, the inferior thoracic aperture is bounded anteriorly by the costal cartilages of ribs VII to X, laterally by ribs XI and XII, and posteriorly by vertebra TXII.

The **abdomen** lies between the thorax and pelvis. The abdominal cavity is separated from the thoracic cavity by the diaphragm and from the pelvis by an imaginary line at the **pelvic inlet**. The abdominal cavity is, in a broad sense, continuous with the pelvic cavity. The abdominal and pelvic organs encroach on and share parts of their respective cavities.

The abdominal cavity contains most of the gastrointestinal organs (stomach, intestines, liver, pancreas, and part of the colon), part of the urinary system (kidneys and ureters), the spleen, and the suprarenal glands. It is lined with a serous membrane – the **peritoneum.**

For descriptive and diagnostic purposes, the anterior abdominal wall is divided into a grid-like pattern with nine regions (Fig. 25.2). The **umbilical region** containing the umbilicus is at the center. Superior to the umbilical region is the **epigastric region**, inferior to it is the **pubic region**. Laterally, from superior to inferior, are the left and right hypochondria, the flanks and the groins. The anterior abdominal wall is often described as four quadrants, again centered around the umbilicus (left and right upper quadrants, and left and right lower quadrants).

The abdominal wall is supported posteriorly by the five lumbar vertebrae, the crura of the diaphragm, the psoas major and minor muscles, and the quadratus lumborum muscle.

The **pelvis** is the part of the trunk below and behind the abdomen. It contains the lower part of the gastrointestinal tract, the urinary bladder, the inferior parts of the ureters, and parts of the male and female reproductive organs.

The skeletal framework for the pelvis is a ring of bone formed by the sacrum, ilium, and pubis. This bony girdle transmits the weight of the trunk to the lower limbs through the hip joint.

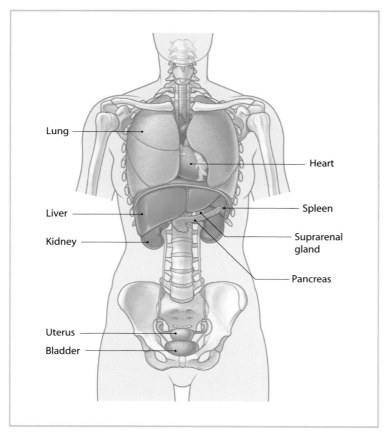

Figure 25.1 Organs of the upper trunk

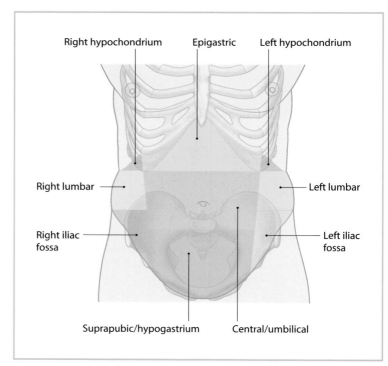

Figure 25.2 Nine regions of the abdomen

The **back** is the posterior part of the trunk and includes the posterior skin and muscles, the vertebral column, the spinal cord, and the neurovascular structures.

BONES

The bony **vertebral column** extends from the base of the skull to the coccyx. It protects the spinal cord and supports the weight of the trunk, transferring it to the pelvis and lower limbs. As most of the weight of the trunk is anterior to it, the vertebral column is supported by layers of muscles, which act as levers and strong extensors and rotators to maintain stability and enable movement. There are 33 vertebrae – 7 cervical, 12 thoracic, 5 lumbar, 5 sacral, and 4 coccygeal. The sacrum and coccyx are formed from fused sacral and coccygeal vertebrae, respectively.

MUSCLES

The muscles of the trunk are at the periphery of the chest, abdomen, pelvis, and back, and are subdivided into chest wall, back, and abdominal muscles, and muscular support for the pelvis. They:

- facilitate respiration (breathing);
- support the internal abdominal organs;
- maintain stability.

NERVES

The nerve supply to the trunk is provided by the segmental spinal nerves, which emerge from the spinal canal at the intervertebral foramina of the vertebral column (Fig. 25.3). The **posterior** and **anterior roots** for each **spinal nerve** combine and intertwine to produce peripheral nerves, which provide cutaneous (Fig. 25.4) and motor innervation to structures at the periphery of the trunk; **autonomic nerves** supply the internal structures (e.g. heart, lungs, gastrointestinal tract). Points of innervation that can be clinically significant in patients with major injury or illness involving the nervous system include:

- spinal nerve T4 innervation of the nipple;
- spinal nerve T10 innervation of the umbilicus;
- ilio-inguinal and iliohypogastric nerve (both derivatives of T12) innervation of the lower anterior abdominal wall, groin, and anterior scrotum.

The pelvis also contains segmental spinal nerves, but in this region they unite in an organized fashion to form the **lumbosacral plexus** of nerves. Within the pelvis this branching network gives rise to nerves that supply the entire pelvis, reproductive organs, genitalia, anus, and entire lower limb.

Both sympathetic and parasympathetic parts of the **autonomic division** innervate the trunk.

Sympathetic preganglionic nerve fibers leave the spinal cord and pass to a **ganglion** (collection of nerve cell bodies) just a few centimeters from the vertebral column, where they synapse with the **postganglionic nerve fibers**. The postganglionic nerve fibers that leave a particular ganglion are oriented in a row and are connected to nerve fibers from other – superior and inferior – ganglia. A row of ganglia (the sympathetic trunk) is therefore formed along the lateral margins of the vertebral column. The sympathetic trunk extends from the neck to the pelvis (see Chapter 1). It sends out

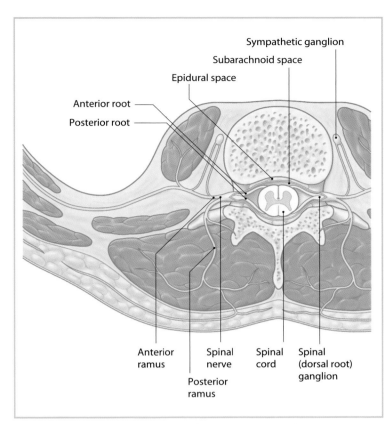

Figure 25.3 Spinal nerves emerging from the spinal canal

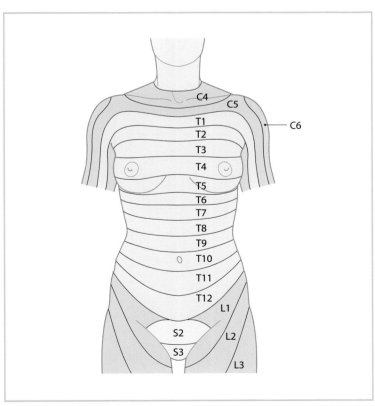

Figure 25.4 Cutaneous nerve distribution of the trunk (dermatomes)

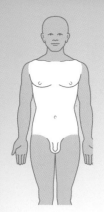

sympathetic nerve fibers, which usually run alongside other nerves and arteries to the rest of the body. Sympathetic stimulation increases respiratory and heart rate, slows digestion, and contracts urethral and anal sphincters.

Parasympathetic preganglionic nerve fibers leave the spinal cord for ganglia outside the spinal cord, where they synapse with postganglionic nerve fibers that travel to the target organ or region (like the sympathetic system). The parasympathetic ganglia are further from the spinal cord than the sympathetic ganglia and, unlike the sympathetic system, they do not send fibers to the entire body. Instead, parasympathetic fibers innervate the solid organs of the thorax, abdomen, pelvis, and gastrointestinal tract. The exceptions to this are those parasympathetic fibers that innervate structures in the head and neck (e.g. the lacrimal glands). Parasympathetic stimulation decreases respiratory and heart rates, increases digestive rate, stimulates gland secretion, and relaxes urethral and anal sphincters.

ARTERIES

Blood is pumped from the left ventricle of the heart into the **ascending aorta**, from which arise the arteries that supply the heart itself (coronary arteries). At the level of the second costal cartilage the aorta enters the superior mediastinum, where it is referred to as the **arch of the aorta** (Fig. 25.5). The arteries that supply the head and neck and the upper limbs – the brachiocephalic trunk, and the left common carotid and left subclavian arteries – branch from its superior border. The arch of the aorta then turns leftward and descends inferiorly as the **thoracic aorta**. This gives off visceral

branches to the bronchi, esophagus, and diaphragm, and parietal branches (the intercostal arteries).

At the level of vertebra TXII the thoracic aorta passes through the diaphragm at the aortic hiatus and is referred to as the **abdominal aorta**. From the aortic hiatus at TXII to its termination at LIV where it bifurcates to form the common iliac arteries, the abdominal aorta gives off nine branches. The three unpaired visceral branches are the main arteries to the digestive tract:

- the **celiac artery** and its three branches supply the organs of the foregut (inferior esophagus, stomach, upper duodenum, liver, pancreas, and spleen);
- the **superior mesenteric artery** and its five branches supply the midgut (lower duodenum, rest of small intestine, and proximal half of the large intestine);
- the **inferior mesenteric artery** and its three branches supply the hindgut (distal half of large intestine to the superior part of the rectum).

The three paired (right and left) visceral branches are:

- the **middle suprarenal arteries** to the suprarenal glands;
- the **renal arteries** to the kidneys;
- the gonadal arteries – **testicular** (in men) and **ovarian** (in women).

The three parietal arteries are:

- the paired **inferior phrenic arteries** to the underside of the diaphragm;
- the **lumbar arteries** (usually four pairs) to the posterior abdominal muscles;
- the single **median sacral artery** descending on the anterior sacrum down to the coccygeal area.

At the level of vertebra LIV, the abdominal aorta divides into **left** and **right common iliac arteries**, which descend into the pelvis, where they divide into external and internal branches. The **internal iliac artery** supplies the lateral and posterior pelvis and gluteal region, and the **external iliac artery** supplies the anterior and superior part of the pelvis. The external iliac artery leaves the pelvis by passing deep to the inguinal ligament; its name then changes to the femoral artery and it supplies blood to the entire lower limb.

VEINS

Venous drainage of the trunk is towards the right atrium of the heart (Fig. 25.6). In the thorax, venous drainage is to small **intercostal veins**, which drain the anterior, lateral, and posterior chest walls. These vessels drain into the azygos system of veins (**azygos, hemi-azygos,** and **accessory hemi-azygos veins**) along the internal surface of the posterior chest wall. The azygos vein drains into the **superior vena cava** in the upper chest.

The superior vena cava receives blood from the upper chest and the head and neck and drains into the superior part of the right atrium of the heart. Within the thorax, oxygenated venous blood passes from the lungs to the heart through the **pulmonary veins**. The heart has a system of **coronary veins**, which empty into the right atrium.

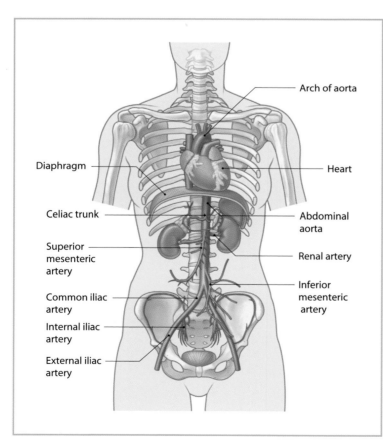

Figure 25.5 Major arteries of the trunk

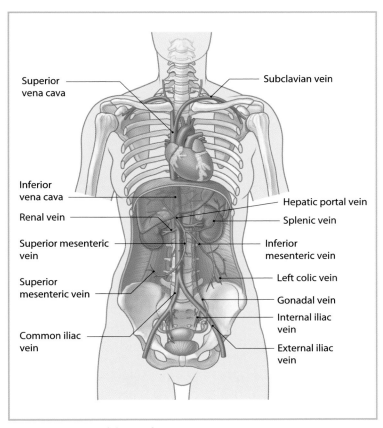

Figure 25.6 Veins of the trunk

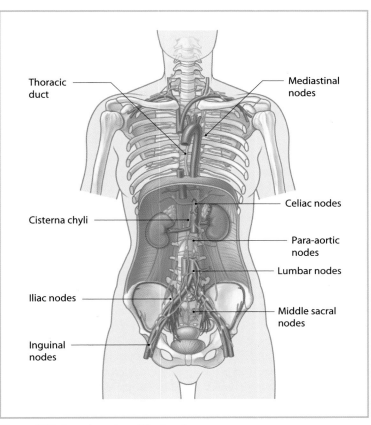

Figure 25.7 Lymph nodes of the trunk

The inferior vena cava, which empties into the inferior part of the right atrium, receives blood from the inferior trunk, pelvis, and both lower limbs.

The portal system of veins receives blood from the abdominal viscera supplied by the celiac trunk, superior mesenteric artery, and inferior mesenteric arteries (which supply blood to the gastrointestinal tract from the inferior esophagus to the rectum). The **hepatic portal vein** is formed by the **splenic** and **superior mesenteric veins**. The venous blood within these veins is rich in absorbed digestive products, and flows via the hepatic portal vein into the liver, from where **short hepatic veins** drain to the inferior vena cava.

LYMPHATICS

Lymph from the trunk drains to several locations (Fig. 25.7). In general, lymph node groups are:

- at sites of internal organs (e.g. spleen, kidneys);
- along the intrathoracic, intra-abdominal, and intrapelvic surfaces of the vertebrae.

Lymphatic drainage of the thorax is to lymph node groups at the axilla, within the middle mediastinum, and at the root of each lung.

The abdominal wall has unique lymphatic drainage in that lymph from above the umbilicus flows toward the **axillary lymph nodes** whereas lymph from below the umbilicus flows to the **superficial inguinal nodes**. The internal structures of the abdomen drain toward lymph node groups along the posterior abdominal wall. Many of these groups are along large arteries and each is named after the closest structure (e.g. pre- and postaortic nodes, lumbar nodes, celiac nodes). This principle is also true for lymph node groups within the pelvis (e.g. presacral lymph nodes).

26 Vertebral column

The vertebral column is a series of bones (**vertebrae**) stacked on top of each other to support the weight of the body. It is a central attachment point for muscles and bones of the appendicular skeleton. There are 33 vertebrae: 7 cervical, 12 thoracic, 5 lumbar, 5 fused sacral, and 4 fused coccygeal vertebrae.

Typically, a vertebra has a **vertebral body**, two **pedicles**, two **laminae**, two **transverse processes**, and a single **spinous process**. The **vertebral foramen** is the space between the vertebral body, pedicles, and laminae. Consecutive foramina create the **vertebral canal**, which contains the spinal cord and meninges. Most vertebrae possess a pair of **superior and inferior articular processes** (Fig. 26.1). The **facet joints** between these confer an interlocking arrangement that limits anterior and posterior dislocation of the spinal column.

The vertebral bodies are united by fibrocartilage **intervertebral discs**. The outer part of a disc is the tough **anulus fibrosus** (ring) and the soft inner part is the **nucleus pulposus**. The combination of these two parts is such that the intervertebral disc can act as a shock absorber for the vertebral column and provide some flexibility.

At birth the vertebral column is concave anteriorly in the thoracic and sacral regions. These are the primary curves of the spine. The secondary (convex) curves of the cervical and lumbar regions develop after birth with the elevation and extension of the infant's head and when the child assumes an erect position when learning to walk. The joints, ligaments, and muscles of the back (see Chapter 28) stabilize and facilitate movement of the vertebral column. Several ligaments provide support to the vertebral column (Fig. 26.2, Table 26.1), including:

- the **anterior longitudinal** and **posterior longitudinal ligaments** on the anterior and posterior surfaces of the vertebral body, which together with the intervertebral discs make up the **joints between vertebral bodies**;
- the **ligamentum flavum** between adjacent laminae;
- the **supraspinous ligaments**, which connect the tips of the spinous processes;
- the **interspinous ligaments** between the spinous processes.

VERTEBRAL TYPES

The **cervical vertebrae** are distinguished from other vertebrae by their small vertebral bodies, bifid spinous processes (except CVII), and **transverse foramina** within the transverse processes (which allow the passage of the vertebral artery).

The **atlas** (CI) has no body or spinous process, but it has two lateral masses connected by the **anterior** and **posterior arches**. It articulates with the occipital bone of the skull through the **atlanto-occipital joint**, which enables flexion, extension, and lateral bending (flexion) of the head. The **axis** (CII) has a unique finger-like projection – the **dens** (odontoid process) – which articulates with the anterior arch of the atlas (CI). This unique articulation allows rotation of the head. There are also two joints between the lateral masses of the atlas and axis, the **atlantoaxial joints**.

Vertebra CVII has a large palpable spinous process and is known as the **vertebra prominens**.

Thoracic vertebrae are characterized by articular facets on their vertebral bodies and transverse processes for articulation with the ribs (except TXI and TXII) at the **costovertebral joints**. Their broad

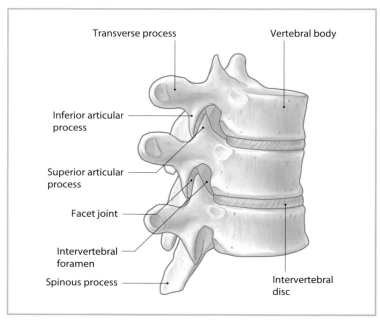

Figure 26.1 Anterolateral view of the vertebral column

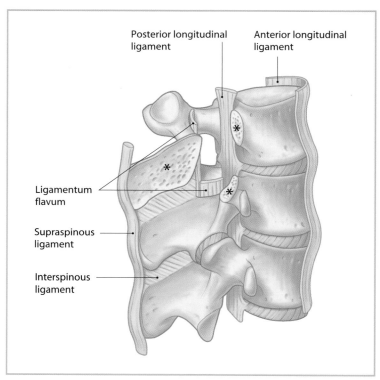

Figure 26.2 Ligaments of the spine. Asterisks indicate cut surfaces

laminae and downward-projecting spinous processes overlap with those of the vertebra beneath and increase rigidity in this region.

Each **lumbar vertebra** (Fig. 26.3) has a large vertebral body to withstand the accumulated weight of the body. The superior articular processes (the **mammillary process**) are enlarged.

The **sacrum**, a fusion of five vertebrae, is a triangular-shaped bone that forms the concave posterior wall of the pelvis. It is

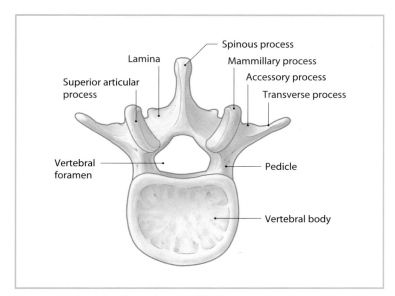

Figure 26.3 Superior view of a typical lumbar vertebra

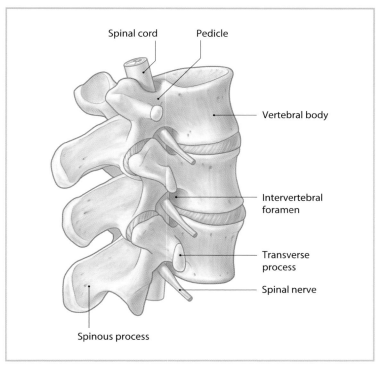

Figure 26.4 Posterolateral view of the vertebral column

weightbearing and has foramina for nerves from the lumbosacral plexus (see Chapter 32). At the inferior end of the vertebral column is the small **coccyx** (tail bone), made up of four fused vertebrae. It serves as an attachment point for pelvic ligaments and muscles.

NERVES
Innervation to the vertebrae, ligaments, joints, and muscles and skin of the vertebral column is from the posterior rami of spinal nerves as they exit from their respective intervertebral foramina (Fig. 26.4).

ARTERIES
Blood is supplied to the vertebrae by segmental spinal branches of the ascending cervical, vertebral, intercostal, lumbar, and lateral sacral arteries.

VEINS AND LYMPHATICS
Venous drainage of the external vertebral column is provided by a network of valveless veins that envelops each vertebra. These veins connect superiorly with the venous dural sinuses from the skull and brain, and inferiorly with the pelvic veins. In the thorax, the **external vertebral venous plexus** connects with the azygos vein and with the superior and inferior vena cavae.

Within the spinal canal is the **internal vertebral venous plexus**. This system extends from the base of the skull to the coccyx and drains structures within the spinal canal (i.e. the spinal cord and meninges). Venous blood can flow in either direction in the venous plexuses, depending on the relative pressure within each region. This arrangement facilitates tumor metastasis.

SPINAL CORD AND MENINGES
Within the vertebral canal the spinal cord is invested by the meninges and is continuous with the medulla oblongata of the brainstem. Inferiorly, in adults it ends at the level of vertebra LII by forming the **conus medullaris**. In children it can extend as far inferiorly as vertebra LIV.

The spinal cord gives rise to 31 pairs of spinal nerves formed by the union of **posterior** (sensory) and **anterior** (motor) **rootlets**, which arise from the dorsolateral and ventrolateral aspects of the

cord, respectively (see Fig. 25.3). These mixed (sensory and motor) spinal nerves exit the vertebral canal through the intervertebral foramen and then divide into posterior and anterior rami:

- the **posterior rami** segmentally supply the deep muscles of the back and overlying skin;
- the **anterior rami** segmentally supply the anterolateral body wall and regionally contribute to the formation of the cervical, brachial, lumbar, and sacral plexuses, which allow several segments of the spinal cord to unite, divide, and travel to a specific region as a peripheral nerve (e.g. the sciatic nerve).

Arteries
Blood is supplied to the spinal cord by a network of arteries that surrounds the vertebral column. The **anterior spinal artery** and two **posterior spinal arteries** are longitudinally oriented vessels that run the length of the spinal cord and receive blood from the vertebral, deep cervical, intercostal, and lumbar arteries:

- the anterior spinal artery provides blood to the anterior two-thirds of the spinal cord and the vertebral body;
- the posterior spinal arteries supply blood to the posterior one-third of the spinal cord and the vertebral body.

An additional source of blood to the spinal cord is from the **radicular arteries**, a set of segmental arteries originating from the vertebral, deep cervical, ascending cervical, posterior intercostal, lumbar, and lateral sacral arteries. These arteries, which are paired (left and right), enter the spinal canal through the intervertebral foramina and are the primary source of blood for the spinal cord, vertebrae, and meninges.

The **anterior radicular artery** (artery of Adamkiewicz) is a large radicular artery that supplies the inferior thoracic and lumbar region

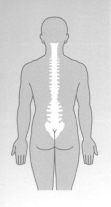

of the spinal cord and is the primary blood source to the anterior spinal artery along the inferior two-thirds of the spinal cord.

Veins and lymphatics

Venous drainage of the spinal cord is through the internal vertebral venous plexus described above. The spinal cord has no lymphatic vessels.

■ CLINICAL CORRELATION

Lumbar intervertebral disc herniation

Back pain is a common symptom of lumbar disc herniation. Many patients recall at least one or a series of events, such as a car accident, heavy lifting and twisting, or other trauma that caused it. The pain is exacerbated by heavy lifting or strenuous activity, originates in the lower back, and may radiate to the gluteal region and posterior thigh. If the lumbar disc herniation is compressing a nerve root, the pain often extends inferiorly to the knee joint. Sometimes, sitting for prolonged periods of time can worsen the pain.

The reason for disc herniation is unknown, but may be multifactorial and related to repetitive trauma, unstable or weak back musculature, or genetic defects.

The most common locations for disc herniation are at the LIV/LV and LV/S1 discs. Nucleus pulposus, the softer material within a disc, herniates or protrudes from the disc and exerts pressure on nearby structures. If the herniated disc applies pressure to a spinal nerve root, a syndrome of symptoms consistent with the distribution of the involved nerve root result (Fig. 26.5): herniation of the disc between LIV and LV compresses the L5 nerve root; herniation of the disc between LV and SI compresses the S1 nerve root.

Features of **L4 nerve root compression** are:

- weakness of quadriceps femoris and hip adductors;
- loss or diminishment of the patellar reflex;
- decreased sensation along the posterior thigh, anterior knee, and medial leg and medial malleolus of ankle (Fig. 26.4).

Features of **L5 nerve root compression** are:

- weakness of gluteus medius, extensor hallucis longus, and extensor digitorum brevis muscles;
- no loss of reflexes;
- decreased sensation along the anterolateral leg, dorsum of foot, and first web space between toes I and II.

Features of **S1 nerve root compression** are:

- weakness of gluteus maximus, gastrocnemius, fibularis longus, fibularis brevis, and fibularis tertius muscles;
- loss of the Achilles' reflex.
- decreased sensation along the lateral malleolus of the ankle, lateral foot, and dorsum of fifth toe.

Symptoms caused by disc herniation can be diagnosed by careful history and examination. Magnetic resonance imaging (MRI) scans of the involved region of the vertebral column are also helpful in identifying the extent of the disease process.

In general, treatment of mild disc herniation symptoms involves a short period of rest, relaxation, and physical therapy as necessary to decrease back pain and facilitate early return to normal daily activities. Painkillers are occasionally prescribed for patient comfort.

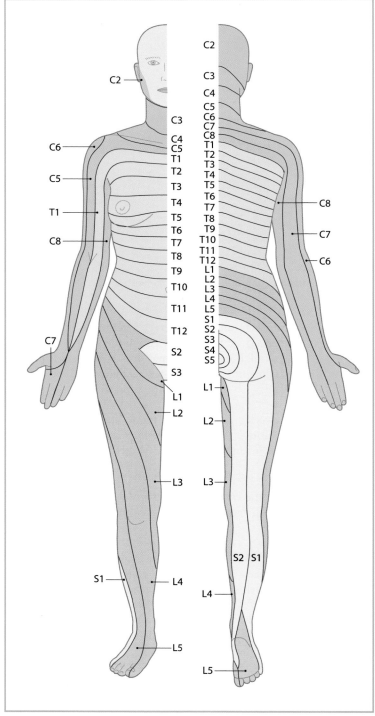

Figure 26.5 Cutaneous nerve distribution (dermatomes)

Occasionally, a large central herniation of an intervertebral disc applies great pressure to both left and right nerve roots. This can cause paralysis of both lower limbs, loss of bladder and anal sphincter control, and loss of bilateral (left and right) ankle reflexes, with numbness in the gluteal and perianal areas. This constellation of symptoms indicates a serious disc protrusion or other disorder that requires immediate medical treatment. In some cases, it is necessary to remove the herniated disc surgically to alleviate the pressure on the spinal nerve roots.

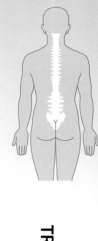

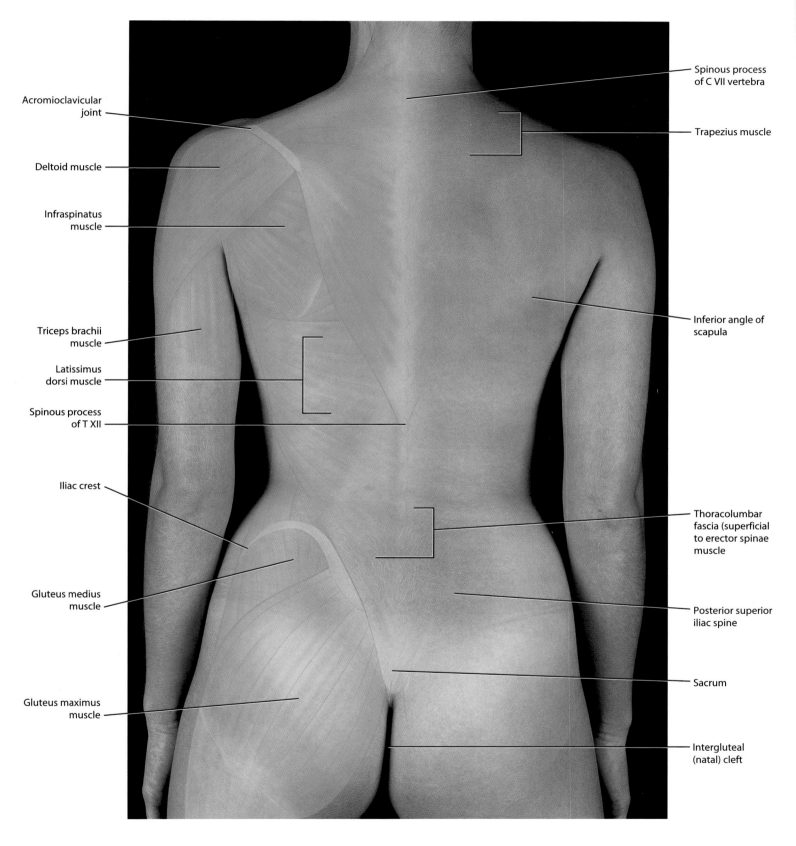

Acromioclavicular joint

Deltoid muscle

Infraspinatus muscle

Triceps brachii muscle

Latissimus dorsi muscle

Spinous process of T XII

Iliac crest

Gluteus medius muscle

Gluteus maximus muscle

Spinous process of C VII vertebra

Trapezius muscle

Inferior angle of scapula

Thoracolumbar fascia (superficial to erector spinae muscle)

Posterior superior iliac spine

Sacrum

Intergluteal (natal) cleft

Figure 26.6 Vertebral column – surface anatomy. Posterior view of the back of a young woman. Observe the anatomical landmarks, which help delineate various levels of the spine (e.g. iliac crest corresponds to vertebra LIV level)

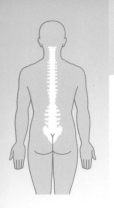

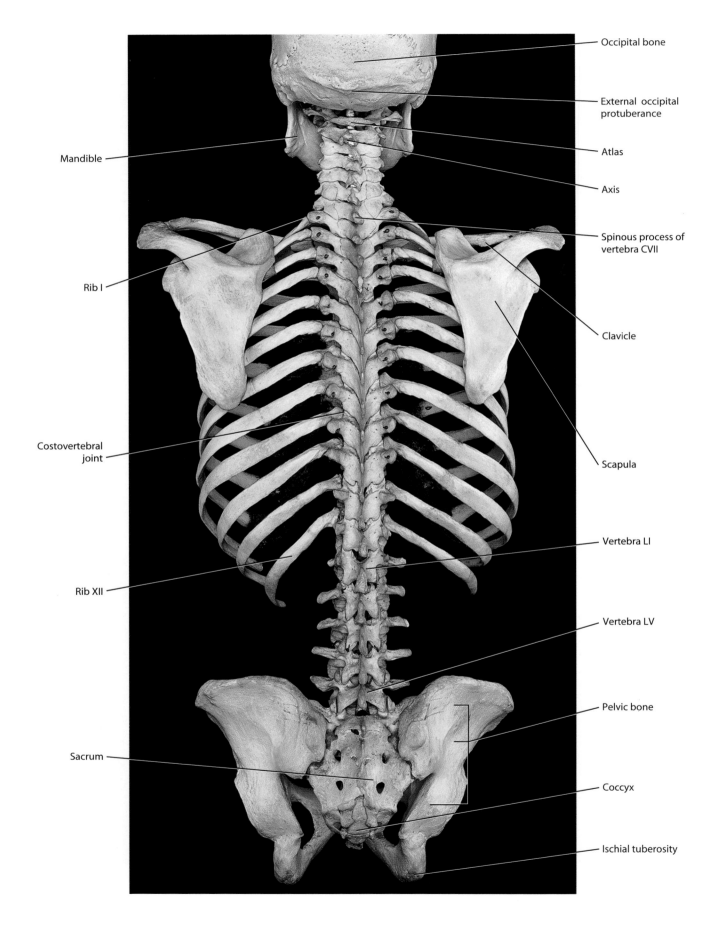

Occipital bone

External occipital protuberance

Atlas

Axis

Spinous process of vertebra CVII

Clavicle

Scapula

Vertebra LI

Vertebra LV

Pelvic bone

Coccyx

Ischial tuberosity

Mandible

Rib I

Costovertebral joint

Rib XII

Sacrum

Figure 26.7 Axial skeleton – articulated 1. Posterior view of the entire vertebral column articulated with the complete axial skeleton showing the bony support for the head, neck, back, and pelvis. Observe the differences in the posterior view of the cervical, thoracic, and lumbar vertebrae

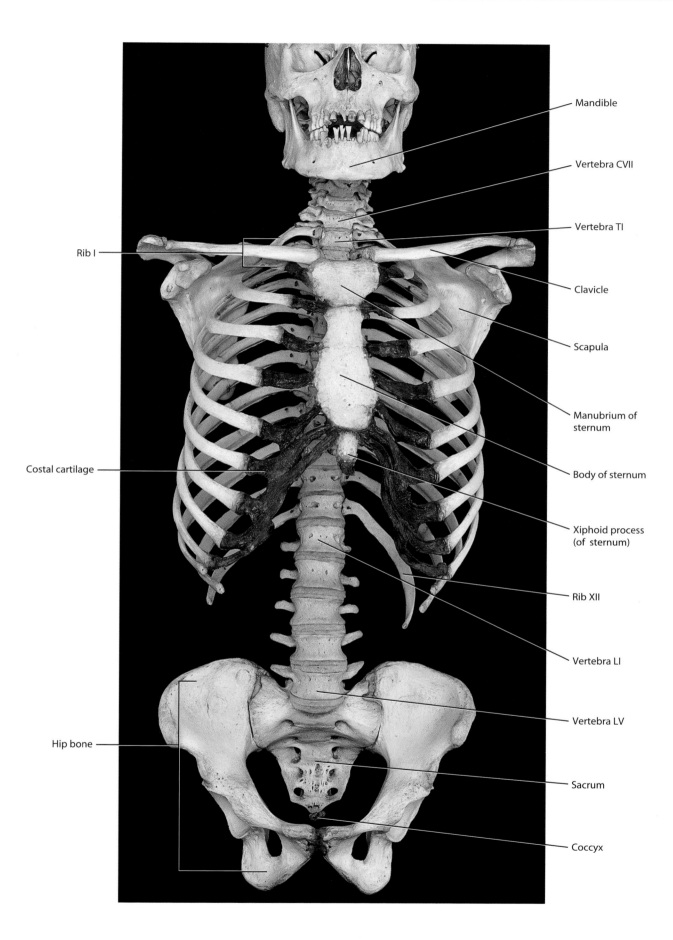

Mandible

Vertebra CVII

Vertebra TI

Rib I

Clavicle

Scapula

Manubrium of sternum

Costal cartilage

Body of sternum

Xiphoid process (of sternum)

Rib XII

Vertebra LI

Hip bone

Vertebra LV

Sacrum

Coccyx

Figure 26.8 Axial skeleton – articulated 2. Anterior view of the articulated vertebral column with the complete axial skeleton included for reference and showing the bony support for the head, neck, thorax, and pelvis. Observe how vertebra LV joins to the sacrum

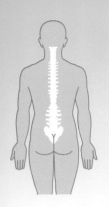

TRUNK

Vertebral column

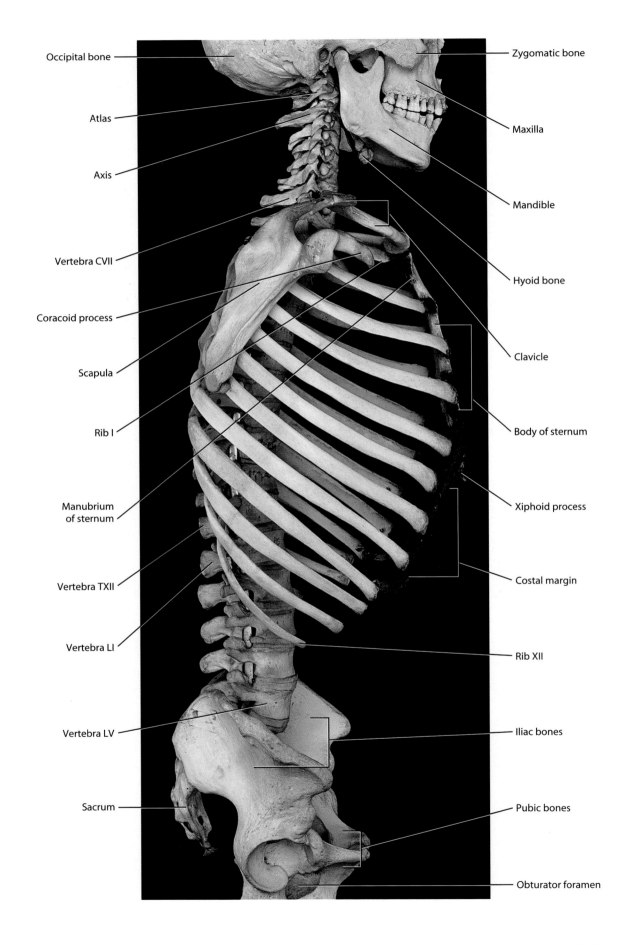

Occipital bone

Atlas

Axis

Vertebra CVII

Coracoid process

Scapula

Rib I

Manubrium
of sternum

Vertebra TXII

Vertebra LI

Vertebra LV

Sacrum

Zygomatic bone

Maxilla

Mandible

Hyoid bone

Clavicle

Body of sternum

Xiphoid process

Costal margin

Rib XII

Iliac bones

Pubic bones

Obturator foramen

Figure 26.9 Axial skeleton – articulated 3. Lateral view of the vertebral column articulated with the complete axial skeleton showing the bony support of the head, neck, back, thorax, and pelvis. Note the spinal curvatures. Observe the relationships of the ribs to the thoracic vertebrae

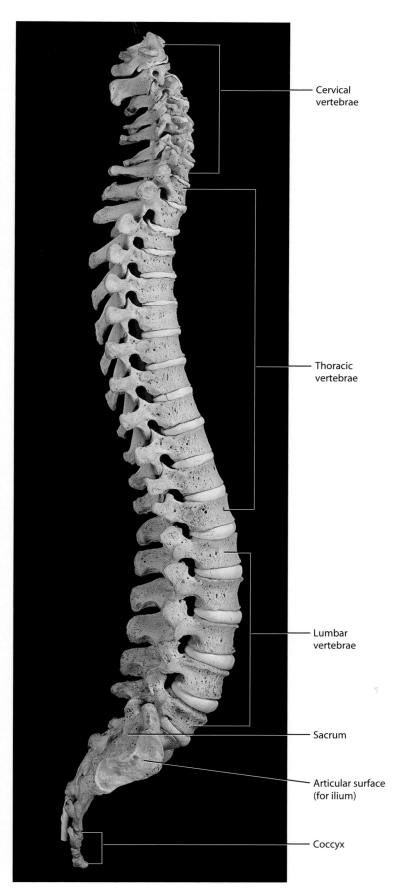

Cervical
vertebrae

Thoracic
vertebrae

Lumbar
vertebrae

Sacrum

Articular surface
(for ilium)

Coccyx

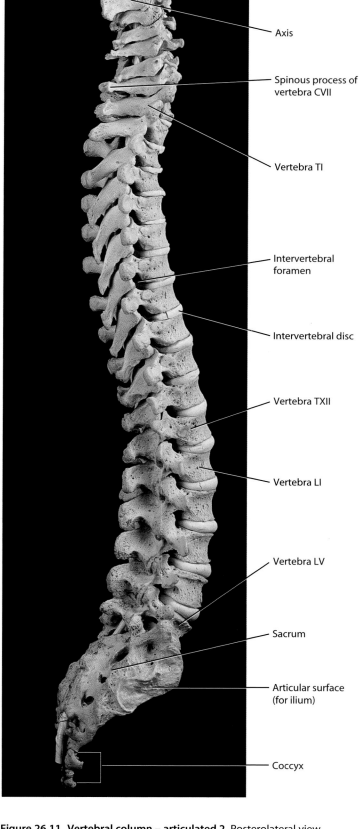

Atlas

Axis

Spinous process of
vertebra CVII

Vertebra TI

Intervertebral
foramen

Intervertebral disc

Vertebra TXII

Vertebra LI

Vertebra LV

Sacrum

Articular surface
(for ilium)

Coccyx

TRUNK Vertebral column

Figure 26.10 Vertebral column – articulated 1. Lateral view of the vertebral column showing the subdivisions and curvatures. This is the right side of the articulated vertebral column with all supporting bones removed. Observe the curvatures of the spine, which have been reconstructed here. This is the vertebral column of an elderly person

Figure 26.11 Vertebral column – articulated 2. Posterolateral view showing the right side of an articulated vertebral column with specific vertebrae and anatomical landmarks. This view shows the facet joints, which are most easily seen in the lumbar region (see facet joints between LIII and LIV)

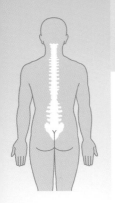

Vertebral column **TRUNK**

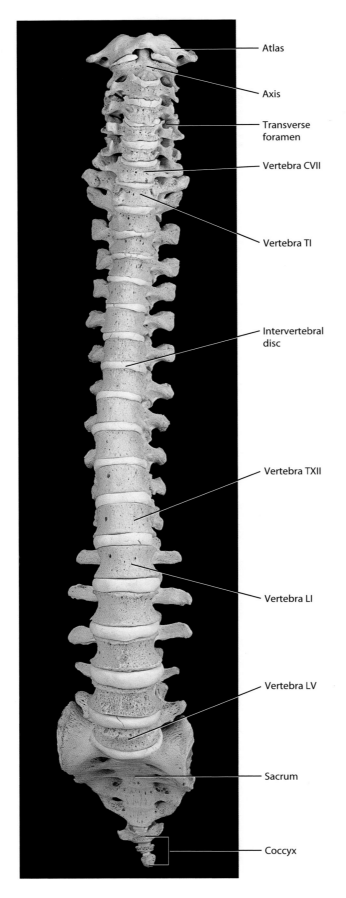

Atlas

Axis

Transverse foramen

Vertebra CVII

Vertebra TI

Intervertebral disc

Vertebra TXII

Vertebra LI

Vertebra LV

Sacrum

Coccyx

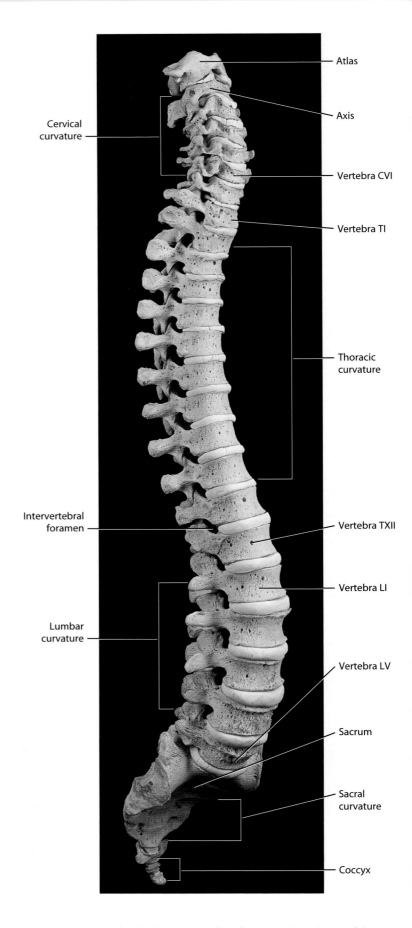

Cervical curvature

Atlas

Axis

Vertebra CVI

Vertebra TI

Thoracic curvature

Intervertebral foramen

Vertebra TXII

Vertebra LI

Lumbar curvature

Vertebra LV

Sacrum

Sacral curvature

Coccyx

Figure 26.12 Vertebral column – articulated 3. Anterior view of the vertebral column showing specific vertebrae and anatomical landmarks. Observe the transverse foramina, which are present only in the cervical vertebrae (see vertebra CI, the atlas)

Figure 26.13 Vertebral column – articulated 4. Anterolateral view of the right side of the vertebral column. This views shows the intervertebral foramina. Spinal nerves leave the spinal cord through these foramina and travel laterally to innervate the body

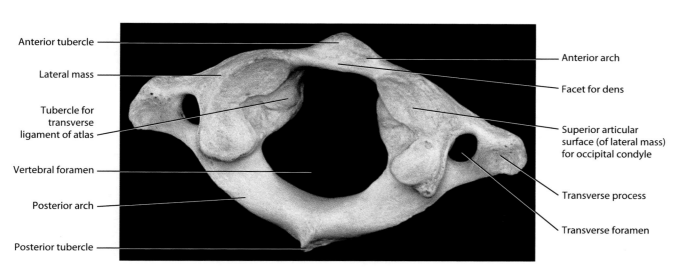

Anterior tubercle

Lateral mass

Tubercle for transverse ligament of atlas

Vertebral foramen

Posterior arch

Posterior tubercle

Anterior arch

Facet for dens

Superior articular surface (of lateral mass) for occipital condyle

Transverse process

Transverse foramen

Figure 26.14 Vertebra CI. Superior view of vertebra CI (atlas). The skull, which rests on the atlas, articulates with the superior articular surfaces of the atlas. Observe the transverse foramina, which are present only in the cervical vertebrae

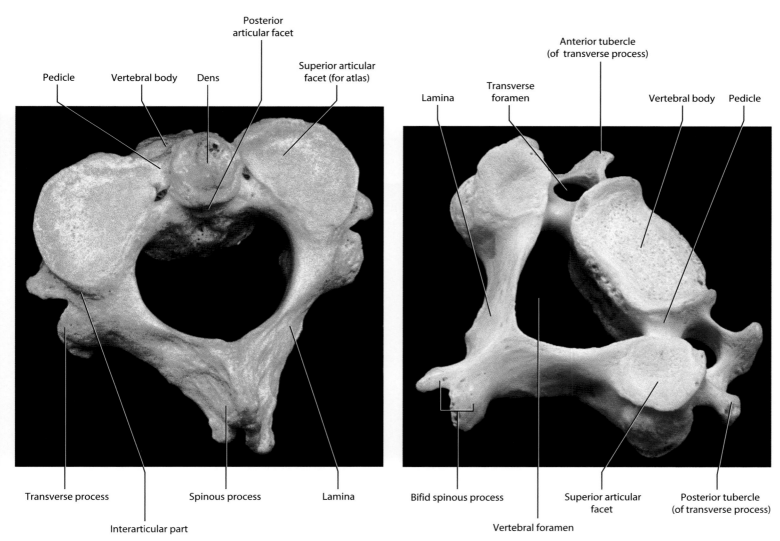

Posterior articular facet

Pedicle   Vertebral body   Dens

Superior articular facet (for atlas)

Anterior tubercle (of transverse process)

Lamina

Transverse foramen

Vertebral body   Pedicle

Transverse process

Spinous process   Lamina

Interarticular part

Bifid spinous process

Vertebral foramen

Superior articular facet

Posterior tubercle (of transverse process)

Figure 26.15 Vertebra CII. Superior view of vertebra CII (axis). The weight of the skull and atlas is transmitted onto the superior articular facets. In the center of the anterior part of the axis is an osseous protuberance (the dens), which acts as a pivot point, allowing left and right rotation of the skull

Figure 26.16 Cervical vertebra. Superior view of a typical cervical vertebra. Notice the bifid spinous process and the transverse foramina for passage of the vertebral artery on its course to the brain

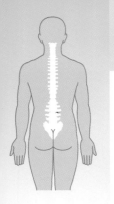

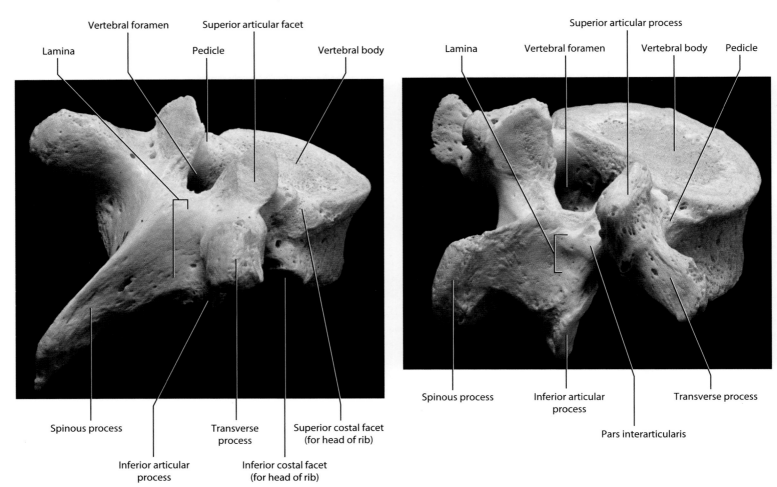

Vertebral foramen Superior articular facet

Lamina Pedicle Vertebral body

Spinous process Transverse process Superior costal facet (for head of rib)

Inferior articular process Inferior costal facet (for head of rib)

Superior articular process

Lamina Vertebral foramen Vertebral body Pedicle

Spinous process Inferior articular process Transverse process

Pars interarticularis

Figure 26.17 Thoracic vertebra. Posterolateral view of a typical thoracic vertebra. Ribs attach to the thoracic vertebrae by facet joints on the transverse processes. A typical thoracic vertebra also has a long downward-pointing spinous process

Figure 26.18 Lumbar vertebra. Posterolateral view of a typical lumbar vertebra. These are the largest vertebrae and have large articular processes and thickened spinous processes

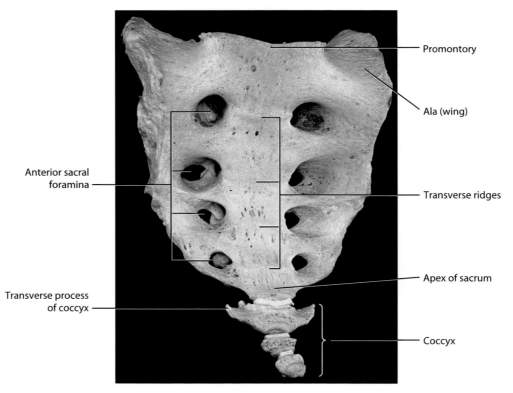

Promontory

Ala (wing)

Anterior sacral foramina

Transverse ridges

Transverse process of coccyx

Apex of sacrum

Coccyx

Figure 26.19 Sacrum and coccyx. Anterior view of the sacrum and coccyx. Observe the sacral foramina through which the terminal nerves of the spinal cord leave the spinal canal to innervate structures of the pelvis and lower limb. Also observe the coccyx, which is formed from four small vestigial vertebrae

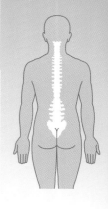

TABLE 26.1 LIGAMENTS OF THE VERTEBRAL COLUMN		
Ligament	**Attachments**	**Function**
Anterior longitudinal	Covers the anterior part of the vertebral bodies and the intervertebral discs. Extends from anterior tubercle of CI (atlas) to the sacrum.	Limits extension of the vertebral column, maintains stability of the intervertebral discs
Posterior longitudinal	Attached to the posterior aspect of the intervertebral discs (within the vertebral canal). Runs from CII vertebra to the sacrum	Restricts flexion of the vertebral column and posterior herniation of the discs
Intertransverse	Runs between adjacent transverse processes	Limits lateral bending to the contralateral side
Interspinous	Connects adjacent spinous processes	Limits flexion of the vertebral column
Supraspinous	Accessory ligament to the interspinous ligament. Runs between the tips of adjacent spinous processes	Limits flexion of the vertebral column
Ligamenta flava	Unites laminae of adjacent vertebrae (paired ligaments)	Resist flexion of the vertebral column
Ligamentum nuchae	In cervical region the supraspinous and interspinous ligaments thicken to form this ligament. Extends from spine of CVII to external occipital protuberance	Provides muscle attachment for trapezius and rhomboid minor. Supports neck and prevents hyperflexion

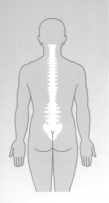

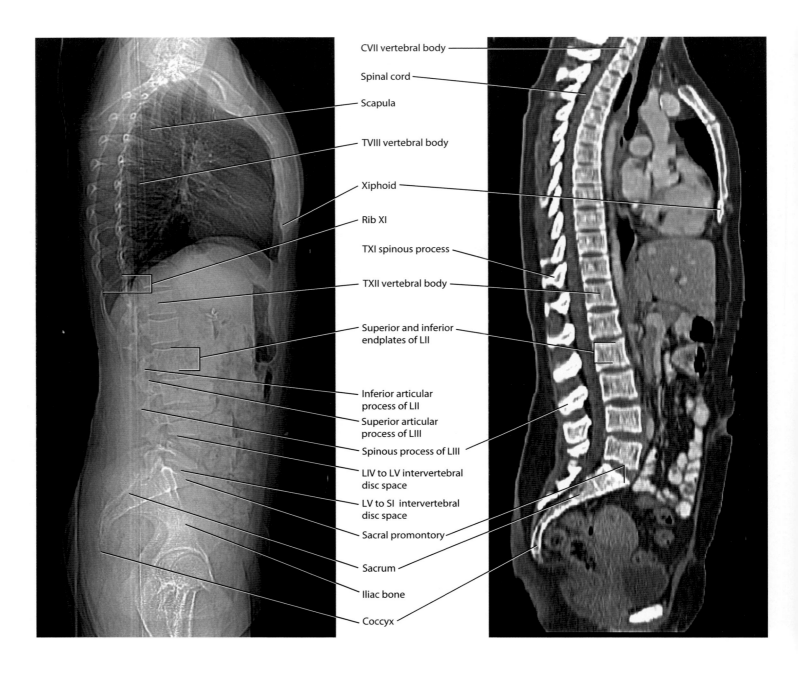

CVII vertebral body

Spinal cord

Scapula

TVIII vertebral body

Xiphoid

Rib XI

TXI spinous process

TXII vertebral body

Superior and inferior endplates of LII

Inferior articular process of LII

Superior articular process of LIII

Spinous process of LIII

LIV to LV intervertebral disc space

LV to SI intervertebral disc space

Sacral promontory

Sacrum

Iliac bone

Coccyx

Figure 26.20 Vertebral column – CT scan (lateral view). Note the orientation of the air fluid level in the stomach, indicating that the image was taken with the patient lying supine. The vertebral bodies of the thoracic and lumbar regions are visible as is the sacrum and coccyx. Observe the curvatures of this normal spine

Figure 26.21 Vertebral column – CT scan (sagittal view). This scan shows the relationship of the vertebral column to the aorta, heart, liver, and small bowel. Observe how the lumbar vertebrae are located posterior to the abdominal contents

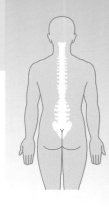

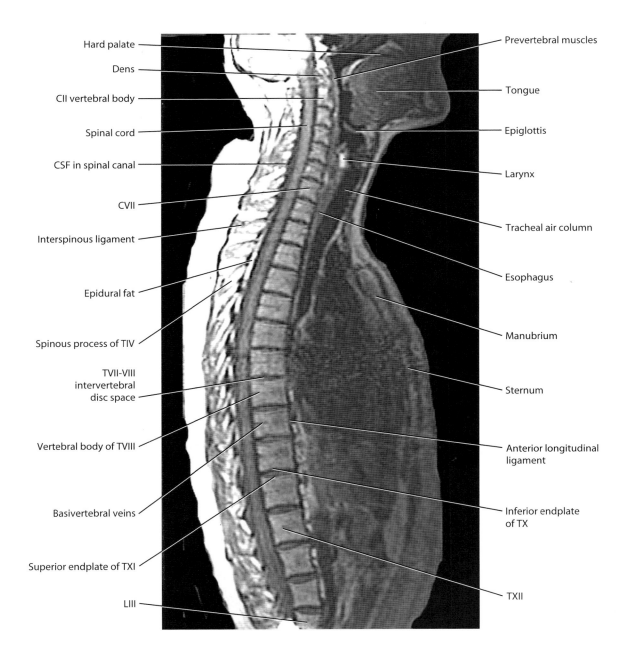

Hard palate

Dens

CII vertebral body

Spinal cord

CSF in spinal canal

CVII

Interspinous ligament

Epidural fat

Spinous process of TIV

TVII-VIII intervertebral disc space

Vertebral body of TVIII

Basivertebral veins

Superior endplate of TXI

LIII

Prevertebral muscles

Tongue

Epiglottis

Larynx

Tracheal air column

Esophagus

Manubrium

Sternum

Anterior longitudinal ligament

Inferior endplate of TX

TXII

Figure 26.22 Vertebral column – MRI scan (sagittal view). Observe the size of the vertebral bodies and their relationship to the spinal cord

The suboccipital region is in the upper part of the posterior neck just below the occipital bone and deep to the trapezius, splenius capitis, and semispinalis capitis muscles. The suboccipital triangle contains the **vertebral artery**, the **suboccipital nerve** (C1), and the **suboccipital venous plexus**. The skeletal support for this region is provided by the occipital bone, the atlas (CI), and the axis (CII). These three bony structures form the atlanto-occipital and atlanto-axial joints. These articulations allow flexion, extension, and rotation of the head.

MUSCLES

The four muscles of the suboccipital region lie deep to the semispinalis capitis muscle (Fig. 27.1 and Table 27.1). Three of these muscles form the borders of the suboccipital triangle:

- the inferolateral border is formed by the **obliquus capitis inferior** muscle;
- the superolateral border by the **obliquus capitis superior** muscle;
- the superomedial border by the **rectus capitis posterior major** muscle.

The fourth muscle, the **rectus capitis posterior minor**, does not take part in formation of the triangle, but it can be observed just medial to the rectus capitis posterior major muscle.

The main function of these muscles is to hold the head in the neutral position, but they also extend and rotate the head. They are innervated by branches of C1 (the suboccipital nerve).

NERVES

The posterior rami of the first four cervical nerves (C1 to C4) are in the suboccipital region (Fig. 27.1). The suboccipital nerve (C1) enters the region by piercing the atlanto-occipital membrane and supplies all four suboccipital muscles. The **greater occipital nerve** (C2) passes inferiorly to the obliquus capitis inferior muscle and supplies sensation to the skin of the posterior scalp. The posterior rami of C3 and C4 supply the upper cervical muscles, scalp, and skin of the posterior neck.

ARTERIES

The structures in the suboccipital region receive blood from branches of the vertebral, occipital, and deep cervical arteries.

- The **vertebral artery** arises from the first part of the subclavian artery and ascends through the transverse foramina of the upper six cervical vertebrae on its way to the brain; its suboccipital part provides **muscular branches** to each of the suboccipital muscles.
- The **occipital artery** branches from the external carotid artery. In the suboccipital region, it lies on the obliquus capitis superior and semispinalis capitis muscles. Accompanied by the greater occipital nerve, the occipital artery pierces the trapezius muscle and ascends and divides into numerous branches to the skin of the posterior scalp.
- The **deep cervical artery**, a branch of the costocervical trunk, is in the suboccipital region just deep to the semispinalis capitis muscle. Here, branches of the deep cervical artery anastomose with branches of the occipital artery.

VEINS AND LYMPHATICS

The **deep cervical veins** drain the suboccipital region and are deep to the semispinalis capitis muscle within the suboccipital triangle. They connect with the **suboccipital venous plexus**, which is part of the vertebral venous system, a valveless network connected superiorly to the intracranial dural sinuses and inferiorly to the pelvic veins. In the neck and trunk, the vertebral venous system joins with the azygos and caval veins (see Chapter 29). Because this venous network is valveless, blood can flow in both directions and so provide a route for the spread of cancer, emboli, and infection.

Lymphatic vessels from the suboccipital region drain to the **occipital**, **spinal accessory**, and **superior cervical nodes**.

■ CLINICAL CORRELATIONS
Neck muscle strain ('whiplash')

Cervical (neck) muscle strain is caused by hyperextension of the neck. A common cause is a motor vehicle accident in which the patient's vehicle is struck from the rear. The momentum of the impact can cause hyperextension of the neck muscles, ligaments, or other soft tissues, and is commonly known as 'whiplash'. Cervical nerve root compression (radiculopathy) as a result of cervical strain injuries may cause unique signs and symptoms, depending on the level of injury (Table 27.2). These are often caused by cervical intervertebral disc herniation, and they often resolve spontaneously.

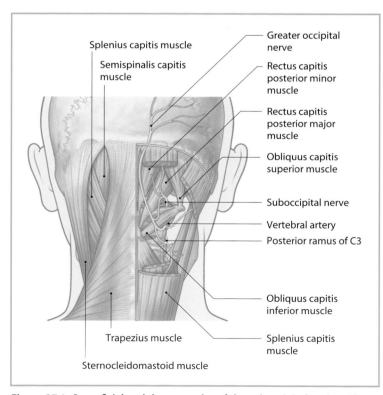

Figure 27.1 Superficial and deep muscles of the suboccipital region. These are shown cut away to reveal the posterior ramus of nerve C3.

Splenius capitis muscle

Semispinalis capitis muscle

Greater occipital nerve

Rectus capitis posterior minor muscle

Rectus capitis posterior major muscle

Obliquus capitis superior muscle

Suboccipital nerve

Vertebral artery

Posterior ramus of C3

Obliquus capitis inferior muscle

Splenius capitis muscle

Trapezius muscle

Sternocleidomastoid muscle

Radiographs are usually obtained after neck trauma to rule out a fracture or other serious injury to the neck. Consultation with a neurosurgeon is necessary if cervical intervertebral disc injury, neck fracture, or any other serious injury is suspected. For many patients with non-serious injuries, initial treatment is aimed at alleviating pain and using nonsurgical modalities such as heat and cold treatments and/or physiotherapy.

Cervical spine fractures

The cervical spine comprises seven vertebrae with articulations that allow the neck to move in several different planes (i.e. flexion, extension, lateral flexion, and rotation). Fractures of the cervical spine occur when forces applied to the head cause abnormal movements of the neck that exceed the strength of the vertebrae. In the cervical spine, fractures of CI are usually secondary to compression injuries to the cervical column, whereas injuries to CII tend to occur secondary to hyperextension. Jefferson's fracture is the most frequently seen and has at least two fracture lines on the ring of CI (Fig. 27.2). The hangman's fracture (Fig. 27.3) involves two fracture lines through the pedicles of CII.

Patients with upper cervical spine fractures usually complain of neck pain after a traumatic event. Some do not have any neurological deficit because the spinal canal at this level is so large. Treatment is aimed at stabilizing the cervical spine and can sometimes be accomplished with external fixation using a halo device or by open reduction and internal fixation (ORIF) in the operating room. Lower cervical spine fractures are treated similarly. Disc herniations and radiculopathy are common with lower cervical spine injury (Table 27.2). Most cervical disc herniations heal spontaneously.

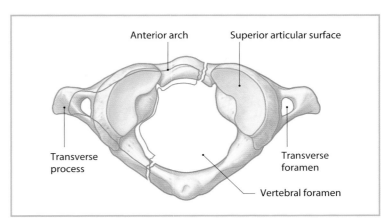

Figure 27.2 Jefferson's fracture of vertebra CI

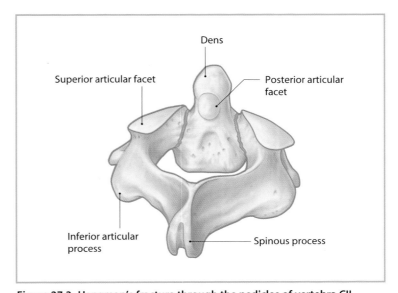

Figure 27.3 Hangman's fracture through the pedicles of vertebra CII

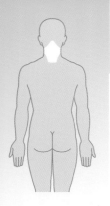

TRUNK

Suboccipital region

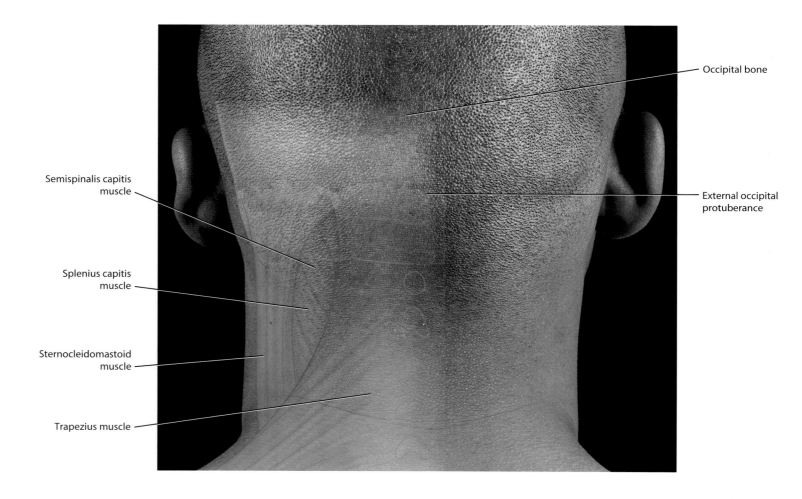

Occipital bone

External occipital protuberance

Semispinalis capitis muscle

Splenius capitis muscle

Sternocleidomastoid muscle

Trapezius muscle

Figure 27.4 Suboccipital region – surface anatomy. Posterior view of the base of the neck of a young man who has shaved his head. Observe the nuchal line visible as a slight shadow joining the ears

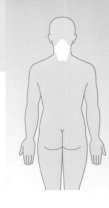

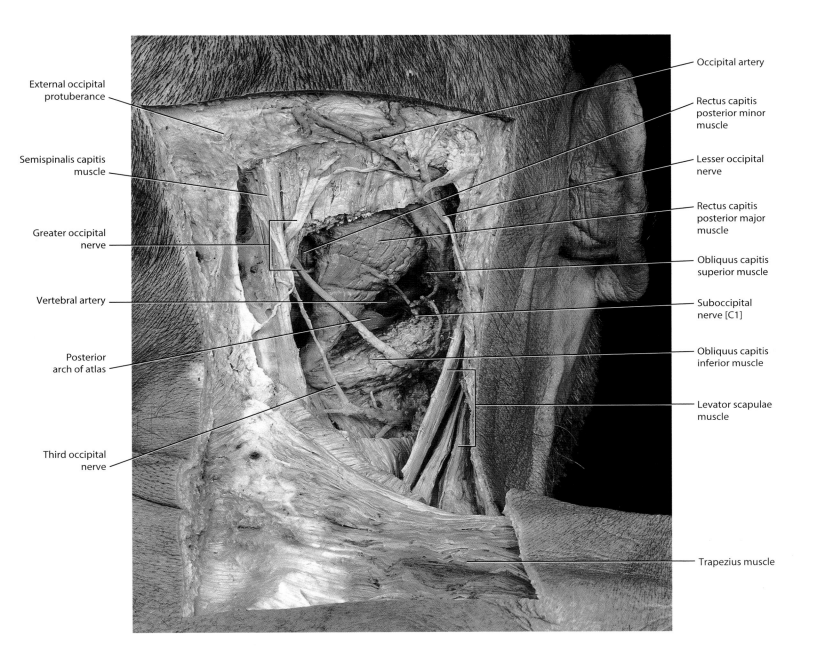

External occipital protuberance

Semispinalis capitis muscle

Greater occipital nerve

Vertebral artery

Posterior arch of atlas

Third occipital nerve

Occipital artery

Rectus capitis posterior minor muscle

Lesser occipital nerve

Rectus capitis posterior major muscle

Obliquus capitis superior muscle

Suboccipital nerve [C1]

Obliquus capitis inferior muscle

Levator scapulae muscle

Trapezius muscle

Figure 27.5 Suboccipital region – superficial dissection. Posterior view of the right suboccipital region. The splenius capitis, semispinalis cervicis, splenius cervicis, and trapezius muscles have been cut and removed to show the structures of the suboccipital region

313

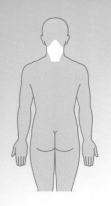

TABLE 27.1 MUSCLES OF THE SUBOCCIPITAL REGION

Muscle	Origin	Insertion	Innervation	Action	Blood supply
Rectus capitis posterior major	Spinous process of axis (CII)	Inferior nuchal line	Extends and rotates head	Suboccipital nerve (C1)	Vertebral and occipital arteries
Rectus capitis posterior minor	Posterior tubercle of atlas (CI)	Inferior nuchal line	Extends head	Suboccipital nerve (C1)	Vertebral and occipital arteries
Obliquus capitis superior	Transverse process of atlas (CI)	Occipital bones between nuchal lines	Lateral flexion	Suboccipital nerve (C1)	Vertebral and occipital arteries
Obliquus capitis inferior	Spinous process of axis (CII)	Transverse process of atlas (CI)	Rotates atlas (CI) and head	Suboccipital nerve (C1)	Vertebral and occipital arteries
Splenius capitis Splenius cervicis	Ligamentum nuchae and spinous processes of CVII to TIII or TIV	Mastoid process and lateral third of superior nuchal line, tubercles of transverse processes of CI to CIII or CIV	Together they extend the head and neck, alone they laterally bend and rotate head to same side	Posterior rami of spinal nerves	Occipital and transverse cervical arteries
Semispinalis cervicis	Transverse processes TI to TVI, articular processes TV to TVIII	Spinous processes of CII to CV	Extension and lateral flexion of vertebral column	Posterior rami (C6 to C8)	Posterior intercostals, occipital and deep cervical branch of costocervical trunk
Semispinalis capitis	Transverse processes CVII and TI to TVI, articular processes CIV to CVI	Occipital bones, fossa between superior and inferior nuchal lines	Extension and lateral flexion of cervical column, extension of the head	Posterior rami (C1 to C6)	Occipital and deep cervical branch of costocervical trunk
Spinalis cervicis	Spinous processes CVII, TI and TII, and ligamentum nuchae	Spinous processes of CII to CIV	Extension, lateral flexion and rotation of vertebral column	Posterior rami, segmental	Posterior intercostals, deep branch of costocervical trunk
Spinalis capitis	Transverse processes CVII to TVI, articular processes CIV to CVI	Occipital bone between superior and inferior nuchal lines	Extension, lateral flexion and rotation of vertebral column	Posterior rami segmental	Posterior intercostals, deep branch of costocervical trunk

TABLE 27.2 CERVICAL RADICULOPATHY FINDINGS

C4	Decreased ability to retract, rotate, and elevate the scapula
C5	Weakness of the deltoid muscle and biceps brachii, decreased biceps brachii tendon reflex
C6	Weakness of forearm flexion, decreased shoulder adduction, decreased biceps brachii tendon and brachioradialis reflexes. Pain from neck to radial side of forearm and thumb
C7	Weakness of the triceps brachii muscle and finger extensor muscles, decreased triceps brachii reflex. Weakness of forearm, extension of pain from the neck to the posterior arm and index/middle fingers
C8	Weakness of intrinsic hand flexor muscles, weakness of elbow extension, pain in ring and little fingers

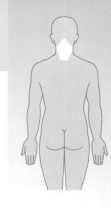

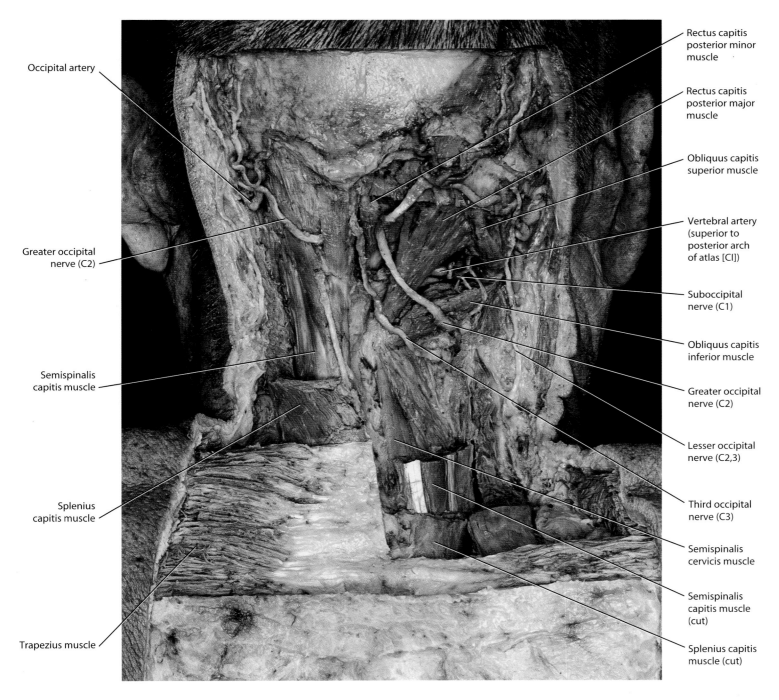

Occipital artery

Greater occipital
nerve (C2)

Semispinalis
capitis muscle

Splenius
capitis muscle

Trapezius muscle

Rectus capitis
posterior minor
muscle

Rectus capitis
posterior major
muscle

Obliquus capitis
superior muscle

Vertebral artery
(superior to
posterior arch
of atlas [CI])

Suboccipital
nerve (C1)

Obliquus capitis
inferior muscle

Greater occipital
nerve (C2)

Lesser occipital
nerve (C2,3)

Third occipital
nerve (C3)

Semispinalis
cervicis muscle

Semispinalis
capitis muscle
(cut)

Splenius capitis
muscle (cut)

Figure 27.6 Suboccipital region – intermediate dissection. Posterior view of the right suboccipital region. Part of the trapezius muscle is visible in the lower part of the dissection, but the splenius and semispinalis muscles have been cut and removed. Observe the vertebral artery, which is visible deep in the dissection

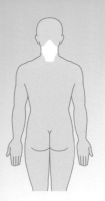

Rectus capitis
posterior major
muscle

Sternocleidomastoid
muscle

Vertebral artery

Obliquus capitis
inferior muscle

Lesser occipital
nerve (C3)

Vertebral artery

C4

Occipital artery

Greater
occipital nerve
(C2)

Posterior arch
of atlas (CI)

Posterior arch
of axis (CII)

Spinal cord

Rootlets of
dorsal root of
spinal nerve

Dorsal root of
spinal nerve

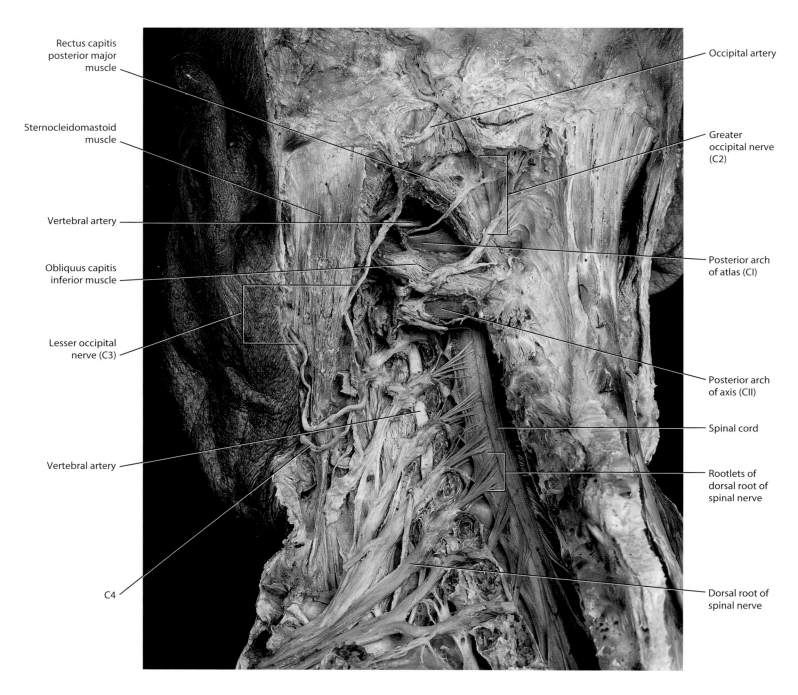

Figure 27.7 Suboccipital region – deep dissection. All of the bone and soft tissue of the left side of the posterior neck have been removed to show the spinal cord and the way in which small nerve roots emerge from the spinal cord and combine to form spinal nerves. The muscles of the suboccipital region have been preserved to show the anatomical relationships

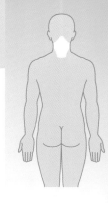

Occipital bone

Atlanto-occipital membrane

Tectorial membrane

Superior longitudinal band of cruciate ligament

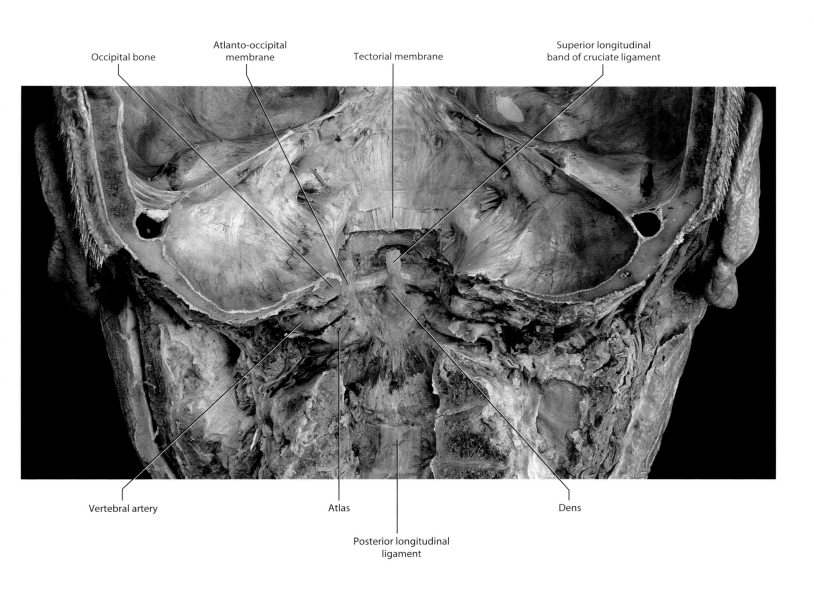

Vertebral artery

Atlas

Dens

Posterior longitudinal ligament

Figure 27.8 Suboccipital region – coronal section. This coronal section through the head shows vertebrae CI and CII and the dens. Imagine how the head would rotate as it pivoted around the dens

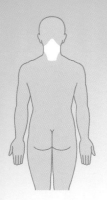

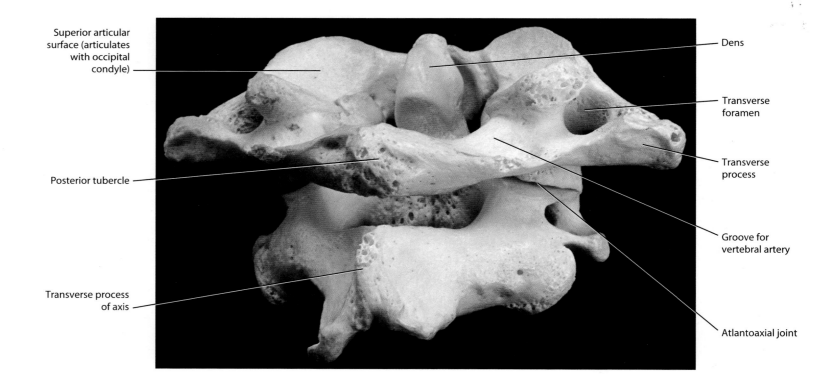

Superior articular surface (articulates with occipital condyle)

Dens

Transverse foramen

Posterior tubercle

Transverse process

Groove for vertebral artery

Transverse process of axis

Atlantoaxial joint

Figure 27.9 Suboccipital region – osteology 1. Posterior view of articulated vertebrae CI (atlas) and CII (axis). Note the superior surface of CI, which articulates with the occipital bones of the skull at the atlanto-occipital joint, and how the dens of CII articulates with CI at the atlanto-axial joint

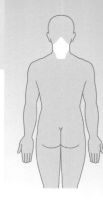

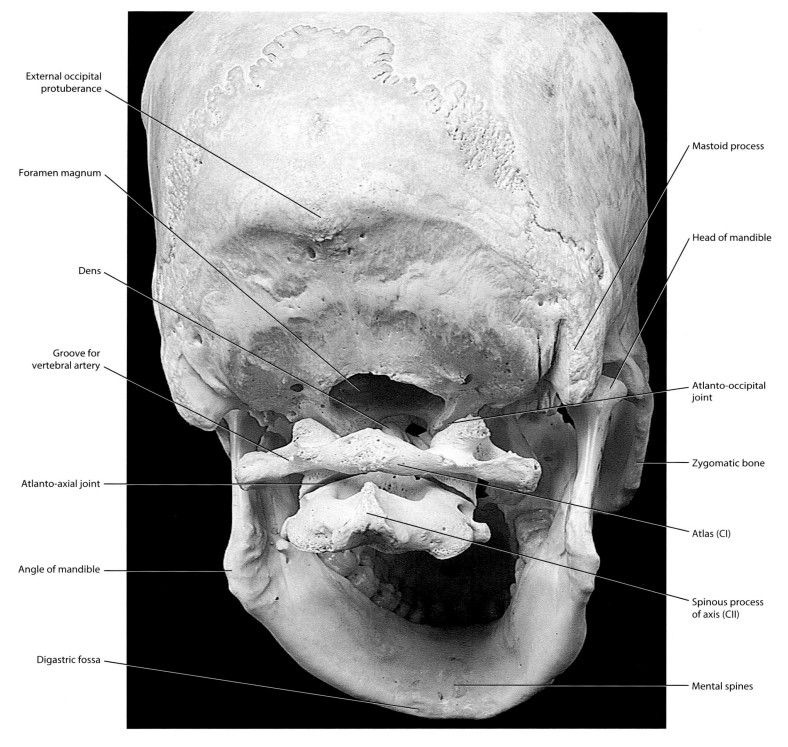

External occipital protuberance

Foramen magnum

Dens

Groove for vertebral artery

Atlanto-axial joint

Angle of mandible

Digastric fossa

Mastoid process

Head of mandible

Atlanto-occipital joint

Zygomatic bone

Atlas (CI)

Spinous process of axis (CII)

Mental spines

Figure 27.10 Suboccipital region – osteology 2. Posterior view of the suboccipital region with all the major bony elements (skull, CI and CII) articulated. Note how the atlanto-occipital joint has been partly opened to show the relative position of the foramen magnum

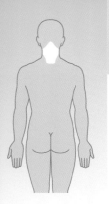

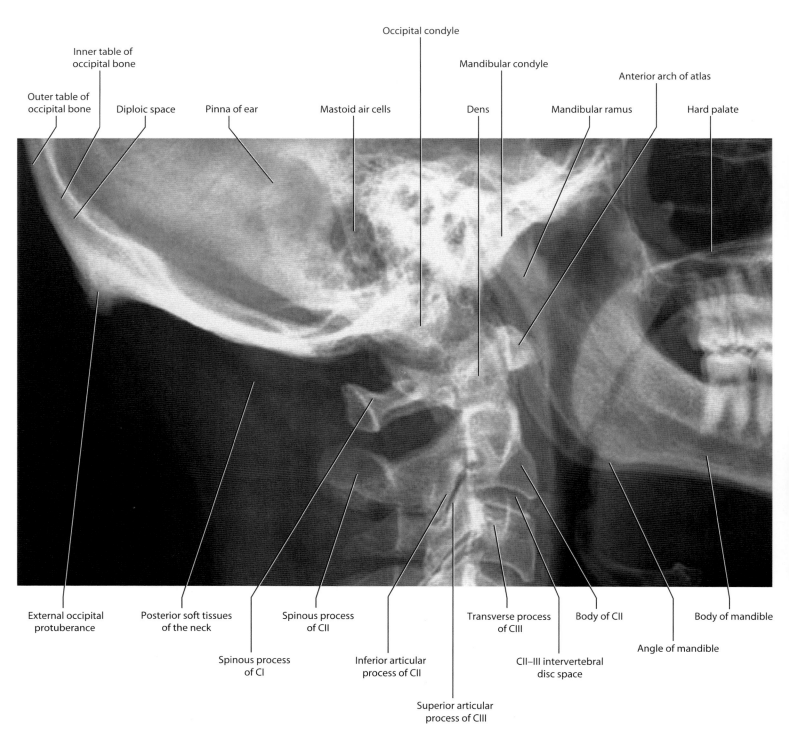

Inner table of
occipital bone

Occipital condyle

Mandibular condyle

Anterior arch of atlas

Outer table of
occipital bone

Diploic space

Pinna of ear

Mastoid air cells

Dens

Mandibular ramus

Hard palate

External occipital
protuberance

Posterior soft tissues
of the neck

Spinous process
of CII

Transverse process
of CIII

Body of CII

Body of mandible

Spinous process
of CI

Inferior articular
process of CII

CII–III intervertebral
disc space

Angle of mandible

Superior articular
process of CIII

Figure 27.11 Suboccipital region – plain film radiograph (lateral view). Note the position of the dens of CII directly posterior to the anterior arch of the atlas (CI). The spinal cord is located directly posterior to the dens (odontoid process of CII). Also observe the location of the occipital protuberance, which is the superior boundary of the attachment of the upper back and neck muscles (semispinalis capitis, semispinalis cervicis) that cover and protect the suboccipital region

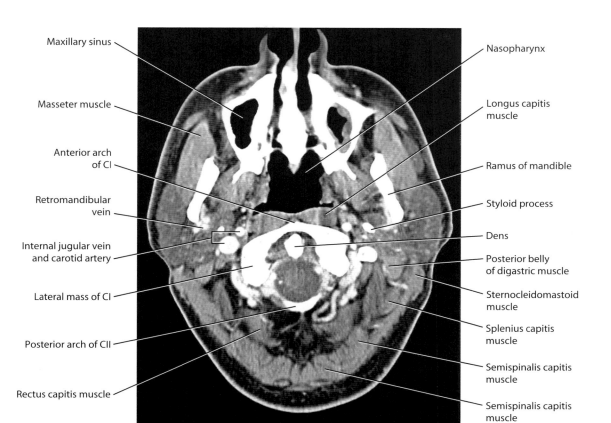

Maxillary sinus

Masseter muscle

Anterior arch of CI

Retromandibular vein

Internal jugular vein and carotid artery

Lateral mass of CI

Posterior arch of CII

Rectus capitis muscle

Nasopharynx

Longus capitis muscle

Ramus of mandible

Styloid process

Dens

Posterior belly of digastric muscle

Sternocleidomastoid muscle

Splenius capitis muscle

Semispinalis capitis muscle

Semispinalis capitis muscle

Figure 27.12 Suboccipital region – CT scan (axial view). This scan is at the level of CI. Observe how large the spinal canal (located posterior to the dens) is at this level

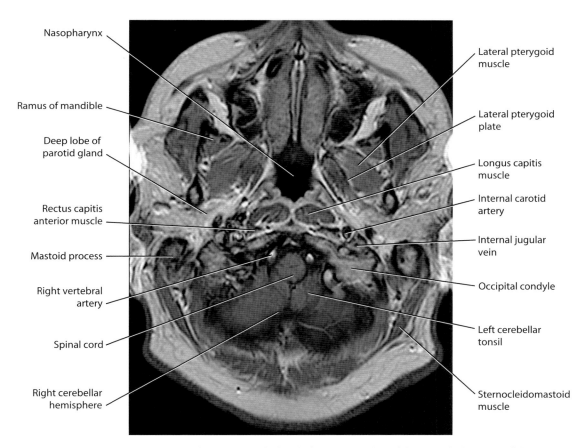

Nasopharynx

Ramus of mandible

Deep lobe of parotid gland

Rectus capitis anterior muscle

Mastoid process

Right vertebral artery

Spinal cord

Right cerebellar hemisphere

Lateral pterygoid muscle

Lateral pterygoid plate

Longus capitis muscle

Internal carotid artery

Internal jugular vein

Occipital condyle

Left cerebellar tonsil

Sternocleidomastoid muscle

Figure 27.13 Suboccipital region – MRI scan (axial view). This scan is at the level of the occipital condyle. Note the location of the vertebral artery, which is deep within the suboccipital region

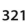

Back muscles

The back is the posterior part of the trunk extending from the neck to the pelvis and includes the skin, fascia, muscles, vertebral column, spinal cord, and supporting neurovasculature.

BONES

The bony support for the back comes from the **vertebral column** and **posterior rib cage**. The vertebral column extends from the base of the skull down to the tip of the coccyx (see Chapter 26). It protects the spinal cord, supports the weight of the trunk, and transmits this weight to the pelvis and lower limbs. The back is also supported posteriorly by many strong muscles, which attach to the vertebral column. The vertebrae, their processes, and the ribs are attachment sites for the back muscles.

The **thoracolumbar fascia**, like the **nuchal fascia** in the neck region, is a thick downward extension of fascia and is attached to each of the vertebral spines inferior to TVII, the supraspinous ligaments, the medial crest of the sacrum, and the ribs. It splits into two layers (**anterior** and **posterior layers**) and supports and provides attachment for the deep back muscles.

MUSCLES

The muscles of the back (Table 28.1) are divided into three groups.

- The **superficial extrinsic back muscles** (trapezius, latissimus dorsi, levator scapulae, and the rhomboids, Fig. 28.1) connect the upper limbs to the trunk and control limb movements (see Chapter 17).
- The **intermediate extrinsic back muscles** (serratus posterior, Fig. 28.2) are superficial respiratory muscles.
- The **deep intrinsic back muscles** (postvertebral muscles) maintain posture and control movements of the vertebral column and head. These 'true' (intrinsic) back muscles are grouped according to their relationship to the surface of the body: the superficial layer of splenius muscles, the intermediate layer of erector spinae muscles (iliocostalis, longissimus, and spinalis), and the deep tranversospinales muscles (semispinalis, multifidus, and rotatores) (Fig. 28.3).

The **splenius** muscles are divided into **capitis** and **cervicis** groups. They originate from the nuchal ligament and spinous processes of TI to TVI and insert onto the superior nuchal line, mastoid process, and posterior tubercles of transverse processes of CII to CIV. As a group, they extend, laterally flex, and rotate the head and neck.

The intermediate layer of **erector spinae** muscles form a broad thick muscle mass, which is attached to the sacrum, iliac crest of the pelvis, and lumbar spinous processes. Just inferior to rib XII the group splits into three columns – iliocostalis, longissimus, and spinalis muscles (from lateral to medial). These three columns ascend and insert onto spinous and transverse processes of more superior vertebrae, ribs, and the posterior base of the skull. They extend the vertebral column and head, and assist in rotational and lateral movements of the spine.

The deep or **transversospinales** muscle group is deep to the erector spinae muscles and runs obliquely from the transverse process of one vertebra to the spinous process of the preceding vertebra. They stabilize, extend, and rotate the vertebral column, and include the **semispinalis** (spanning four to six segments),

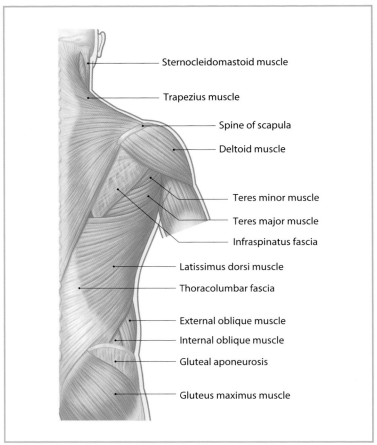

Figure 28.1 Superficial muscles of the back

multifidus (spanning three segments), and **rotatores** (spanning four to six segments) muscles.

The deep layer also includes a small group of segmental muscles (**interspinales**, **intertransversarii**, and **levatores costarum** muscles), which aid in extending and laterally flexing the vertebral column.

NERVES

The superficial extrinsic back muscles are innervated by branches of the **brachial plexus**, except trapezius, which is innervated by the spinal part of the **accessory nerve [XI]**.

The intermediate extrinsic back muscles are innervated by segmental **anterior rami** of T1 to T4 and T9 to T12.

The three layers of deep intrinsic back muscles are innervated by **posterior rami** of spinal nerves.

ARTERIES

The back receives its blood supply in the cervical region from muscular branches of the occipital, ascending cervical, vertebral, and deep cervical arteries (see Chapter 27).

The thoracic and lumbar back receives blood from muscular branches of the posterior intercostal, subcostal, and lumbar arteries (see Chapter 29).

The pelvic part of the back receives blood from the iliolumbar and lateral sacral branches of the internal iliac artery. Meningeal and spinal arteries also arise from these vessels.

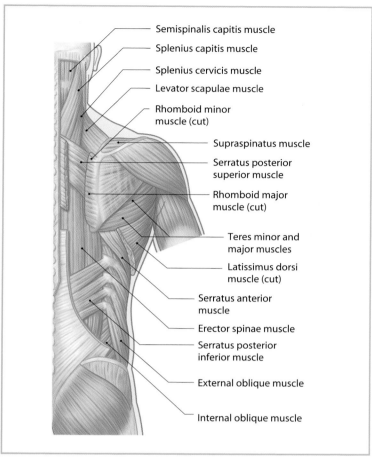

Figure 28.2 Intermediate layer muscles of the back

VEINS AND LYMPHATICS

The veins of the back muscles drain to the **vertebral venous plexus**, which is a group of veins that connects the cranial venous dural sinuses to the pelvic veins. This venous plexus also connects with the azygos vein and vena cavae in the neck and trunk. It is a valveless system, allowing blood to flow in either direction dependent on relative changes in intra-abdominal, intrathoracic, and intracranial pressures. Infection, cancer, and emboli can therefore spread along this system and affect or obstruct any part of it.

Deep structures of the back are drained by lymphatics that run primarily alongside the veins. Lymphatics in the neck drain to the **anterior cervical**, **lateral cervical** and **deep cervical nodes**.

Lymph vessels of the trunk above the umbilicus drain to the **axillary lymph nodes**; lymph vessels inferior to the umbilicus drain to the **superficial inguinal nodes**.

■ CLINICAL CORRELATIONS
Low back muscle strain

Low back muscle strain is minor damage to the muscles of the lower back that occurs during overexertion of the spinal column muscles. It is one of the most common reasons for people to seek urgent medical attention. The back can become weakened by prolonged inactivity, which leads to degeneration of the back muscles and surrounding joints. A small task such as bending over or twisting to pick something up off the floor can then result in excruciating lower back muscle pain. The pain is described as 'sharp and stabbing' or a 'dull ache' at the site of the muscle strain. Frequently, patients complain of muscle spasm in the involved muscle groups. Pain is

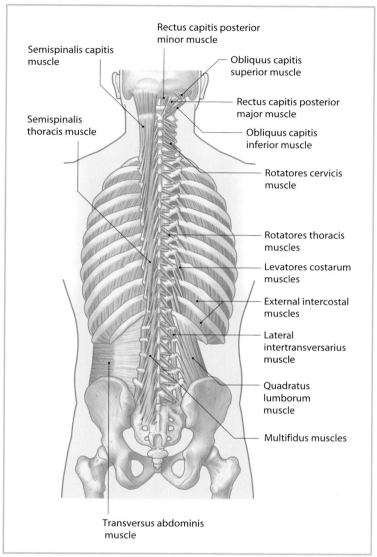

Figure 28.3 Deep muscles of the back

present mainly along the back, but can radiate to structures in the gluteal region and posterior thigh. If there is muscle strain without disc injury, the pain does not radiate inferiorly to the knee joint (see Chapter 26 for a discussion of intervertebral disc herniation with neurologic symptoms).

On examination, the pain is usually localized to the lumbar paraspinal muscles and thoracolumbar fascia. Tenderness over the affected region is common, without overlying skin bruising or edema. Patellar and Achilles' reflexes are normal, as is sensation in both lower limbs.

Treatment of low back muscle strain is usually nonsurgical, with immediate rest followed by a slow return to normal daily activities. Medications and adjunctive physical treatments usually bring about return to normal function within six months.

MNEMONICS	
Deep muscles of the back:	**I Love Spaghetti – Some More Ragu** (Iliocostalis, Longissimus, Spinalis – Semispinalis, Multifidus, Rotatores)
Erector spinae group:	**I Like Standing** (Iliocostalis, Longissimus, Spinalis)

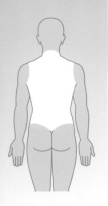

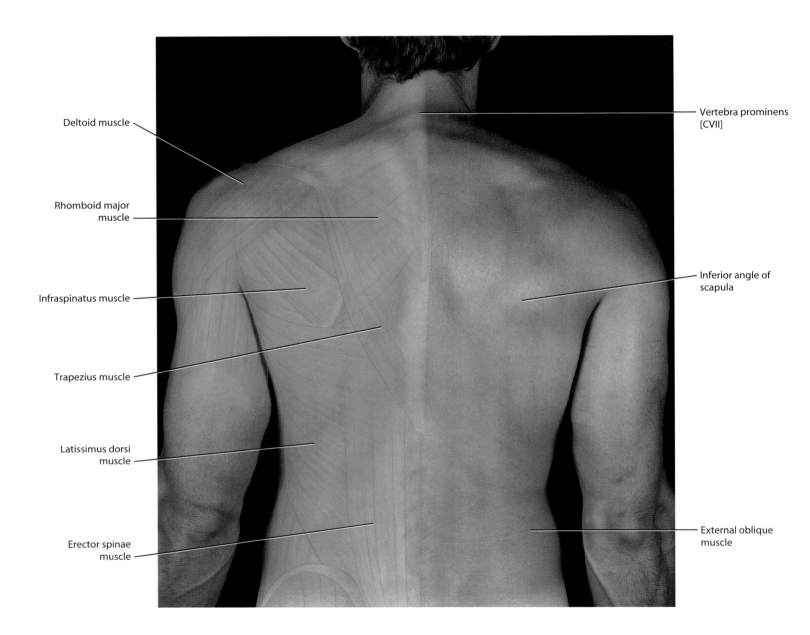

Deltoid muscle

Rhomboid major
muscle

Infraspinatus muscle

Trapezius muscle

Latissimus dorsi
muscle

Erector spinae
muscle

Vertebra prominens
[CVII]

Inferior angle of
scapula

External oblique
muscle

Figure 28.4 **Back muscles – surface anatomy.** Observe the prominences created by the muscles of the back as the muscles are partially flexed

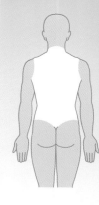

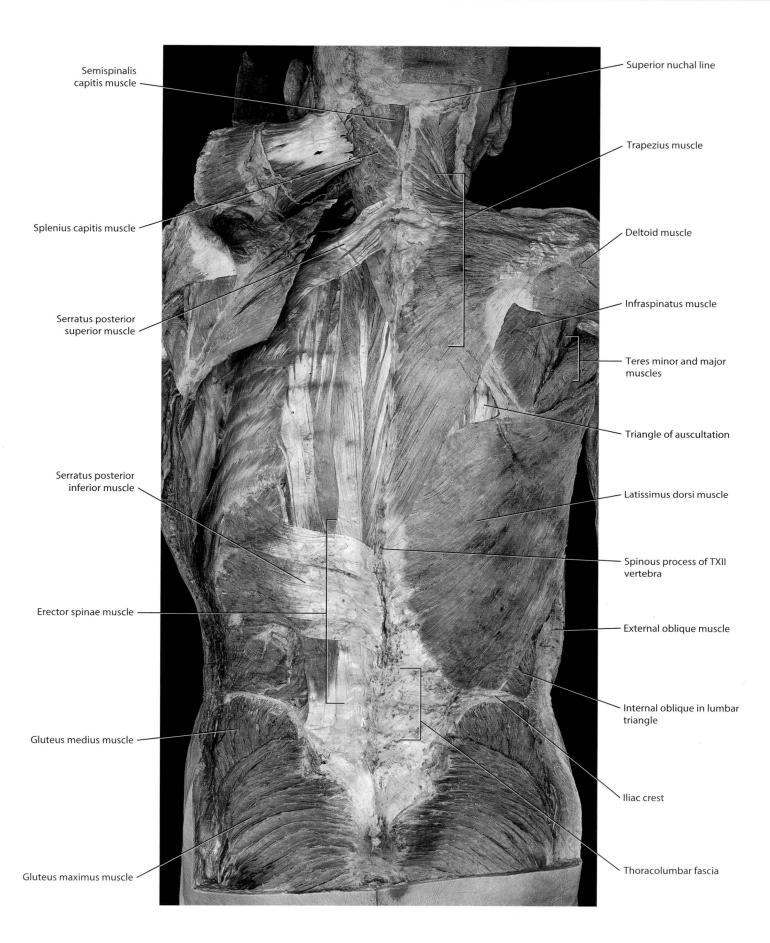

Semispinalis capitis muscle

Splenius capitis muscle

Serratus posterior superior muscle

Serratus posterior inferior muscle

Erector spinae muscle

Gluteus medius muscle

Gluteus maximus muscle

Superior nuchal line

Trapezius muscle

Deltoid muscle

Infraspinatus muscle

Teres minor and major muscles

Triangle of auscultation

Latissimus dorsi muscle

Spinous process of TXII vertebra

External oblique muscle

Internal oblique in lumbar triangle

Iliac crest

Thoracolumbar fascia

Figure 28.5 Back muscles – superficial dissection 1. Observe how on the left side the trapezius muscle and the scapula have been lifted to show additional back muscles that lie beneath

325

TRUNK Back muscles

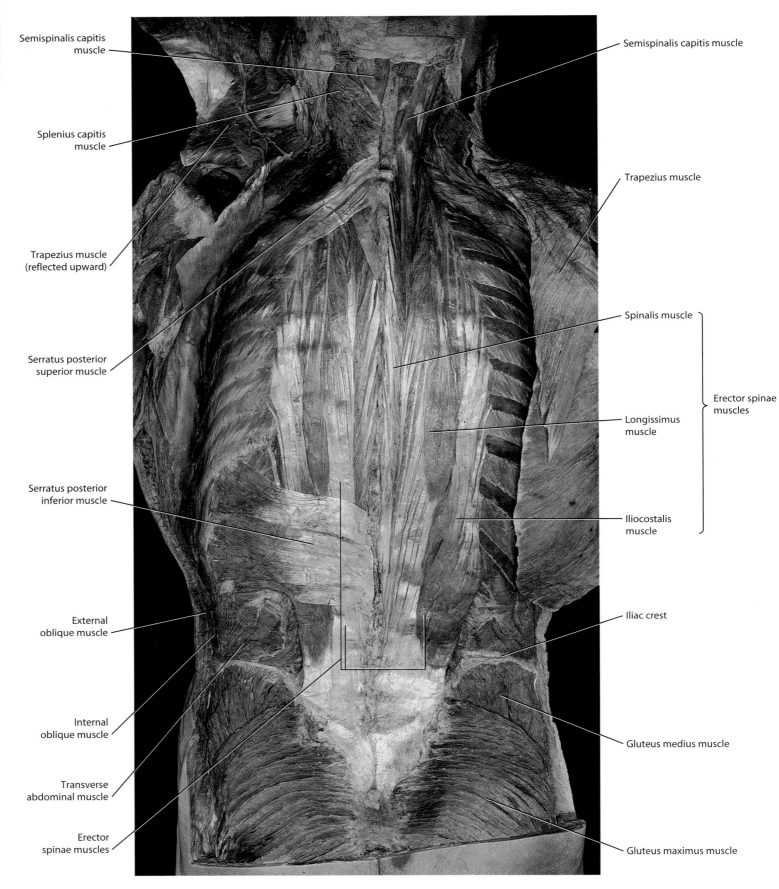

Semispinalis capitis muscle

Splenius capitis muscle

Trapezius muscle (reflected upward)

Serratus posterior superior muscle

Serratus posterior inferior muscle

External oblique muscle

Internal oblique muscle

Transverse abdominal muscle

Erector spinae muscles

Semispinalis capitis muscle

Trapezius muscle

Spinalis muscle

Longissimus muscle

Iliocostalis muscle

Erector spinae muscles

Iliac crest

Gluteus medius muscle

Gluteus maximus muscle

Figure 28.6 Back muscles – superficial dissection 2. Both sides of the back have been dissected to show the erector spinae muscles. The serratus posterior superior and inferior muscles are also visible on the left side

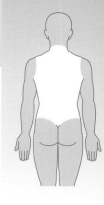

TABLE 28.1 DEEP INTRINSIC BACK MUSCLES

Muscle	Origin	Insertion	Action	Nerve supply	Blood supply
Superficial layer Splenius capitis	Lower half ligamentum nuchae, spinous processes of CVII, TIII and TIV	Mastoid process and lateral superior nuchal line	Extends and laterally flexes head and neck, rotates head	Posterior rami of C4 to C8	Muscular and descending branches of occipital artery, superficial branch of transverse cervical artery
Splenius cervicis	Spinous processes of TIII to TVI	Posterior tubercles of transverse processes of CI to CVI	Extends and laterally flexes head and neck, rotates head		
Intermediate layer Erector spinae (sacrospinalis)	Sacrum, crest of ilium, spinous processes of TXI and TXII and lumbar vertebrae	Iliocostalis (lumborum, thoracis, and cervicis) – angles of lower ribs and cervical transverse processes			
		Longissimus (thoracis, cervicis, and capitis) – transverse processes in thoracic and cervical regions and mastoid process of temporal bone	Extends, and laterally flexes and rotates vertebral column	Posterior rami of spinal nerves (segmental)	Muscular branches of vertebral, deep cervical, intercostal and lumbar arteries
		Spinalis (thoracis, cervicis, and capitis) – spinous processes of upper thoracic vertebrae to skull			
Deep layer Transversospinales	Semispinalis – transverse processes of CIV to TXII	Occipital bone and spinous processes in thoracic and cervical regions, span 4–6 segments	Extends and laterally flexes vertebral column, extends head, ribs, and pelvis	Posterior rami of spinal nerves (segmental)	Muscular branches of posterior intercostals, descending branch of occipital, deep cervical branch of costocervical trunk
	Multifidi – sacrum and ilium, transverse processes TI to TIII and articular processes of CIV to CVII	Spinous process of vertebra above, span 2–4 segments	Extends laterally, flexes and rotates vertebral column; extends and laterally moves pelvis	Posterior rami of spinal nerves (segmental)	Muscular branches of posterior intercostals, descending branch of occipital, deep cervical branch of costocervical trunk
	Rotatores – transverse processes of thoracic vertebrae	Lamina of vertebra directly above vertebra of origin (span 1–2 segments)	Assists in rotating vertebral column	Posterior rami of spinal nerves (segmental)	Muscular branches of posterior intercostals
Minor deep layer Interspinales	Superior aspect of spinous processes of cervical and lumbar vertebrae	Inferior aspect of spinous process of vertebra directly above	Aid in extension and rotation of vertebral column	Posterior rami of spinal nerves (segmental)	Posterior intercostals, lumbar, deep cervical branch of costocervical trunk
Intertransversarii	Transverse processes of cervical and lumbar vertebrae	Transverse process of adjacent vertebra	Lateral bending, stabilize vertebral column	Posterior and anterior rami of spinal nerves (segmental)	Deep cervical branch of costocervical trunk, muscular branches of posterior intercostal and lumbar arteries
Levatores costarum	Tips of transverse processes of CVII and TI and TXI	Insert on rib below between its tubercle and angle	Elevate ribs, assists with lateral bending	Posterior rami of spinal nerves (C8 to C11)	Posterior intercostal arteries

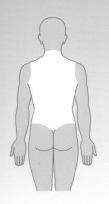

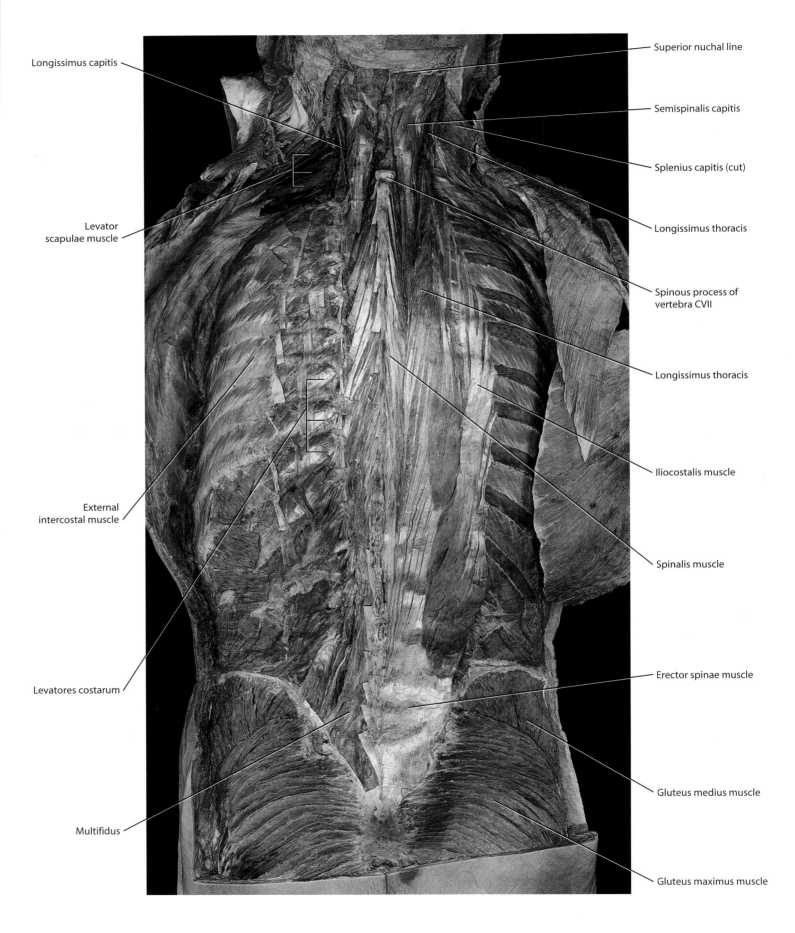

Longissimus capitis

Levator
scapulae muscle

External
intercostal muscle

Levatores costarum

Multifidus

Superior nuchal line

Semispinalis capitis

Splenius capitis (cut)

Longissimus thoracis

Spinous process of
vertebra CVII

Longissimus thoracis

Iliocostalis muscle

Spinalis muscle

Erector spinae muscle

Gluteus medius muscle

Gluteus maximus muscle

Figure 28.7 Back muscles – intermediate dissection 1. The superficial back muscles have been removed as well as part of the erector spinae muscles on the left side to show the levator costarum muscles

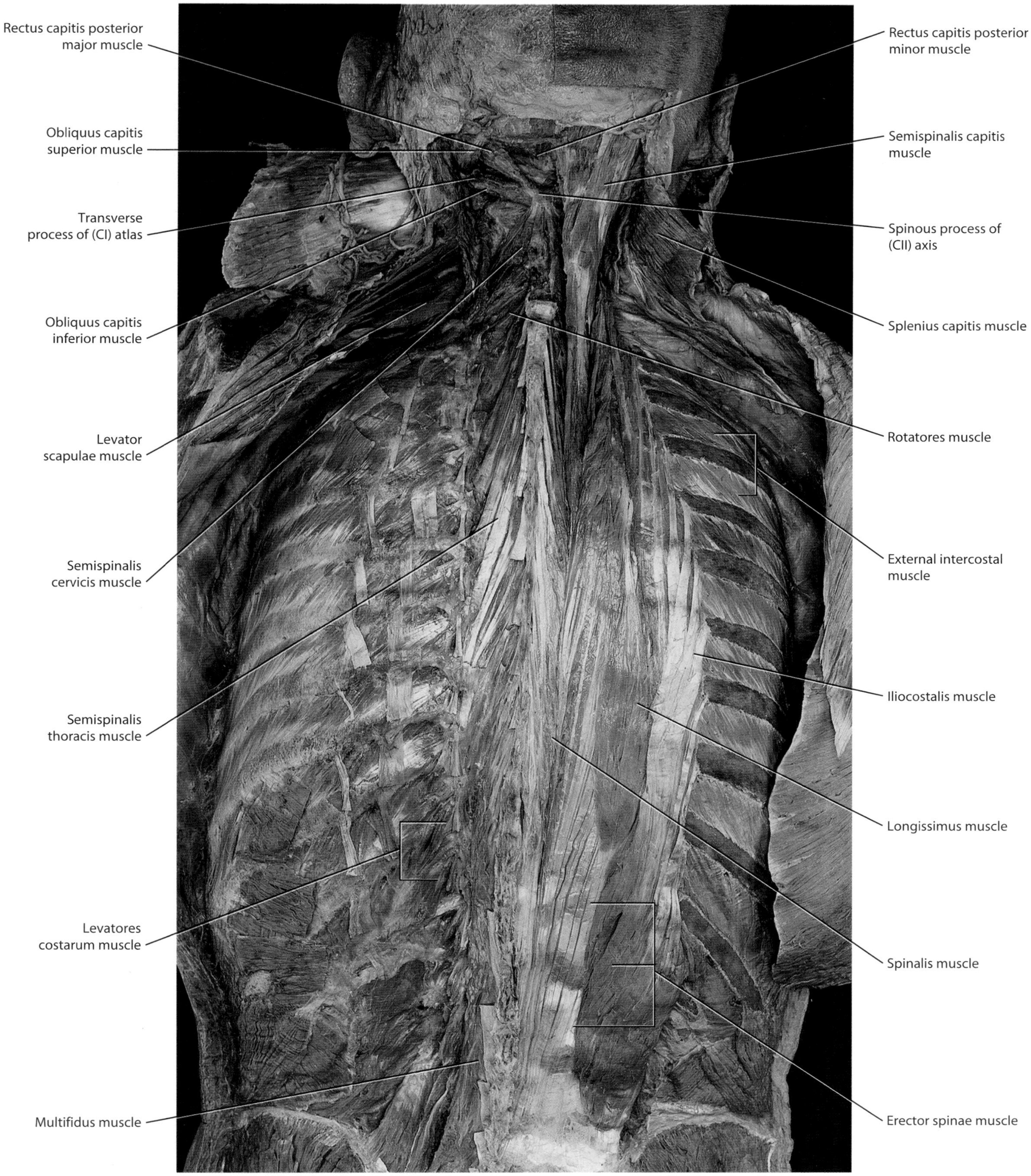

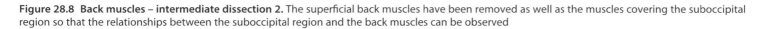

Rectus capitis posterior major muscle

Obliquus capitis superior muscle

Transverse process of (CI) atlas

Obliquus capitis inferior muscle

Levator scapulae muscle

Semispinalis cervicis muscle

Semispinalis thoracis muscle

Levatores costarum muscle

Multifidus muscle

Rectus capitis posterior minor muscle

Semispinalis capitis muscle

Spinous process of (CII) axis

Splenius capitis muscle

Rotatores muscle

External intercostal muscle

Iliocostalis muscle

Longissimus muscle

Spinalis muscle

Erector spinae muscle

TRUNK Back muscles

Figure 28.8 Back muscles – intermediate dissection 2. The superficial back muscles have been removed as well as the muscles covering the suboccipital region so that the relationships between the suboccipital region and the back muscles can be observed

329

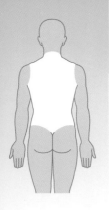

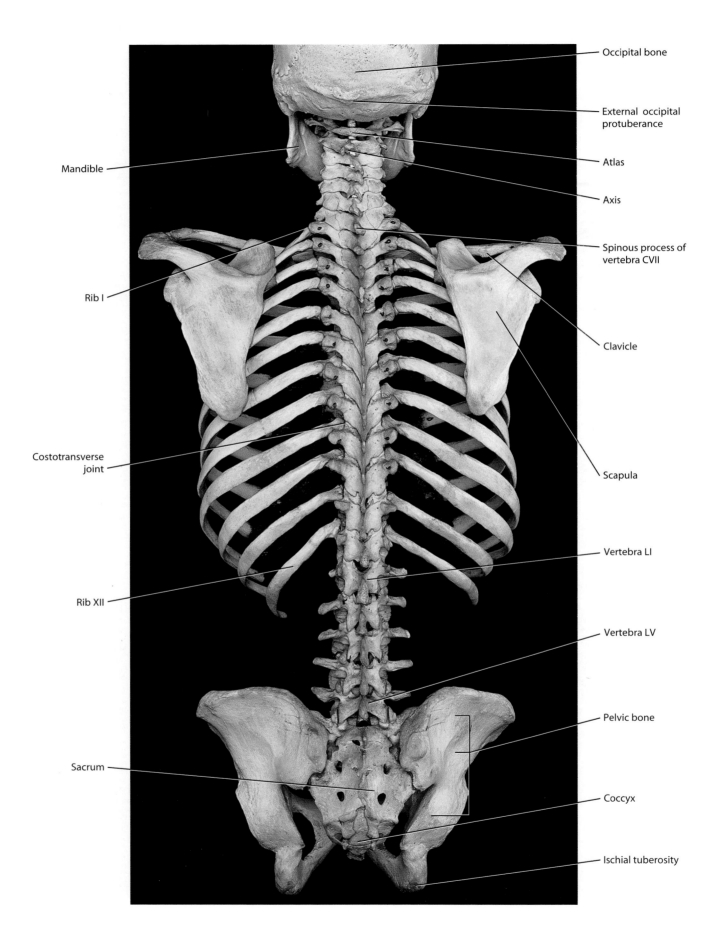

Occipital bone

External occipital protuberance

Atlas

Mandible

Axis

Spinous process of vertebra CVII

Rib I

Clavicle

Costotransverse joint

Scapula

Vertebra LI

Rib XII

Vertebra LV

Pelvic bone

Sacrum

Coccyx

Ischial tuberosity

Figure 28.9 Back muscles – osteology. Posterior view of the elements of the articulated skeleton that support the back muscles

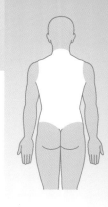

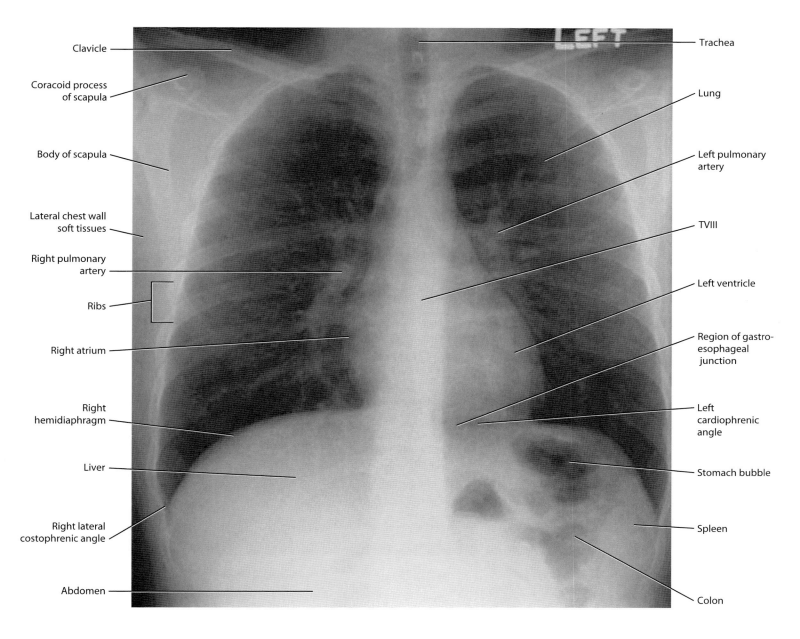

Clavicle

Coracoid process
of scapula

Body of scapula

Lateral chest wall
soft tissues

Right pulmonary
artery

Ribs

Right atrium

Right
hemidiaphragm

Liver

Right lateral
costophrenic angle

Abdomen

Trachea

Lung

Left pulmonary
artery

TVIII

Left ventricle

Region of gastro-
esophageal
junction

Left
cardiophrenic
angle

Stomach bubble

Spleen

Colon

Figure 28.10 Upper back – plain film radiograph (posteroanterior view). Observe the thoracic vertebrae and ribs with respect to the scapulae and compare with Figure 28.9. See also Figure 33.15 for the radiographic appearance of the mid and low back. Note that in clinical practice, both anteroposterior and posteroanterior radiographs are viewed as though looking from anterior to posterior, hence the orientation shown here. To obtain a posteroanterior radiograph, the X-rays are projected from behind the patient to a plate that is touching the patient's chest; structures close to the plate appear very close to actual size, and structures further away appear larger. In anteroposterior views the heart therefore appears much larger (and less distinct) than in this posteroanterior view

331

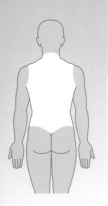

TRUNK

Back muscles

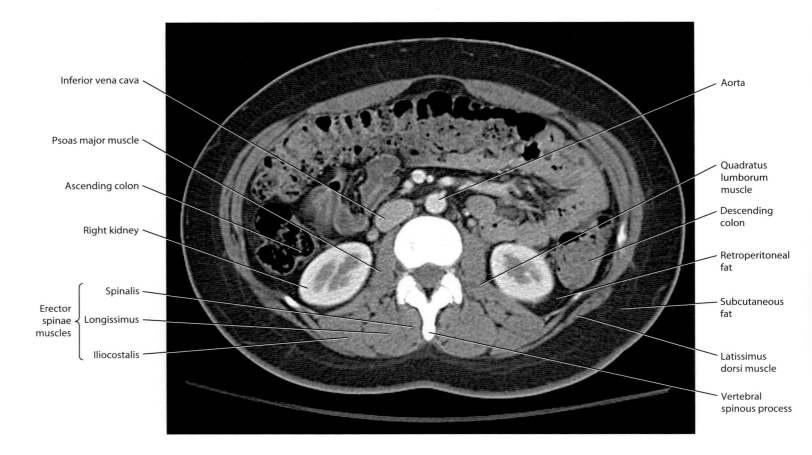

Inferior vena cava

Psoas major muscle

Ascending colon

Right kidney

Erector spinae muscles

Spinalis

Longissimus

Iliocostalis

Aorta

Quadratus lumborum muscle

Descending colon

Retroperitoneal fat

Subcutaneous fat

Latissimus dorsi muscle

Vertebral spinous process

Figure 28.11 **Back muscles – CT scan (axial view).** Note the definition of the erector spinae muscles in this scan at the level of the upper lumbar vertebrae

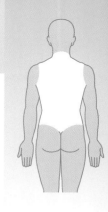

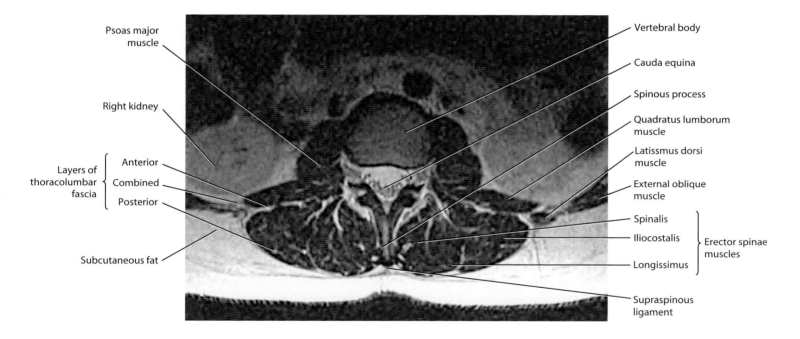

Psoas major muscle

Right kidney

Layers of thoracolumbar fascia
- Anterior
- Combined
- Posterior

Subcutaneous fat

Vertebral body

Cauda equina

Spinous process

Quadratus lumborum muscle

Latissmus dorsi muscle

External oblique muscle

Spinalis
Iliocostalis — Erector spinae muscles
Longissimus

Supraspinous ligament

Figure 28.12 Back muscles – MRI scan (axial view). In this at the level of the middle lumbar vertebrae, note how close the back muscles are to the kidneys

29 Chest wall and mediastinum

The chest wall and mediastinum are parts of the thorax. The thorax has a bony and cartilaginous skeleton and contains the principal organs of respiration and circulation. The 12 thoracic vertebrae make up the posterior wall of the thorax. The 12 pairs of ribs, with their costal cartilages and intercostal muscles, comprise the lateral and anterolateral wall. In the midline, the sternum is the anterior wall. The thorax is approximately conical in shape, with a relatively narrow superior inlet (**superior thoracic aperture**) and a broader inferior outlet (**inferior thoracic aperture**).

The thoracic cavity is divided into the right and left pleural cavities by the mediastinum (Fig. 29.1). The mediastinum is bounded anteriorly by the sternum and posteriorly by the vertebral column; its floor is formed by the diaphragm. Superiorly it is continuous with the structures of the neck through the superior thoracic aperture, which forms the boundary of the superior mediastinum.

MUSCLES

The muscles of the thorax (Table 29.1) are arranged in three layers:

- the **external intercostal** muscles (Fig. 29.2) form the external layer and are contained within the 11 intercostal spaces; the muscles extend from the tubercle of the ribs to the costochondral junction;
- the **internal intercostal** muscles form the middle layer and occupy the 11 intercostal spaces from the border of the sternum to the angle of the ribs;
- the **innermost intercostal**, **subcostales**, and **transversus thoracis** muscles form the internal layer of the chest wall muscles.

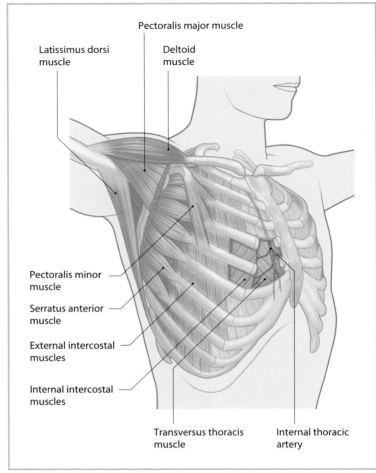

Figure 29.2 Muscles of the chest wall

These muscles pull on the ribs to enable the changes in thoracic volume needed for breathing and help maintain the rigidity of the chest wall.

The **levatores costarum** muscles arise from the transverse processes of vertebrae CVII to TXI and insert into the external surface of the rib below. They are innervated by the posterior rami of the spinal nerves and, as their name suggests, elevate the ribs.

NERVES

The anterior rami of thoracic spinal nerves TI to TXI supply the overlapping segmental innervation of the skin and tissues of the chest wall. Spinal nerve TXII forms the subcostal nerve. Collectively these nerves are the **intercostal nerves**. They pass laterally from their origin at the spinal cord into the costal groove of each rib, and they continue anteriorly around the chest wall, running between the internal and the innermost intercostal muscles. Anteriorly they terminate as cutaneous branches which provide sensation to the skin of the chest wall (see Fig. 26.5).

ARTERIES

The **internal thoracic artery** (Fig. 29.3) is a branch of the subclavian artery. It descends toward the abdomen posterior to the first six costal cartilages and:

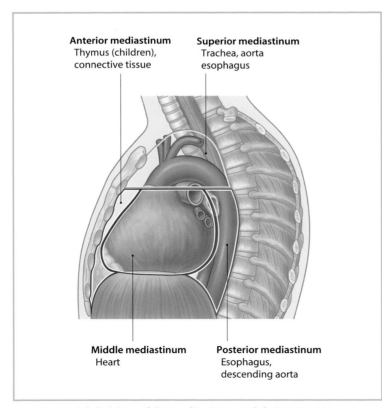

Figure 29.1 Subdivisions of the mediastinum and their contents

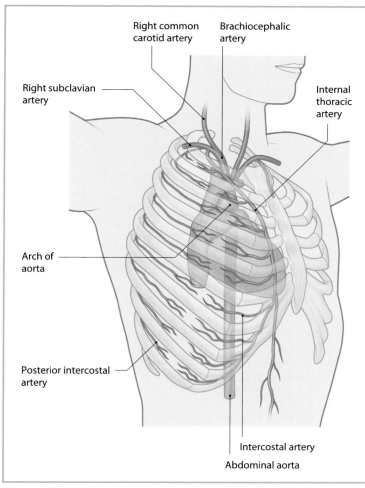

Figure 29.3 **Arterial supply to the chest wall**

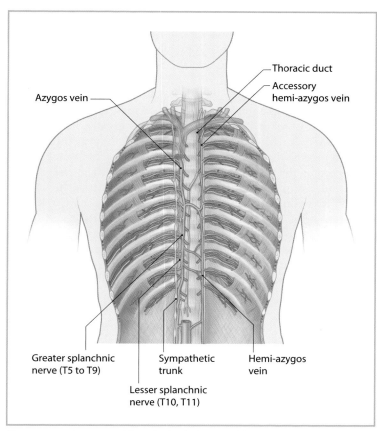

Figure 29.4 **Venous and lymphatic drainage of the posterior chest wall**

- supplies blood to the upper part of the anterior chest wall;
- gives off anterior intercostal arteries to the first six intercostal spaces;
- at the sixth intercostal space divides into two terminal branches – the **superior epigastric artery**, which supplies the lower intercostal spaces and anterior abdominal wall, and the **musculophrenic artery**, which supplies the peripheral part of the diaphragm.

The first two posterior intercostal spaces receive their blood supply from the **supreme intercostal artery**, a branch of the costocervical trunk from the subclavian artery. The remaining nine posterior intercostal spaces are supplied by the **posterior intercostal arteries**, which are branches of the thoracic aorta.

VEINS AND LYMPHATICS

The azygos system of veins is a group of veins on the anterior surfaces of the thoracic vertebrae. It drains the back and the wall of the thorax and abdomen (Fig. 29.4). The terminal veins of the system are the azygos, hemi-azygos, and accessory hemi-azygos veins.

The **azygos vein** is formed by the right ascending lumbar and right subcostal veins. It ascends through the posterior mediastinum to the right of the thoracic vertebrae, arches over the root of the right lung, and empties into the superior vena cava. Tributaries of the azygos vein are the right supreme intercostal vein, right fourth to eleventh posterior intercostal veins, and either or both of the hemi-azygos and accessory hemi-azygos veins.

The **hemi-azygos vein** is formed by the union of the left ascending lumbar and subcostal veins. From its origin, it ascends the posterior chest wall and empties into the azygos vein. Along its route it receives tributaries from the inferior posterior intercostal, mediastinal, and esophageal veins.

The **accessory hemi-azygos vein** begins at the fourth intercostal space and ascends the posterior chest wall, receiving blood from the adjacent intercostal spaces and the bronchial and mediastinal veins. It empties into the hemi-azygos or azygos vein.

Lymphatic drainage of the chest wall is through the **thoracic duct**, which is the largest lymphatic vessel in the body and arises in the abdomen from the **cisterna chyli**. The thoracic duct ascends the posterior abdominal wall, passing through the diaphragm at the aortic hiatus, where it is on the right side of the vertebrae between the aorta and azygos vein at the level of vertebra TXII. Anterior to vertebra TV, the thoracic duct crosses to the left side of the posterior chest wall and ascends to vertebra CVII. In the neck, it passes posteriorly to the carotid sheath to enter the venous system at the junction of the left internal jugular and left subclavian veins. The thoracic duct drains lymph from the whole body, except the right upper limb and the right face and neck, which are drained by the **right lymphatic duct**. On the right side, lymph enters the venous system at the junction of the right internal jugular and right subclavian veins.

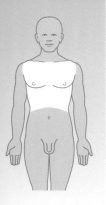

ESOPHAGUS

The esophagus is a narrow, muscular tube that connects the oropharynx and the stomach. It is usually 25–30 cm long and it is divided into cervical, thoracic, and abdominal parts.

AUTONOMIC NERVES

The posterior mediastinum contains two separate sets of autonomic nerves. The first set of autonomic nerves is the **greater, lesser,** and **least splanchnic nerves**, which are branches off the sympathetic trunk (a collection of nerves and ganglia that emerges from the spinal cord on the posterior internal thoracic wall). The greater, lesser, and least splanchnic nerves are preganglionic branches of the fifth to twelfth thoracic sympathetic ganglia. They enter the abdomen and synapse in the **celiac, superior mesenteric,** and **aorticorenal ganglia**, respectively. Postganglionic nerves emerge from these abdominal ganglia to innervate the organs of the abdomen. Sympathetic innervation of the abdomen follows the course of blood vessels and regulates peristalsis and vasodilation.

The second set of autonomic nerves are the **vagus nerves [X]** in the thorax. These nerves carry parasympathetic preganglionic nerve fibers, which contribute to the **cardiac, pulmonary,** and **esophageal plexuses**. Postganglionic nerve fibers from these plexuses terminate at the blood vessels, conducting system of the heart, esophagus, and bronchiolar walls. Parasympathetic activity therefore regulates vasoconstriction of coronary vessels, heart rate, esophageal peristalsis, and bronchoconstriction.

■ CLINICAL CORRELATIONS

Rib fractures

Any excessive force to the chest wall can cause rib fracture, resulting in extreme pain on deep inspiration. On examination, a slight pressure applied to the rib cage elicits a very painful response (barrel test). In addition there is tenderness at the fracture site and ecchymosis (bruising).

Most rib fractures occur in the posterolateral chest wall (Fig. 29.5) and can sometimes be seen on chest radiography. A computed tomography (CT) scan is helpful in delineating some types of rib fracture. Fractures of ribs I and II are significant because a tremendous force is needed to fracture these ribs, so usually there is an additional thoracic injury requiring immediate treatment. Fracture of the lower ribs (X to XII) also warrant further diagnostic investigation (e.g. CT) because they are associated with a high incidence of liver and spleen injury.

Treatment of rib fractures is aimed at reducing pain by oral medication. Admission to hospital and further treatment may be necessary for very severe pain.

Sometimes, fractured ribs puncture the pleura and lung parenchyma, causing a pneumothorax (see Chapter 31). This requires treatment by insertion of a chest tube to prevent tension pneumothorax and to facilitate healing of the lung parenchyma. The tube should be placed through the intercostal tissues, usually in the midaxillary line, and over the top of a rib to avoid iatrogenic damage to the neurovascular structures in the costal groove at the inferior margin of the rib.

Sternal fracture

A sternal fracture (Fig. 29.6) results from a force applied directly to the sternum, and causes chest pain with or without movement. It

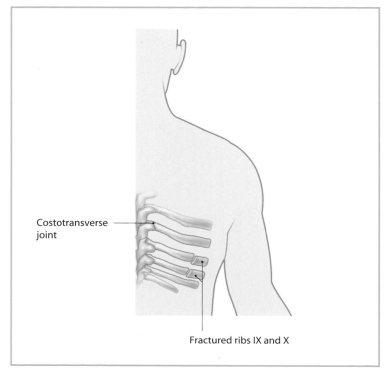

Figure 29.5 Fractures of ribs IX and X

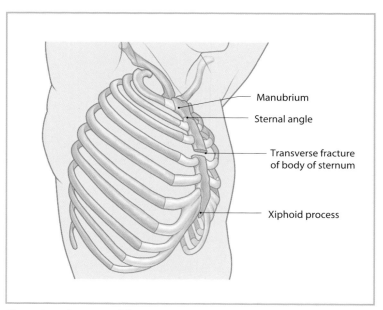

Figure 29.6 Fracture of the sternum

cannot been seen on a standard anteroposterior chest radiograph because of the masking effect of the vertebral column; a lateral chest radiograph is necessary for a suspected sternal fracture.

A sternal fracture is significant because a large force is required to cause the fracture, which means that vital intrathoracic structures may also be injured. Any patient with a sternal fracture should be evaluated to rule out other injuries. An unstable sternal fracture may require surgical treatment, using wire sutures to stabilize the fracture.

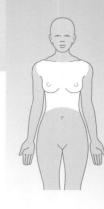

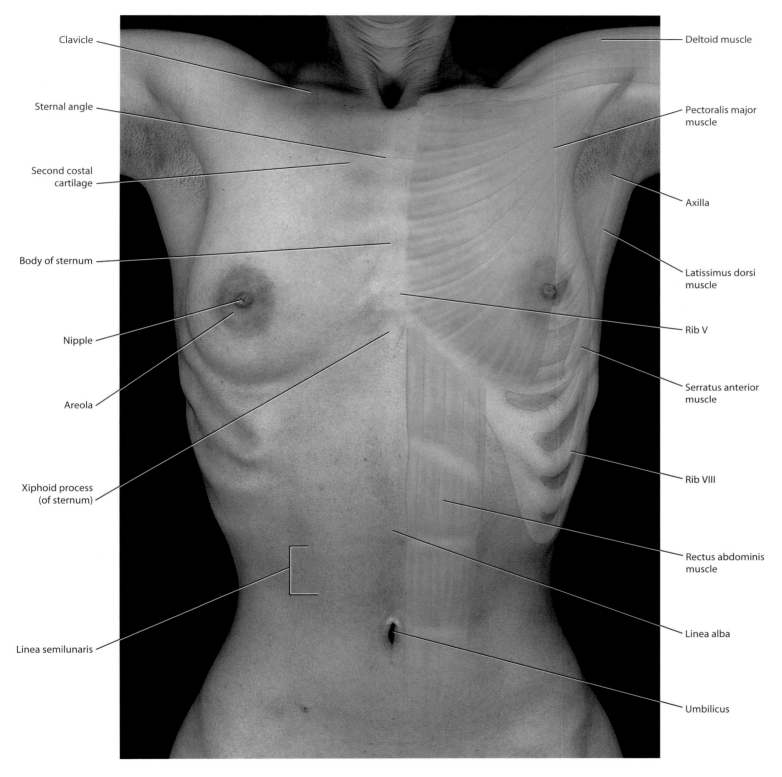

Clavicle

Sternal angle

Second costal
cartilage

Body of sternum

Nipple

Areola

Xiphoid process
(of sternum)

Linea semilunaris

Deltoid muscle

Pectoralis major
muscle

Axilla

Latissimus dorsi
muscle

Rib V

Serratus anterior
muscle

Rib VIII

Rectus abdominis
muscle

Linea alba

Umbilicus

Figure 29.7 Chest wall – surface anatomy. Observe the individual ribs and how they form the shape of the chest wall

337

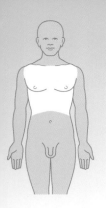

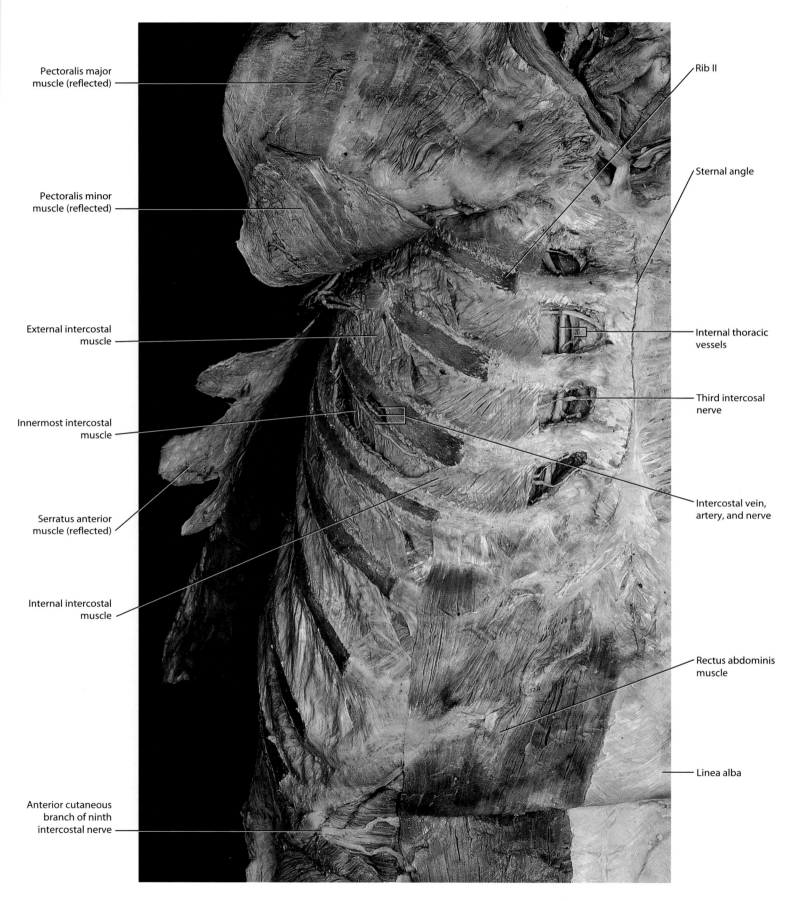

Pectoralis major
muscle (reflected)

Pectoralis minor
muscle (reflected)

External intercostal
muscle

Innermost intercostal
muscle

Serratus anterior
muscle (reflected)

Internal intercostal
muscle

Anterior cutaneous
branch of ninth
intercostal nerve

Rib II

Sternal angle

Internal thoracic
vessels

Third intercosal
nerve

Intercostal vein,
artery, and nerve

Rectus abdominis
muscle

Linea alba

Figure 29.8 Chest wall – superficial dissection. The pectoralis major and minor muscles as well as the serratus anterior muscle have been reflected off the chest wall. Observe the intercostal muscles and the internal thoracic artery

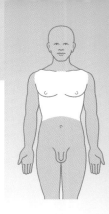

TABLE 29.1 MUSCLES OF THE CHEST WALL

Muscle	Origin	Insertion	Action	Innervation	Blood supply
External intercostals	11 pairs, inferior border of rib, rib tubercle to external intercostal membrane	Superior border of rib below	Maintain intercostal spaces during inspiration and expiration, elevate ribs in inspiration	Intercostal nerves	Aorta, posterior intercostals and their collaterals, costocervical trunk, anterior intercostals of internal thoracic and musculophrenic arteries
Internal intercostals	11 pairs, superior surface of costal cartilages and ribs, sternum to angle of ribs to internal intercostal membrane	Costal cartilage and rib above	Maintain intercostal spaces during inspiration and expiration, depress ribs in forced expiration	Intercostal nerves	Anterior intercostals, posterior intercostals, musculophrenic artery and costocervical trunk
Innermost intercostals	Mid-portion of inferior border of rib	Mid-portion of superior border of rib below	Assist in inspiration and expiration by elevating and depressing ribs	Intercostal nerves	Posterior intercostals and their collaterals
Subcostales	Inner surface of ribs near their angles	Superior border of rib below origin	Aid in depressing ribs	Intercostal nerves	Posterior intercostals, musculophrenic artery
Transversus thoracis	Posterior surface sternum and xiphoid process	Inner surfaces of costal cartilages of ribs II to VI	Depresses costal cartilages; muscle of expiration	Upper six intercostal nerves	Anterior intercostals, internal thoracic artery
Levatores costarum	12 pairs, transverse processes of CVII to TXI	Between tubercle and angle of rib below	Elevate rib, rotators and lateral flexors of vertebral column, assist in inspiration	Posterior rami of C8 to T11	Posterior intercostals
Serratus posterior superior	Ligamentum nuchae and spinous processes of CVII to TIII	Superior border ribs II to V distal to angle	Elevates ribs; inspiration	T1 to T4 intercostal nerves	Highest intercostals, posterior intercostals
Serratus posterior inferior	Spinous processes TXI and TXII, and LI and LII	Inferior border lower four ribs distal to angle	Fixes and depresses lower ribs, acts in expiration	T9 to T12 intercostal nerves	Posterior intercostals
Diaphragm	Sternal part – inner surface of xiphoid process Costal part – costal cartilages and lower 6 ribs Lumbar part – medial and lateral arcuate ligaments right (LI to LIII) and left (LI to LII) lumbar vertebrae	Central tendon	Respirations increase capacity of thoracic cage	Phrenic nerve (C3 to C5)	Superior and inferior phrenic arteries, musculophrenic, and pericardiacophrenic arteries

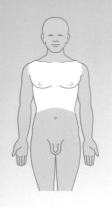

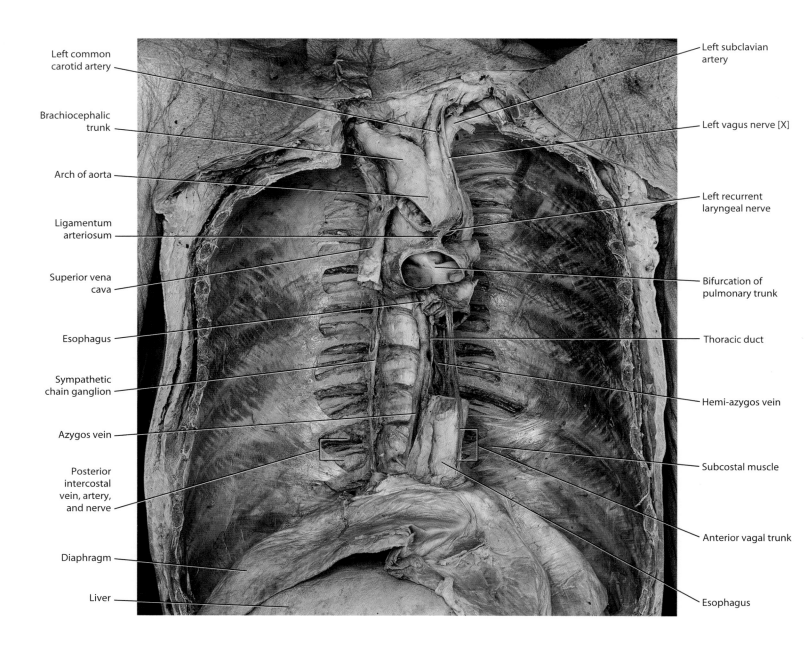

Left common carotid artery

Brachiocephalic trunk

Arch of aorta

Ligamentum arteriosum

Superior vena cava

Esophagus

Sympathetic chain ganglion

Azygos vein

Posterior intercostal vein, artery, and nerve

Diaphragm

Liver

Left subclavian artery

Left vagus nerve [X]

Left recurrent laryngeal nerve

Bifurcation of pulmonary trunk

Thoracic duct

Hemi-azygos vein

Subcostal muscle

Anterior vagal trunk

Esophagus

Figure 29.9 Mediastinum – superficial dissection. The anterior half of the rib cage (cuirass) has been removed along with the heart and lungs and a section of the esophagus to show the ribs and other structures visible along the posterior chest wall, including those which pass through the thorax en route from the head and neck to the abdomen. Observe the greater, lesser, and least splanchnic nerves

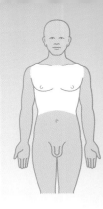

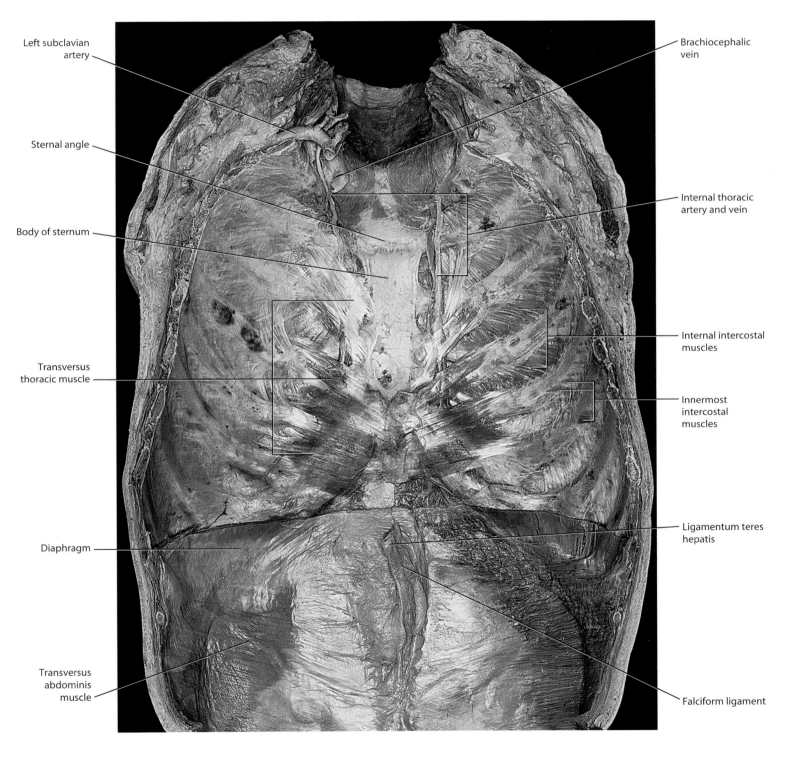

Left subclavian artery

Sternal angle

Body of sternum

Transversus thoracic muscle

Diaphragm

Transversus abdominis muscle

Brachiocephalic vein

Internal thoracic artery and vein

Internal intercostal muscles

Innermost intercostal muscles

Ligamentum teres hepatis

Falciform ligament

Figure 29.10 Chest wall – deep dissection. The internal surface of the anterior chest wall

341

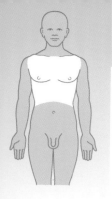

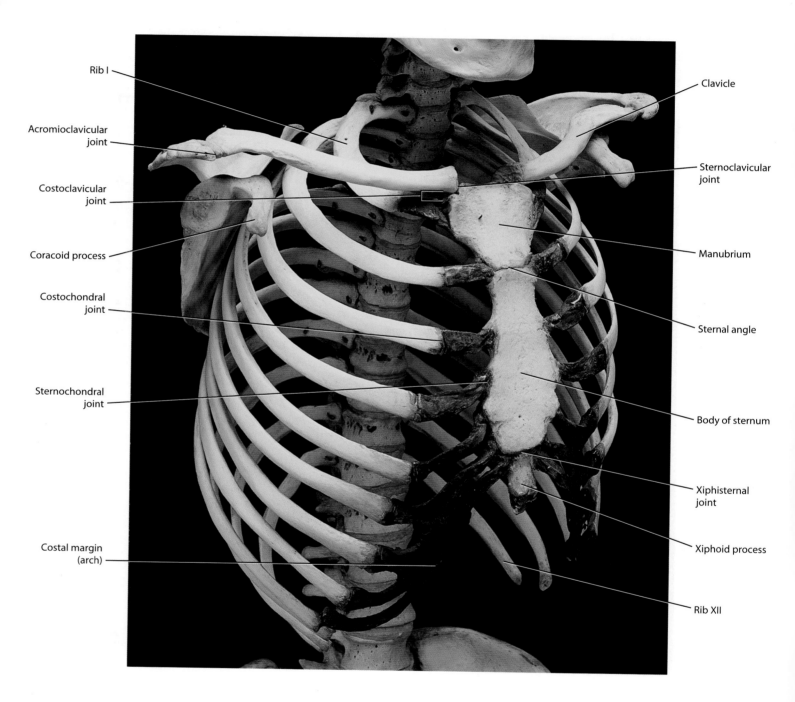

Rib I

Acromioclavicular joint

Costoclavicular joint

Coracoid process

Costochondral joint

Sternochondral joint

Costal margin (arch)

Clavicle

Sternoclavicular joint

Manubrium

Sternal angle

Body of sternum

Xiphisternal joint

Xiphoid process

Rib XII

Figure 29.11 Chest wall and mediastinum – osteology. Anterolateral view of the articulated chest wall and mediastinum. The ribs are joined to the sternum by the costal cartilages. This specimen has the actual costal cartilages; it is not a plastic reproduction

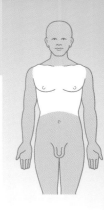

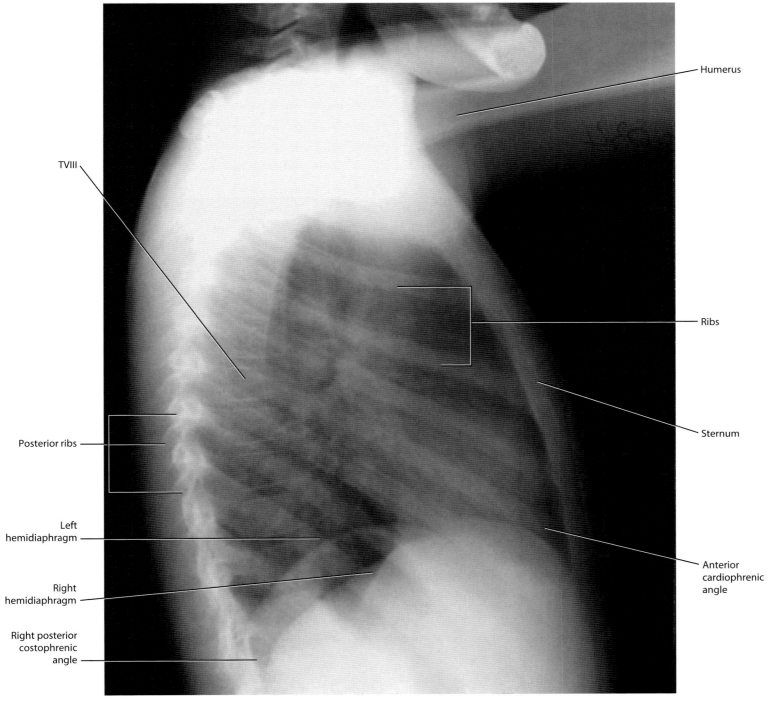

Humerus

TVIII

Ribs

Sternum

Posterior ribs

Anterior
cardiophrenic
angle

Left
hemidiaphragm

Right
hemidiaphragm

Right posterior
costophrenic
angle

Figure 29.12 Chest wall and mediastinum – plain film radiograph (lateral view). Note the diagonal orientation of the ribs on a lateral view, and the dome shape of the left and right hemidiaphragms. The thoracic vertebrae are visible and can be assessed for abnormalities in this lateral chest x-ray. The heart is visible as a gray zone located immediately superior to the hemidiaphragms and in the anterior half of the chest cavity

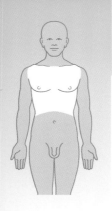

Chest wall and mediastinum **TRUNK**

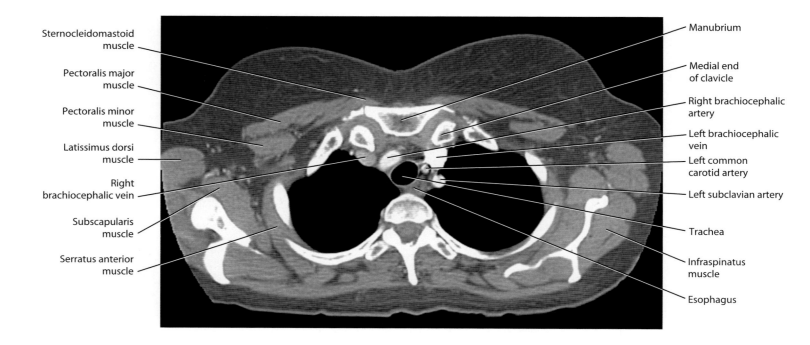

Sternocleidomastoid muscle

Pectoralis major muscle

Pectoralis minor muscle

Latissimus dorsi muscle

Right brachiocephalic vein

Subscapularis muscle

Serratus anterior muscle

Manubrium

Medial end of clavicle

Right brachiocephalic artery

Left brachiocephalic vein

Left common carotid artery

Left subclavian artery

Trachea

Infraspinatus muscle

Esophagus

Figure 29.13 Chest wall and mediastinum – CT scan (axial view). The mediastinal compartments are well evaluated on CT. Observe the muscles that surround and protect the chest wall. This image is taken at the level of the trachea and brachiocephalic vessels within the upper mediastinum

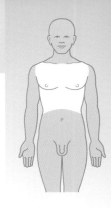

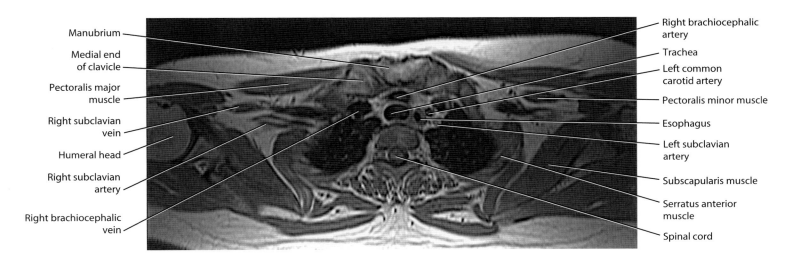

Manubrium

Medial end
of clavicle

Pectoralis major
muscle

Right subclavian
vein

Humeral head

Right subclavian
artery

Right brachiocephalic
vein

Right brachiocephalic
artery

Trachea

Left common
carotid artery

Pectoralis minor muscle

Esophagus

Left subclavian
artery

Subscapularis muscle

Serratus anterior
muscle

Spinal cord

Figure 29.14 Chest wall and mediastinum – MRI scan (axial view). The muscles of the chest wall are well visualized in this scan at the level of the upper mediastinum

The heart is a specialized pump that propels blood to the body. It lies between the lungs in the **mediastinum**, which is subdivided into the **superior** and **inferior mediastinum** by an imaginary horizontal line drawn from the sternal angle to the inferior border of vertebra TIV. The inferior mediastinum is further subdivided into **anterior, middle**, and **posterior mediastinum**.

Support for the heart comes from surrounding structures:

- the ribs, costal cartilages, and sternum anteriorly;
- the vertebral bodies of the middle thoracic vertebrae posteriorly;
- the central tendon of the diaphragm inferiorly; and
- the connection of the heart to the great vessels – the aorta, pulmonary trunk, and superior vena cava superiorly.

Embryologically the heart develops as a midline structure, but in the adult it is oriented obliquely and shifted to the left side of the chest. It is a cone-shaped muscular pump with its apex inferior, at the fifth intercostal space in the midclavicular line, and its base superior, near its junction with the great vessels.

The four chambers of the heart have a multilayered lining – the **endocardium**, the **myocardium** (or middle muscular layer), and the **epicardium** (a superficial layer that includes the visceral layer of the pericardium).

The **pericardium** (pericardial sac) is a strong double-layered sac around the heart and roots of the great vessels. It has a thick, tough outer part (the **fibrous pericardium**) and an inner **serous pericardium**. The serous pericardium has two layers (the **parietal** and **visceral layers**), which form a potential space – the **pericardial cavity**. This cavity is filled with a thin film of serous fluid to reduce friction as the heart pumps and moves within the sac. The pericardium is innervated by branches of the **vagus nerve [X]**, **sympathetic nerve fibers** that follow the route of the blood vessels, and the **phrenic nerves**.

CHAMBERS OF THE HEART

The heart has four chambers – the right atrium, right ventricle, left atrium, and left ventricle (Fig. 30.1). The right atrium receives deoxygenated blood from the body. It pumps it to the right ventricle, which then pumps it to the lungs; this is the **pulmonary circulation**. The left atrium receives oxygenated blood from the lungs. It pumps it to the left ventricle, which then pumps it to the body; this is **systemic circulation**. The atria operate under relatively low pressure and therefore have thinner walls than the ventricles which operate at much higher pressures.

Right atrium

Deoxygenated blood from the head, neck, and upper limbs drains into the right atrium through the superior vena cava; blood draining from the abdomen, pelvis, and lower limbs flows into the right atrium through the inferior vena cava during ventricular rest (diastole).

The right atrium forms the right border of the heart. Its walls are thin and contain an internal muscular ridge (the **crista terminalis**), which is oriented vertically between the superior and inferior venae cavae. Externally, this ridge is visible as a shallow groove (the **sulcus terminalis cordis**). The internal surface of the right atrium also has many small ridges known as **pectinate muscles (musculi pectinati)**.

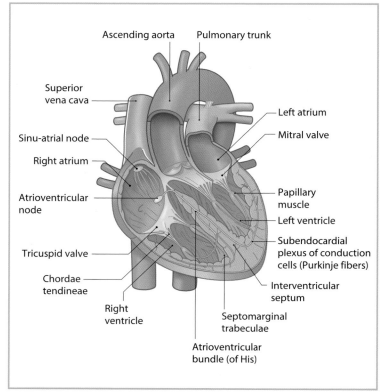

Figure 30.1 The four chambers of the heart and the cardiac conduction system

Within the right atrium, on the interatrial septum there is a shallow depression (the **fossa ovalis**) which marks the site of the fetal foramen ovale.

Right ventricle

Blood leaving the right atrium passes through the **tricuspid valve** (right atrioventricular valve) into the right ventricle, which is the most anterior chamber of the heart. The tricuspid valve consists of three **cusps** (or leaflets) held in place by **chordae tendineae**, which are slender fibrous threads that connect the valve cusps to the **papillary muscles**. The papillary muscles originate from the internal wall of the right ventricle. The valve cusps, chordae tendineae, and papillary muscles prevent the valve from 'blowing out' or leaking under the high pressures created during ventricular contraction.

The internal surface of the right ventricle is roughened by many muscular ridges and projections (the **trabeculae carneae**). One of these muscular ridges, the **septomarginal trabeculae** (moderator band), carries the right branch of the atrioventricular bundle, which is part of the conduction system of the heart. Another muscular ridge – the **supraventricular crest** – separates the inflow (venous) and outflow (**conus arteriosus** or infundibulum) tracts of the right ventricle.

The right ventricle contracts under moderate pressure during ventricular systole. As it does, the tricuspid valve closes and the **pulmonary valve** opens. Blood flows through the pulmonary valve, which has three cusps, and passes through the pulmonary arteries to the lungs. The simultaneous closing of the mitral and tricuspid valves and the opening of the pulmonary valve creates the first heart sound heard over the precordium (anterior chest wall) when examining a patient with a stethoscope.

Left atrium

Blood that has been oxygenated in the lungs returns to the left atrium through the **pulmonary veins**. The left atrium, which forms most of the **base of heart**, is posterior to the right atrium. The esophagus, left pulmonary bronchus, and descending aorta are posterior to the left atrium. The four valveless pulmonary veins enter the left atrium on its posterior wall.

Internally, the left atrium, like the right atrium, contains pectinate muscles. On the **interatrial septum** there is a fossa ovalis corresponding with that of the right atrium. Blood flows through the **mitral valve** (left atrioventricular valve) into the left ventricle during diastole. The mitral valve is composed of only two cusps, and like the tricuspid valve, is supported by chordae tendineae and papillary muscles.

Left ventricle

The left ventricle makes up a substantial part of the **apex of heart** and also forms the left border of the heart. Its internal surface is smoother than that of the right ventricle, and it has a much thicker wall because it has to generate a high pressure to pump blood to the entire body. As the left ventricle contracts (ventricular systole), the mitral valve closes and the **aortic valve** opens. Blood is pumped through the aortic valve, which consists of three cusps, into the aorta. When the left ventricle relaxes (ventricular diastole), the simultaneous closure of the aortic and pulmonary valves creates the second heart sound.

NERVES

Nerve supply to the heart is provided by the **superficial** and **deep cardiac plexuses**, which are composed of parasympathetic nerve fibers from the **vagus nerve [X]** and sympathetic nerve fibers from the **superior thoracic** and **cervical sympathetic ganglia**. These fibers follow the course of the coronary arteries. Parasympathetic stimulation slows the heart rate, whereas sympathetic stimulation increases heart rate. Pain fibers to the heart follow the route of the sympathetic fibers.

CORONARY ARTERIES

The coronary arteries supply blood to the myocardium (cardiac muscle) (Table 30.1 and Fig. 30.2). The **left coronary artery** branches off the **left coronary sinus** of the aorta and after approximately 1 cm, divides into:

- the **anterior interventricular branch** (left anterior descending artery), which supplies the anterior two-thirds of the interventricular septum of the heart and the anterior wall and apex of the heart.
- the **circumflex branch**, which is within the left atrioventricular groove and continues around the left side of the heart as **marginal branches** leave it to supply blood to the left ventricle.

The **right coronary artery** arises from the **right coronary sinus** and lies within the coronary groove between the right atrium and right ventricle. A small branch from it supplies blood to the sinu-atrial (SA) node; other small arterial branches (the acute marginal

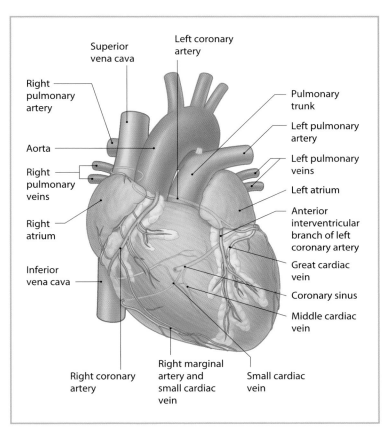

Figure 30.2 Coronary arteries and veins

branches) provide blood to the right ventricle. The right coronary artery continues around the heart to the **posterior interventricular sulcus**, where it terminates, branching to take blood to the atrioventricular node. Now known as the **posterior interventricular branch** (posterior descending artery), it supplies blood to the posterior third of the interventricular septum and the apex of heart.

VEINS AND LYMPHATICS

Most of the cardiac veins, which follow the path of the coronary arteries described above, drain to the **coronary sinus** in the atrioventricular sulcus on the posterior surface of the heart, which drains into the right atrium. The **great cardiac vein**, adjacent to the anterior interventricular artery, drains blood superiorly from the apex of the heart towards the base and around to the coronary sinus. The **middle cardiac vein** begins on the posterior surface of the heart next to the posterior interventricular artery and drains to the coronary sinus. The **small cardiac vein** runs alongside the right marginal artery in the atrioventricular groove and also drains to the coronary sinus.

Veins from the anterior wall of the heart drain directly to the right atrium. Many small veins of the heart drain directly to the adjacent chamber of the heart. These are known as thebesian veins.

Lymphatic drainage of the heart is to the **subepicardial** and **mediastinal tracheobronchial lymph node groups**.

CONDUCTION SYSTEM OF THE HEART

The heart contains a specialized set of muscle fibers that regulate contraction of the atria, and then transfer this impulse to the

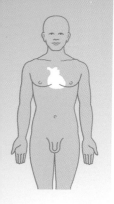

ventricles and the rest of the heart. These muscle fibers are affected by sympathetic and parasympathetic stimulation. The **sinu-atrial (SA) node**, in the wall of the right atrium at the junction of the superior vena cava and right atrium, is composed of a group of these specialized fibers and is the 'pacemaker' of the heart because it initiates the heart beat by stimulating atrial contraction. From the SA node, the cardiac impulse is sent to the **atrioventricular (AV) node**, which is a smaller group of specialized cells in the inferior part of the **interatrial septum**. The AV node directs impulses from both atria to the **atrioventricular bundle** (the 'bundle of His'). From here, the impulse spreads out into the **left** and **right bundle branches**, which are composed of subendocardial plexuses of conduction cells (Purkinje fibers). The left and right bundle branches enter the respective ventricles and initiate ventricular contraction. Disruption of this electrical pathway can cause a cardiac arrhythmia (irregular heart beat).

■ CLINICAL CORRELATIONS
Auscultation of heart sounds
There are usually two heart sounds: S1 and S2 (often referred to as 'lub' and 'dup'). The first (lub) is caused by closure of the mitral and tricuspid valves as the ventricles contract (systole). The second heart sound (dup) results from closure of the aortic and pulmonary valves at the end of ventricular contraction (diastole). The sounds of the four valves closing can be auscultated (listened to) at the locations shown in Figure 30.3. Careful auscultation may reveal a heart murmur that may warrant further evaluation.

Myocardial infarction
Complete occlusion (blockage) of a coronary artery deprives the myocardium of oxygen and causes death (infarction) of the tissue (Fig. 30.4). This usually causes severe chest pain, which may radiate to the left arm, left neck, jaw, and various other sites. This is known as a 'heart attack'.

Chest pain is also caused by decreased (as opposed to completely blocked) blood supply to the myocardium, and this condition is angina pectoris. The primary reason for decreased blood flow is a narrowing or partial obstruction of the coronary arteries. Risk factors for such coronary artery disease include smoking, diabetes mellitus, high blood pressure, high cholesterol and triglyceride levels, advanced age, obesity, and a genetic predispostion.

Treatment of myocardial injury is aimed at restoring blood flow to the area of the heart involved. This can sometimes be accomplished by procedures such as coronary angioplasty with possible stent placement or coronary artery bypass grafting. Chest pain is a common symptom of myocardial disease, but it has many other causes including trauma, infection, dyspepsia, gastro-esophageal reflux disease, arthritis, muscle spasm, and tumor.

MNEMONIC

Position of tricuspid valve: **TRy to be Right**
(**T**ricuspid is between **R**ight atrium and ventricle)

TABLE 30.1 ARTERIAL SUPPLY TO THE HEART

Artery/Branch	Origin	Course	Distribution	Anastomoses
Right coronary artery	Right aortic sinus	Follows coronary (AV) sulcus between the atria and ventricles	Right atrium, SA and AV nodes, and posterior part of IV septum	Circumflex and anterior branches of left coronary artery
Sinu-atrial (SA) nodal branch	Right coronary artery near its origin (in 60%)	Ascends to SA node	Pulmonary trunk and SA node	
Right marginal branch	Right coronary artery	Passes to the inferior margin of heart and apex of heart	Right ventricle and apex of heart	IV branches
Posterior interventricular (IV) branch	Right coronary artery	Runs from posterior IV sulcus to apex of heart	Right and left ventricles and IV septum	Circumflex and anterior branches of left coronary artery
Atrioventricular (AV) nodal branch	Right coronary artery near origin of posterior IV branch	Passes to AV node	AV node	
Left coronary artery	Left aortic sinus	Runs in coronary sulcus and gives off anterior IV and circumflex branches	Most of left atrium and ventricle, IV septum, and AV bundles; may supply AV node	Right coronary artery
SA nodal branch	Circumflex branch (in 40%)	Ascends on posterior surface of left atrium to SA node	Left atrium and SA node	
Anterior interventricular branch	Left coronary artery	Passes along anterior IV sulcus to apex of heart	Right and left ventricles and IV septum	Posterior IV branch of right coronary artery
Circumflex branch	Left coronary artery	Passes to left in coronary sulcus and runs to posterior surface of heart	Left atrium and left ventricle	Right coronary artery
Left marginal artery	Circumflex branch	Follows left border of heart	Left ventricle	IV branches

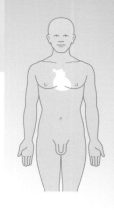

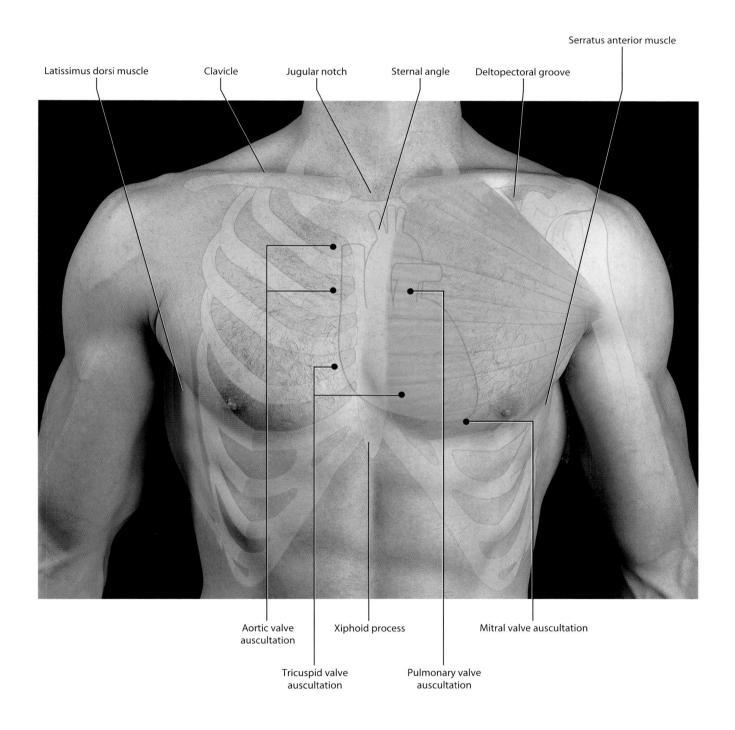

Serratus anterior muscle

Latissimus dorsi muscle   Clavicle   Jugular notch   Sternal angle   Deltopectoral groove

Aortic valve
auscultation

Xiphoid process

Mitral valve auscultation

Tricuspid valve
auscultation

Pulmonary valve
auscultation

Figure 30.3 Heart – surface anatomy. Anterior view of the surface landmarks of the anterior thorax in relation to the heart

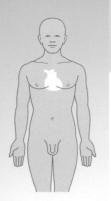

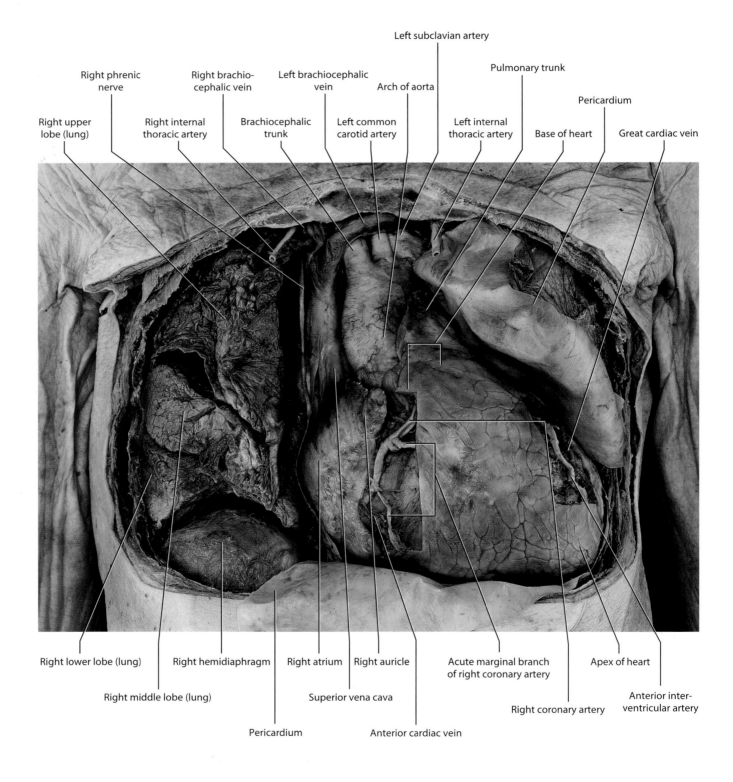

Left subclavian artery

Right phrenic
nerve

Right brachio-
cephalic vein

Left brachiocephalic
vein

Arch of aorta

Pulmonary trunk

Pericardium

Right upper
lobe (lung)

Right internal
thoracic artery

Brachiocephalic
trunk

Left common
carotid artery

Left internal
thoracic artery

Base of heart

Great cardiac vein

Right lower lobe (lung)

Right hemidiaphragm

Right atrium

Right auricle

Acute marginal branch
of right coronary artery

Apex of heart

Right middle lobe (lung)

Superior vena cava

Anterior inter-
ventricular artery

Right coronary artery

Pericardium

Anterior cardiac vein

Figure 30.4 Heart – in situ. In this anterior view layers of pericardium have been reflected away from the surface of the heart to reveal coronary arteries. Note that in this image the heart is hypertrophic

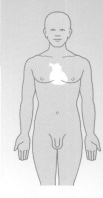

Right pulmonary
artery

Right lung

Right phrenic
nerve

Right internal
thoracic
artery

Right
brachiocephalic
vein

Superior vena
cava

Trachea

Left brachiocephalic
vein

Left
common
carotid
artery

Left
vagus
nerve [X]

Left internal
thoracic artery

Arch of aorta

Left primary
bronchus

Left phrenic
nerve

Left pulmonary
artery

Right
hemidiaphragm

Right superior
pulmonary vein

Opening of inferior
vena cava

Reflected
pericardium

Left inferior
pulmonary vein

Thoracic aorta

Left
hemidiaphragm

Right inferior
pulmonary vein

Right primary
bronchus

Esophagus

Left superior
pulmonary vein

Anterior surface of
thoracic vertebra

Figure 30.5 Pericardium – opened. The heart has been removed to reveal the openings in the pericardium

351

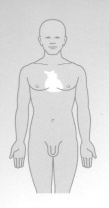

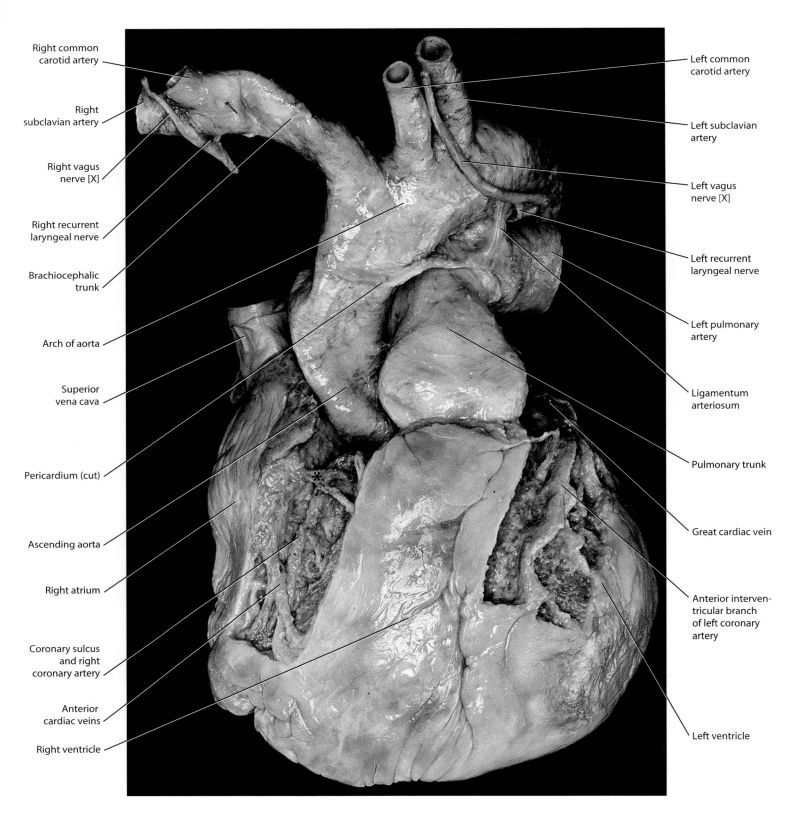

Right common
carotid artery

Right
subclavian artery

Right vagus
nerve [X]

Right recurrent
laryngeal nerve

Brachiocephalic
trunk

Arch of aorta

Superior
vena cava

Pericardium (cut)

Ascending aorta

Right atrium

Coronary sulcus
and right
coronary artery

Anterior
cardiac veins

Right ventricle

Left common
carotid artery

Left subclavian
artery

Left vagus
nerve [X]

Left recurrent
laryngeal nerve

Left pulmonary
artery

Ligamentum
arteriosum

Pulmonary trunk

Great cardiac vein

Anterior interven-
tricular branch
of left coronary
artery

Left ventricle

Figure 30.6 Heart – isolated 1. Anterior view of the heart and its attachments to the great vessels, dissected to reveal coronary and cardiac arteries and veins. An anterior cardiac vein is marked with an asterisk

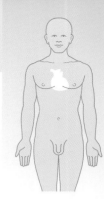

Circumflex branch of
left coronary artery

Right auricle

Pulmonary trunk

Anterior interventricular
branch of
left coronary artery

Superior vena
cava

Aorta

Base of heart

Great cardiac
vein

Right atrium

Acute marginal
branch of right
coronary artery

Right coronary
artery

Right ventricle

Great cardiac
vein

Left ventricle

Anterior
cardiac vein

Septal branches of anterior
interventricular branch
of left coronary artery

Apex of heart

Figure 30.7 Heart – isolated 2. Anterior view of the heart dissected to reveal coronary and cardiac arteries and veins

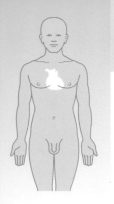

TRUNK

Heart

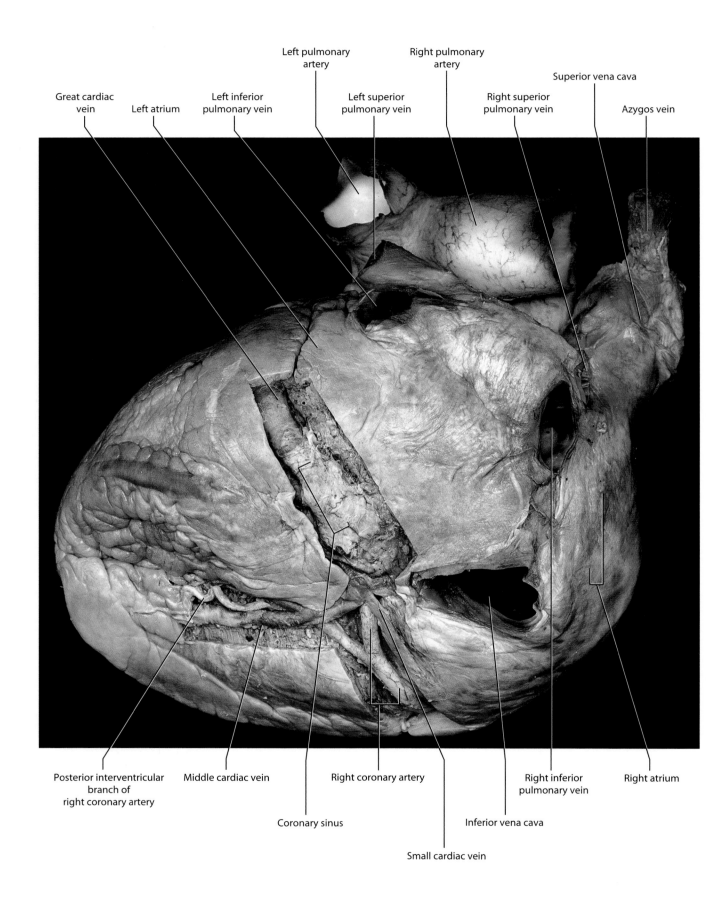

Left pulmonary artery

Right pulmonary artery

Superior vena cava

Great cardiac vein

Left atrium

Left inferior pulmonary vein

Left superior pulmonary vein

Right superior pulmonary vein

Azygos vein

Posterior interventricular branch of right coronary artery

Middle cardiac vein

Right coronary artery

Right inferior pulmonary vein

Right atrium

Coronary sinus

Inferior vena cava

Small cardiac vein

354 **Figure 30.8 Heart – isolated 3.** Posterior view of the heart dissected to reveal coronary and cardiac arteries and veins

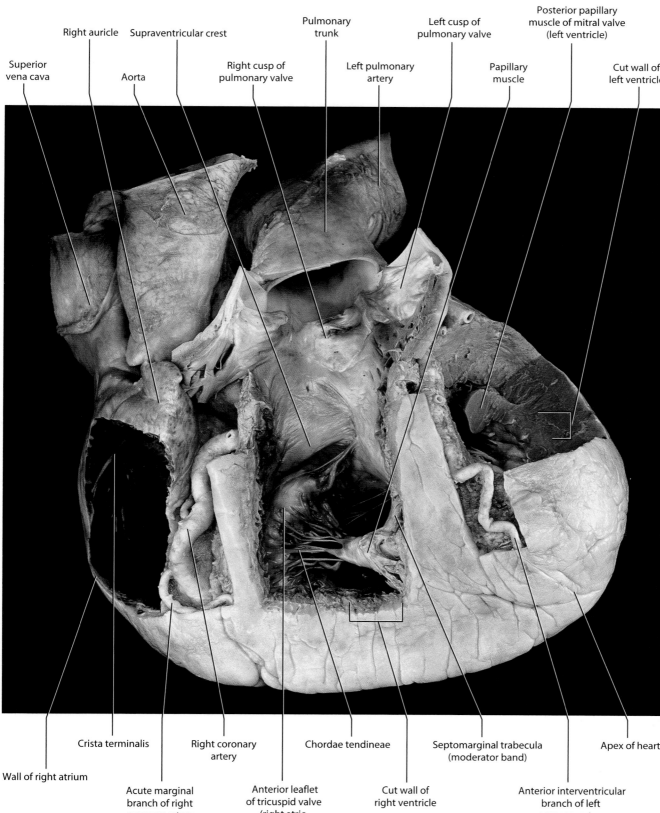

Superior
vena cava

Right auricle

Supraventricular crest

Aorta

Right cusp of
pulmonary valve

Pulmonary
trunk

Left pulmonary
artery

Left cusp of
pulmonary valve

Papillary
muscle

Posterior papillary
muscle of mitral valve
(left ventricle)

Cut wall of
left ventricle

Wall of right atrium

Crista terminalis

Acute marginal
branch of right
coronary artery

Right coronary
artery

Anterior leaflet
of tricuspid valve
(right atrio-
ventricular valve)

Chordae tendineae

Cut wall of
right ventricle

Septomarginal trabecula
(moderator band)

Anterior interventricular
branch of left
coronary artery

Apex of heart

Figure 30.9 Heart – isolated 4. Anterior view of the heart. The myocardium has been partially cut away to reveal the internal structure of the isolated right atrium, right ventricle, and left ventricle

355

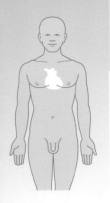

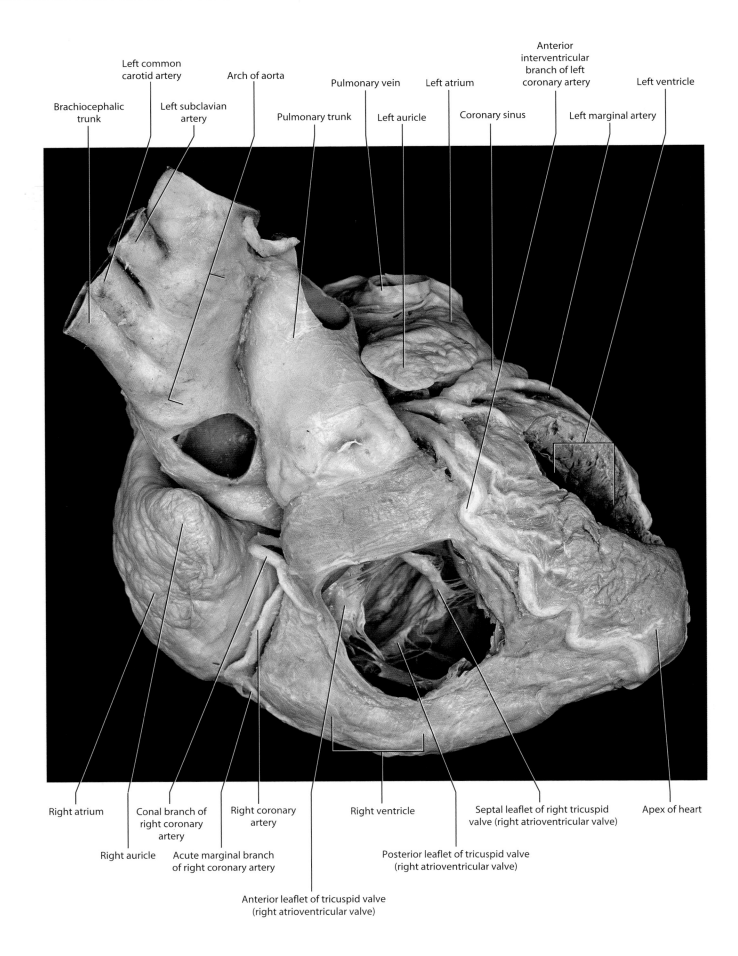

Left common
carotid artery

Arch of aorta

Anterior
interventricular
branch of left
coronary artery

Brachiocephalic
trunk

Left subclavian
artery

Pulmonary trunk

Pulmonary vein

Left auricle

Left atrium

Coronary sinus

Left ventricle

Left marginal artery

Right atrium

Conal branch of
right coronary
artery

Right coronary
artery

Right ventricle

Septal leaflet of right tricuspid
valve (right atrioventricular valve)

Apex of heart

Right auricle

Acute marginal branch
of right coronary artery

Posterior leaflet of tricuspid valve
(right atrioventricular valve)

Anterior leaflet of tricuspid valve
(right atrioventricular valve)

Figure 30.10 Heart – isolated 5. Superior view of the heart. The myocardium has been partially cut away to reveal the internal structure of the right ventricle

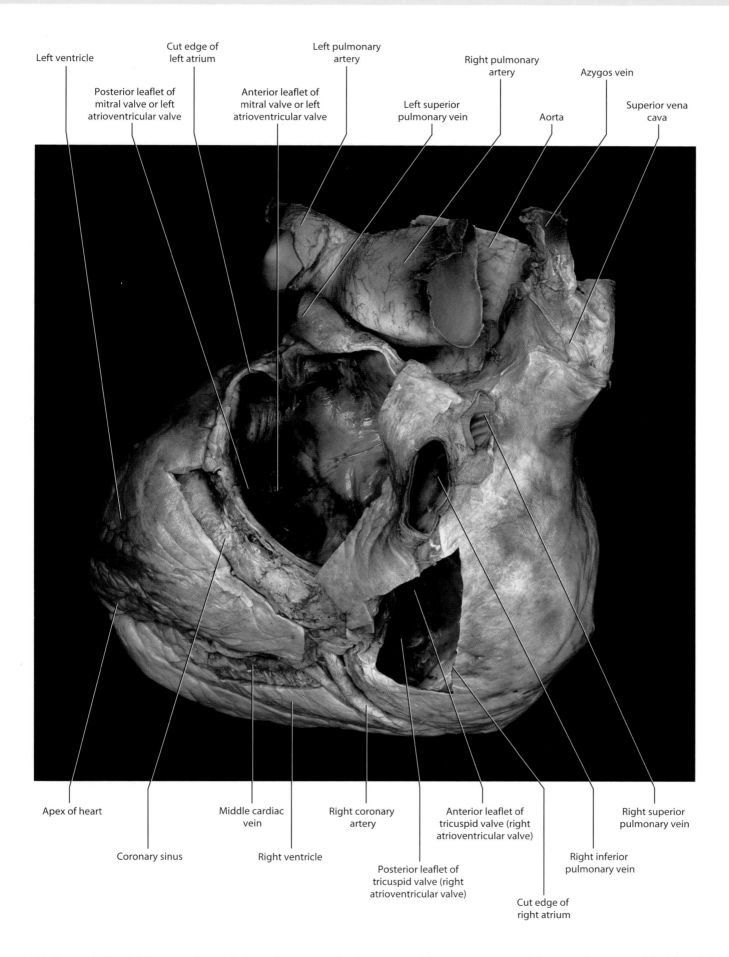

Left ventricle

Cut edge of
left atrium

Left pulmonary
artery

Right pulmonary
artery

Azygos vein

Posterior leaflet of
mitral valve or left
atrioventricular valve

Anterior leaflet of
mitral valve or left
atrioventricular valve

Left superior
pulmonary vein

Aorta

Superior vena
cava

Apex of heart

Middle cardiac
vein

Right coronary
artery

Anterior leaflet of
tricuspid valve (right
atrioventricular valve)

Right superior
pulmonary vein

Coronary sinus

Right ventricle

Posterior leaflet of
tricuspid valve (right
atrioventricular valve)

Right inferior
pulmonary vein

Cut edge of
right atrium

Figure 30.11 Heart – isolated 6. Posterior view of the heart. The myocardium has been partially cut away to reveal the internal structure of the left and right atria

357

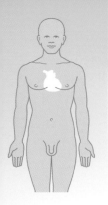

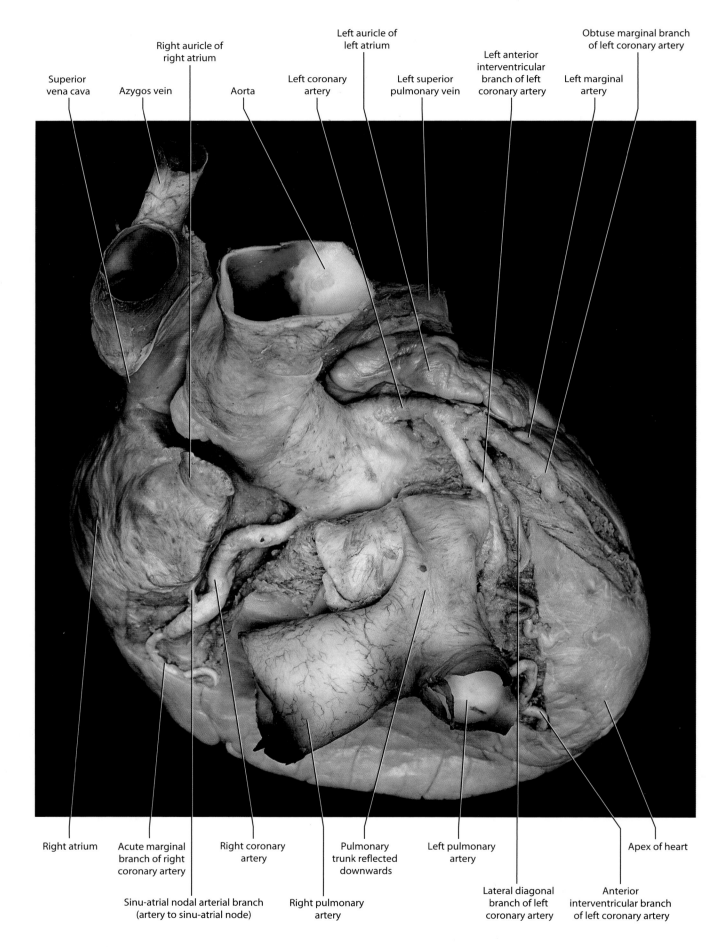

Superior
vena cava

Azygos vein

Right auricle of
right atrium

Aorta

Left coronary
artery

Left auricle of
left atrium

Left superior
pulmonary vein

Left anterior
interventricular
branch of left
coronary artery

Obtuse marginal branch
of left coronary artery

Left marginal
artery

Right atrium

Acute marginal
branch of right
coronary artery

Right coronary
artery

Pulmonary
trunk reflected
downwards

Left pulmonary
artery

Apex of heart

Sinu-atrial nodal arterial branch
(artery to sinu-atrial node)

Right pulmonary
artery

Lateral diagonal
branch of left
coronary artery

Anterior
interventricular branch
of left coronary artery

Figure 30.12 Heart – isolated 7. Superior view of the heart. Note the aorta, venae cavae, and coronary arteries. The pulmonary arterial trunk has been reflected downwards to reveal the coronary arteries as they branch off the aorta

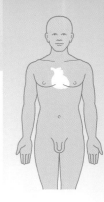

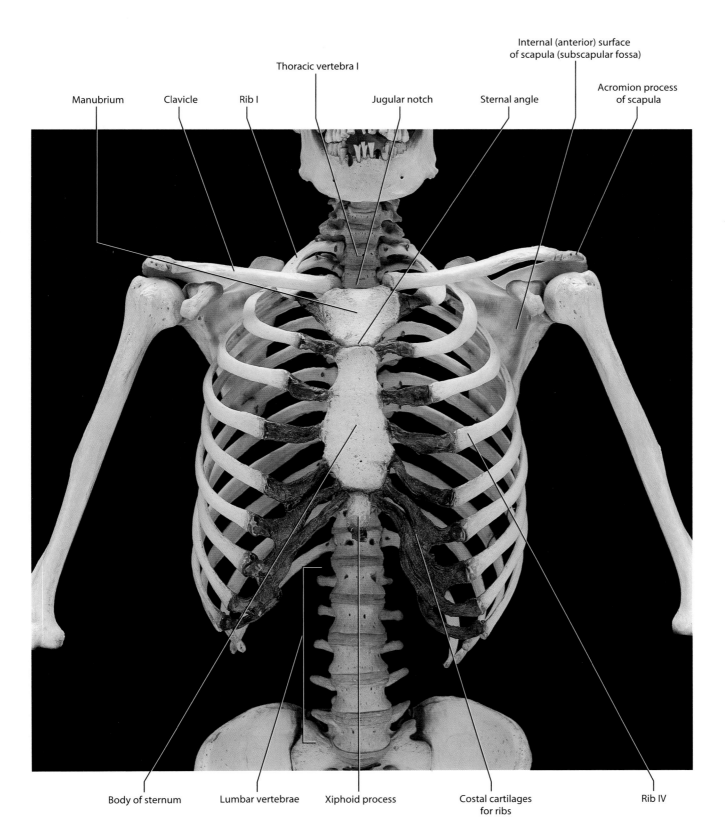

Figure 30.13 Heart – osteology. Anterior view of the bony framework of the thorax

HEART – PLAIN FILM RADIOGRAPH (POSTEROANTERIOR VIEW)

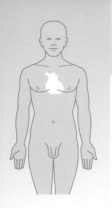

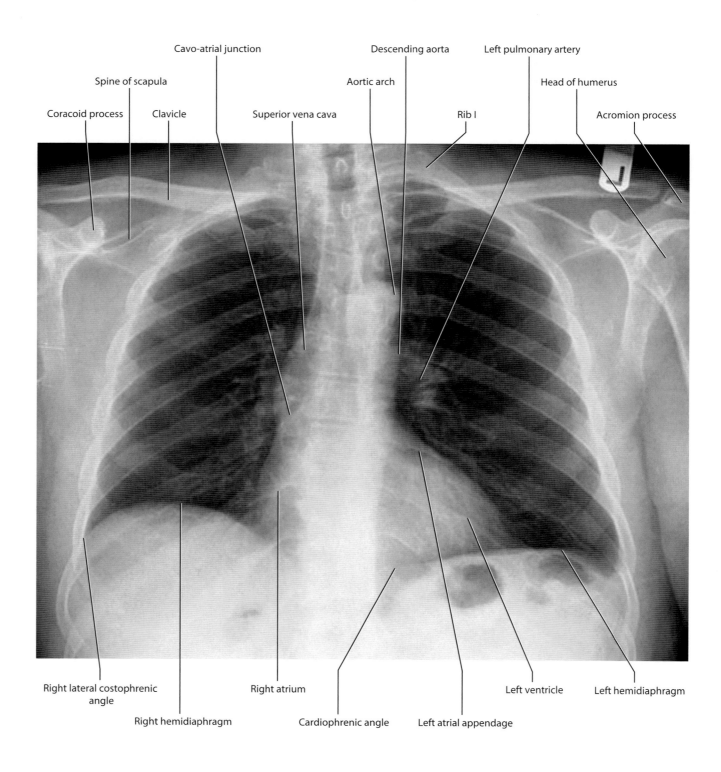

Cavo-atrial junction

Spine of scapula

Coracoid process   Clavicle

Superior vena cava

Descending aorta   Left pulmonary artery

Aortic arch

Head of humerus

Rib I

Acromion process

Right lateral costophrenic angle

Right atrium

Left ventricle   Left hemidiaphragm

Right hemidiaphragm   Cardiophrenic angle   Left atrial appendage

Figure 30.14 Heart – plain film radiograph (posteroanterior view). Note that the right border of the heart on posteroanterior chest radiographs is the right atrium, and the left border is the left ventricle. In clinical practice, both anteroposterior and posteroanterior radiographs are viewed as though looking from anterior to posterior, hence the orientation shown here. To obtain a posteroanterior radiograph, the X-rays are projected from behind the patient to a plate that is touching the patient's chest; structures close to the plate appear very close to actual size, and structures further away appear larger. In anteroposterior views the heart therefore appears much larger (and less distinct) than in this posteroanterior view

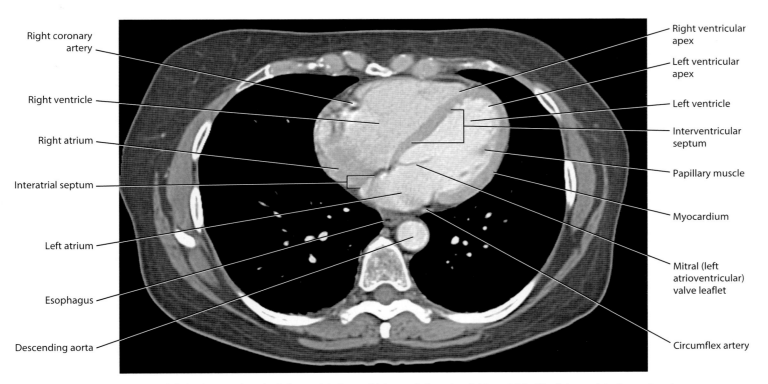

Right coronary artery

Right ventricle

Right atrium

Interatrial septum

Left atrium

Esophagus

Descending aorta

Right ventricular apex

Left ventricular apex

Left ventricle

Interventricular septum

Papillary muscle

Myocardium

Mitral (left atrioventricular) valve leaflet

Circumflex artery

Figure 30.15 Heart – CT scan (axial view). Note that the left ventricle has a thicker wall than the right ventricle. The interventricular septum is seen as a diagonal band which divides the heart at this level. Because of the special technique implemented to enhance the heart structures in this scan, the lung tissues are not well visualized

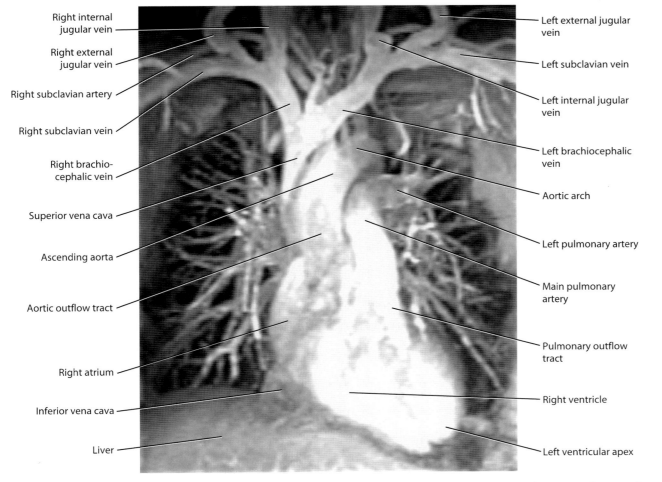

Right internal jugular vein

Right external jugular vein

Right subclavian artery

Right subclavian vein

Right brachio-cephalic vein

Superior vena cava

Ascending aorta

Aortic outflow tract

Right atrium

Inferior vena cava

Liver

Left external jugular vein

Left subclavian vein

Left internal jugular vein

Left brachiocephalic vein

Aortic arch

Left pulmonary artery

Main pulmonary artery

Pulmonary outflow tract

Right ventricle

Left ventricular apex

Figure 30.16 Heart – MRA scan (coronal view). Magnetic resonance angiograms (MRA) have the advantage of visualizing the veins at the same time as the arteries, whereas conventional angiography usually shows only the arteries or only the veins

31 Lungs

The lungs, situated in the right and left thorax (Fig. 31.1), are the site of gas exchange. Each lung is enclosed by a two-layered serous membrane:

- the outer membrane – the **parietal pleura** – is attached to the inner surface of the thoracic wall by the **endothoracic fascia**, receives segmental sensory innervation from branches of the **intercostal nerves** and is supplied with blood by branches of the **internal thoracic, superior phrenic**, and **intercostal arteries**;
- the inner membrane – the **visceral pleura** – attaches directly to the lungs, is innervated by **vagal fibers** that originate in the **pulmonary plexus** of nerves, and is supplied with blood from the **bronchial arteries**.

The parietal and visceral pleurae are normally in close contact, separated by a thin film of serous fluid.

Structural support for the lungs is from the flexible bony cartilaginous thoracic wall (see Chapter 29).

Air from the mouth and nose enters the lungs through the **trachea**, which lies in the midline of the neck, anterior to the esophagus. The trachea begins just inferior to the cricoid cartilage (at vertebra CVI) and extends downward for 9–15 cm. It is composed of a series of backward-facing, C-shaped hyaline cartilaginous rings. The trachea divides into the **left** and **right main bronchi** at the level of the sternal angle and the junction of vertebrae TIV/TV.

Each main bronchus enters the lung at the hilum and further subdivides. The right main bronchus divides into three lobar

bronchi, the left into two. These secondary bronchi further divide into tertiary bronchi (Table 31.1). The part of a lung supplied by a tertiary **segmental bronchus** is a **bronchopulmonary segment**. This is clinically significant because a complete bronchopulmonary segment can be surgically removed without compromising the function of the remaining parts of that lung.

Each **hilum of the lung** contains a main bronchus, a pulmonary artery, two pulmonary veins, the autonomic pulmonary plexus of nerves, bronchial arteries, and lymph nodes. These structures are surrounded by a sleeve of pleura that extends inferiorly as the **pulmonary ligament**. On both sides, the main bronchus lies posterior to the pulmonary artery and the pulmonary veins lie anteroinferior to the main bronchus and pulmonary artery.

The **right lung** is larger than the **left lung** because the heart occupies space in the left chest cavity. There are three **lobes** in the right lung – the superior, middle, and inferior lobes – whereas the left lung has only two – the superior and inferior lobes (Fig. 31.2). These lobes are separated by fissures. In the right lung, the **oblique fissure** separates the superior and middle lobes and the **horizontal fissure of right lung** separates the middle and inferior lobes; the two lobes in the left lung are separated by the oblique fissure. The inferior part of the superior lobe of the left lung is the **lingula of the left lung** and is the anatomical counterpart of the middle lobe of the right lung.

ARTERIES
The **bronchial arteries** supply oxygenated blood to the tissue (parenchyma) of the lung (Fig. 31.3). The right lung is supplied by one bronchial artery and the left lung by two. These bronchial arteries arise from the aorta.

Deoxygenated blood for gas exchange is carried to the lungs by the **pulmonary arteries**.

NERVES
The lungs are innervated by the autonomic pulmonary plexus of nerves on the surface of the primary bronchus at the hilum of each lung. Each pulmonary plexus receives:

- parasympathetic innervation from both vagus nerves [X];
- sympathetic innervation from the sympathetic trunk and cardiac plexus.

Sympathetic stimulation dilates the bronchi; parasympathetic stimulation constricts the bronchi and increases respiratory glandular secretions.

The left and right phrenic nerves are anterior to the hilum of each lung. The left and right vagus nerves [X] are posterior to the hila and are more closely associated with the esophagus.

VEINS AND LYMPHATICS
The superior and inferior pulmonary veins transport oxygenated blood from the lungs to the heart. The **right superior pulmonary vein** of the right lung drains the right superior and middle lobes; the **right inferior pulmonary vein** drains the inferior lobe. On the left side, the **left superior pulmonary vein** drains the left superior lobe and the lingula, and the **left inferior pulmonary vein** drains

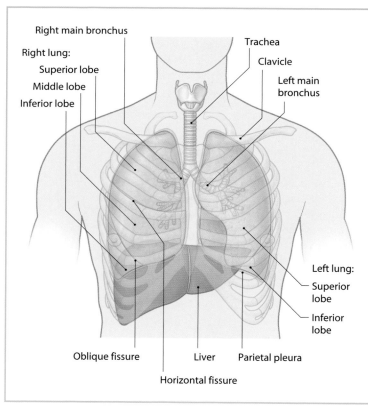

Figure 31.1 The lungs

Right main bronchus

Right lung:
Superior lobe
Middle lobe
Inferior lobe

Trachea
Clavicle
Left main bronchus

Left lung:
Superior lobe
Inferior lobe

Oblique fissure   Liver   Parietal pleura
Horizontal fissure

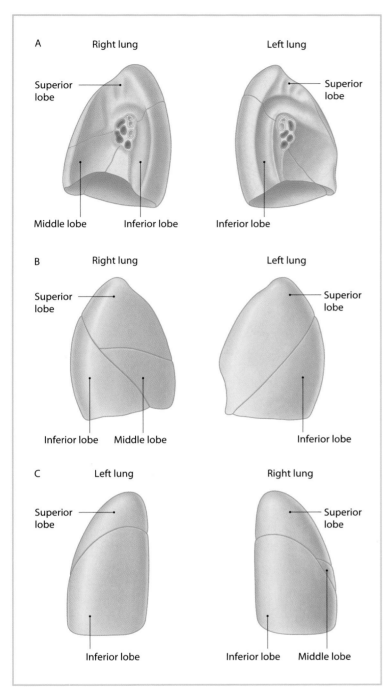

Figure 31.2 Lobes of the lungs: hilar (A), lateral (B), and posterior (C) views

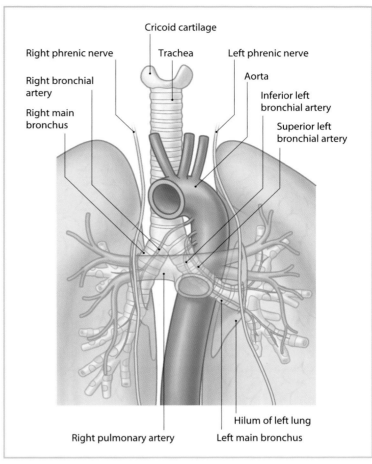

Figure 31.3 Hilar region of the lungs

the left inferior lobe. These four pulmonary veins empty into the left atrium.

The **bronchial veins** drain blood from the parenchyma of the lung and, on the right, empty into the **azygos vein**; on the left they drain into the **accessory hemi-azygos vein**.

Lymph drainage is provided by a superficial plexus and a deep plexus of lymph vessels. Both plexuses accompany the bronchial tree and the pulmonary arteries and veins, and drain to **hilar lymph nodes** and **tracheobronchial nodes** around the tracheal bifurcation. From here, lymph drains to the bronchomediastinal lymph trunks.

■ CLINICAL CORRELATIONS
Pneumonia
Pneumonia (Fig. 31.4) is an infectious inflammatory process within the parenchyma of the lung. The most common cause is infection with the bacteria *Streptococcus pneumoniae* or *Haemophilus influenzae*. Pneumonia can also be caused by a variety of viruses, among them influenza and para-influenza viruses and enteroviruses. The infection spreads rapidly and can involve an entire lobe of a lung.

Most patients have tachypnea (increased respiratory rate), fever, and a cough that often produces purulent sputum. Some also have chest pain or a feeling of 'tightness' in the chest, chills, and symptoms of upper respiratory tract infection (rhinorrhea, pharyngitis, sinus congestion).

On examination, patients are usually febrile and have an increased respiratory rate. Inspiratory rales and rhonchi can be heard on auscultation of the chest, and it might be possible to detect decreased breath sounds over the infected lobe. Diagnosis can also be made from the chest radiograph – patchy or homogeneous infiltrates in the involved lobe show up as whitened areas. A sputum specimen should be obtained and sent for analysis and confirmation of the cause of the infection.

Commonly, treatment is started with broad-spectrum antibiotics directed at the most likely causative agents, and this is changed as necessary when the sputum culture results are available.

363

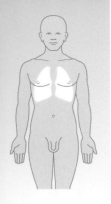

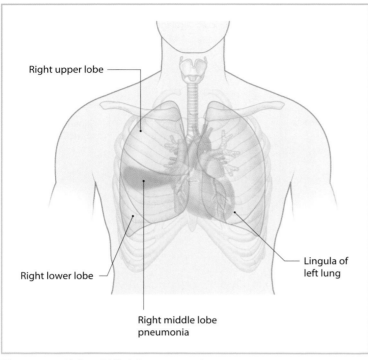

Right upper lobe

Right lower lobe

Right middle lobe
pneumonia

Lingula of
left lung

Figure 31.4 Right middle lobe pneumonia

Lung abscess

A lung abscess is defined as the presence of purulent material contained within the parenchyma of the lung. The most common cause is aspiration pneumonia. This is usually caused by anaerobic bacteria that originate in the digestive tract (*Bacteroides*, *Fusobacterium*, and *Peptostreptococcus* spp.). As these bacteria multiply within the lung, the body defends itself by producing pus. Patients report a cough with purulent sputum, fever, pain, and fatigue.

Lung abscess is diagnosed by chest radiography, which shows an air fluid level in the region of the abscess; computed tomography and bronchoscopy can also be useful in diagnosis.

Treatment of lung abscess comprises high-dose intravenous antibiotics, aggressive pulmonary toilet (coughing, chest physiotherapy), and bronchoscopy to remove purulent material. This treatment does not always eradicate the infection and surgical drainage is sometimes necessary.

Pneumothorax

A pneumothorax is a puncture or other injury to the lung that causes air to be released into the pleural space. Patients report shortness of breath, weakness, pain, and anxiety. A tension pneumothorax is a condition in which air enters (but does not leave) the pleural space through the defect in the lung with every breath. A pneumothorax increases the size of the pleural space and displaces the lung. Eventually the involved lung is unable to function normally (Fig. 31.5). This places direct pressure on the heart and can result in death.

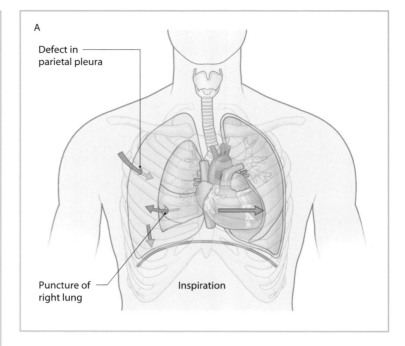

A

Defect in
parietal pleura

Puncture of
right lung

Inspiration

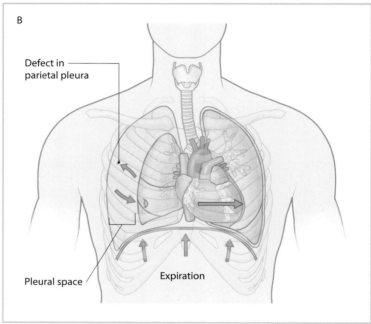

B

Defect in
parietal pleura

Pleural space

Expiration

Figure 31.5 Tension pneumothorax. During inspiration (A) air enters the pleural space. During expiration (B) air cannot escape through the defect in the parietal pleura; this causes the pleural space to become larger and applies pressure to the heart and lungs

Immediate decompression of a pneumothorax is carried out by placing a needle device into the second intercostal space in the midclavicular line of the affected side. This is followed by placing a chest tube (thoracostomy) into the pleural space, usually through the fourth intercostal space at the midaxillary line.

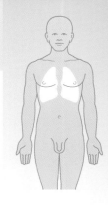

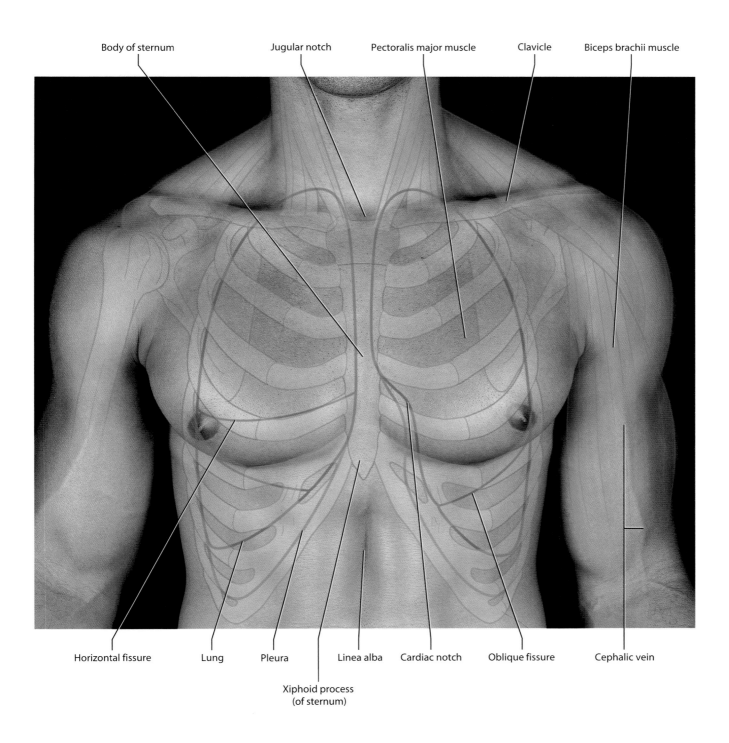

Body of sternum

Jugular notch

Pectoralis major muscle

Clavicle

Biceps brachii muscle

Horizontal fissure

Lung

Pleura

Linea alba

Cardiac notch

Oblique fissure

Cephalic vein

Xiphoid process
(of sternum)

Figure 31.6 Lungs – surface anatomy. Anterior view showing the surface topography of the chest in relation to the lungs

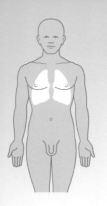

Right pulmonary
artery

Right brachiocephalic
vein

Brachiocephalic
artery

Trachea and
bifurcation of trachea

Arch of aorta

Left brachiocephalic
vein

Left common
carotid artery

Left subclavian artery

Left vagus nerve [X]

Left pulmonary
artery

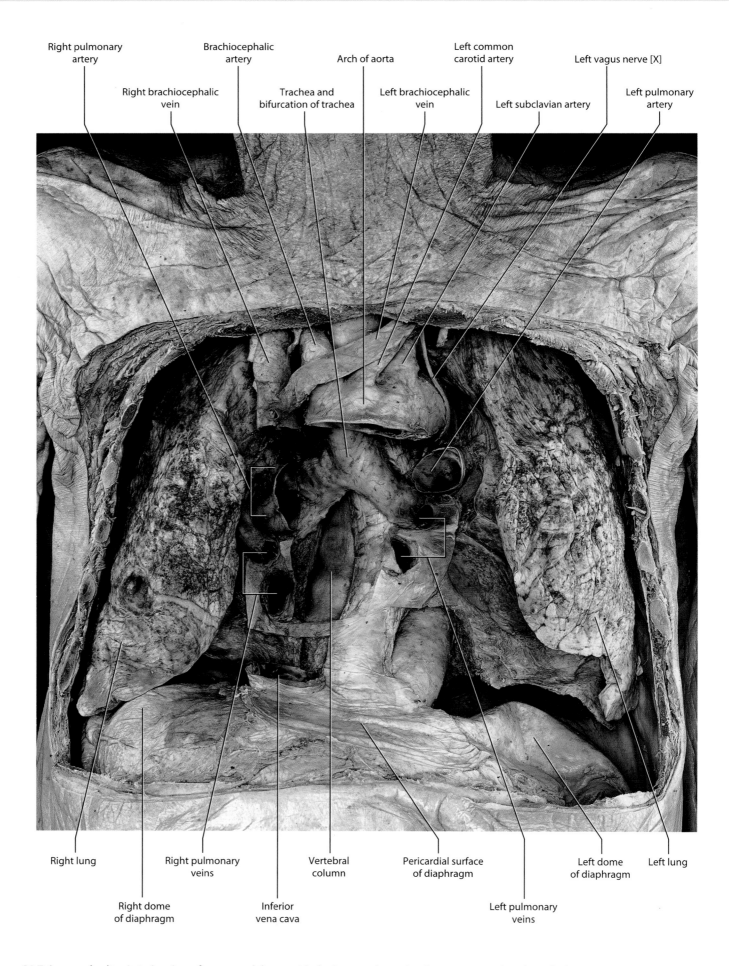

Right lung

Right pulmonary
veins

Right dome
of diaphragm

Inferior
vena cava

Vertebral
column

Pericardial surface
of diaphragm

Left pulmonary
veins

Left dome
of diaphragm

Left lung

Figure 31.7 Lungs – in situ. Anterior view of an opened thorax with the heart and anterior rib cage removed to show the lungs

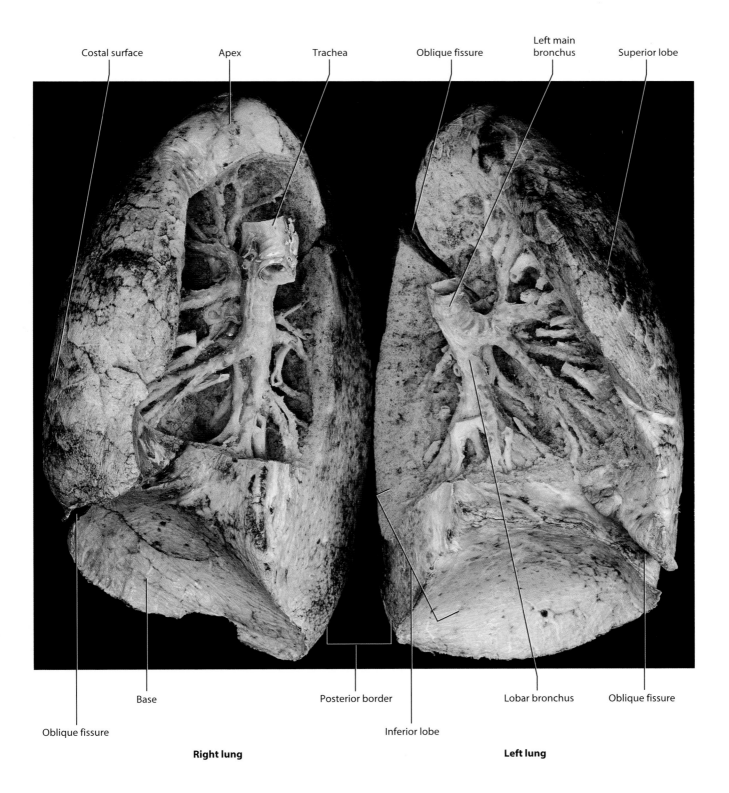

Costal surface   Apex   Trachea   Oblique fissure   Left main bronchus   Superior lobe

Base   Posterior border   Lobar bronchus   Oblique fissure

Oblique fissure   Inferior lobe

Right lung   **Left lung**

Figure 31.8 Lungs – isolated. Dissection of the bronchial tree of the right and left lungs. Observe how the primary bronchus of the right lung is more vertically oriented than the left; this is why more small aspirated objects are found in the right lung rather than in the left lung

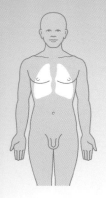

TABLE 31.1 LUNGS – BRONCHOPULMONARY SEGMENTS*

Lobe	Right lung		Left lung	
Superior lobe	SI	Apical segment	SI	Apical segment**
	SII	Posterior segment	SII	Posterior segment**
	SIII	Anterior segment	SIII	Anterior segment
			SIV	Superior lingular segment ⎱ lingula
			SV	Inferior lingular segment ⎰
Middle lobe	SIV	Lateral segment		
	SV	Medial segment		
Inferior lobe	SVI	Superior (apical) segment	SVI	Superior (apical) segment
	SVII	Medial basal segment	SVII	Medial basal segment #
	SVIII	Anterior basal segment	SVIII	Anterior basal segment #
	SIX	Lateral basal segment	SIX	Lateral basal segment
	SX	Posterior basal segment	SX	Posterior basal segment

* Bronchopulmonary segment: a segment of lung supplied independently by a segmental (tertiary) bronchus and a tertiary branch of the pulmonary artery. Its name is taken from the segmental bronchus that supplies it. Intersegmental veins in the connective septa drain adjacent segments to pulmonary veins.

** Frequently combined into apicoposterior. (SI + SII)

\# Frequently combined into anteromedial basal.

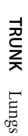

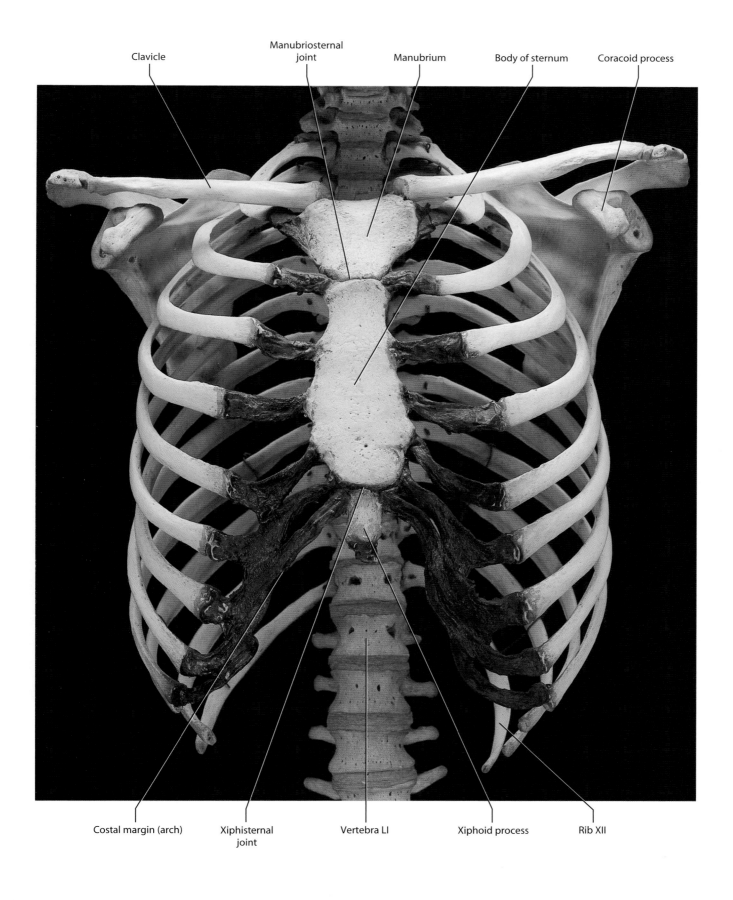

Clavicle

Manubriosternal joint

Manubrium

Body of sternum

Coracoid process

Costal margin (arch)

Xiphisternal joint

Vertebra LI

Xiphoid process

Rib XII

Figure 31.9 Lungs – osteology. Anterior view of the thorax (rib cage). The costal cartilages add to the flexibility of the rib cage and enable deep breathing. The costal cartilages in this photograph are real

369

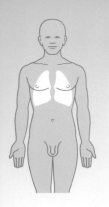

LUNGS – PLAIN FILM RADIOGRAPH (POSTEROANTERIOR VIEW)

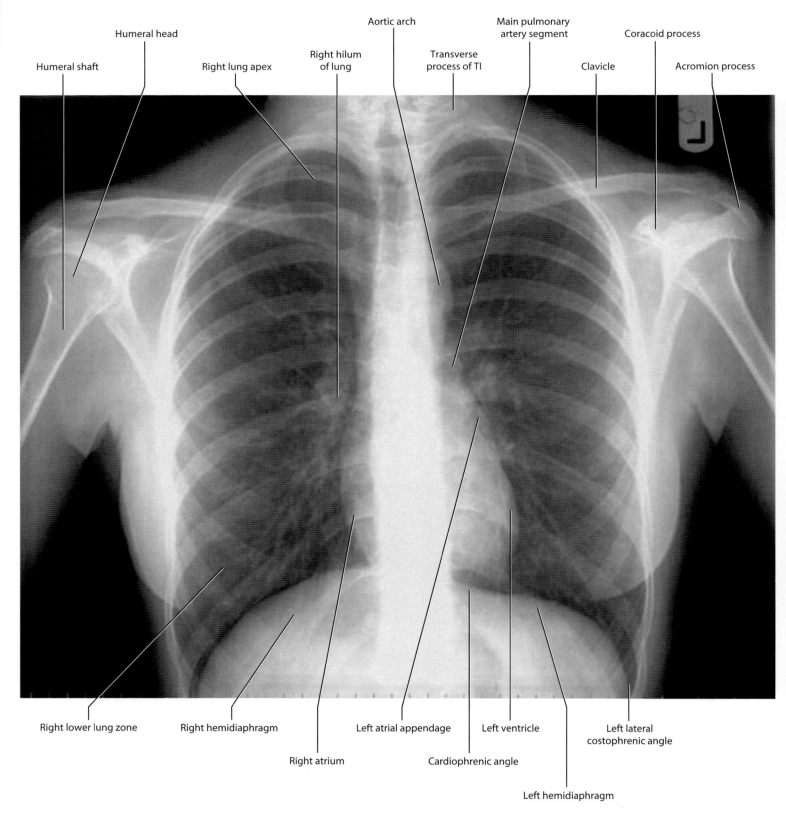

Humeral head

Humeral shaft

Right lung apex

Right hilum
of lung

Aortic arch

Transverse
process of TI

Main pulmonary
artery segment

Coracoid process

Clavicle

Acromion process

Right lower lung zone

Right hemidiaphragm

Left atrial appendage

Left ventricle

Left lateral
costophrenic angle

Right atrium

Cardiophrenic angle

Left hemidiaphragm

Figure 31.10 Lungs – plain film radiograph (posteroanterior view). The lungs contain air, which appears dark in radiographs, however the larger pulmonary vessels and bronchi are visible as lighter lung markings within the left and right pleural spaces. These lung markings extend to the periphery of the pleural space in a normal individual (as seen here). In pneumothorax, lung tissues are displaced creating large dark areas without lung markings. Note that in clinical practice, both anteroposterior and posteroanterior radiographs are viewed as though looking from anterior to posterior, hence the orientation shown here. To obtain a posteroanterior radiograph, the X-rays are projected from behind the patient to a plate that is touching the patient's chest; structures close to the plate appear very close to actual size, and structures further away appear larger. In anteroposterior views the heart therefore appears much larger (and less distinct) than in this posteroanterior view

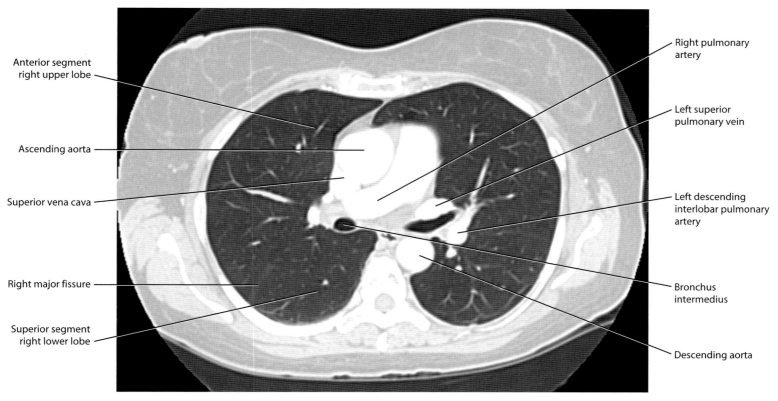

Anterior segment right upper lobe

Ascending aorta

Superior vena cava

Right major fissure

Superior segment right lower lobe

Right pulmonary artery

Left superior pulmonary vein

Left descending interlobar pulmonary artery

Bronchus intermedius

Descending aorta

Figure 31.11 Lungs – CT scan (axial view). A special technique has been used to enhance the visualization of the soft tissues of the lungs in this scan at the level of the great vessels. Small vessels are seen as white markings within the otherwise gray-appearing normal lung tissue. In patients with pneumothorax, the area of the pneumothorax would appear black because air does not give a signal in CT scans

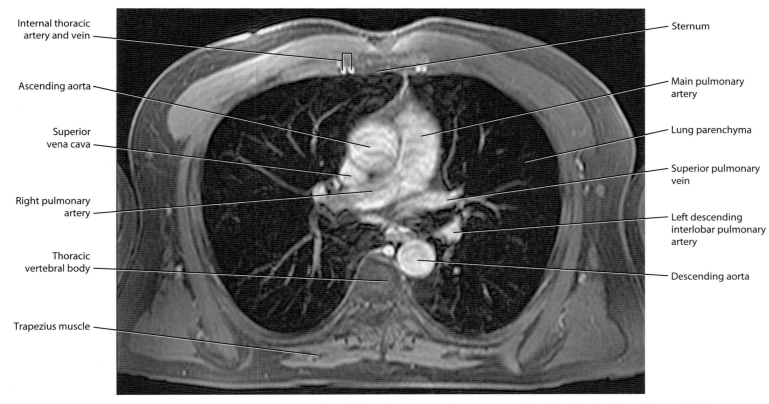

Internal thoracic artery and vein

Ascending aorta

Superior vena cava

Right pulmonary artery

Thoracic vertebral body

Trapezius muscle

Sternum

Main pulmonary artery

Lung parenchyma

Superior pulmonary vein

Left descending interlobar pulmonary artery

Descending aorta

Figure 31.12 Lungs – MRI scan (axial view). Observe how normal lungs fill the chest cavity. MRI is not as good as CT in showing lung defects; this is because more time is required to obtain MRI scans, and movement of the heart and lungs during scanning causes distortion of the image

Diaphragm and posterior abdominal wall

The diaphragm and the posterior abdominal wall are two anatomically linked structures that support and protect the abdominal contents. The diaphragm is the primary muscle of breathing and separates the thorax from the abdomen, whereas the muscles of the posterior abdominal wall aid movements of the vertebral column and lower limb. The posterior abdominal wall extends from the posterior attachment of the diaphragm down to the iliac crests. Bony support is provided by the lower ribs, lower thoracic vertebrae, lumbar vertebrae, and the pelvis.

MUSCLES

The four muscles (Fig. 32.1A) of the posterior abdominal wall are the diaphragm, quadratus lumborum, iliacus, and psoas (Table 32.1).

Diaphragm

The diaphragm is a domed muscle with a central tendinous region. When viewed from the front (anteriorly), it has two upward-curving domes. The right dome passes over the liver, which causes it to be higher than the left dome. In the central tendinous part of the diaphragm are three major openings for the passage of important structures. From anterior to posterior, these openings are at vertebral levels TVIII, TX, and TXII/LI (Table 32.2).

Motor innervation to the diaphragm is provided by the **right** and **left phrenic nerves** (C3 to C5). The phrenic nerves also provide sensory innervation to the central part of the diaphragm. Sensory innervation to the peripheral parts of the diaphragm is provided by the intercostal nerves (T5 to T11) and the subcostal nerves (T12).

Blood is supplied to the diaphragm by the **superior phrenic arteries** (branches of the thoracic aorta), the **musculophrenic** and **pericardiacophrenic arteries** (branches of the internal thoracic arteries), and the **inferior phrenic arteries** (branches of the abdominal aorta).

Venous drainage is provided by the **musculophrenic** and **pericardiacophrenic veins**, which drain to the internal thoracic veins. The **right inferior phrenic vein** drains to the inferior vena cava; the **left inferior phrenic vein** drains to the left suprarenal vein, which then empties into the left renal vein.

Lymphatic drainage of the diaphragm is to lymphatic plexuses on the superior and inferior diaphragmatic surfaces. These lymphatic vessels in turn drain to the posterior mediastinal and superior lumbar lymph node groups.

Quadratus lumborum muscle

The quadratus lumborum muscle (Fig. 32.1A) is a rectangular muscle that fills the space between the most inferior rib (rib XII) and the superior part of the pelvis (the iliac crest). It aids breathing by supporting the diaphragm. It is also a lateral flexor of the trunk (see Table 32.1).

Psoas and iliacus muscles

These muscles originate from the internal surfaces of the lower lumbar vertebrae and pelvis, and join and insert as the iliopsoas muscle onto the lesser trochanter of the femur. The primary action of the iliopsoas muscle is to flex the thigh at the hip joint (see Table 32.1).

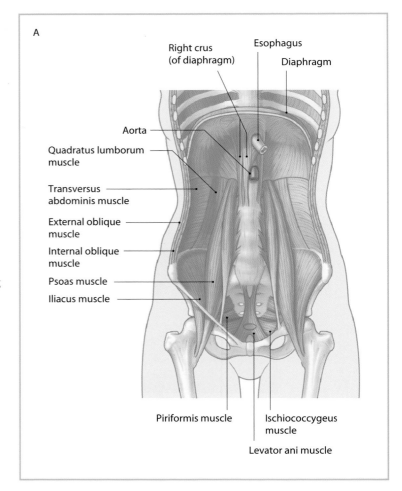

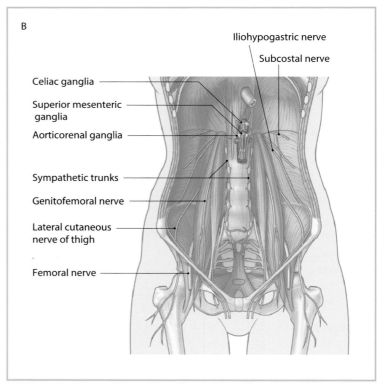

Figure 32.1 Muscles (A) and nerves (B) of the posterior abdominal wall

NERVES OF THE POSTERIOR ABDOMINAL WALL

The subcostal nerve is the anterior ramus of thoracic nerve T12. It enters the posterior wall of the abdomen next to the arcuate ligament of the diaphragm and crosses the quadratus lumborum muscle just posterior to the kidney. The subcostal nerve supplies muscles of the posterior abdominal wall, peritoneum, and the skin of the suprapubic region.

The lumbar part of the lumbosacral plexus of nerves (L1 to S3) is formed within the psoas major muscle by the web-like union of the anterior rami of lumbar nerves L1 to L4. Nerves branch from this part of the plexus to provide sensory and motor innervation to the lower abdomen, pelvis, and lower limb. The iliohypogastric and ilio-inguinal nerves (branches of L1) pass along the posterior abdominal wall.

- The **iliohypogastric nerve** supplies the skin superior to the inguinal ligament and the muscles of the anterior abdominal wall.
- Initially, the **ilio-inguinal nerve** passes parallel to the iliohypogastric nerve from their common origin at L1, and then passes through the internal inguinal ring to innervate the skin and muscles of the anterior abdominal wall and the skin of the external genitalia.
- The **genitofemoral nerve** (L1, L2) is identified as it descends on the anterior surface of the psoas major muscle (Fig. 32.1B). It divides into **genital branches** (which run through the inguinal canal to supply the cremasteric fascia of the scrotum and some of the skin of the genitalia) and **femoral branches** (which pass deep to the inguinal ligament and innervate the skin of the medial thigh).
- The **lateral cutaneous nerve of thigh** (L2, L3) crosses the iliacus muscle and passes deep to the lateral attachment of the inguinal ligament (see Fig. 32.1B). It supplies the peritoneum along its course and the skin of the lateral superior aspect of the thigh.
- The **femoral nerve** (L2 to L4) is identified as it descends along the posterior abdominal wall in a furrow between the psoas major and iliacus muscles. After supplying the iliacus muscle, it passes deep to the inguinal ligament lateral to the femoral artery and supplies the skin and muscles of the anterior compartment of thigh.
- The **obturator nerve** (L2 to L4) passes inferiorly along the medial side of the psoas major muscle and then along the lateral pelvic wall to enter the medial thigh through the obturator foramen. It supplies the skin and adductor muscles of the medial compartment of thigh (see Chapter 40). In the female pelvis the obturator nerve is lateral to the ovary.
- The **lumbosacral trunk** (L4, L5) is medial to the psoas major muscle and descends over the ala of the sacrum to join the sacral part of the lumbosacral plexus of nerves (S2 to S4), which then innervates structures of the pelvis (see Chapter 36).

ARTERIES

The **abdominal aorta** is the main artery supplying the posterior abdominal wall. It is a continuation of the thoracic aorta, which enters the abdomen between the two crura of the diaphragm at the anterior surface of vertebra TXII. It is usually slightly to the left of the midline and ends at vertebra LIV by branching into the **left** and **right common iliac arteries**. Each common iliac artery then divides into the **internal** and **external iliac arteries** (see Chapter 36):

- the internal iliac artery supplies pelvic structures, the gluteal region, and the genitalia;

- the external iliac artery is the main source of blood for the lower limb.

The abdominal aorta gives off visceral (to the organs) and parietal (to the abdominal wall) branches, which may be either single or paired. The unpaired **visceral branches** arise from the anterior aspect of the aorta and include the **celiac trunk** (Fig. 32.2A) and **superior**

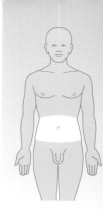

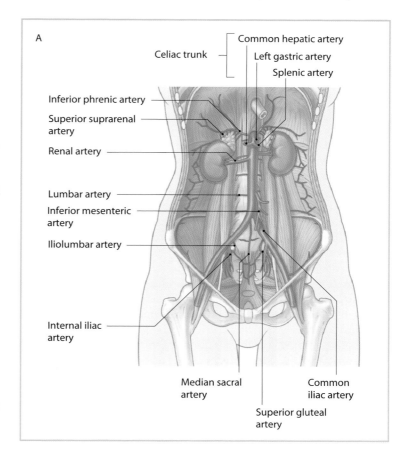

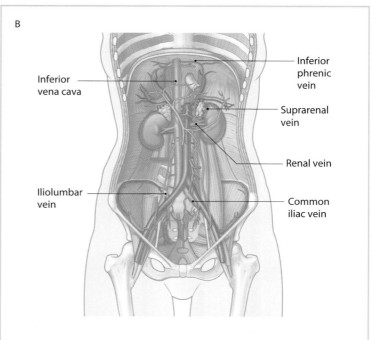

Figure 32.2 Arteries (A) and veins (B) of the posterior abdominal wall

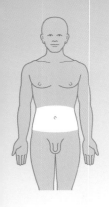

and **inferior mesenteric arteries**. These large vessels supply the lower esophagus, stomach, and the small and large intestines, which are derivatives of the embryonic foregut, midgut, and hindgut, respectively. Branches from these large vessels also supply the three unpaired organs of the abdomen – the liver, pancreas, and spleen.

The **visceral paired arteries** are the **suprarenal**, **renal**, and gonadal (**testicular** and **ovarian**) **arteries**.

The **parietal branches** are the paired **inferior phrenic arteries** (which supply the inferior surface of the diaphragm), the four or five paired **lumbar arteries** (which supply the posterior abdominal wall), and the **median sacral artery** (a single terminal branch that arises from the aorta posterior to its termination to supply the posterior pelvic wall).

There are many anastomoses between the visceral arteries, providing a rich blood supply to the digestive tract and organs.

VEINS AND LYMPHATICS

The largest vein in the posterior abdominal wall is the **inferior vena cava** (Fig. 32.2B), which is formed at vertebral level LIV by the union of the left and right **common iliac veins**. It ascends on the posterior abdominal wall to the right of the midline, passes through the central tendon of the diaphragm at vertebral level TVIII, and empties into the right atrium after a short course through the thoracic cavity.

Venous blood from the abdominal viscera (stomach, small and large intestines, gallbladder, pancreas, and spleen) drains into the **hepatic portal vein**. Subsequently it is processed and detoxified in the liver. It then enters the **hepatic veins**, which empty into the inferior vena cava.

Lymphatic drainage of the abdominal viscera and posterior abdominal wall is to lymph nodes along the origins of the primary arteries that supply the gastrointestinal tract – the **celiac**, **superior mesenteric**, and **inferior mesenteric nodes**. These nodes are **pre-aortic nodes**.

Lymph from the intestines drains along left and right **intestinal trunks**, which empty into the **cisterna chyli** (the root of the thoracic duct) along the midline posterior abdominal wall.

Lymph nodes along the lateral aspects of the aorta drain the posterior abdominal wall, kidneys, suprarenal glands and gonads (testes and ovaries). Their efferents form the **lumbar trunks**.

■ CLINICAL CORRELATIONS
Hiatus hernia and gastro-esophageal reflux disease (GERD)
A hiatus hernia is the abnormal herniation of proximal stomach into the thoracic cavity. This can result from a genetic predisposition, trauma, or other causes.

Under normal circumstances the distal esophagus is attached to the diaphragm and kept in place by ligamentous and membranous soft tissues. Disruption of this attachment can cause part of the distal esophagus to slide superiorly into the posterior mediastinum. There are three types of hiatus hernia (Fig. 32.3).

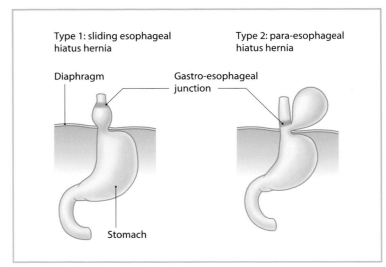

Figure 32.3 Common types of hiatus hernia

- Type I – sliding hiatus hernia – occurs when the distal esophagus and stomach are not adequately secured in place.
- Type II – para-esophageal or rolling hernia – occurs when the phrenico-esophageal ligament is intact, but the proximal stomach is not. The cardiac part of the stomach can slide upward through an abnormally large hiatus. In more severe cases, the spleen and colon may also herniate through the diaphragmatic hiatus into the chest cavity.
- Type III hernia – a combination of types I and II.

Patients with any of these abnormalities usually have a prolonged history of heartburn and dyspepsia. They may also report partial regurgitation of food products shortly after a meal. The pain is burning in nature and can cause chest pain, which is sometimes difficult to distinguish from cardiac chest pain in patients with myocardial infarction. In patients with hiatus hernia the symptoms subside after a time with no immediate sequelae. Sometimes, there are nonesophageal symptoms such as coughing, wheezing, and hoarse voice.

On examination there is usually no specific finding and the examination may be normal.

Initial management of hiatus hernia is medical. Physicians may recommend antacid medications. Some lifestyle changes are recommended, such as smoking cessation, decreasing alcohol and caffeine intake, avoiding illegal drug use, and eating small meals. If a routine course of medical management fails the patient may be referred to a surgeon for further investigation. Moderate-to-severe symptoms that fail to respond to medical management can be treated surgically using procedures to restore the normal position of the distal esophagus and proximal stomach.

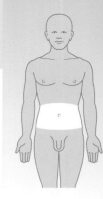

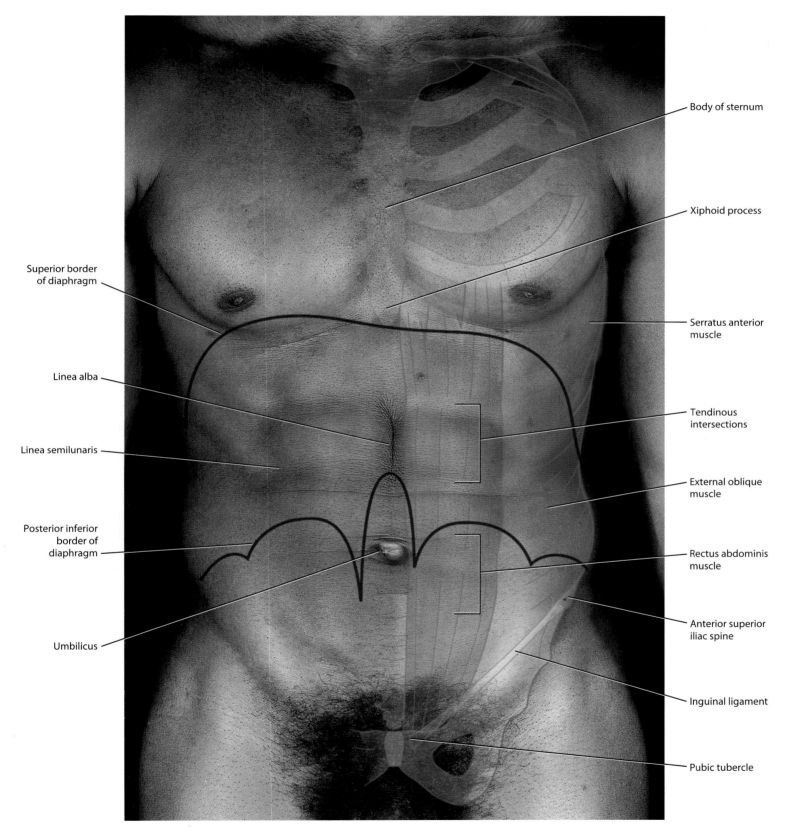

Body of sternum

Xiphoid process

Superior border of diaphragm

Serratus anterior muscle

Linea alba

Tendinous intersections

Linea semilunaris

External oblique muscle

Posterior inferior border of diaphragm

Rectus abdominis muscle

Anterior superior iliac spine

Umbilicus

Inguinal ligament

Pubic tubercle

Figure 32.4 Diaphragm and posterior abdominal wall – surface anatomy. Anterior view of the abdominal wall. The location of the xiphoid process of the sternum approximately delineates the anterior border of the diaphragm

375

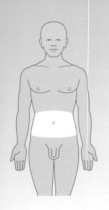

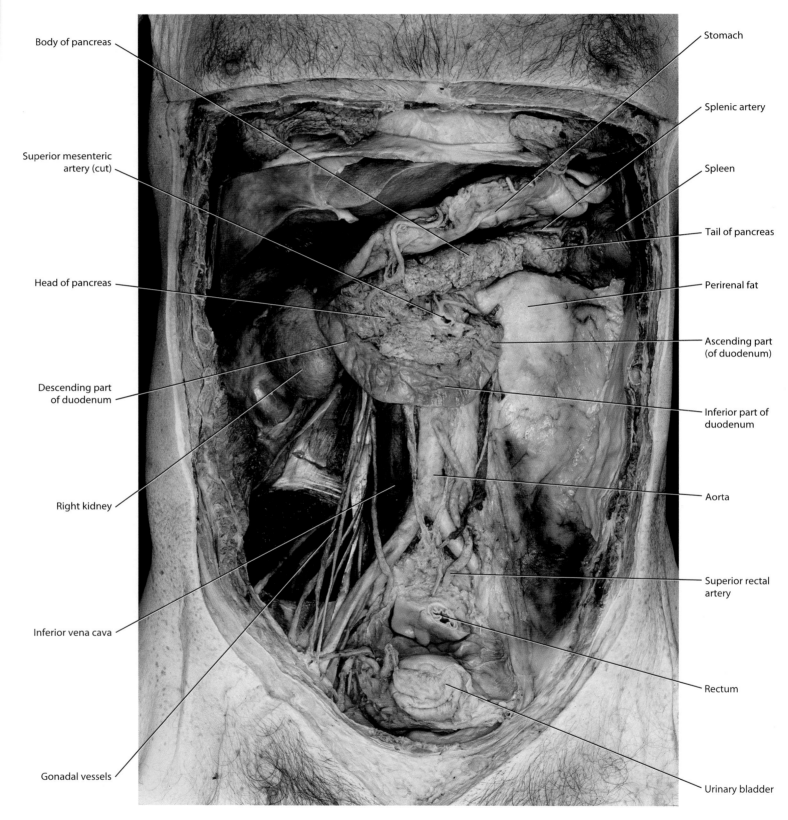

Body of pancreas

Superior mesenteric artery (cut)

Head of pancreas

Descending part of duodenum

Right kidney

Inferior vena cava

Gonadal vessels

Stomach

Splenic artery

Spleen

Tail of pancreas

Perirenal fat

Ascending part (of duodenum)

Inferior part of duodenum

Aorta

Superior rectal artery

Rectum

Urinary bladder

Figure 32.5 Diaphragm and posterior abdominal organs – superficial dissection. In this dissection the anterior part of the diaphragm is visible. Most of the intestine and colon have been removed to show some muscles of the posterior abdominal wall. The right kidney, which is retroperitoneal, is visible

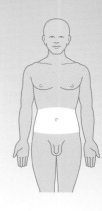

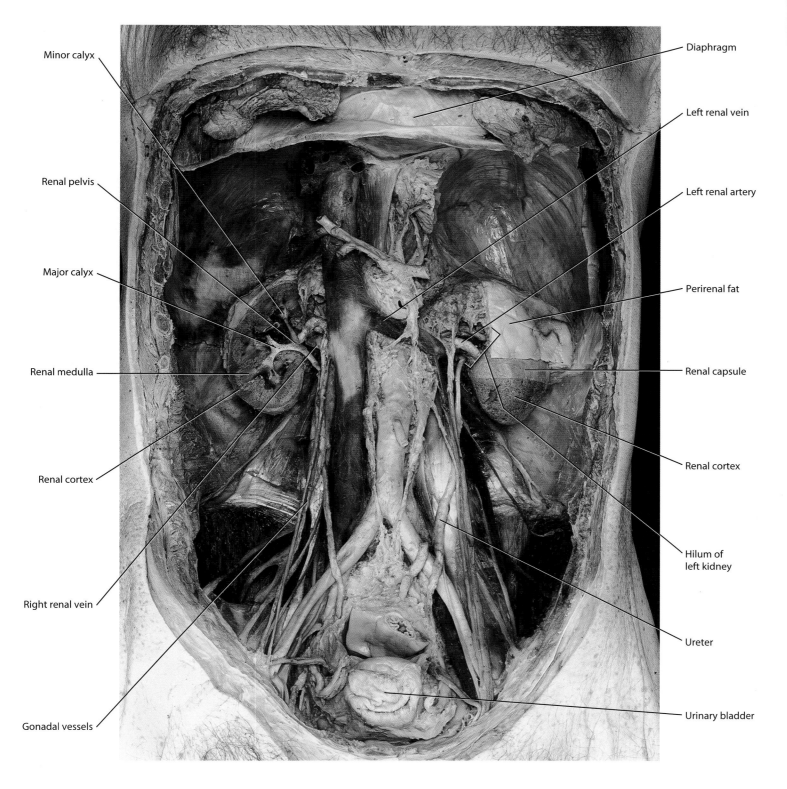

Minor calyx

Renal pelvis

Major calyx

Renal medulla

Renal cortex

Right renal vein

Gonadal vessels

Diaphragm

Left renal vein

Left renal artery

Perirenal fat

Renal capsule

Renal cortex

Hilum of
left kidney

Ureter

Urinary bladder

TRUNK Diaphragm and posterior abdominal wall

Figure 32.6 Diaphragm and posterior abdominal organs – intermediate dissection 1. Anterior view of the posterior abdominal wall. The kidneys are shown in section on the right and the layers of renal fascia on the left. This dissection shows the dome-like structure of the diaphragm and its relationship to the posterior abdominal wall

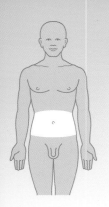

Diaphragm and posterior abdominal wall **TRUNK**

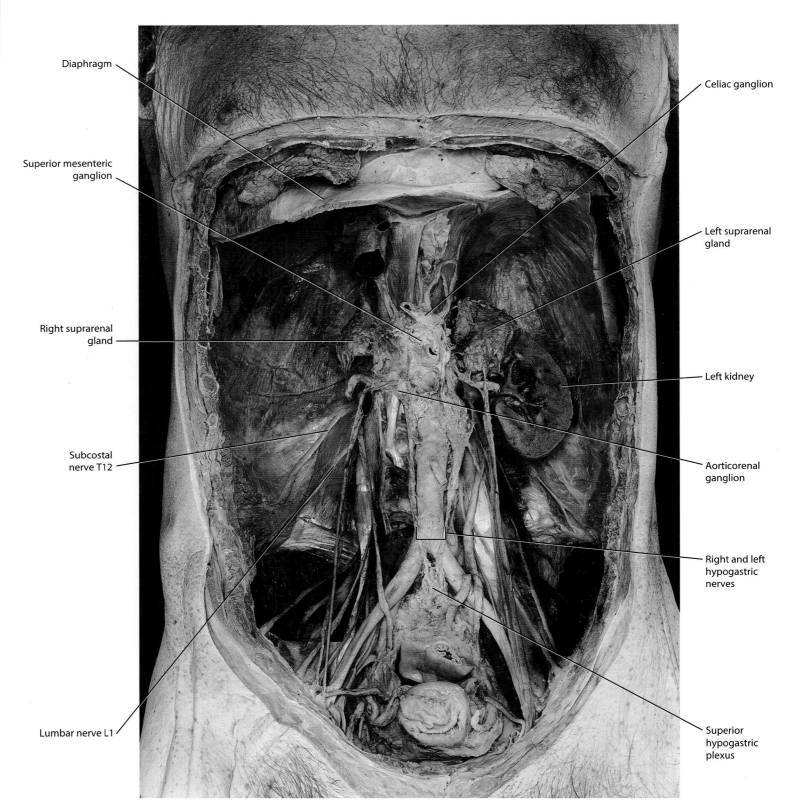

Diaphragm

Celiac ganglion

Superior mesenteric ganglion

Left suprarenal gland

Right suprarenal gland

Left kidney

Subcostal nerve T12

Aorticorenal ganglion

Right and left hypogastric nerves

Lumbar nerve L1

Superior hypogastric plexus

Figure 32.7 Diaphragm and posterior abdominal organs – intermediate dissection 2. Anterior view of the posterior abdominal wall, showing the suprarenal glands. The internal surface of the right posterior abdominal wall is visible. Observe the nerves in this area

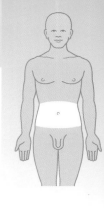

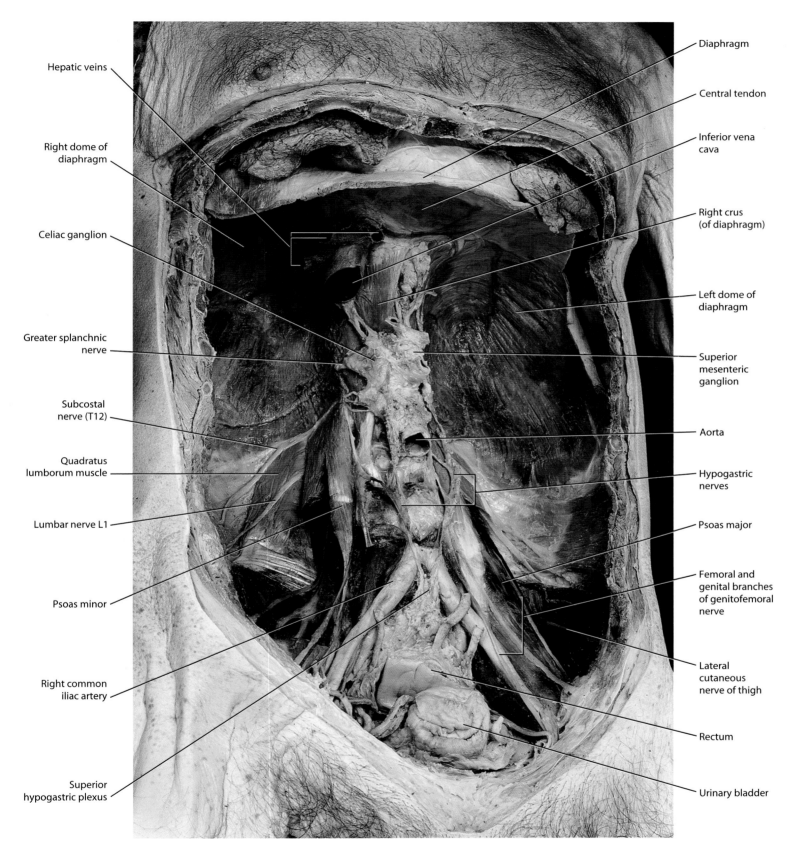

Hepatic veins

Right dome of
diaphragm

Celiac ganglion

Greater splanchnic
nerve

Subcostal
nerve (T12)

Quadratus
lumborum muscle

Lumbar nerve L1

Psoas minor

Right common
iliac artery

Superior
hypogastric plexus

Diaphragm

Central tendon

Inferior vena
cava

Right crus
(of diaphragm)

Left dome of
diaphragm

Superior
mesenteric
ganglion

Aorta

Hypogastric
nerves

Psoas major

Femoral and
genital branches
of genitofemoral
nerve

Lateral
cutaneous
nerve of thigh

Rectum

Urinary bladder

TRUNK Diaphragm and posterior abdominal wall

Figure 32.8 Diaphragm and posterior abdominal wall – deep dissection 1. Anterolateral and slightly inferior view of the posterior abdominal wall showing the posterior abdominal musculature and neurovascular structures. Observe the central tendon and the left and right domes of the diaphragm. Also observe the quadratus lumborum muscle

379

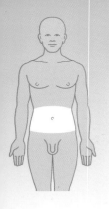

TABLE 32.1 MUSCLES OF THE POSTERIOR ABDOMINAL WALL

Muscle	Origin	Insertion	Nerve supply	Action	Blood supply
Diaphragm	Xiphoid process, lower six costal cartilages, lateral and medial arcuate ligaments, crura (LII and LIII), median arcuate ligaments	Central tendon	Phrenic (C3 to C5)	Chief muscles of respiration	Pericardiacophrenic musculophrenic, superior and inferior phrenic arteries
Quadratus lumborum	Iliolumbar ligament, iliac crest, lower lumbar transverse processes	Rib XII and upper lumbar transverse processes	T12 to L3	Fixes rib XII, flexes trunk, flexes vertebral column laterally	Iliolumbar artery
Psoas major	Lumbar vertebrae	Lesser trochanter	L2 to L4	See iliacus muscle	Lumbar arteries
Iliacus*	Floor of iliac fossa	Tendon of the psoas major muscle and lesser trochanter	Femoral nerve	Flexes and rotates thigh medially, then rotates the thigh laterally, flexes vertebral column	Iliolumbar artery
Psoas minor#	Vertebrae TXII to LI and intervertebral disc	Pectineal ligament and iliac fascia	L1	Helps flex vertebral column	Lumbar arteries

* Joins psoas major to form iliopsoas muscle.
# Frequently absent.

TABLE 32.2 OPENINGS IN THE DIAPHRAGM AND THE STRUCTURES PASSING THROUGH THEM

Openings	Structures	Vertebral levels
Inferior vena cava (central tendon)	Inferior vena cava, right phrenic nerve	TVIII
Esophageal hiatus	Esophagus, vagal trunks, esophageal branches of left gastric artery	TX
Aortic hiatus	Aorta, thoracic duct, azygos, and hemi-azygos veins	TXII (behind the diaphragm, between the crura)
Other structures that pass through the diaphragm	Left phrenic nerve	Left dome of diaphragm
	Splanchnic nerves	Crura of diaphragm
	Sympathetic trunks	Posterior to medial arcuate ligament
	Subcostal nerve and vessels	Posterior to lateral arcuate ligament
	Superior epigastric vessels	Anterior between costal and sternal attachments
	Musculophrenic vessels	Between the seventh and eighth costal cartilages

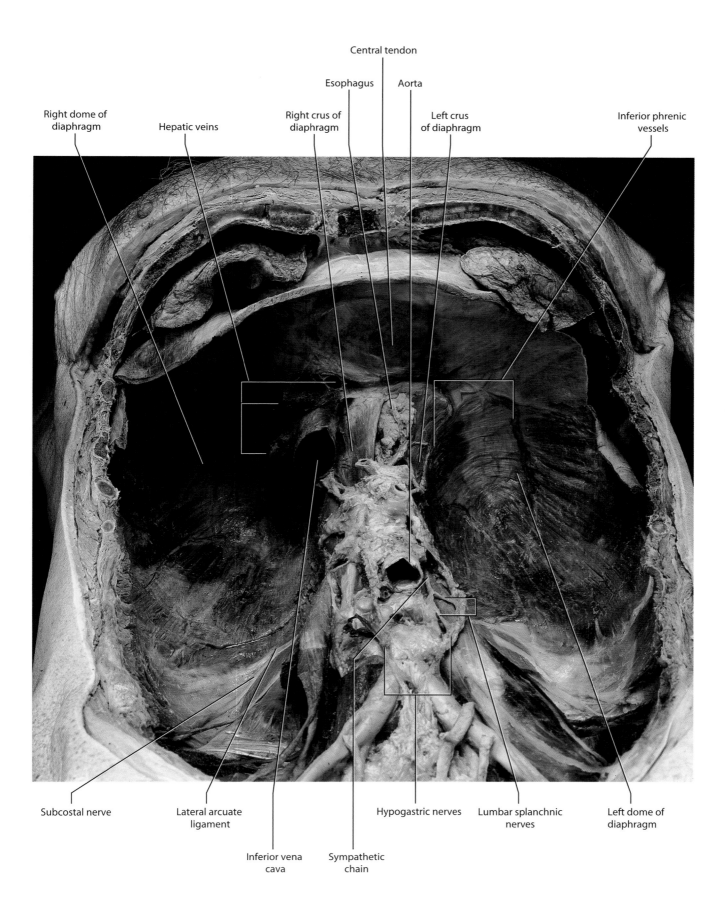

Central tendon

Esophagus   Aorta

Right dome of   Hepatic veins   Right crus of   Left crus   Inferior phrenic
diaphragm   diaphragm   of diaphragm   vessels

Subcostal nerve   Lateral arcuate   Hypogastric nerves   Lumbar splanchnic   Left dome of
                         ligament   nerves   diaphragm

Inferior vena   Sympathetic
cava   chain

TRUNK   Diaphragm and posterior abdominal wall

Figure 32.9 Diaphragm and posterior abdominal wall – deep dissection 2. This view looks up into the diaphragm and demonstrates the domes of the diaphragm and structures that pass through it. The central tendon of the diaphragm is clearly visible

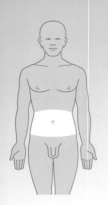

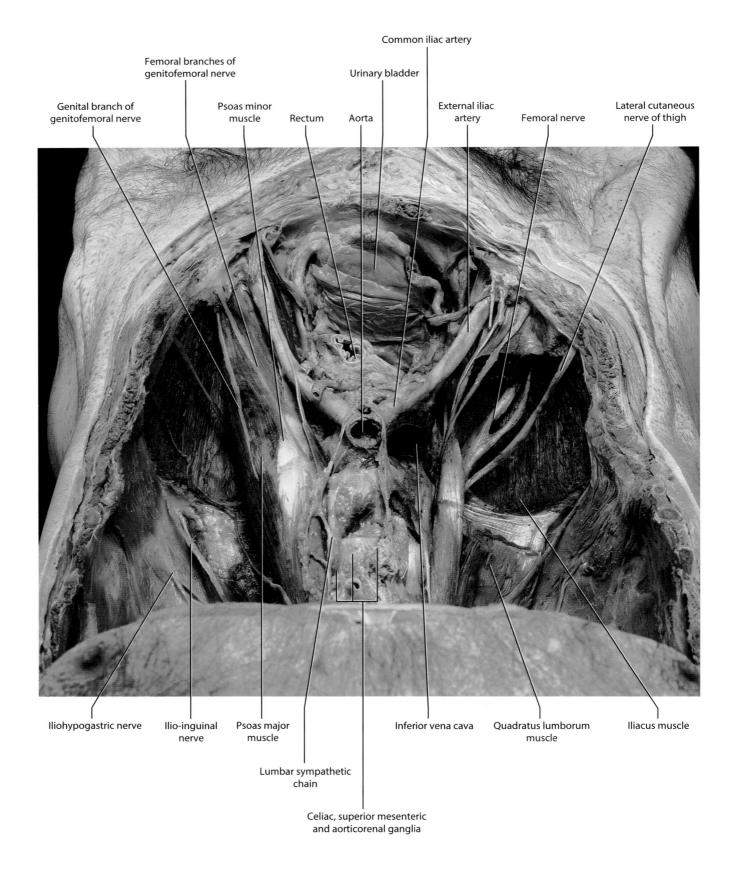

Genital branch of
genitofemoral nerve

Femoral branches of
genitofemoral nerve

Psoas minor
muscle

Rectum

Aorta

Urinary bladder

Common iliac artery

External iliac
artery

Femoral nerve

Lateral cutaneous
nerve of thigh

Iliohypogastric nerve

Ilio-inguinal
nerve

Psoas major
muscle

Inferior vena cava

Quadratus lumborum
muscle

Iliacus muscle

Lumbar sympathetic
chain

Celiac, superior mesenteric
and aorticorenal ganglia

Figure 32.10 Diaphragm and posterior abdominal wall – deep dissection 3. Anterior superior view, looking down into the pelvis at components of the lumbar plexus. Observe the quadratus lumborum muscles and how they are related to the iliacus muscles

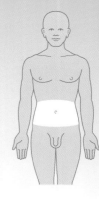

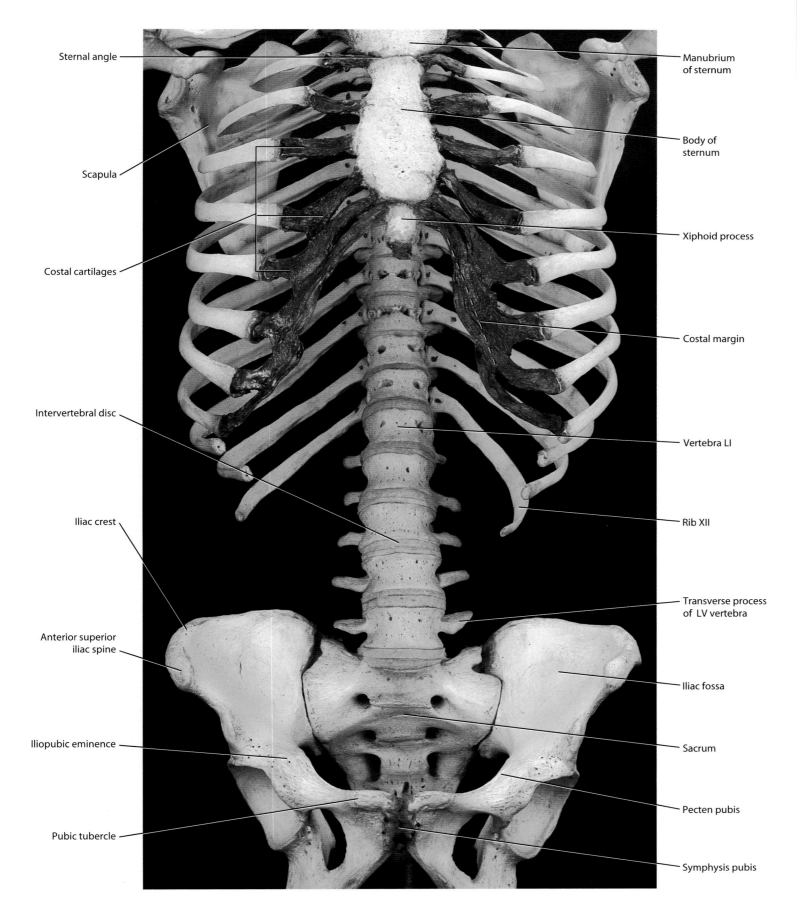

Sternal angle

Scapula

Costal cartilages

Intervertebral disc

Iliac crest

Anterior superior
iliac spine

Iliopubic eminence

Pubic tubercle

Manubrium
of sternum

Body of
sternum

Xiphoid process

Costal margin

Vertebra LI

Rib XII

Transverse process
of LV vertebra

Iliac fossa

Sacrum

Pecten pubis

Symphysis pubis

Figure 32.11 Diaphragm and posterior abdominal wall – osteology. Anterior view of the articulated skeleton, which encloses the diaphragm and posterior abdominal wall

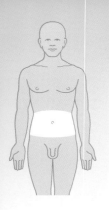

TRUNK

Diaphragm and posterior abdominal wall

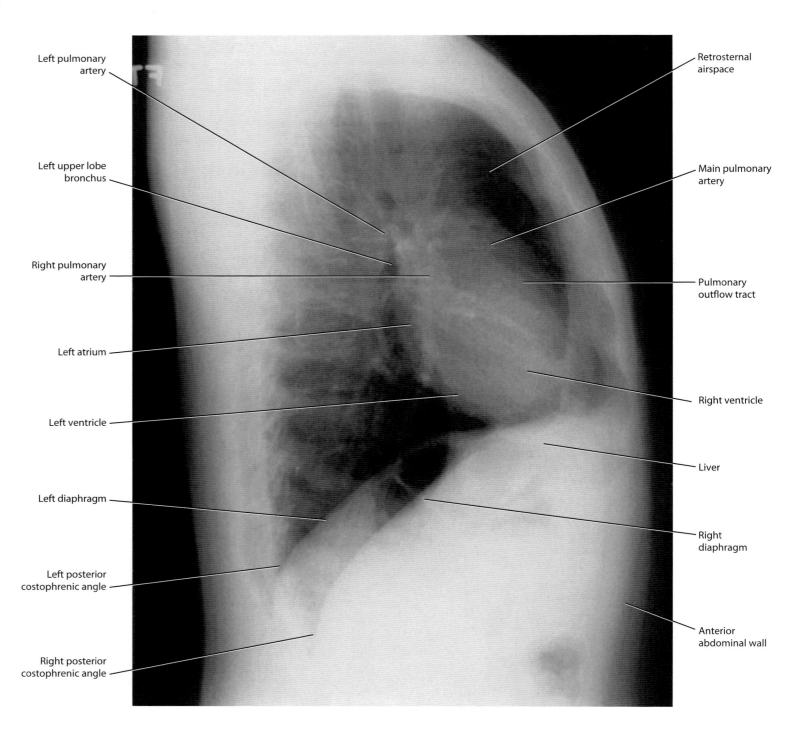

Left pulmonary artery

Left upper lobe bronchus

Right pulmonary artery

Left atrium

Left ventricle

Left diaphragm

Left posterior costophrenic angle

Right posterior costophrenic angle

Retrosternal airspace

Main pulmonary artery

Pulmonary outflow tract

Right ventricle

Liver

Right diaphragm

Anterior abdominal wall

Figure 32.12 Diaphragm and posterior abdominal wall – plain film radiograph (lateral view). Note that the posterior aspect of the lungs projects well below the apex of the diaphragm. This is clinically important because a posteroanterior radiograph will not show abnormalities of the lower parts of both lungs; both views should be requested when assessing the lungs radiographically. The heart shadow is clearly visible as a gray zone located superior to the diaphragm in the anterior chest cavity. This is in contrast with Figure 29.12. Both films are normal films, however the radiographic technicians have utilized different methods in obtaining the film. The differences demonstrate the difficulty in assessing a single radiograph. In many cases several views are obtained and correlated with the physical examination of the patient before a clinical diagnosis is made

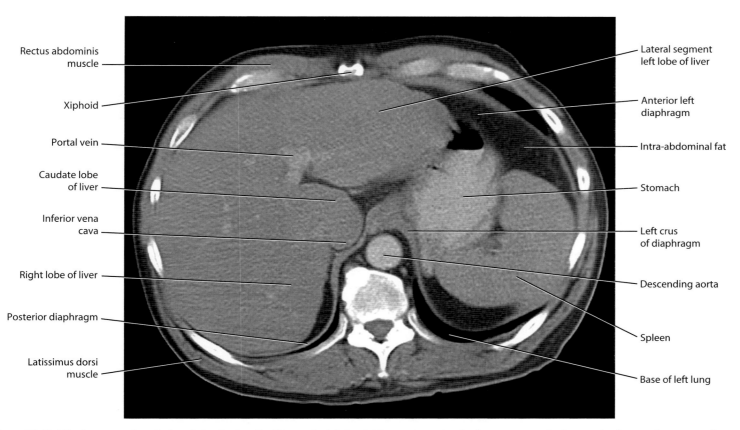

Rectus abdominis muscle

Xiphoid

Portal vein

Caudate lobe of liver

Inferior vena cava

Right lobe of liver

Posterior diaphragm

Latissimus dorsi muscle

Lateral segment left lobe of liver

Anterior left diaphragm

Intra-abdominal fat

Stomach

Left crus of diaphragm

Descending aorta

Spleen

Base of left lung

Figure 32.13 Diaphragm and posterior abdominal wall – CT scan (axial view). Observe how the diaphragm covers the liver and spleen and separates them from the lungs. Compare this image with Figure 32.09 to see the left and right crus of the diaphragm, which are posterior attachment points that permit passage of the esophagus from the chest to the abdomen and also help join the diaphragm to the posterior body wall

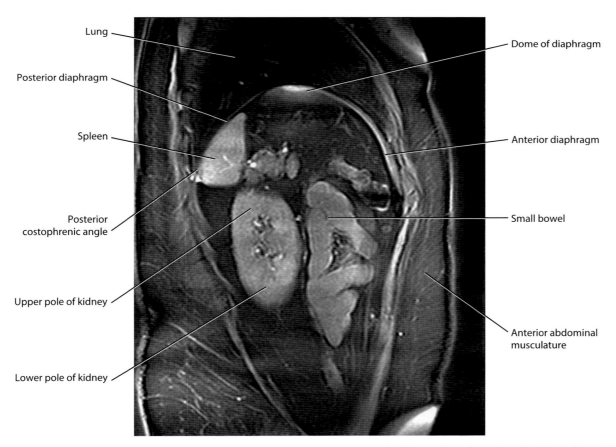

Lung

Posterior diaphragm

Spleen

Posterior costophrenic angle

Upper pole of kidney

Lower pole of kidney

Dome of diaphragm

Anterior diaphragm

Small bowel

Anterior abdominal musculature

Figure 32.14 Diaphragm and posterior abdominal wall – MRI scan (sagittal view). This scan left of the midline shows how the dome shape of the diaphragm is better appreciated in a sagittal view. Note how the spleen is closely apposed to the diaphragm and the upper part of the left kidney

The **abdominopelvic cavity** contains a large proportion of the digestive (see Chapter 34) and urogenital organs (see Chapter 37) and their supporting neurovascular structures. It is enclosed by:

- the musculotendinous thoracic diaphragm superiorly (see Chapter 32);
- the muscular abdominal wall anterolaterally (see Chapter 35);
- a bony and muscular wall posteriorly;
- the fibromuscular pelvic diaphragm inferiorly.

The abdominopelvic cavity contains the abdominal organs – the liver, gallbladder, spleen, pancreas, kidneys, and suprarenal glands. The liver, gallbladder, and spleen are contained in the **peritoneal cavity**. The **retroperitoneal space** – the area posterior to the peritoneal cavity – houses the pancreas, kidneys, and suprarenal glands (Fig. 33.1).

Bony support for the abdominopelvic cavity is provided by the inferior ribs, the thoracic and lumbar vertebrae, and the superior part of the pelvis. The muscles described in Chapters 25, 32, and 36 also support this region.

LIVER

The liver (Fig. 33.2) is the largest glandular organ in the body and is in the right upper quadrant of the peritoneal cavity of the abdomen. It is subphrenic and is protected by the lower right ribs.

The liver receives blood from the hepatic portal vein (see Chapter 34), which carries nutrients from the gastrointestinal tract. Within the liver, these substances are metabolized by the appropriate pathway.

The superior surface of the liver (the **diaphragmatic surface**) interfaces with the diaphragm, and the inferior surface (the **visceral surface**) interfaces with the gastrointestinal tract. The liver is enclosed in peritoneum, except a small part of the diaphragmatic surface (the **bare area**). The **triangular**, **falciform**, and **coronary** ligaments, which are at the ends of the bare area, tether the liver to the diaphragm. The falciform ligament, which is between the left and right anatomical lobes of the liver, extends anteriorly from the liver to insert onto the internal surface of the anterior abdominal wall. Embryologically, the **round ligament of liver** contains the umbilical vessels as they enter the abdomen and traverse the liver to provide blood directly to the heart.

On the right side of the visceral surface of the liver are the gallbladder and inferior vena cava. On the left side the **fissure for round ligament**, **falciform ligament**, and **ligamentum venosum** divide the liver into left and right lobes. At the midpoint between the gallbladder and inferior vena cava is the **porta hepatis**, which is the entrance and exit point for the hepatic arteries, hepatic portal vein, hepatic ducts, autonomic nerves, and lymphatic vessels.

The liver is subdivided into **left**, **right**, **quadrate**, and **caudate lobes**:

- the division into left and right lobes is defined by the falciform ligament and the round ligament of liver;
- the quadrate lobe is bounded by the fossa for the gallbladder, round ligament of liver, fissure for ligamentum venosum, and the porta hepatis;

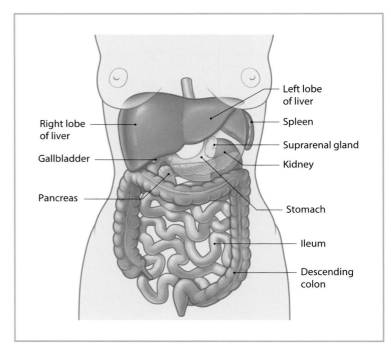

Figure 33.1 Solid abdominal organs in situ

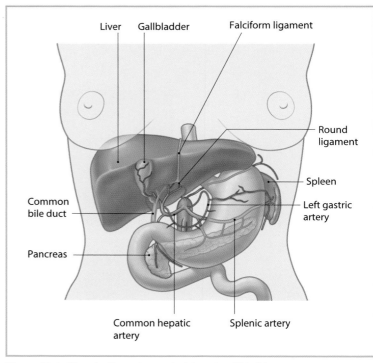

Figure 33.2 Liver (reflected superiorly) and gallbladder

- the caudate lobe is bounded by the **groove for the inferior vena cava**, fissure for the ligamentum venosum, and the porta hepatis.

The liver is innervated by the **hepatic plexus** of nerves, a subdivision of the celiac plexus, along the abdominal aorta. Autonomic nerve fibers follow the course of the hepatic arteries and portal veins to the liver. Sympathetic innervation is postganglionic from the **celiac ganglion**; parasympathetic innervation is from the **vagus nerve [X]**.

Approximately 30% of the blood supply to the liver is from the **left** and **right hepatic arteries**, which enter the liver at the porta hepatis. The remaining 70% is from the hepatic portal vein, which carries blood poor in oxygen but rich in absorbed digestive products.

Venous drainage of the liver is provided by **left**, **intermediate**, and **right hepatic veins**, which empty into the inferior vena cava along the posterior border of the liver.

Lymphatic drainage of the liver is through vessels that exit the liver at the porta hepatis and drain to abdominal lymph node groups at the liver and along the abdominal aorta.

GALLBLADDER

The gallbladder (Fig. 33.1) is a pear-shaped green reservoir that stores approximately 30–50 ml of bile. It lies on the visceral (inferior) surface of the liver, suspended by peritoneal attachments. The gallbladder receives bile from the liver through the **common hepatic duct** and **cystic duct**. It concentrates the bile by absorbing water and salts. During digestion, as fats enter the small intestine, the gallbladder secretes concentrated bile into the cystic duct, which empties into the **bile duct**. From here the bile enters the duodenum at the **major duodenal papilla**. Secreted bile contains enzymes that continue the digestion of fats in the partially digested food.

Innervation of the gallbladder is autonomic and from the **hepatic plexus**. Blood supply is from the **cystic artery**, which is usually a branch of the right hepatic artery. Venous drainage is by the **cystic vein** to the hepatic portal vein. Lymphatic drainage is to nodes at the porta hepatis and **celiac lymph nodes**.

PANCREAS

The pancreas (Fig. 33.3) is a slender yellow gland that has both exocrine and endocrine functions. It is in the retroperitoneal space

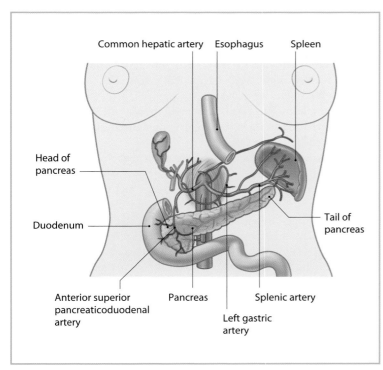

Head of pancreas

Duodenum

Common hepatic artery   Esophagus   Spleen

Tail of pancreas

Anterior superior pancreaticoduodenal artery

Pancreas

Splenic artery

Left gastric artery

Figure 33.3 Pancreas and spleen in situ

and has three parts – the **head of pancreas** with the **uncinate process**, the **body of pancreas**, and the **tail of pancreas**. The **main pancreatic duct** resides within the tail of the pancreas and empties towards the bile duct. The **accessory pancreatic duct** usually drains sequentially into the duodenum.

The exocrine function of the pancreas involves the production of pancreatic enzymes, which are secreted into the bile duct and enter the duodenum through the hepatopancreatic ampulla. These enzymes, in conjunction with bile, digest the food that enters the small intestine from the stomach.

The endocrine function of the pancreas is the secretion of the hormones insulin and glucagon, which play a role in blood glucose homeostasis.

Innervation to the pancreas is provided by the sympathetic **splanchnic nerves** along the posterior thoracic wall and the vagus nerves [X] through the **celiac** and **superior mesenteric plexuses**. Blood is supplied by the **superior** and **inferior pancreaticoduodenal arterial arcades** and the **splenic artery**. Venous drainage is through the **splenic vein**, which empties into the hepatic portal vein. Lymphatic drainage is through vessels that follow the course of the splenic artery to the **celiac** and **pre-aortic nodes**.

SPLEEN

The spleen (Fig. 33.3) is the largest lymphoid organ in the body and is in the left upper quadrant of the abdomen deep to the ribs. Within the peritoneum, it is suspended by two ligaments named after the sites to which they attach:

- the **splenorenal ligament** attaches the spleen to the left kidney;
- the **gastrosplenic ligament** attaches the spleen to the stomach.

The spleen breaks down 'worn-out' blood cells and monitors the blood for antigen–antibody complexes, which indicate the presence of infectious agents. Nerves and blood vessels enter and exit the spleen at the **splenic hilum** on the medial border of the spleen.

Innervation to the spleen is by autonomic nerves from the **celiac plexus**. Blood is supplied by the **splenic artery**, a branch from the celiac trunk. Venous drainage is through the **splenic vein**, which empties into the hepatic portal vein. Lymphatic drainage is to nodes along the course of the splenic artery and lymph nodes along the aorta (e.g. pre-aortic nodes).

KIDNEY

The kidneys (Fig. 33.4) are a pair of 'bean-shaped' organs deep and inferior to the pancreas along either side of the vertebral column in the retroperitoneal space at vertebral levels TXI to LI/LII. They are the filtration center for the body, removing impurities such as nitrogenous waste (urea) from the blood and controlling intravascular volume. The fluid and metabolic byproducts filtered out of the blood enter the **renal pelvis** where they become part of the **urine**, which flows along the **ureters** to the **urinary bladder** and subsequently leaves the body through the **urethra**.

Neurovascular structures enter the kidney at the medially facing **hilum of kidney**. The kidney is innervated by sympathetic nerves derived from T12 and L1 spinal nerves; the **vagus nerves [X]** provide parasympathetic innervation. Blood is supplied by the **renal arteries**, which are direct branches off the abdominal aorta at vertebral level LII (Table 33.1). The **left renal vein**, which receives the left gonadal vein and suprarenal veins, exits the hilum and

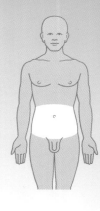

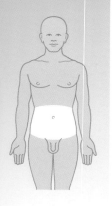
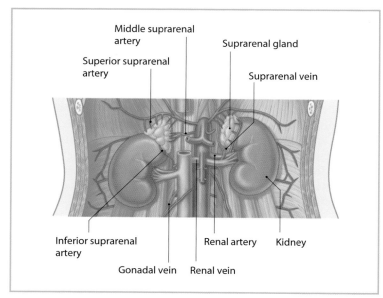

Figure 33.4 Kidneys

crosses the aorta anteriorly to enter the inferior vena cava. The **right renal vein** empties into the inferior vena cava. Lymphatics drain to the **renal**, **lumbar**, and **para-aortic lymph node groups**.

SUPRARENAL GLANDS

Resting on the superior surface of each kidney are the pyramid-shaped suprarenal (adrenal) glands. These endocrine glands have an outer **cortex** and inner **medulla**:

- the cortex secretes hormones that affect general metabolism, sexual development, electrolyte balance, and regulation of blood pressure;
- the medulla secretes the hormones epinephrine (adrenaline) and norepinephrine (noradrenaline), which are components of the sympathetic nervous system and play a role in the 'fight or flight' response.

The suprarenal glands are innervated by the **aorticorenal plexus**, which contains both parasympathetic and sympathetic fibers. The blood supply is from the **superior**, **middle**, and **inferior suprarenal arteries** that arise from the inferior phrenic artery, the aorta, and the renal arteries, respectively. The veins follow the course of the arteries but empty into a single **suprarenal vein** on each side; on the left side this empties into the renal vein and on the right side into the inferior vena cava.

■ CLINICAL CORRELATIONS

Gallstones

Gallstones (cholelithiasis) are stone-like deposits within the gallbladder. The gallbladder stores and concentrates bile secreted by the liver, and abnormal metabolism of bile can result in gallstones – cholesterol and pigment stones are the two most common types.

Gallstones typically cause pain in the epigastric region or right upper quadrant of the abdomen after eating a meal containing a

large amount of fat. The pain may be constant or may come and go in waves (biliary colic), occasionally radiating to the right shoulder or tip of the scapula. Associated symptoms include nausea and vomiting. Intermittent episodes of biliary colic may occur over a long period of time until at some point a painful episode occurs that does not resolve. This prolonged pain, which is usually more intense, is often what causes the patient to seek medical advice.

On examination, the patient is tender to palpation in the right hypochondrium of the abdomen. A positive Murphy's sign is elicited if the patient experiences a sharp increase in pain during inspiration with the examiner's hand palpating the right hypochondrium. This physical finding is unique to cholecystitis (inflammation of the gallbladder). In addition, some patients are pyrexic and jaundiced as a result of obstruction to the biliary output from the gallbladder and the resultant entry of bile into the blood.

Ultrasound is the imaging modality of choice in evaluating biliary dysfunction. In patients with cholecystitis (inflammation of the gallbladder) ultrasound may demonstrate an enlarged gallbladder with thickened walls and demonstrate stones within the gallbladder or biliary duct system.

If the patient's condition does not resolve spontaneously, the usual recommendation is a course of antibiotics and cholecystectomy (removal of the gallbladder) to prevent further complications such as infection, sepsis, and other abdominal sequelae.

Kidney stones

Kidney stones (nephrolithiasis) are quite common. Like gallstones, a genetic predisposition is a causal factor, but there is also a positive correlation with eating certain foods (e.g. those resulting in hypercalcemia). Stones may develop secondary to a variation in the metabolism and secretion of substances by the kidney. Approximately 80 to 90% of large kidney stones (such as calcium oxalate stones) are radiopaque and are visible on radiography, but uric acid stones are not.

Typically, kidney stones cause a sudden onset of flank and back pain with some radiation to the lateral abdomen. The pain is intense and may come and go in waves. There may be blood in the urine. Patients with such intense pain frequently go to the emergency room for treatment.

On examination there is usually tenderness at the costophrenic angle, where the ribs meet the diaphragm, and microscopic hematuria (blood in the urine).

A diagnosis of kidney stones is best confirmed by computed tomography (CT) without intravenous contrast, although intravenous pyelograms (an older diagnostic method) and other diagnostic modalities, such as ultrasound, may also be used. The kidney stones are visible as small white objects on the film.

Management of kidney stones includes analgesia for patient comfort. Stones filtered from the urine are sent for analysis and the results then guide the clinician in assisting the patient to prevent further stone formation. Rarely, the stones are too large to pass through the urinary system. Referral to a urologist for further evaluation is then necessary and the stones can be surgically removed by lithotripsy.

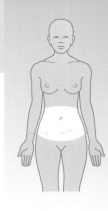

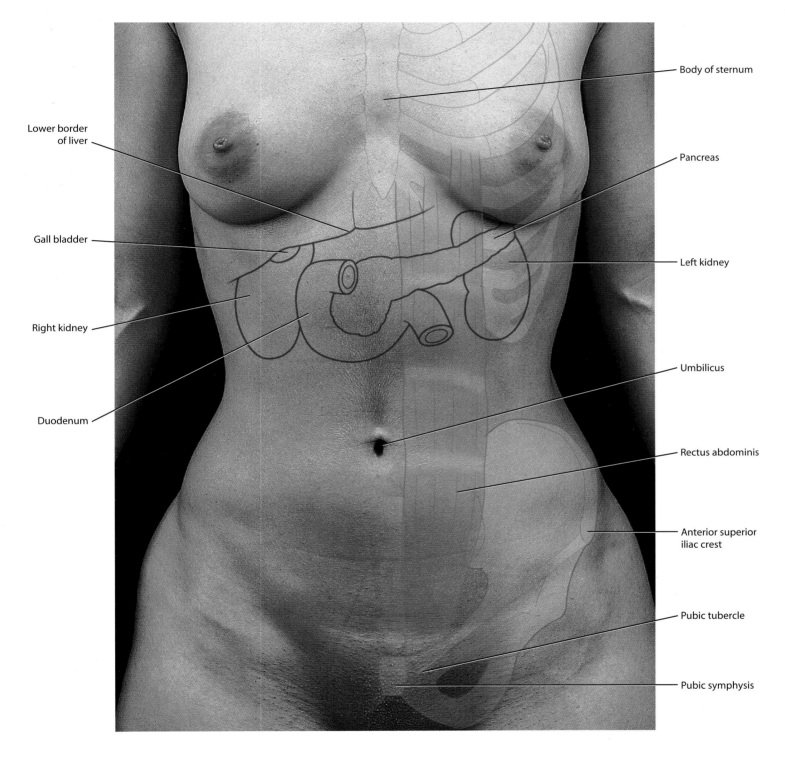

Body of sternum

Lower border of liver

Pancreas

Gall bladder

Left kidney

Right kidney

Duodenum

Umbilicus

Rectus abdominis

Anterior superior iliac crest

Pubic tubercle

Pubic symphysis

Figure 33.5 Abdomen – surface anatomy. Observe the umbilicus, which is usually located at the level of the bifurcation of the aorta in thin individuals

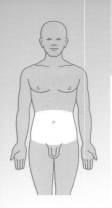

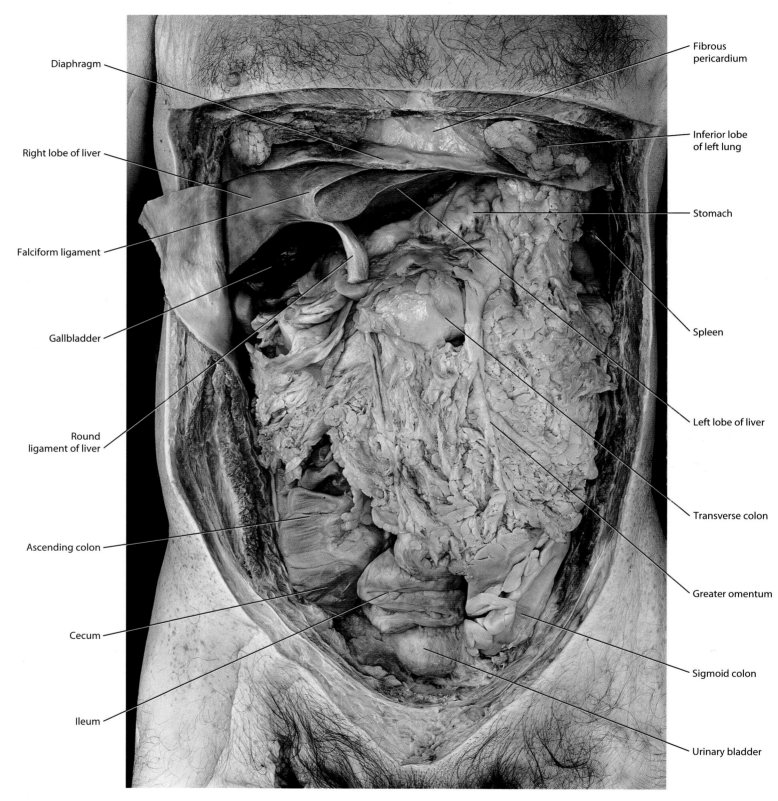

Diaphragm

Right lobe of liver

Falciform ligament

Gallbladder

Round
ligament of liver

Ascending colon

Cecum

Ileum

Fibrous
pericardium

Inferior lobe
of left lung

Stomach

Spleen

Left lobe of liver

Transverse colon

Greater omentum

Sigmoid colon

Urinary bladder

Figure 33.6 Abdominal organs – superficial dissection 1. The anterior abdominal wall has been removed to show the entire abdomen as it appears undissected. Observe the location of the stomach and the greater omentum, which is suspended from the greater curvature of the stomach. Also note the terminal ileum and ascending colon in the right lower quadrant of the abdomen

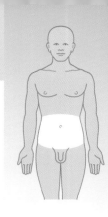

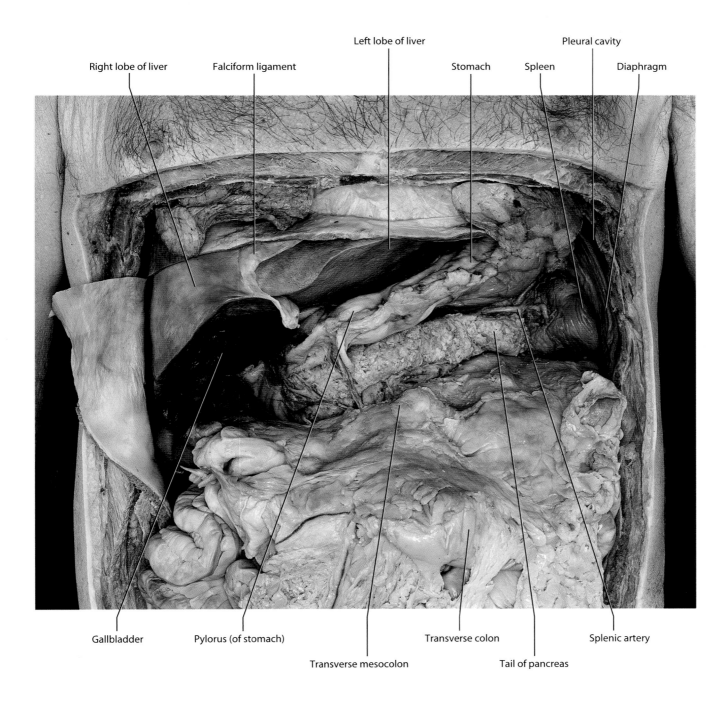

Right lobe of liver   Falciform ligament   Left lobe of liver   Stomach   Spleen   Pleural cavity   Diaphragm

Gallbladder   Pylorus (of stomach)   Transverse mesocolon   Transverse colon   Tail of pancreas   Splenic artery

Figure 33.7 Abdominal organs – superficial dissection 2. Anterior view of the supracolic (superior to the colon) compartment showing the interrelationships between the liver, gallbladder, pancreas, spleen, and transverse colon. The anterior abdominal wall has been removed to show the liver and spleen as they lie in relationship to the stomach and greater omentum

391

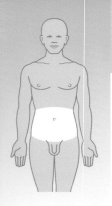

TABLE 33.1 BRANCHES OF THE ABDOMINAL AORTA				
Vessel	**Vertebral level**	**Paired**	**Single**	**Distribution**
Inferior phrenic	TXII	√		Crura and inferior surface of diaphragm and the suprarenal gland
Celiac trunk	TXII		√	Esophagus (lower), stomach, duodenum, liver, pancreas, spleen
Superior mesenteric	LI		√	Pancreas, duodenum, jejunum, ileum, cecum, appendix, ascending colon, and transverse colon
Suprarenal	LI	√		Suprarenal glands
Renal	LII	√		Kidneys, ureter, and suprarenal gland
Gonadal (ovarian/testicular)	LIII	√		Ovary/testis, ureter
Inferior mesenteric	LIII		√	Transverse, descending, and sigmoid colon, rectum
Lumbar (four pairs)	LI to LIV	√		Vertebral column, spinal cord, posterior abdominal wall
Median sacral	LIV		√	Rectum, sacrum

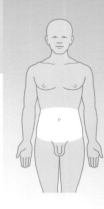

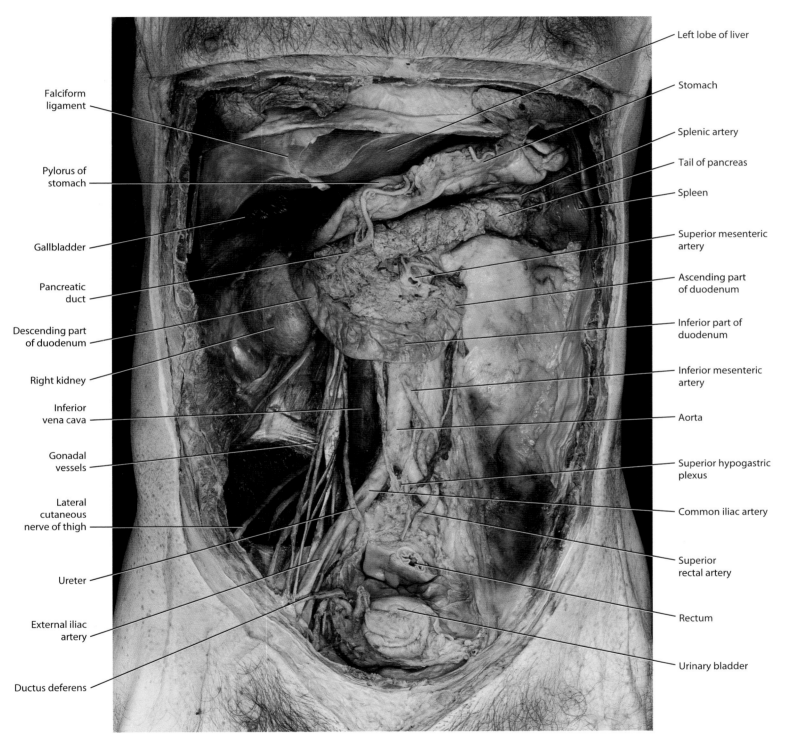

Falciform ligament

Pylorus of stomach

Gallbladder

Pancreatic duct

Descending part of duodenum

Right kidney

Inferior vena cava

Gonadal vessels

Lateral cutaneous nerve of thigh

Ureter

External iliac artery

Ductus deferens

Left lobe of liver

Stomach

Splenic artery

Tail of pancreas

Spleen

Superior mesenteric artery

Ascending part of duodenum

Inferior part of duodenum

Inferior mesenteric artery

Aorta

Superior hypogastric plexus

Common iliac artery

Superior rectal artery

Rectum

Urinary bladder

Figure 33.8 Abdominal organs – deep dissection 1. In this dissection, the small and large intestines have been removed to show the liver, gallbladder, pancreas, spleen, and kidneys. Observe how the abdominal aorta is to the left of the inferior vena cava

393

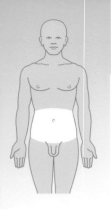

TRUNK

Abdominal organs

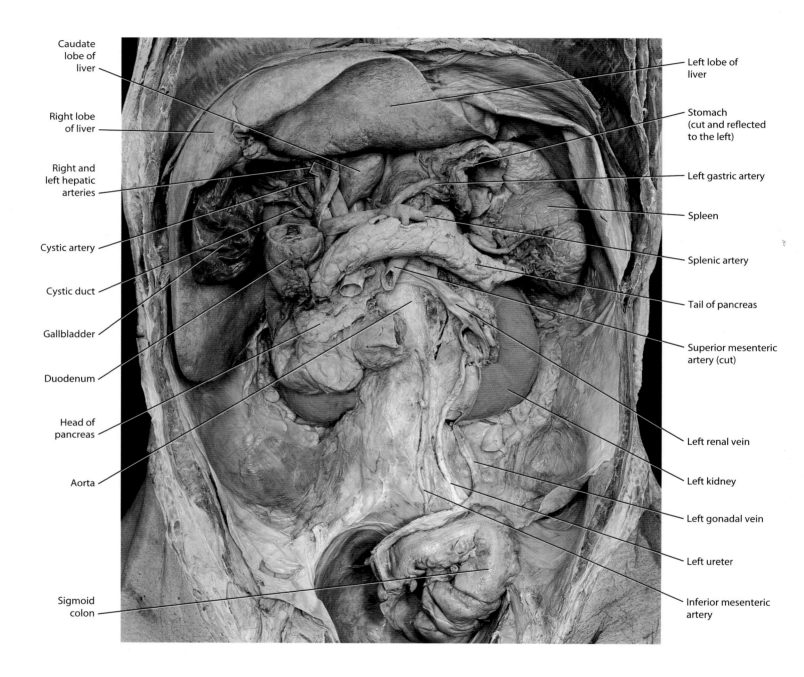

Caudate
lobe of
liver

Right lobe
of liver

Right and
left hepatic
arteries

Cystic artery

Cystic duct

Gallbladder

Duodenum

Head of
pancreas

Aorta

Sigmoid
colon

Left lobe of
liver

Stomach
(cut and reflected
to the left)

Left gastric artery

Spleen

Splenic artery

Tail of pancreas

Superior mesenteric
artery (cut)

Left renal vein

Left kidney

Left gonadal vein

Left ureter

Inferior mesenteric
artery

Figure 33.9 Abdominal organs – deep dissection 2. The small intestine and colon have been removed, but the fatty tissue covering the aorta is intact.
Observe the C-shaped duodenum and how it is related to the head of the pancreas

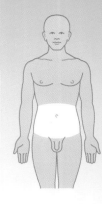

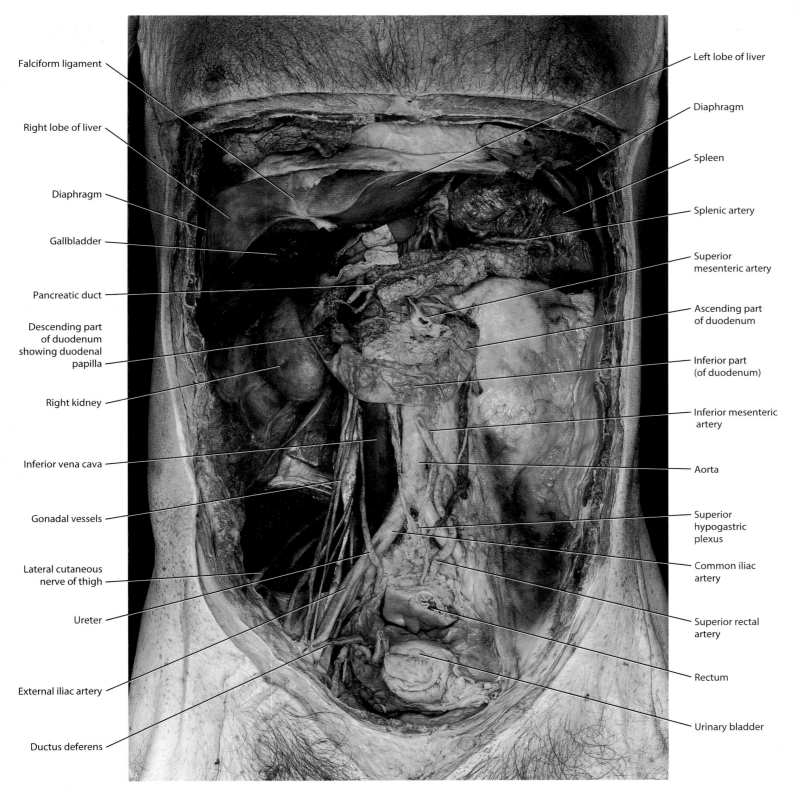

Falciform ligament

Right lobe of liver

Diaphragm

Gallbladder

Pancreatic duct

Descending part
of duodenum
showing duodenal
papilla

Right kidney

Inferior vena cava

Gonadal vessels

Lateral cutaneous
nerve of thigh

Ureter

External iliac artery

Ductus deferens

Left lobe of liver

Diaphragm

Spleen

Splenic artery

Superior
mesenteric artery

Ascending part
of duodenum

Inferior part
(of duodenum)

Inferior mesenteric
artery

Aorta

Superior
hypogastric
plexus

Common iliac
artery

Superior rectal
artery

Rectum

Urinary bladder

Figure 33.10 Abdominal organs – deep dissection 3. Dissection to show the ducts of the pancreas. In addition, a square-shaped window has been created in the duodenum to visualize the major duodenal papilla, which is where the main pancreatic duct empties into the intestinal tract

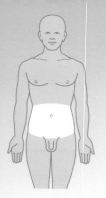

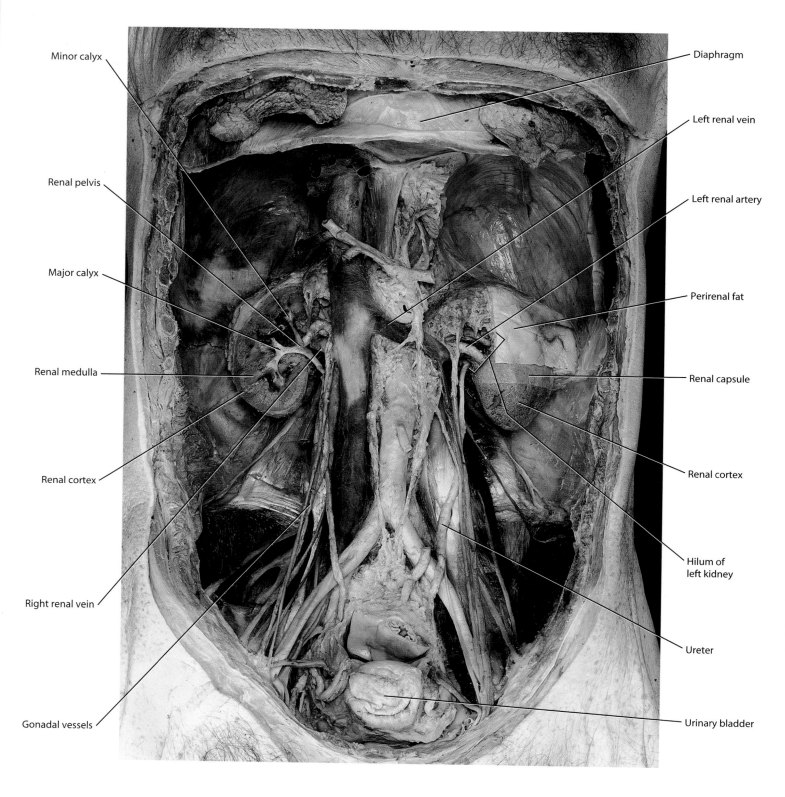

Minor calyx

Renal pelvis

Major calyx

Renal medulla

Renal cortex

Right renal vein

Gonadal vessels

Diaphragm

Left renal vein

Left renal artery

Perirenal fat

Renal capsule

Renal cortex

Hilum of left kidney

Ureter

Urinary bladder

Figure 33.11 Kidneys – in situ. Dissection to the kidneys as they appear within the body. The right kidney has been partly dissected to show the pelvis of the kidney and the first part of the ureter

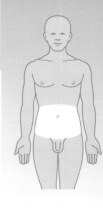

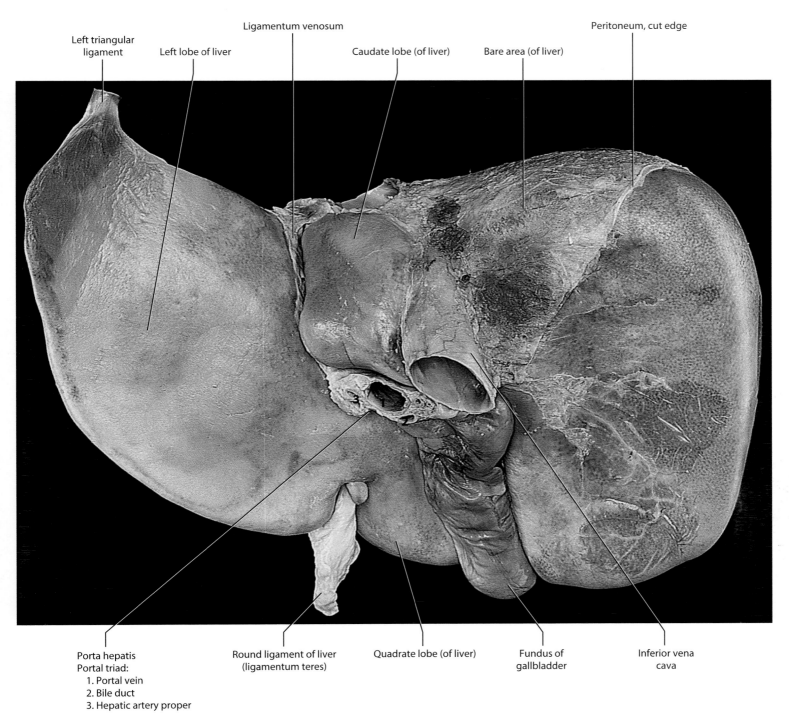

Left triangular ligament

Left lobe of liver

Ligamentum venosum

Caudate lobe (of liver)

Bare area (of liver)

Peritoneum, cut edge

Porta hepatis
Portal triad:
1. Portal vein
2. Bile duct
3. Hepatic artery proper

Round ligament of liver (ligamentum teres)

Quadrate lobe (of liver)

Fundus of gallbladder

Inferior vena cava

Figure 33.12 Liver – isolated. Inferior view of the liver. Observe the porta hepatis and gallbladder

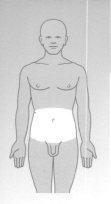

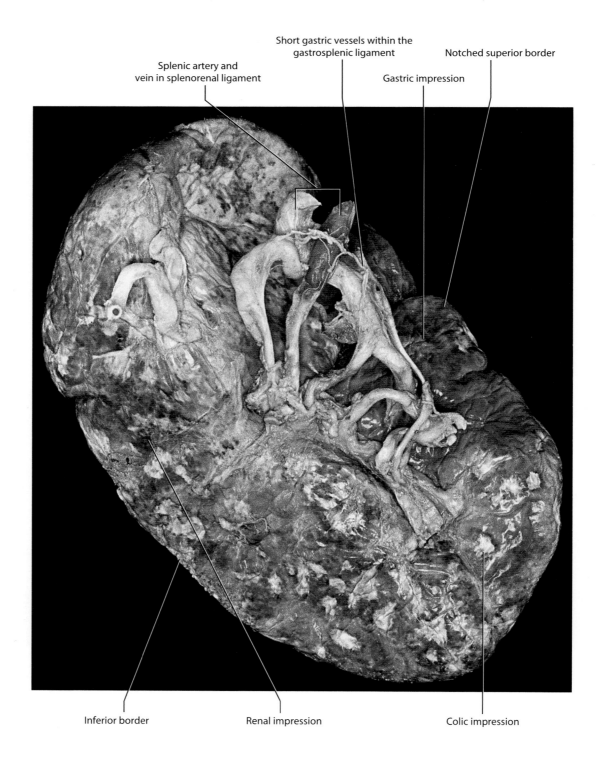

Short gastric vessels within the
gastrosplenic ligament

Splenic artery and
vein in splenorenal ligament

Notched superior border

Gastric impression

Inferior border

Renal impression

Colic impression

Figure 33.13 Spleen – isolated. Hilar (medial) view of the spleen showing where vessels enter it. Observe the splenic hilum with ligaments, nerves, and vessels, and the contact impressions

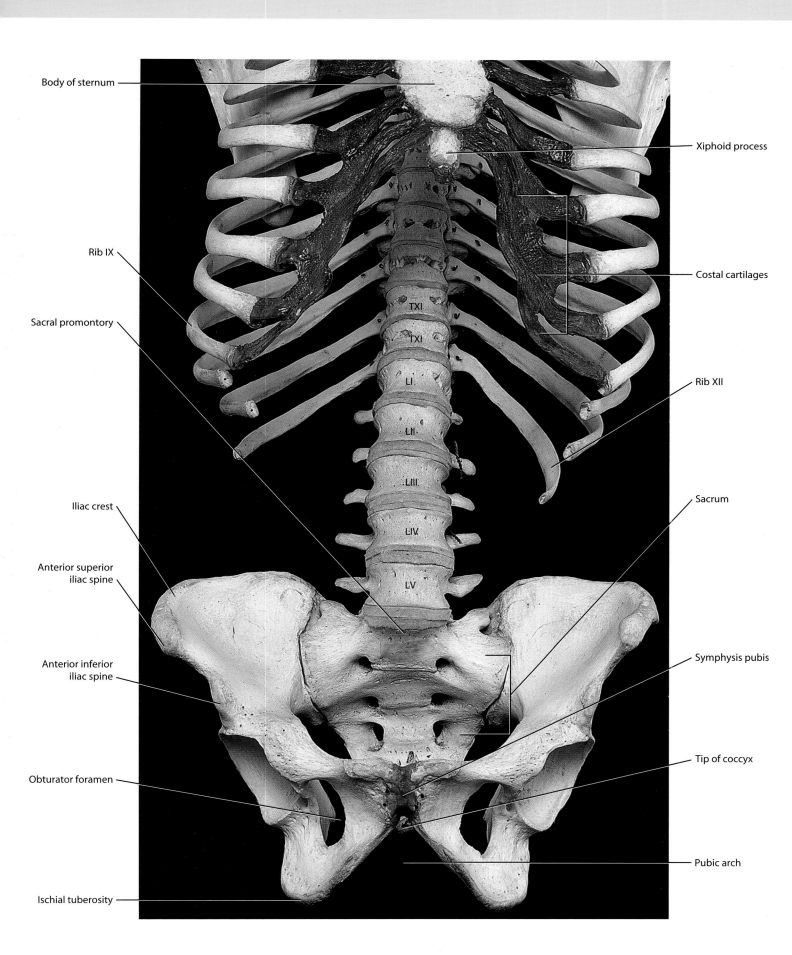

Body of sternum

Xiphoid process

Rib IX

Costal cartilages

Sacral promontory

TXI

TXI

LI

Rib XII

LII

LIII

Iliac crest

LIV

Sacrum

Anterior superior
iliac spine

LV

Anterior inferior
iliac spine

Symphysis pubis

Obturator foramen

Tip of coccyx

Pubic arch

Ischial tuberosity

Figure 33.14 Abdomen – osteology. Anterior view of the articulated skeleton that supports the abdominal organs. The pancreas is usually at the level of vertebra LI.

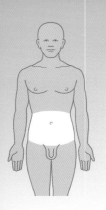

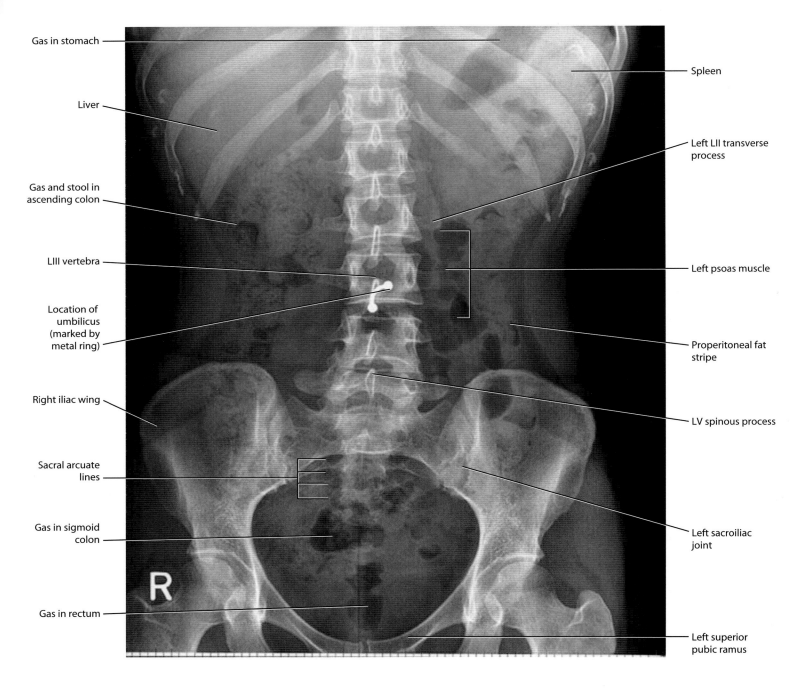

Gas in stomach

Liver

Gas and stool in ascending colon

LIII vertebra

Location of umbilicus (marked by metal ring)

Right iliac wing

Sacral arcuate lines

Gas in sigmoid colon

Gas in rectum

Spleen

Left LII transverse process

Left psoas muscle

Properitoneal fat stripe

LV spinous process

Left sacroiliac joint

Left superior pubic ramus

R

Figure 33.15 Abdominal organs – plain film radiograph (anteroposterior view). The small intestine is usually located in the vicinity of the umbilicus in this view. The colon is visible at the periphery of the abdominal cavity as a series of sponge-like markings (stool) amidst dark markings (gas). This is a normal bowel gas pattern. It is also important to note the presence of gas in the rectum. Patients with complete bowel obstruction usually do not have this finding. Note the subtle outlines of the left psoas muscle in this supine radiograph

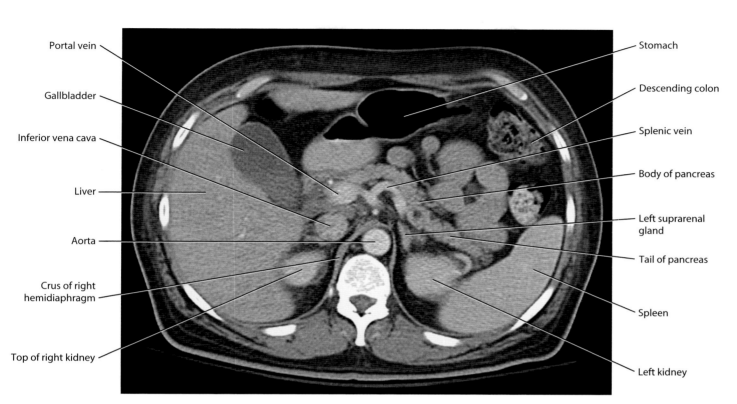

Portal vein

Gallbladder

Inferior vena cava

Liver

Aorta

Crus of right
hemidiaphragm

Top of right kidney

Stomach

Descending colon

Splenic vein

Body of pancreas

Left suprarenal
gland

Tail of pancreas

Spleen

Left kidney

Figure 33.16 Abdominal organs – CT scan (axial view). In this scan of the upper abdomen, the solid organs of the abdomen are well visualized. Note that the right adrenal gland is not visible at this level because it is at a level superior to that of the left adrenal gland

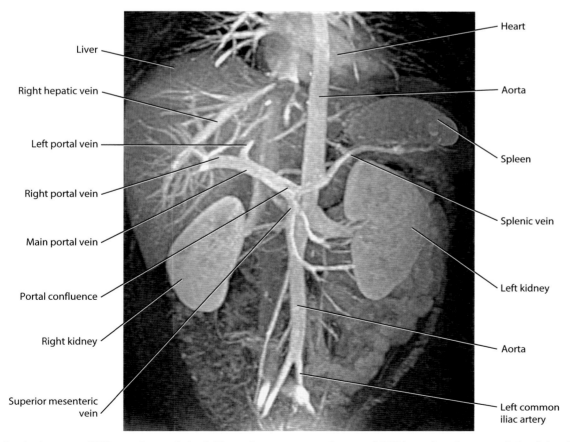

Liver

Right hepatic vein

Left portal vein

Right portal vein

Main portal vein

Portal confluence

Right kidney

Superior mesenteric
vein

Heart

Aorta

Spleen

Splenic vein

Left kidney

Aorta

Left common
iliac artery

Figure 33.17 Abdominal organs – MRA scan (coronal view). Magnetic resonance angiograms (MRA) have the advantage of visualizing the veins at the same time as the arteries, whereas conventional angiography usually shows only the arteries or only the veins. Observe how the splenic vein joins the superior mesenteric vein to become the portal vein

The abdominal cavity contains the accessory abdominal organs (see Chapter 33) and the hollow tube of the gastrointestinal (GI) tract. The GI tract extends from the mouth to the anus and is subdivided structurally and functionally into several organs that specialize in processing ingested food (Fig. 34.1). These gastrointestinal organs are discussed here in the order that food passes through them.

ESOPHAGUS

The first part of the GI tract is the **oral cavity** (see Chapter 9) where food is formed into a bolus, which is propelled posteriorly by the tongue and oral cavity muscles into the **oropharynx**. From here, the bolus is transferred to the **esophagus**, which transports food and swallowed substances to the stomach. In the chest the esophagus runs slightly to the left of the vertebral bodies and posterior to the trachea (Fig. 34.2). It enters the abdomen through a hiatus in the diaphragm at level TX. The abdominal esophagus is approximately 2–3 cm long and joins the stomach at the **esophagogastric sphincter** (lower esophageal sphincter). This muscular sphincter prevents regurgitation of stomach contents into the esophagus. Innervation of the esophagus is by:

- **parasympathetic nerve fibers**, which travel with the **vagus nerves** [X];
- **sympathetic nerve fibers** that originate from the **greater** and **lesser splanchnic nerves**.

Blood is supplied to the esophagus by several vessels – the **subclavian artery**, **thoracic aorta**, **inferior phrenic artery**, **and left gastric artery**. Venous drainage of the distal thoracic esophagus is to the **azygos venous system**, whereas the short abdominal esophagus

drains to the **hepatic portal venous system**. This forms clinically significant portal-systemic anastomoses. Lymphatic drainage of the lower esophagus is via the **left gastric** and **celiac nodes**.

STOMACH

The stomach breaks down large food particles into smaller pieces so that they can be processed more easily (Fig. 34.3). The stomach also

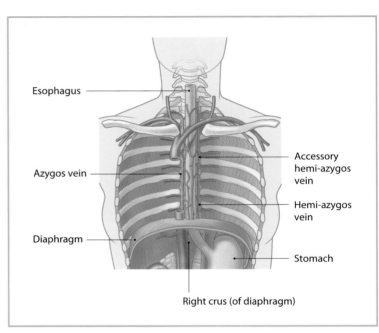

Figure 34.2 Esophagus

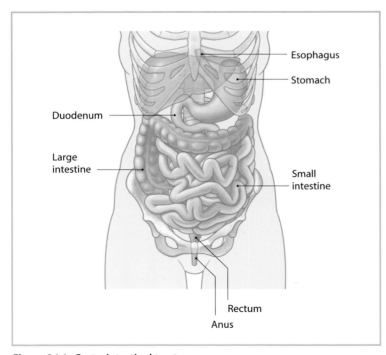

Figure 34.1 Gastrointestinal tract

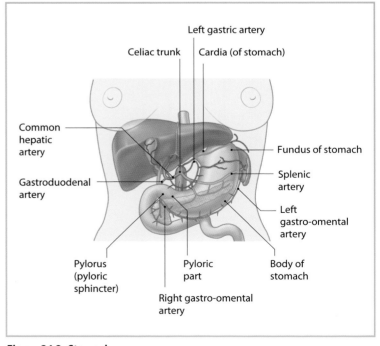

Figure 34.3 Stomach

secretes digestive enzymes, such as pepsin, which break down proteins and starches. The stomach is entirely intraperitoneal and is in the left hypochrondrium and epigastric regions of the abdomen. It is subdivided into four parts – the cardia, fundus, body, and pylorus. It also has anterior and posterior surfaces covered with peritoneum and two curvatures (the greater and the lesser curvatures).

The gastric **cardia** is the part of the stomach that receives swallowed food. It contains the esophagogastric sphincter (see above). The second part of the stomach is the domed **fundus of stomach**; when seen on an upright chest radiograph this usually contains gas. The **body of stomach** is the longest part of the stomach and is where most of the gastric digestion of proteins and starches occurs. It is rich in glands that produce hydrochloric acid, which facilitates the breakdown of food products. The **pyloric part** is the distal, funnel-like part of the stomach. Its proximal part, the **pyloric antrum**, leads into the narrow **pyloric canal** and **pyloric sphincter**, which controls the release of stomach contents into the duodenum (small intestine).

Sensory and autonomic (parasympathetic and sympathetic) innervation to the stomach is provided by the **celiac plexus** of nerves near the origin of the celiac artery. Blood is supplied by the **celiac trunk** and its branches – the **left gastric**, **splenic**, and **common hepatic arteries**. Venous drainage of the stomach is to the **gastric** and **gastro-omental veins** (Table 34.1). Lymphatic drainage is to the celiac nodes and also lymph node groups adjacent to the spleen and pancreas.

SMALL INTESTINE

The small intestine (small bowel) is the longest part of the gastrointestinal tract (usually around 5.5 m long), and comprises three major regions – the duodenum, jejunum, and ileum. It joins the stomach at the pyloric sphincter and terminally joins the large intestine at the **ileocecal fold** or **valve** (Fig. 34.4).

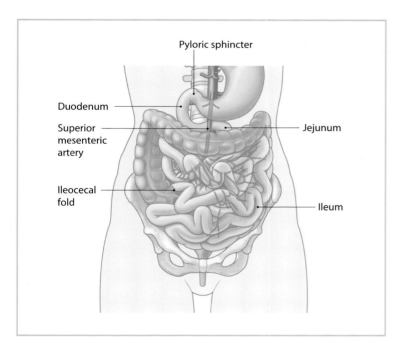

Figure 34.4 Small intestine

The short **duodenum** is the first part of the small intestine and has four parts – the superior, descending, inferior, and ascending parts. It is almost entirely retroperitoneal, except for part of its superior and ascending parts. The duodenum is approximately 25–27 cm long and encircles the head of the pancreas. It is in the epigastric and umbilical regions of the abdomen at vertebral levels LI to LIII just anterior to the inferior vena cava, aorta, and right kidney.

The **superior part** of the duodenum passes toward the right side of the abdomen from the pylorus. The **descending part** passes inferiorly to the right of vertebra LII. The hepatic and pancreatic ducts open into the duodenal lumen at the midpoint of the descending section through the **major duodenal papilla** and **minor duodenal papilla**. This is important clinically because damage to or pathology of this part of the duodenum prevents hepatic and pancreatic secretions from entering the digestive system and so inhibits digestion.

The **inferior part** of the duodenum then passes to the left, crossing the inferior vena cava and aorta before curving superiorly to become the **ascending part**. The duodenum terminates at the **duodenojejunal flexure**, where it joins the jejunum. The duodenojejunal flexure is suspended from the abdominal wall by the **suspensory ligament of duodenum**. Abnormalities in embryological rotation of the gut may occur at this site.

The duodenum is innervated by autonomic nerves from the celiac plexus. Blood supply is provided by branches of the celiac trunk and superior mesenteric arteries (Table 34.2). Venous drainage is to the hepatic portal system through veins that follow the route of the arteries. Lymphatic drainage is to the lymph node group near the head of the pancreas.

The second part of the small intestine is the **jejunum**, in the left hypochrondrium of the abdomen. The jejunum accounts for approximately 2 m of the small intestine and is held in place by a posterior mesentery. The jejunum is a location for lipid and protein digestion; primary starch digestion occurs in the oral cavity and stomach. Internally the jejunum has **plica circulares**, which are circular rings created by the musculature within the jejunal walls. The jejunum usually has thicker walls and a larger diameter than the ileum (Table 34.3).

The **ileum** begins at the distal jejunum. It is the longest part of the small intestine, accounting for around 3 m of the total length. It is here that most digested nutrients are absorbed. The ileum is in the umbilical and right lower quadrants of the abdomen.

The jejunum and ileum are innervated by autonomic nerves around the superior mesenteric artery. Blood is supplied by the superior mesenteric artery and venous drainage is to the superior mesenteric vein, which joins the splenic vein to form the hepatic portal vein. Lymphatic drainage is to the superior mesenteric nodes and the posterior mesentery.

The ileum joins the large intestine at the **ileocecal fold**, a sphincterless valve through which the bolus of food passes into the first part of the large intestine – the cecum.

The small intestine has stretch receptors within its wall, which produce a sensation of pain when the lumen distends.

LARGE INTESTINE

The large intestine (large bowel) extends from the ileocecal fold to the anus and is approximately 1.5 m long. It consists of the cecum, appendix, colon (which has four parts – ascending, transverse,

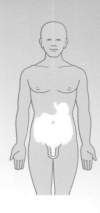

In Figure 34.4, the following labels appear:

- Pyloric sphincter
- Duodenum
- Superior mesenteric artery
- Ileocecal fold
- Jejunum
- Ileum

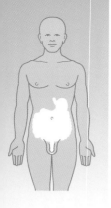
descending, and sigmoid), rectum, and anal canal, which complete the gastrointestinal tube within the pelvis (Fig. 34.5). Parts of the colon are intraperitoneal, others are retroperitoneal.

The large intestine has three longitudinal bands of smooth muscle (**taeniae coli**) which, because they are shorter than the rest of the colonic wall, produce sacculations (**haustra**). Peritoneum-covered **omental appendices** (fatty tags) extend from the external wall of the colon. The diameter of the colon is much larger than that of the small intestine. The ascending and descending colon are usually retroperitoneal whereas the transverse and sigmoid colon are intraperitoneal and are suspended by mesentery. The colon possesses two flexures – the **right** and **left colic flexures**.

At the start of the large intestine is the **cecum**, a blind-ending pouch in the right groin. The cecum is intraperitoneal and receives intestinal contents from the ileum through the ileocecal fold. Suspended from the inferior part of the cecum is the **appendix**, which is a blind diverticulum of the intestine. The appendix is usually around 8–10 cm long, although this is variable, and has a small lumen. It can be retrocecal (behind the cecum) and suspended from the ileum by the **meso-appendix**. Blood supply to, and venous drainage from, the appendix is by the **appendicular artery** and **appendicular vein**, respectively, which are derived from the superior mesenteric vessels. The appendix contains concentrated lymphoid tissue.

The **ascending colon** arises from the cecum along the right lateral side of the abdominal cavity toward the liver. It is covered anteriorly and on both sides with peritoneum, which fixes it to the posterior abdominal wall forming the **right paracolic gutter**. This gutter extends between the right **subphrenic space** to the pelvis.

On reaching the liver the ascending colon turns left at the right colic flexure and becomes the **transverse colon**. This horizontally oriented part of the colon is intraperitoneal and suspended from the posterior abdominal wall by the transverse **mesocolon**, making

it the most mobile part of the large intestine. Its course is towards the spleen and it becomes the **descending colon** at the left colic flexure.

The descending colon runs inferiorly from the left colic flexure to the left groin where it becomes the **sigmoid colon**, so named because of its 'S' shape. For descriptive purposes the sigmoid colon begins at the **pelvic inlet** and descends to the level of SIII where it becomes the **rectum**. The sigmoid colon is attached by a mesentery (**sigmoid mesocolon**) to the pelvic wall.

The colon is innervated by autonomic nerves from plexuses along the abdominal aorta – the superior mesenteric, inferior mesenteric, and aortic plexuses. These nerve groups are derived from the vagus [X] and splanchnic nerves, which originate from the sympathetic trunk.

The colon's blood supply is from branches of the **superior mesenteric** and **inferior mesenteric arteries**. The superior mesenteric artery has many small arterial branches divided into two main groups – **jejunal and ileal arteries**. Some of the distal ileal branches of the superior mesenteric artery supply the right colon. The inferior mesenteric artery has several branches (**left colic**, and **sigmoid** and **rectal branches**), which supply the region after which they are named.

Venous drainage of the colon is through veins that pass alongside the arteries and empty into the hepatic portal vein through the superior and inferior mesenteric veins. Lymphatic drainage of the colon is regional in that each region drains towards lymph node groups along the corresponding side of the aorta.

The large intestine absorbs water, salts, and bile fats, so preserving the body's nutrients while preparing undigested matter for elimination.

RECTUM AND ANAL CANAL

The rectum is the part of the gastrointestinal tract that extends from the sigmoid colon to the anal canal; it has no mesentery (Fig. 34.6). The dilated terminal part of the rectum is the **rectal ampulla**, which supports and retains the fecal mass before defecation.

Figure 34.5 Large intestine and its blood supply

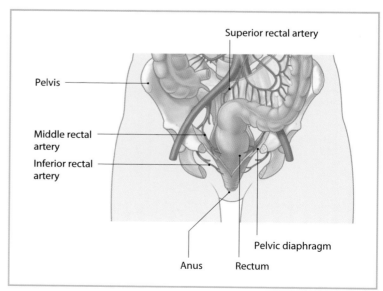

Figure 34.6 Rectum and anus

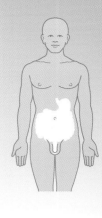

The anal canal is the terminal part of the gastrointestinal tract and is approximately 4 cm long. Internally it has an upper and lower part separated by a line (**pectinate line**) formed by the joining of anal skin with rectal mucosa. Each part has a unique innervation (see below). The anal canal is surrounded by **internal** (under involuntary control) and **external** (under voluntary control) **anal sphincters**, which regulate the passage of fecal material.

The rectum is innervated by sympathetic and parasympathetic nerve fibers emerging from the **sacral plexus**. The sympathetic nerve fibers are derived from the **lumbar sympathetic trunk**; the **superior hypogastric plexus** at the root of the inferior mesenteric artery carries the parasympathetic fibers. Sensory innervation is provided by the **pelvic splanchnic** or **lumbar splanchnic nerves**.

The rectum and superior anal canal are sensitive to stretching. Sympathetic and parasympathetic innervation to the upper anal canal is through the **inferior hypogastric plexus**. The inferior part of the anal canal, below the pectinate line, is sensitive to pain, touch, and temperature because it receives somatic innervation from the branches of the **pudendal nerve**.

Blood is supplied to the proximal, middle, and distal rectum, and the upper anal canal superior to the pectinate line by:

- the **superior rectal artery**, a continuation of the inferior mesenteric artery;
- the **middle rectal arteries** arising from the inferior vesical artery (in men) and **uterine artery** (in women), which are branches of the internal iliac arteries;
- the **inferior rectal arteries** arising from the internal pudendal arteries, which are branches of the internal iliac arteries.

The anal canal inferior to the pectinate line receives blood from the **internal pudendal artery**.

Venous drainage of the rectum is by the **superior**, **middle**, and **inferior rectal veins**. The superior rectal vein drains to the hepatic portal venous system whereas the middle and inferior rectal veins drain to the systemic system through the internal iliac vein.

Lymphatic drainage from the rectum and upper two-thirds of the anal canal is to the iliac and sacral lymph node groups, which drain toward the **pre-aortic nodes**. The lower third of the anal canal drains lymph to the **superficial inguinal nodes** in the inguinal region.

■ CLINICAL CORRELATIONS
Obstruction of the intestine

Intestinal obstruction is defined as any process that causes cessation of the normal flow of contents within the intestine. This has a variety of causes, such as a foreign body (a large swallowed object) within the intestinal lumen or twisting of the intestine, which can occur secondary to postoperative adhesions (bands of fibrous scar tissue). Hernias, inflammatory bowel disease, and cancer are other causes.

Obstruction of the small intestine usually causes intermittent and short episodes of vague abdominal pain. The pain may be described as sharp and spasm-like, a dull ache, or crampy. It may resolve spontaneously for brief periods or it may progress to more intense and constant abdominal pain, depending on whether the obstruction is partial or complete. A complete obstruction causes nausea, vomiting, and abnormal abdominal distention, and it is usually this that causes patients to seek medical advice.

On examination the patient usually lies very still because subtle movements in the abdomen can exacerbate the pain. Auscultation of the abdomen may reveal hyperactive bowel sounds because of the increased activity in the proximal intestine as it attempts to push food material beyond the site of obstruction. Later in the time course of an obstruction and before rupture of the bowel, the bowel sounds decrease or are completely absent.

Abdominal examination of a patient with bowel obstruction should be carried out carefully. Gentle palpation of the abdomen causes generalized intra-abdominal pain. Pain due to pressure applied to the abdomen by the examiner's hand may increase when the examiner removes the hand from the abdomen (rebound tenderness); gentle shaking of the patient's trunk may also illicit pain (jar tenderness). Rebound and jar tenderness are sensitive indicators of peritoneal irritation because the peritoneum is richly innervated. Any pressure applied to inflamed or infected peritoneum causes pain.

Peritoneal irritation is a sign that an obstruction requires evaluation by a surgeon and blood tests to determine whether there is any infection. Untreated, a bowel obstruction will cause distention of the abdomen and the resulting fluid sequestration within the intestine (Fig. 34.7) will cause intravascular volume depletion, manifested by decreased blood pressure and fever as infection spreads.

Patients usually seek medical care early in the course of the obstruction and can be admitted to hospital for nonsurgical bowel rest and decompression (by passing a nasogastric tube into the stomach and removing stomach acids and any undigested food material proximal to the obstruction site). Severe bowel obstruction must be evaluated by a surgeon for possible intraoperative repair.

Appendicitis

Appendicitis is inflammation and infection of the appendix. The appendiceal lumen may be obstructed by a swallowed foreign object, an appendicolith (appendix stone), or an intestinal infection causing appendiceal edema. It usually takes some time for the inflammatory process to manifest clinically. Infection ensues as a result of bacterial growth stasis within the lumen.

Appendicitis classically causes vague peri-umbilical pain, which over the course of several hours seems to move to the right lower quadrant. In addition, there is a lack of appetite, which precedes nausea and vomiting. Irritation of the peritoneum in the right lower quadrant results as the appendix becomes more edematous and the infection spreads to the surface of the appendix. If left untreated the infection can lead to perforation of the appendix (a process usually taking at least 1 to 2 days, though the exact time course is variable).

The patient lies still on the examining table because of the peritoneal irritation. Pain in the right lower quadrant of the abdomen is manifested by exquisite tenderness to light palpation. Pressure applied to the left lower quadrant of the abdomen, followed by release of the pressure, causes right-sided abdominal pain (Rovsing's sign). Rebound and jar tenderness are present in severe appendicitis. An increased white blood cell count is indicative of infection.

Early in the course of appendicitis surgical evaluation of the need for appendectomy (surgical removal of the appendix) is required.

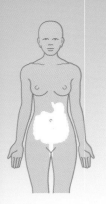

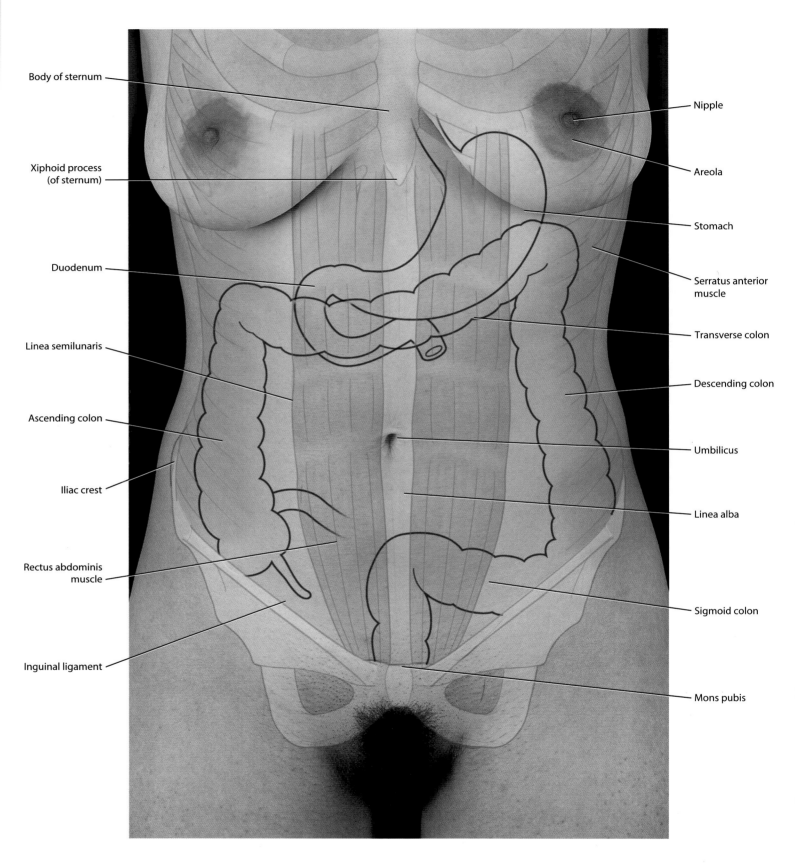

Body of sternum

Xiphoid process
(of sternum)

Duodenum

Linea semilunaris

Ascending colon

Iliac crest

Rectus abdominis
muscle

Inguinal ligament

Nipple

Areola

Stomach

Serratus anterior
muscle

Transverse colon

Descending colon

Umbilicus

Linea alba

Sigmoid colon

Mons pubis

Figure 34.7 Gastrointestinal tract – surface anatomy. Anterior view of the abdominal region of a young woman. Observe the location of the umbilicus in relationship to the iliac crest

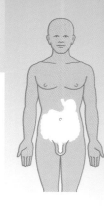

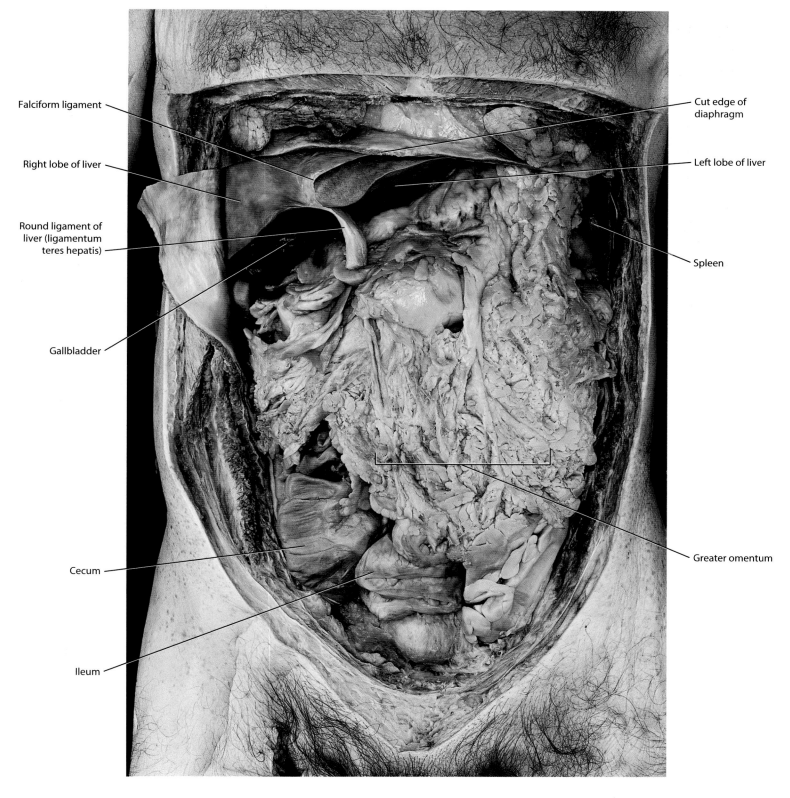

Falciform ligament

Right lobe of liver

Round ligament of liver (ligamentum teres hepatis)

Gallbladder

Cecum

Ileum

Cut edge of diaphragm

Left lobe of liver

Spleen

Greater omentum

Figure 34.8 Gastrointestinal tract – superficial dissection 1. The anterior abdominal wall has been removed. The greater omentum covering the intestine is intact

407

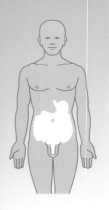

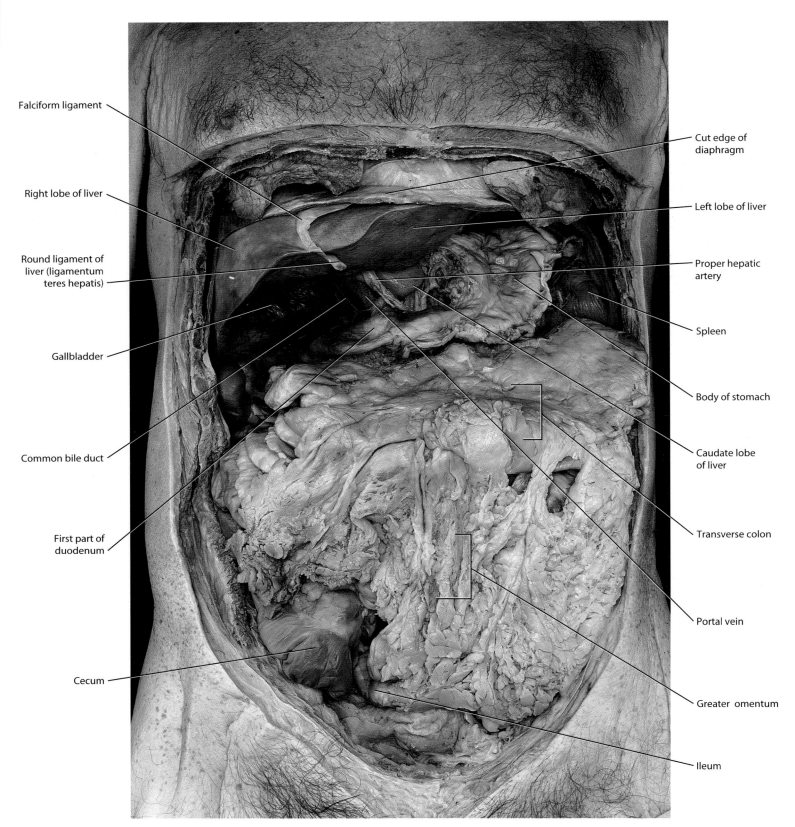

Falciform ligament

Right lobe of liver

Round ligament of liver (ligamentum teres hepatis)

Gallbladder

Common bile duct

First part of duodenum

Cecum

Cut edge of diaphragm

Left lobe of liver

Proper hepatic artery

Spleen

Body of stomach

Caudate lobe of liver

Transverse colon

Portal vein

Greater omentum

Ileum

Figure 34.9 **Gastrointestinal tract – superficial dissection 2.** The liver has been raised superiorly to reveal the gallbladder and stomach

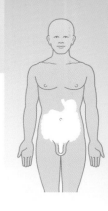

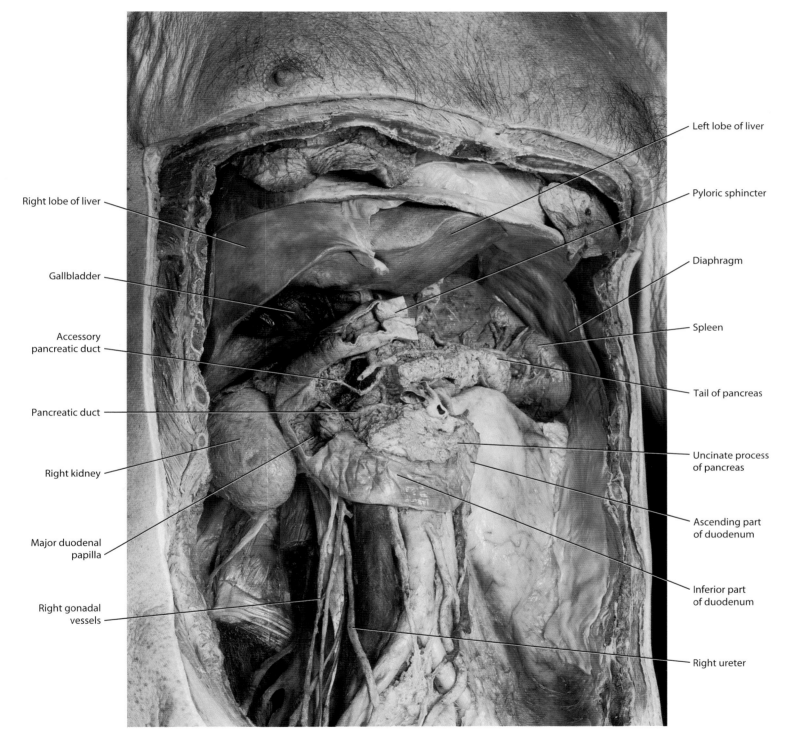

Right lobe of liver

Gallbladder

Accessory
pancreatic duct

Pancreatic duct

Right kidney

Major duodenal
papilla

Right gonadal
vessels

Left lobe of liver

Pyloric sphincter

Diaphragm

Spleen

Tail of pancreas

Uncinate process
of pancreas

Ascending part
of duodenum

Inferior part
of duodenum

Right ureter

Figure 34.10 Gastrointestinal tract – duodenum. The stomach, small intestine and large intestine have been removed to show the duodenum. A small window has been cut out of the duodenum to show the duodenal papilla (papilla of Vater)

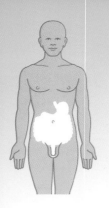

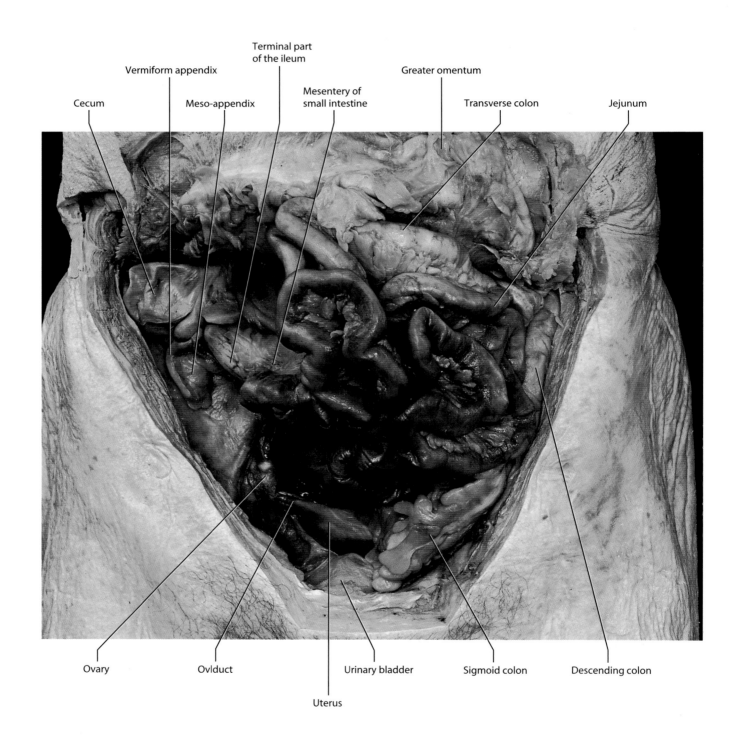

Cecum

Vermiform appendix

Meso-appendix

Terminal part
of the ileum

Mesentery of
small intestine

Greater omentum

Transverse colon

Jejunum

Ovary

Oviduct

Urinary bladder

Sigmoid colon

Descending colon

Uterus

Figure 34.11 Gastrointestinal tract – cecum and appendix. The distal small intestine has been displaced superiorly and to the left side to reveal the cecum and appendix

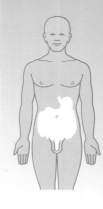

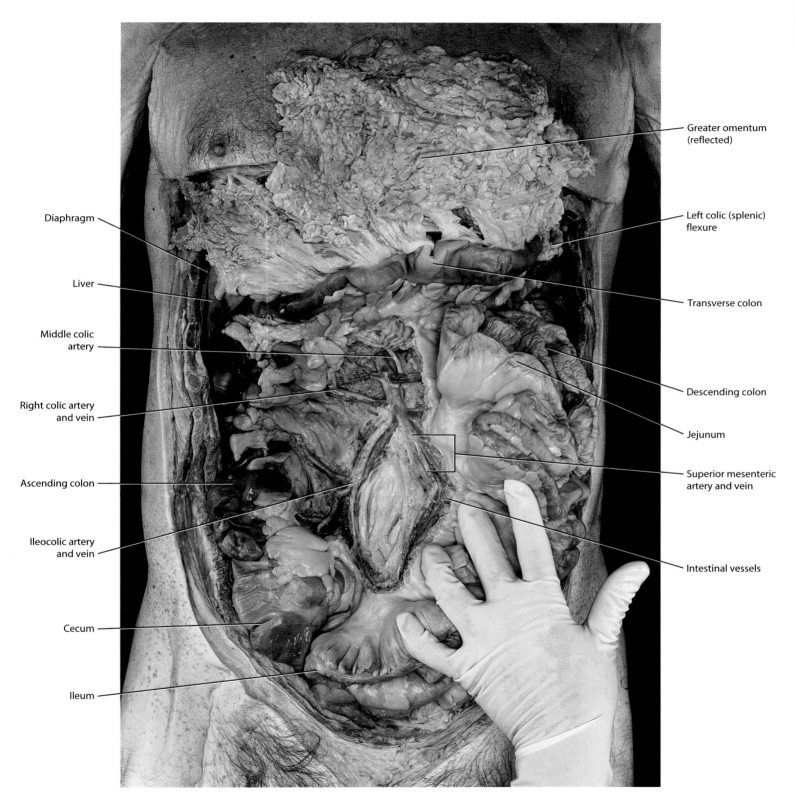

Diaphragm

Liver

Middle colic artery

Right colic artery and vein

Ascending colon

Ileocolic artery and vein

Cecum

Ileum

Greater omentum (reflected)

Left colic (splenic) flexure

Transverse colon

Descending colon

Jejunum

Superior mesenteric artery and vein

Intestinal vessels

Figure 34.12 Gastrointestinal tract – intermediate dissection 1. The greater omentum has been reflected superiorly. The dissector's hand is holding the jejunum and part of the ileum of the small intestine so that the arteries to the small intestine can be seen. Observe the way in which the small intestine is anchored to the posterior body wall from the left upper quadrant to right lower quadrant by the posterior mesentery

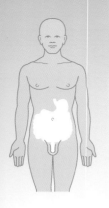

Gastrointestinal tract **TRUNK**

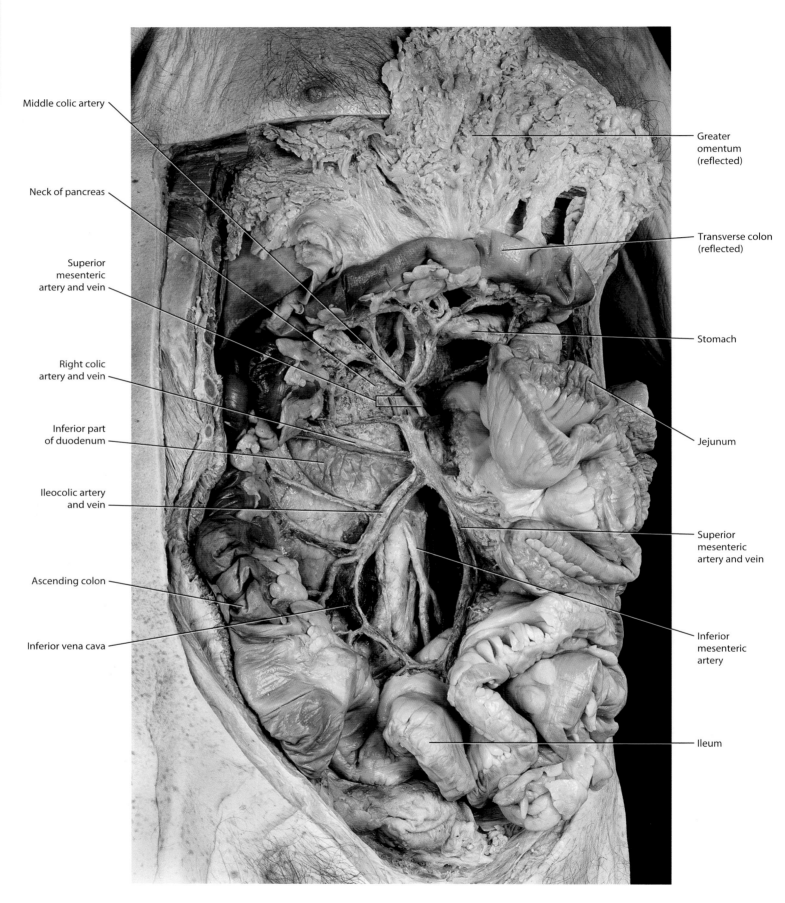

Middle colic artery

Neck of pancreas

Superior mesenteric artery and vein

Right colic artery and vein

Inferior part of duodenum

Ileocolic artery and vein

Ascending colon

Inferior vena cava

Greater omentum (reflected)

Transverse colon (reflected)

Stomach

Jejunum

Superior mesenteric artery and vein

Inferior mesenteric artery

Ileum

Figure 34.13 Gastrointestinal tract – intermediate dissection 2. This dissection shows the arteriovenous anatomy of the right side of the large intestine. The greater omentum, which is attached to the stomach and transverse colon, has been reflected superiorly. The small intestine has been reflected to the left side. The inferior mesenteric artery which supplies blood primarily to the left colon is also visible

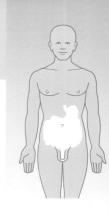

TABLE 34.1 GASTROINTESTINAL TRACT: NEUROVASCULAR SUPPLY					
Abdominal organs	**Arteries**	**Lymphatics**	**Veins**	**Sympathetic fibers**	**Parasympathetic fibers**
Foregut (distal esophagus to mid-duodenum): distal esophagus, stomach, proximal duodenum, liver, gallbladder, pancreas, and spleen	Celiac (TXII) trunk → left gastric (lesser curvature of stomach and esophagus) Common hepatic → right gastric (lesser curvature) Gastroduodenal → gastro-omental (greater curvature) and superior pancreaticoduodenal (head of pancreas and duodenum) Cystic (gallbladder) → right and left hepatic (liver) Splenic → greater pancreatic (pancreas), left gastro-omental (greater omentum and greater curvature), short gastrics (fundus of stomach)	Celiac (pre-aortic) and hepatic nodes and regional nodes adjacent to arteries (splenic, left gastro-omental, pyloric, left gastric) ↓ Cisterna chyli and thoracic duct	Foregut, midgut, and hindgut: all venous blood from the gastrointestinal tract, spleen, and pancreas drains to the liver via the portal vein Venous blood in the liver passes through hepatic sinusoids to the central veins. These unite to form – typically – three hepatic veins, which drain to the inferior vena cava	Preganglionics via the greater splanchnics (T5 to T9) to celiac ganglion. Postganglionics via the peri-arterial plexuses of branches of the celiac trunk	Preganglionics from the anterior and posterior vagal trunks Postganglionics in or near the organs innervated
Midgut (mid-duodenum to just proximal to left colic flexure): distal duodenum, jejunum, ileum, cecum, appendix, ascending colon, and transverse colon just proximal to left colic flexure	Superior mesenteric artery (LI) → inferior pancreaticoduodenal (pancreas and duodenum), right colic (ascending colon), jejunal and ileal branches (jejunum and ileum), ileocolic (ileocecal junction), appendicular (appendix) and middle colic (transverse colon)	Nodes in the mesentery and pre-aortic nodes at origin of superior mesenteric artery ↓ Intestinal lymph trunk ↓ Cisterna chyli and thoracic duct	" "	Preganglionics via the greater and lesser splanchnic nerves (T5 to T9 and T10 to T11, respectively) synapse in celiac and superior mesenteric (prevertebral) ganglia. Postganglionic peri-arterial fibers are delivered via branches of the superior mesenteric artery	Preganglionics from the vagal trunks synapse with postganglionic neurons in the myenteric and submucosal plexuses in the intestinal wall as far as the left colic flexure
Hindgut: left colic flexure, descending colon, sigmoid colon, and rectum to pectinate line	Inferior mesenteric artery (LIII) → left colic (descending colon), sigmoid branches, (sigmoid colon), and superior rectal/hemorrhoidal (upper part of anal canal)	Regional nodes – left colic sigmoid, inferior mesenteric, and pre-aortic nodes ↓ Cisterna chyli and thoracic duct	" "	Preganglionic lumbar splanchnics (L1, L2) travel through plexuses on the inferior mesenteric artery and its branches. Preganglionics synapse in the celiac and superior mesenteric ganglia	Pelvic splanchnic (S2 to S4) preganglionics to postganglionic neurons in the myenteric and submucosal plexuses in the intestinal wall from the left colic flexure to the anal pectinate line

Pain fibers from the abdominal viscera are present in both sympathetic and parasympathetic pathways, enter the central nervous system without synapsing, and pass to the nearest spinal nerve. Their paths are similar to those for somatic pain. Parasympathetic pathways probably carry visceral sensations (nausea, hunger, rectal distension) to the central nervous system.

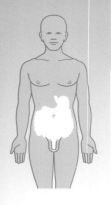

TABLE 34.2 RELATIONSHIPS OF THE DUODENUM							
Part	Anterior	Posterior	Medial	Superior	Inferior	Level	Length
Superior part*	Gallbladder, liver (quadrate lobe)	Bile duct, portal vein, gastroduodenal artery		Neck of gallbladder, lesser omentum, omental foramen	Head of pancreas	LI	2 cm
Descending part	Transverse colon and mesocolon, and small intestine	Right suprarenal gland, hilum of right kidney, right psoas muscle, ureter, renal vessels	Head of pancreas, bile duct, and pancreatico-duodenal vessels**			LII to LIII	8 cm
Inferior part#	Superior mesenteric vessels, root of the mesentery, coils of small intestine	Right ureter, right psoas muscle, gonadal vessels, inferior vena cava, inferior mesenteric artery, aorta		Head and uncinate process (of pancreas)	Coils of small intestine	LIII	10 cm
						LIII	3 cm
Ascending part	Root of mesentery, coils of jejunum	Left psoas muscle, aorta	Head of pancreas	Body of pancreas			

* Site of 95% of duodenal ulcers. Posterior wall ulcers can erode the gastroduodenal artery. Gallstones may form a fistula through the anterior wall.
** A common opening, the major duodenal papilla, for the pancreatic and bile ducts, opens midway down the posteromedial wall. The retroperitoneal (lack of mesentery) nature of this region provides immobility and gives stability to the entering ducts.
# The superior mesenteric vessels, which pass anterior to the duodenum, can produce a 'nutcracker' effect, slowing the passage of digested substances through this region of the gut.

TABLE 34.3 FEATURES OF THE JEJUNUM AND ILEUM		
	Jejunum	Ileum
Length (fraction of combined 3–5 m total)	2/5	3/5
Location	Umbilical region, below the left side of transverse mesocolon	Pubic region and groin; usually extends into pelvis
Diameter	2–4 cm	2–3 cm
Wall	Thick and heavy	Thin and light
Vessels	More, one or two arcades	Less, three to four arcades
Vasa recta (small mesenteric vessels)	Long	Short
Fat	Less, gradient	More, deposited throughout
Mucosal circular folds (plicae circulare)	Larger, numerous, closely set	Smaller, widely separated to absent distally

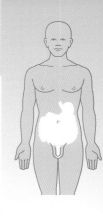

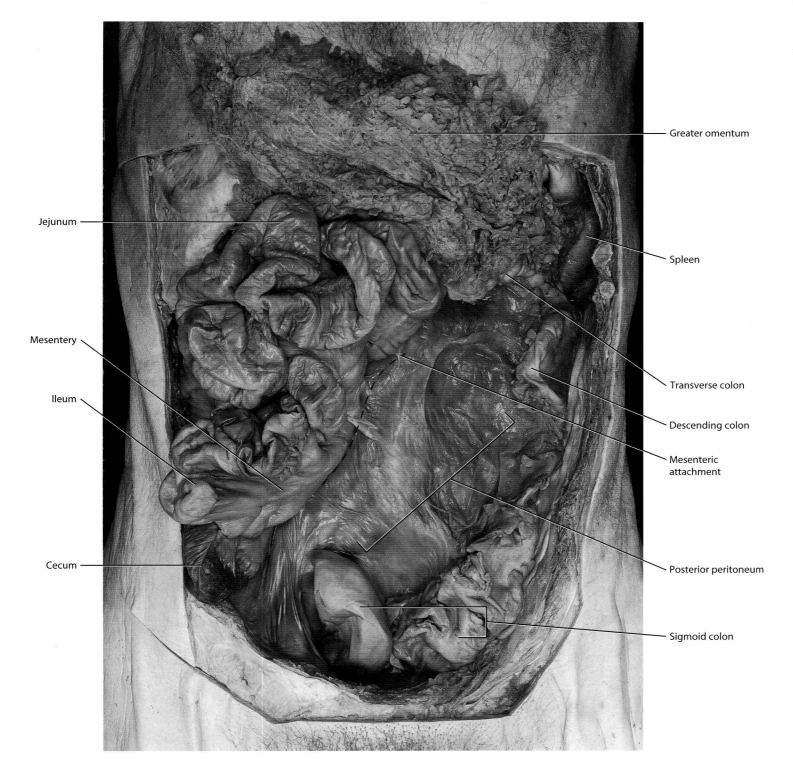

Jejunum

Mesentery

Ileum

Cecum

Greater omentum

Spleen

Transverse colon

Descending colon

Mesenteric attachment

Posterior peritoneum

Sigmoid colon

Figure 34.14 Gastrointestinal tract – mesentery of small intestine 1. The greater omentum has been reflected superiorly and the jejunum and ileum reflected to the right to reveal the diagonal attachment of the mesentery of the small intestine to the posterior abdomen

415

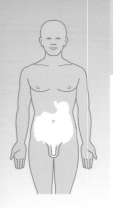

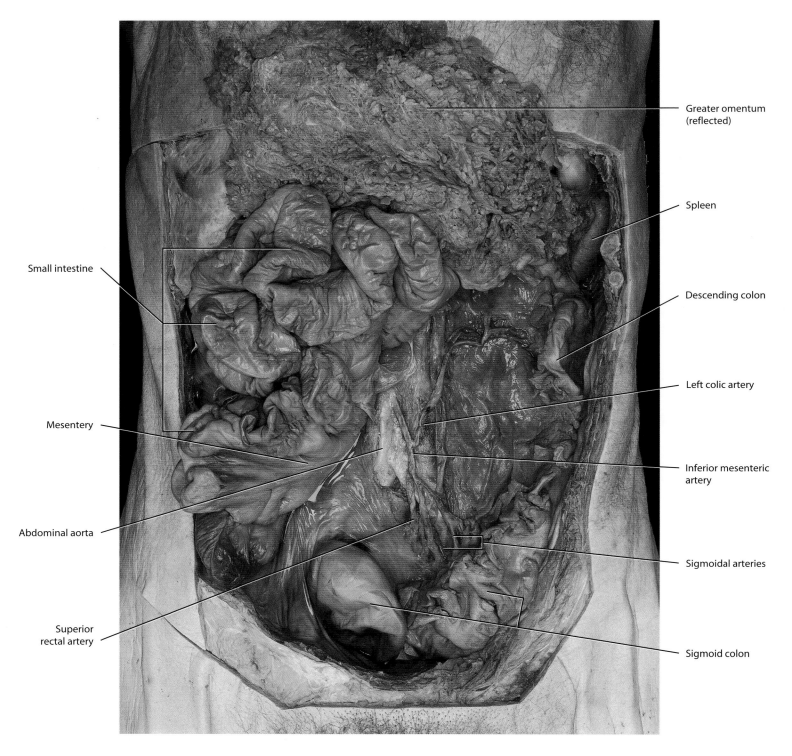

Greater omentum (reflected)

Spleen

Descending colon

Left colic artery

Inferior mesenteric artery

Sigmoidal arteries

Sigmoid colon

Small intestine

Mesentery

Abdominal aorta

Superior rectal artery

Figure 34.15 Gastrointestinal tract – mesentery of small intestine 2. The inferior mesenteric artery is shown supplying the descending artery and sigmoid colon

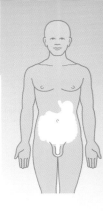

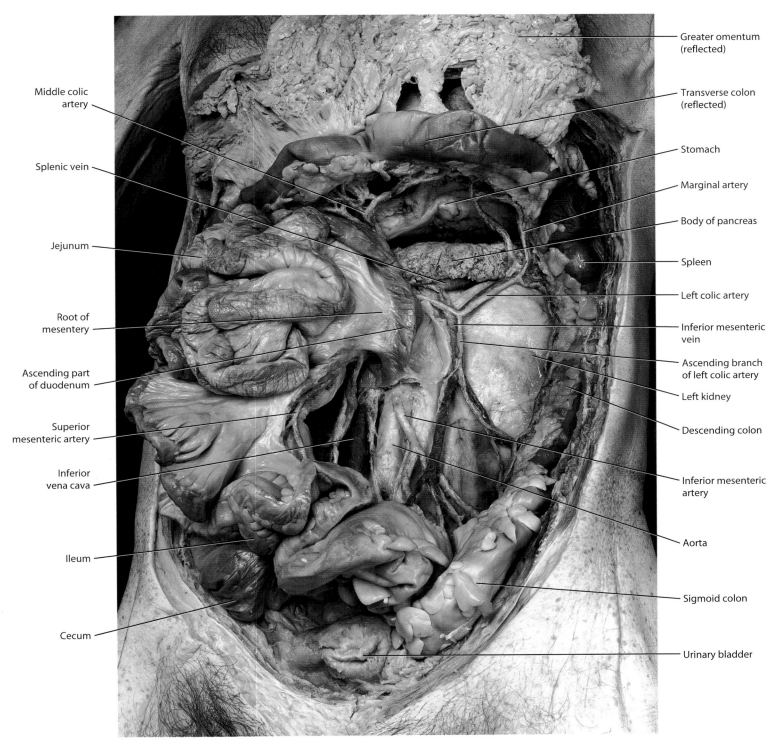

Middle colic artery

Splenic vein

Jejunum

Root of mesentery

Ascending part of duodenum

Superior mesenteric artery

Inferior vena cava

Ileum

Cecum

Greater omentum (reflected)

Transverse colon (reflected)

Stomach

Marginal artery

Body of pancreas

Spleen

Left colic artery

Inferior mesenteric vein

Ascending branch of left colic artery

Left kidney

Descending colon

Inferior mesenteric artery

Aorta

Sigmoid colon

Urinary bladder

Figure 34.16 Gastrointestinal tract – right infracolic compartment. The omentum has been reflected superiorly and the small intestine has been displaced to the right side. This reveals the surgically important relationship between the stomach, distal pancreas, spleen and left kidney. The mesentery of the small intestine and posterior peritoneum have been removed to reveal the left colic and inferior mesenteric arteries

417

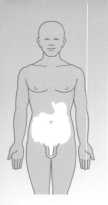

Gastrointestinal tract **TRUNK**

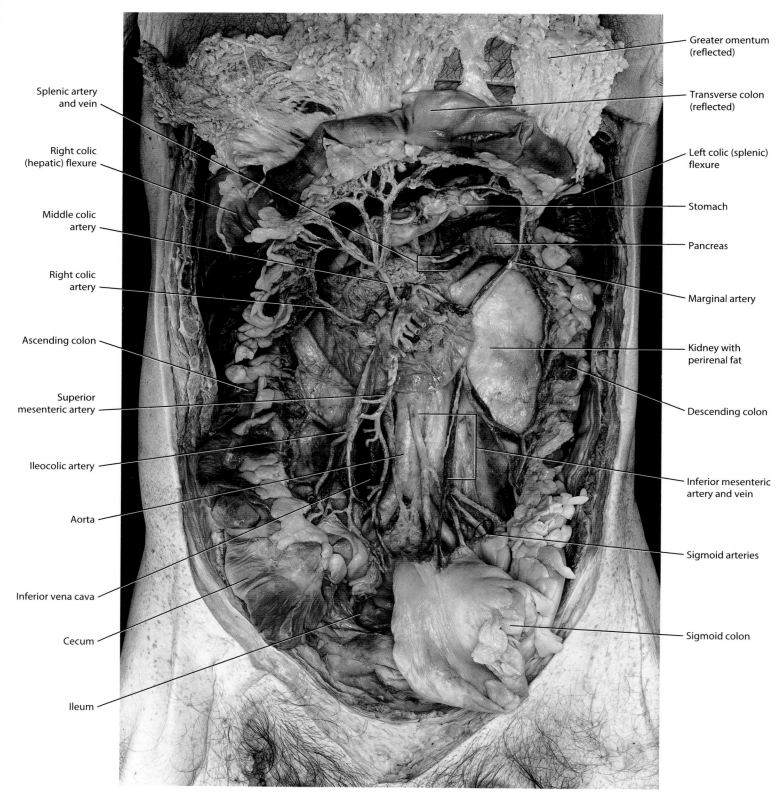

Splenic artery and vein

Right colic (hepatic) flexure

Middle colic artery

Right colic artery

Ascending colon

Superior mesenteric artery

Ileocolic artery

Aorta

Inferior vena cava

Cecum

Ileum

Greater omentum (reflected)

Transverse colon (reflected)

Left colic (splenic) flexure

Stomach

Pancreas

Marginal artery

Kidney with perirenal fat

Descending colon

Inferior mesenteric artery and vein

Sigmoid arteries

Sigmoid colon

Figure 34.17 Gastrointestinal tract – left infracolic compartment. The entire small intestine has been removed. The arteries to the small and large intestines are shown. The left kidney is visible. The transverse mesocolon has been dissected out to show the pancreas and stomach

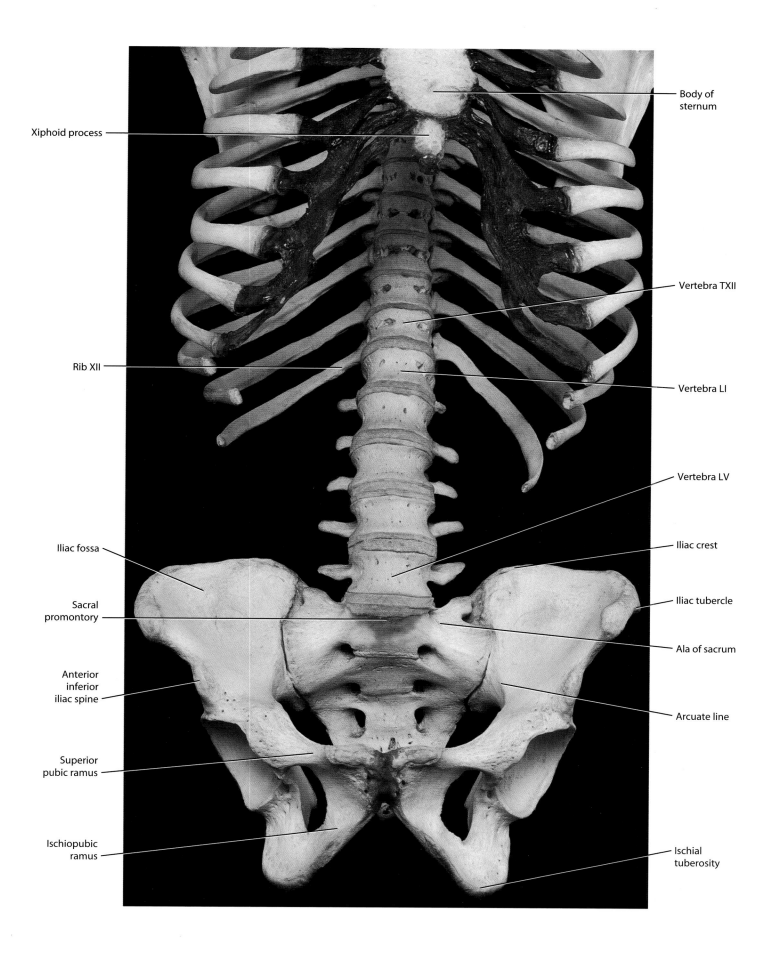

Body of
sternum

Xiphoid process

Vertebra TXII

Rib XII

Vertebra LI

Vertebra LV

Iliac fossa

Iliac crest

Sacral
promontory

Iliac tubercle

Ala of sacrum

Anterior
inferior
iliac spine

Arcuate line

Superior
pubic ramus

Ischiopubic
ramus

Ischial
tuberosity

Figure 34.18 Gastrointestinal tract – osteology. Anterior view of the bones that support the gastrointestinal tract

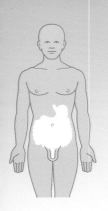

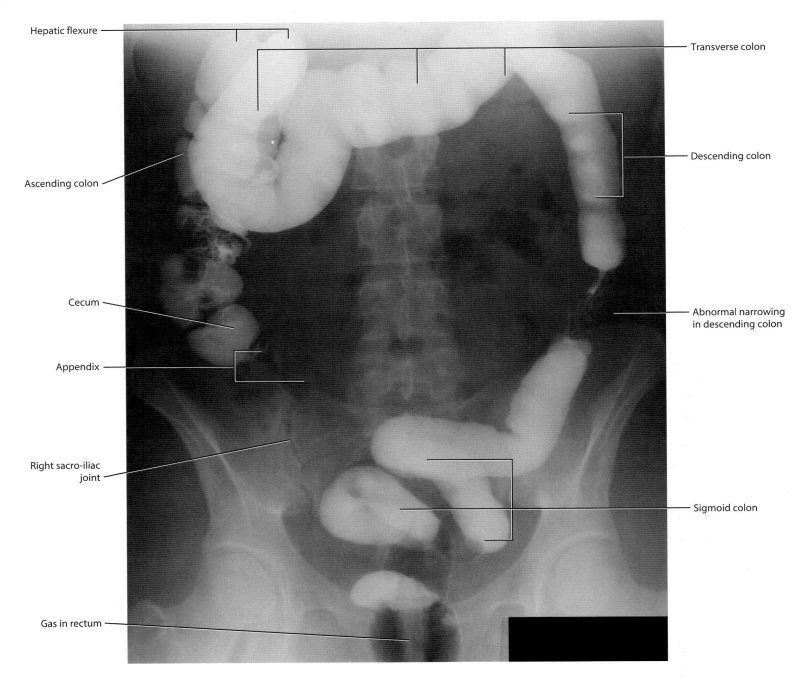

Hepatic flexure

Transverse colon

Ascending colon

Descending colon

Cecum

Abnormal narrowing
in descending colon

Appendix

Right sacro-iliac
joint

Sigmoid colon

Gas in rectum

Figure 34.19 Gastrointestinal tract – barium contrast radiograph (anteroposterior view, supine position). The colon is situated peripherally and the small bowel occupies the central portion of the abdominal cavity, as visualized by use of a barium enema. Note the area of narrowing, which was due to carcinoma of the colon. Also observe the presence of the normal appendix, which has taken up some contrast

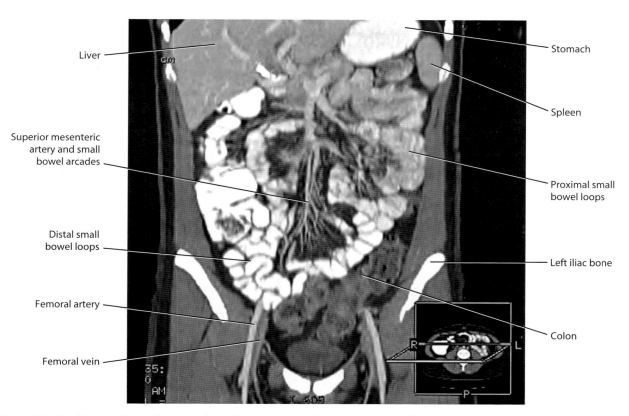

Figure 34.20 Gastrointestinal tract – CT scan (coronal view). This scan was performed some time after administration of oral contrast medium. The contrast medium has moved into the distal small bowel and proximal colon, which appear much enhanced as a result. Note the detail of the venous and arterial arcades extending to the small bowel loop

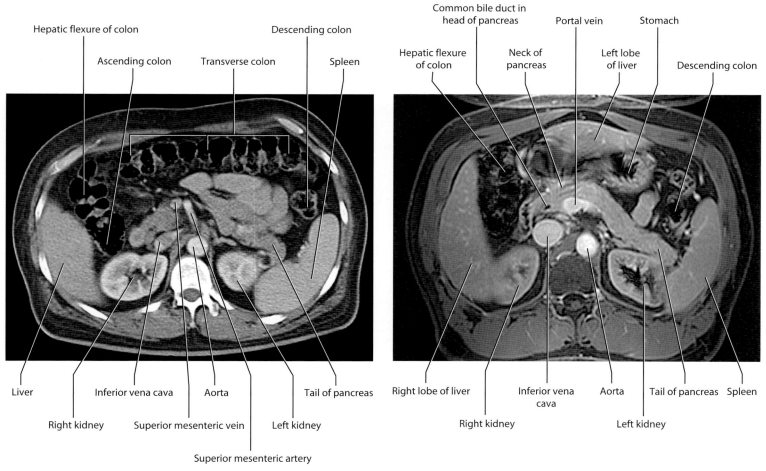

Figure 34.21 Gastrointestinal tract – CT scan (axial view). The patient is supine, as can be inferred from the gas in the transverse colon, rising to the most superior point, and stool in the inferior parts.

Figure 34.22 Gastrointestinal tract – MRI scan (axial view). This view is at approximately at the level of the LI vertebral body

421

35

Anterolateral abdominal wall and groin

The abdomen is the part of the trunk that lies between the diaphragm and pelvis. The abdominal and pelvic cavities are continuous, and the abdominal cavity is lined by a serous membrane (**peritoneum**, see Chapters 33 and 34) and contains most of the organs of the digestive system.

From superficial to deep, the layers covering the anterior and lateral abdomen are skin, subcutaneous tissue, muscles or fascia, extraperitoneal tissue, and peritoneum (Table 35.1). This multilayered musculofascial organization contributes to the anatomy of the groin. During embryological descent of the male gonads, these layers are drawn inferiorly and contribute to the formation of the spermatic cord and scrotum.

Structural support for the abdominal region is provided superiorly by the inferior margin of the rib cage, anteriorly by the muscles of the anterior abdominal wall, inferiorly by the pelvic girdle and pelvic diaphragm (see Chapter 36), and posteriorly by the vertebral column, ribs, and back muscles.

MUSCLES

The anterior abdominal wall contains the **rectus abdominis** muscle, which is a long muscle in the midline that flexes the trunk and extends from the inferior rib cage to the pelvic inlet. The rectus abdominis is covered by several layers of fascia derived from three anterolateral abdominal muscles (Fig. 35.1).

The anterolateral abdominal wall is composed of three sheet-like muscles (Table 35.2): an outer **external oblique**, a middle **internal oblique**, and an inner **transversus abdominis** muscle (Fig. 35.1). Anteriorly, these muscles become aponeurotic, fuse, and form a sheath around the rectus abdominis muscle. They rotate and flex the trunk anteriorly and laterally, and assist in expiration, coughing, vomiting, and defecation.

The **rectus sheath** (Table 35.3) formed by the anterolateral abdominal muscle aponeurosis contains the superior and inferior epigastric vessels, the segmental thoraco-abdominal nerves (T7 to T11), the subcostal (T12) nerves, and lymphatic vessels.

NERVES

Sensory and motor innervation of the anterolateral abdominal wall and groin is by the **thoraco-abdominal nerves** (T7 to T11), the **subcostal nerves** (T12), and the first lumbar nerves (L1, which divides into the **iliohypogastric** and **ilio-inguinal nerves**) (Fig. 35.2). These segmental nerves are oriented transversely over the abdomen in the neurovascular plane between the internal oblique and transversus abdominis muscles.

ARTERIES

The anterolateral abdominal wall is supplied by the **intercostal**, **subcostal**, **superior epigastric** (from the internal thoracic artery), **musculophrenic** (from the superior epigastric artery), and **inferior epigastric** (from the external iliac artery) **arteries** and by branches of the **femoral artery** (Fig. 35.2). The superior and inferior epigastric arteries anastomose in the anterior abdomen to create a collateral circulation between the subclavian and external iliac arteries.

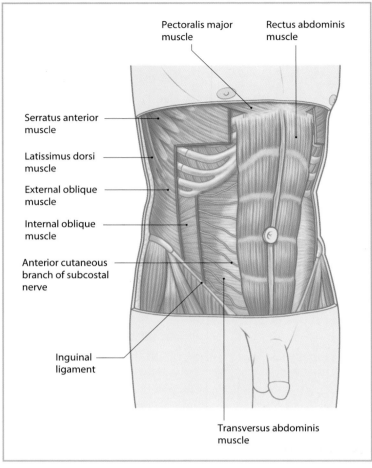

Figure 35.1 Anterior abdominal wall muscles

VEINS AND LYMPHATICS

Venous drainage for the anterolateral abdominal wall is via venae comitantes of the arteries listed above. Lymphatic drainage above the level of the umbilicus flows to the **axillary lymph nodes**; lymph vessels below the umbilicus drain to the **superficial inguinal nodes**. These nodes also receive lymphatic drainage from the external genitalia, the anal region, and the lower limbs.

ABDOMINAL WALL

The internal surface of the anterior abdominal wall inferior to the umbilicus has five ridges of peritoneum, which are derivatives of fetal structures:

- the **median umbilical fold**, produced by the urachus (the remnant of the allantois), extends from the bladder to the umbilicus;
- the **medial umbilical folds**, produced by the obliterated umbilical arteries, extend from the lateral aspect of bladder to the umbilicus;
- the **lateral umbilical fold**, produced by the functional inferior epigastric arteries extends from the medial aspect of the deep inguinal ring to the arcuate line;
- superior to the umbilicus, also on the internal surface of the anterior abdominal wall, the **round ligament of liver** extends from the umbilicus to the visceral surface of the liver.

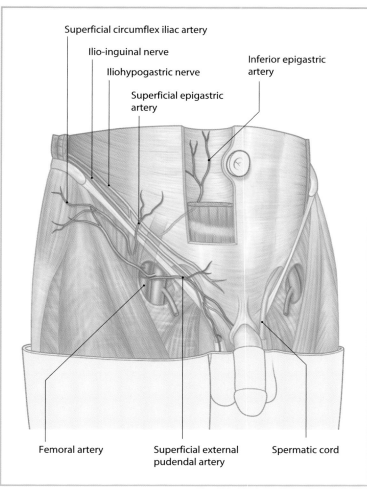

Figure 35.2 Groin

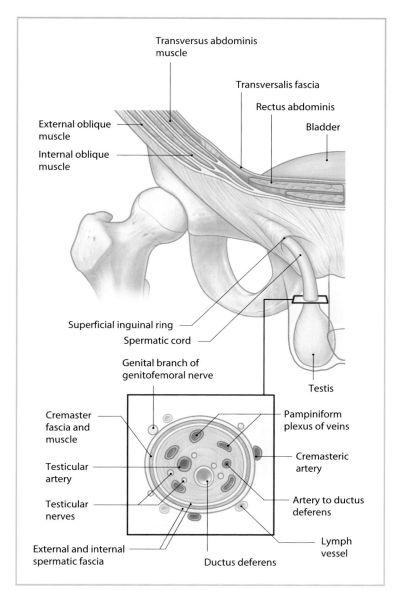

Figure 35.3 Spermatic cord

INGUINAL REGION (GROIN)

Just superior to the inguinal ligament, the **inguinal canal** forms a passage for structures passing through the abdominal wall. It has a deep and a superficial ring. In the male, the **spermatic cord** passes from the abdominal cavity through the inguinal canal to the scrotum (Fig. 35.3). In the female, the **round ligament of uterus** passes from the uterus through the inguinal canal and attaches to the base of the labia majora.

From the **deep inguinal ring** to the **superficial inguinal ring**, the structures that the canal passes through are the peritoneum, the transversalis fascia, the transversus abdominis muscle, the internal oblique muscle, and the external oblique muscle.

In the male, the inguinal canal contains the spermatic cord, the cremasteric vessels, the ilio-inguinal nerve, and the genital branch of the genitofemoral nerve. In the female, the inguinal canal contains the round ligament of uterus and the genital branch of the genitofemoral nerve (see Chapter 32).

SPERMATIC CORD

The spermatic cord begins at the deep inguinal ring superior to the inguinal ligament and lateral to the inferior epigastric vessels. It passes through the inguinal canal (Fig. 35.3) with:

- the **ductus deferens;**
- sympathetic autonomic nerves;

- the **testicular artery** (from the aorta);
- **artery to ductus deferens** (from the inferior vesical artery);
- **cremasteric artery** (from the inferior epigastric artery);
- **pampiniform plexus** of veins (a spiral coiling group of veins that drains the scrotum and testis);
- lymph vessels that drain to the lumbar and pre-aortic lymph nodes;
- **genital branch** of the genitofemoral nerve;
- **cremaster muscle** (from the internal oblique muscle), which elevates the scrotum.

SCROTUM

The scrotum is derived from the anterolateral abdominal wall. It supports the testis, which must remain at a slightly lower temperature than the rest of the body to produce viable sperm.

■ CLINICAL CORRELATIONS
Direct and indirect inguinal and femoral hernias

A hernia is a defect in the abdominal wall resulting in a protrusion of abdominal contents. The most common location for a hernia is

TRUNK Anterolateral abdominal wall and groin

423

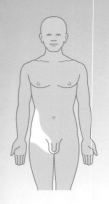
in the groin. At least 5% of people have a hernia during their lifetime. Causes include chronic increased intra-abdominal pressure as a result of cough, constipation, prostate enlargement, or colon cancer.

The defect that forms in the abdominal wall usually occurs at the weakest point; this is the deep inguinal ring, through which pass the spermatic cord in men and the round ligament of uterus in women. Approximately half of all inguinal hernias follow this route through the inguinal canal, and are called **indirect inguinal hernias** (Fig. 35.4). Occasionally, in men, a hernial sac can be seen extending into the scrotum.

Direct inguinal hernias result from an acquired defect of the anterolateral abdominal wall through the **inguinal (Hesselbach's) triangle** (Fig. 35.4), which is bounded:

- inferiorly, by the inguinal ligament;
- laterally, by the inferior epigastric vessels; and
- medially, by the lateral border of the rectus abdominis muscle.

This triangle includes part of the abdominal wall just superior to the inguinal canal. Direct inguinal hernias can also extend to the scrotum, making differentiation by clinical examination difficult.

A third major type of hernia is the **femoral hernia** (see Chapter 40). In general, hernias cause the sensation of a bulge that increases with a Valsalva maneuver (abdominal straining against a closed glottis), and decrease with relaxation (spontaneously reducible hernia). The bulge may remain constant for long periods (incarcerated hernia), indicating that the hernial sac and intestinal contents cannot return to their intra-abdominal location. If the blood flow to the hernia contents is limited, ischemia will ensue (strangulated hernia).

A diagnosis of hernia is clinical and based on the history and physical examination. The hernial sac is palpable as the patient carries out a Valsalva maneuver (for example, by coughing).

Management of inguinal hernia is by elective repair unless there are symptoms and signs of strangulation, in which case immediate surgery for hernia reduction and repair is required.

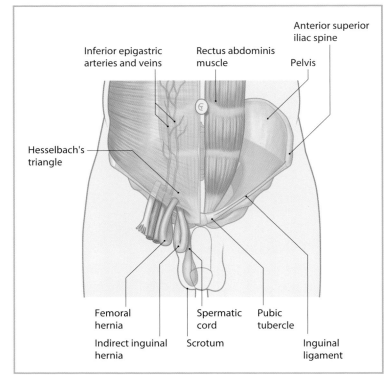

Figure 35.4 Femoral and indirect inguinal hernias

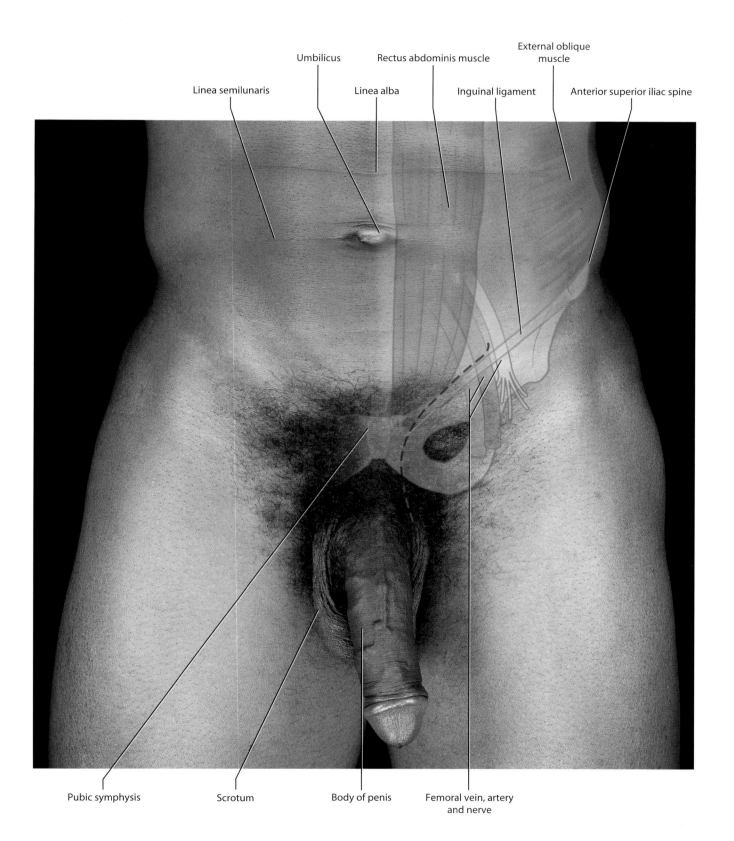

Linea semilunaris

Umbilicus

Linea alba

Rectus abdominis muscle

Inguinal ligament

External oblique muscle

Anterior superior iliac spine

Pubic symphysis

Scrotum

Body of penis

Femoral vein, artery and nerve

TRUNK Anterolateral abdominal wall and groin

Figure 35.5 Anterolateral abdominal wall and groin, male – surface anatomy. Observe the prominence of the area just superior to the inguinal crease, which contains the spermatic cord

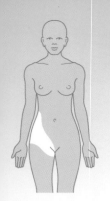

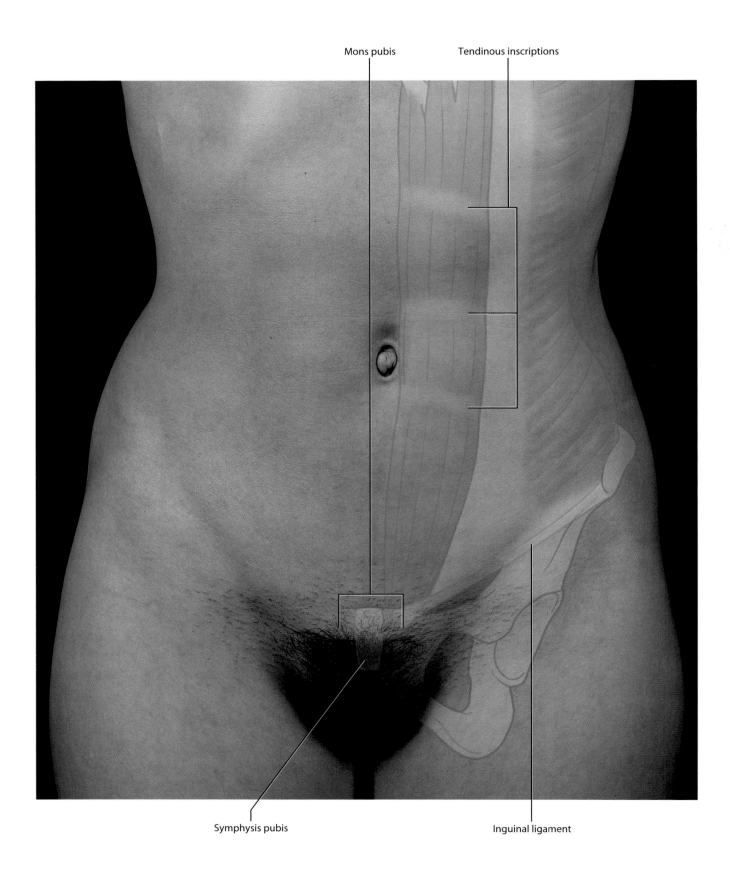

Mons pubis

Tendinous inscriptions

Symphysis pubis

Inguinal ligament

Figure 35.6 **Anterolateral abdominal wall and groin, female – surface anatomy.** Observe the inguinal crease

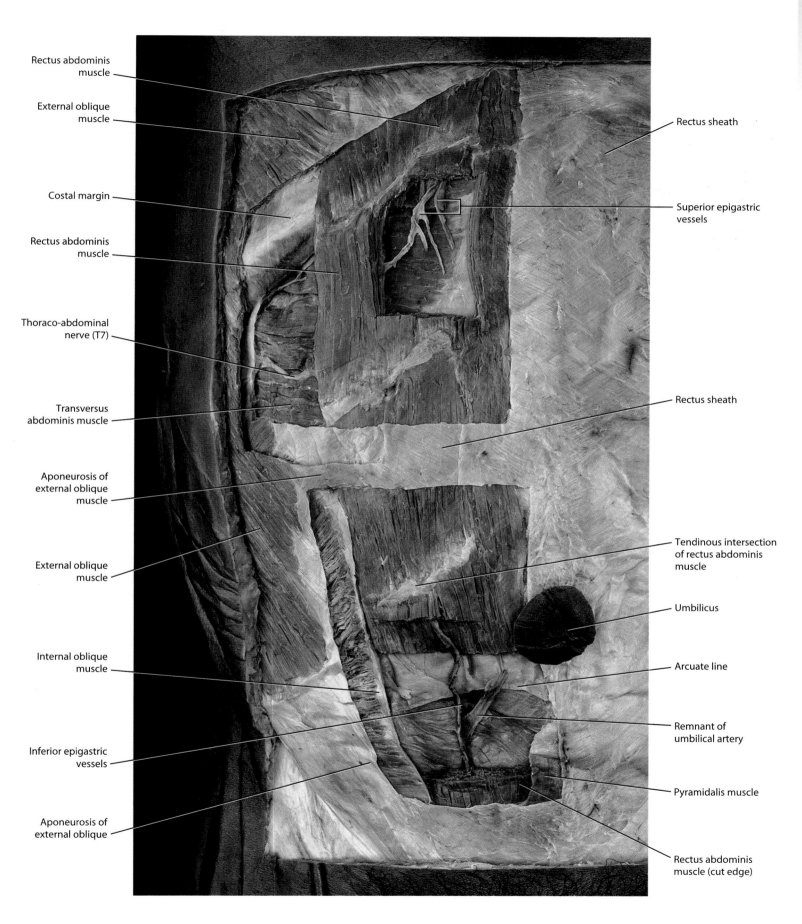

Rectus abdominis muscle

External oblique muscle

Costal margin

Rectus abdominis muscle

Thoraco-abdominal nerve (T7)

Transversus abdominis muscle

Aponeurosis of external oblique muscle

External oblique muscle

Internal oblique muscle

Inferior epigastric vessels

Aponeurosis of external oblique

Rectus sheath

Superior epigastric vessels

Rectus sheath

Tendinous intersection of rectus abdominis muscle

Umbilicus

Arcuate line

Remnant of umbilical artery

Pyramidalis muscle

Rectus abdominis muscle (cut edge)

Figure 35.7 Anterolateral abdominal wall – superficial dissection. Anterior view of the anterolateral abdominal wall. Rectangular-shaped windows have been cut in the rectus sheath and muscles to show deeper structures. Note the superior and inferior epigastric vessels. The umbilicus has been preserved as a point of reference

ANTEROLATERAL ABDOMINAL WALL – INTERMEDIATE DISSECTION

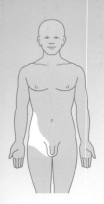

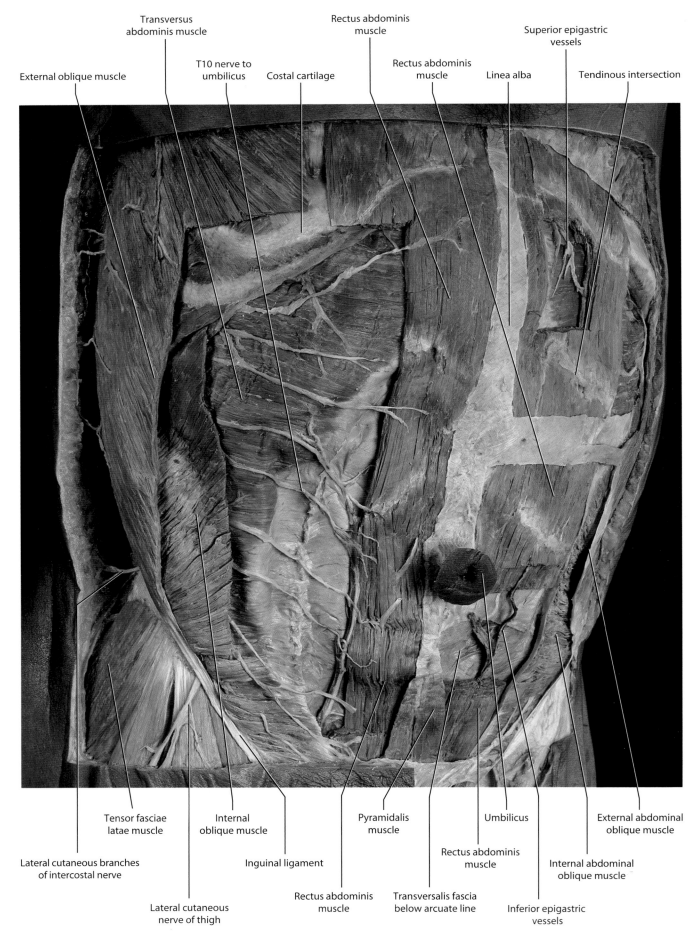

Transversus abdominis muscle

Rectus abdominis muscle

External oblique muscle

T10 nerve to umbilicus

Costal cartilage

Rectus abdominis muscle

Superior epigastric vessels

Linea alba

Tendinous intersection

Tensor fasciae latae muscle

Internal oblique muscle

Pyramidalis muscle

Umbilicus

External abdominal oblique muscle

Lateral cutaneous branches of intercostal nerve

Inguinal ligament

Rectus abdominis muscle

Internal abdominal oblique muscle

Lateral cutaneous nerve of thigh

Rectus abdominis muscle

Transversalis fascia below arcuate line

Inferior epigastric vessels

Figure 35.8 Anterolateral abdominal wall – intermediate dissection. This dissection is deeper than that in Figure 35.7; the external and internal oblique muscles have been almost completely removed on the right side of the body to show the spinal nerves and transversus abdominis muscle

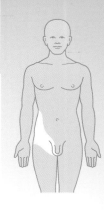

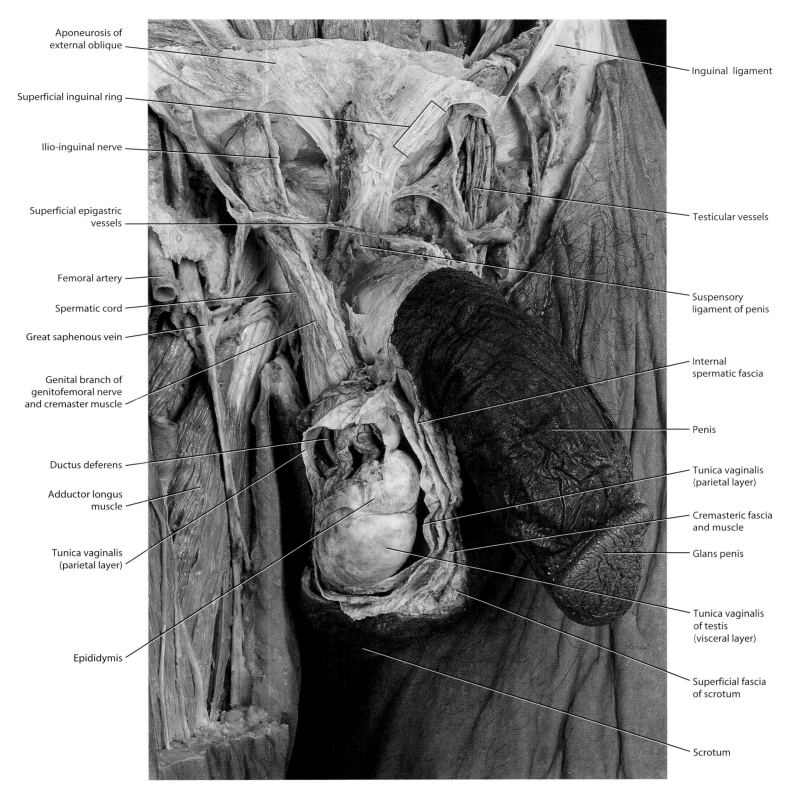

Aponeurosis of external oblique

Superficial inguinal ring

Ilio-inguinal nerve

Superficial epigastric vessels

Femoral artery

Spermatic cord

Great saphenous vein

Genital branch of genitofemoral nerve and cremaster muscle

Ductus deferens

Adductor longus muscle

Tunica vaginalis (parietal layer)

Epididymis

Inguinal ligament

Testicular vessels

Suspensory ligament of penis

Internal spermatic fascia

Penis

Tunica vaginalis (parietal layer)

Cremasteric fascia and muscle

Glans penis

Tunica vaginalis of testis (visceral layer)

Superficial fascia of scrotum

Scrotum

Figure 35.9 Groin, male – intermediate dissection. The spermatic cord and superficial inguinal ring are preserved. Observe the layers of the scrotum and the testis

429

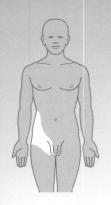

TABLE 35.1 ANTEROLATERAL ABDOMINAL WALL – LAYERS AND DERIVATIVES

Anterior abdominal wall layers	Scrotal layers	Inguinal canal
1. Skin	Skin	
2. Superficial fascia	Dartos fascia and muscle	
3. External abdominal oblique muscle/aponeurosis	External spermatic fascia	Superficial inguinal ring, anterior wall, floor – inguinal and lacunar ligaments
4. Internal abdominal oblique muscle/aponeurosis	Cremaster muscle	Roof and posterior wall via conjoint tendon
5. Transversus abdominis muscle	Cremaster muscle	
6. Transversalis fascia	Internal spermatic fascia	Deep inguinal ring and posterior wall
7. Extraperitoneal connective tissue/fat	Fat	
8. Peritoneum	Tunica vaginalis	

TABLE 35.2 MUSCLES OF ANTEROLATERAL ABDOMINAL WALL

Muscle	Origin	Insertion	Action	Nerve supply	Blood supply
External oblique	External surface lower eight ribs	Iliac crest, pubic tubercle, linea alba, xiphoid process	Rotates and flexes the trunk, compresses abdominal contents	T7 to T11 intercostal nerves, subcostal (T12), iliohypogastric, and ilio-inguinal (L1) nerves	Superior and inferior epigastric arteries
Internal oblique	Inguinal ligament (lateral 2/3), iliac crest, and thoracolumbar fascia	Lower four ribs, linea alba, pubic crest and pectineal line	Rotates and flexes the trunk, compresses abdominal contents	T7 to T11 intercostal nerves, subcostal (T12), iliohypogastric, and ilio-inguinal (L1) nerves	Superior and inferior epigastric and deep circumflex iliac arteries
Transversus abdominis	Lower six costal cartilages, thoracolumbar fascia, iliac crest, inguinal ligament (lateral 1/3)	Xiphoid process, linea alba, pubic crest and pectineal line via conjoint tendon	Compresses abdominal contents with the oblique muscles	T7 to T11 intercostal nerves, subcostal (T12), iliohypogastric, and ilio-inguinal (L1) nerves	Deep circumflex iliac, and inferior epigastric arteries
Rectus abdominis	Pubic crest and pubic symphysis	Xiphoid process, costal cartilages V to VII	Compresses abdominal contents and flexes trunk	T7 to T11 intercostal nerves, subcostal nerve (T12)	Superior and inferior epigastric arteries
Pyramidalis	Body of pubis	Linea alba	Tenses the linea alba	Subcostal nerve (T12)	Inferior epigastric artery

TABLE 35.3 COMPONENTS OF RECTUS SHEATH

Level	Anterior wall	Posterior wall
Above costal margin	Aponeurosis of external oblique muscle	Costal cartilages
Costal margin to lower 1/4 of sheath	Aponeurosis of external oblique muscle and anterior lamina of internal oblique muscle	Posterior lamina of internal oblique, aponeurosis of transversus abdominis and transversalis fascia
Lower 1/4 of sheath	Aponeurosis of external and internal oblique and transversus abdominis muscles	Transversalis fascia

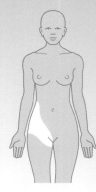

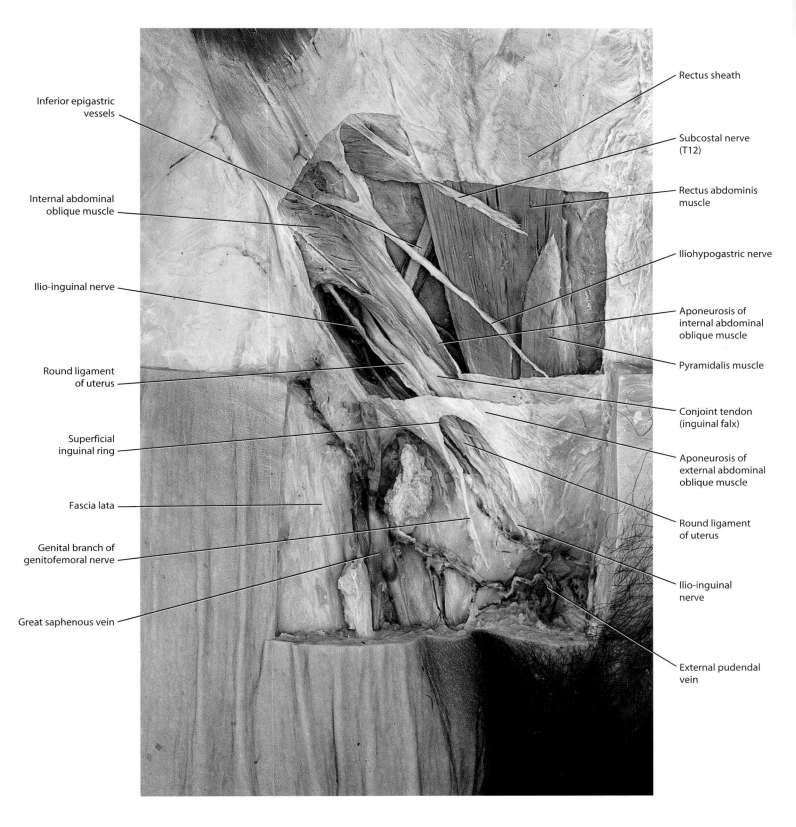

Inferior epigastric vessels

Internal abdominal oblique muscle

Ilio-inguinal nerve

Round ligament of uterus

Superficial inguinal ring

Fascia lata

Genital branch of genitofemoral nerve

Great saphenous vein

Rectus sheath

Subcostal nerve (T12)

Rectus abdominis muscle

Iliohypogastric nerve

Aponeurosis of internal abdominal oblique muscle

Pyramidalis muscle

Conjoint tendon (inguinal falx)

Aponeurosis of external abdominal oblique muscle

Round ligament of uterus

Ilio-inguinal nerve

External pudendal vein

Figure 35.10 Groin, female – intermediate dissection. The round ligament of uterus is seen emerging from the superficial inguinal ring and inserting onto the base of the labia majora

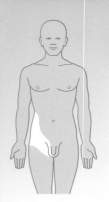

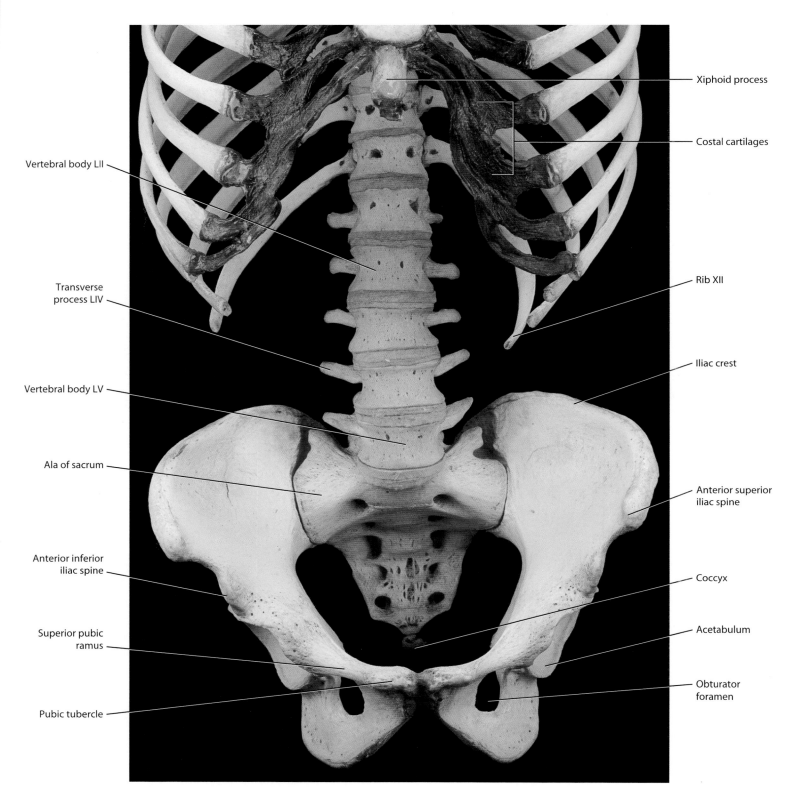

Xiphoid process

Costal cartilages

Vertebral body LII

Transverse
process LIV

Rib XII

Iliac crest

Vertebral body LV

Ala of sacrum

Anterior superior
iliac spine

Anterior inferior
iliac spine

Coccyx

Superior pubic
ramus

Acetabulum

Obturator
foramen

Pubic tubercle

Figure 35.11 Anterolateral abdominal wall and groin – osteology. Anterior view of the articulated bones that support the anterolateral abdominal wall and groin

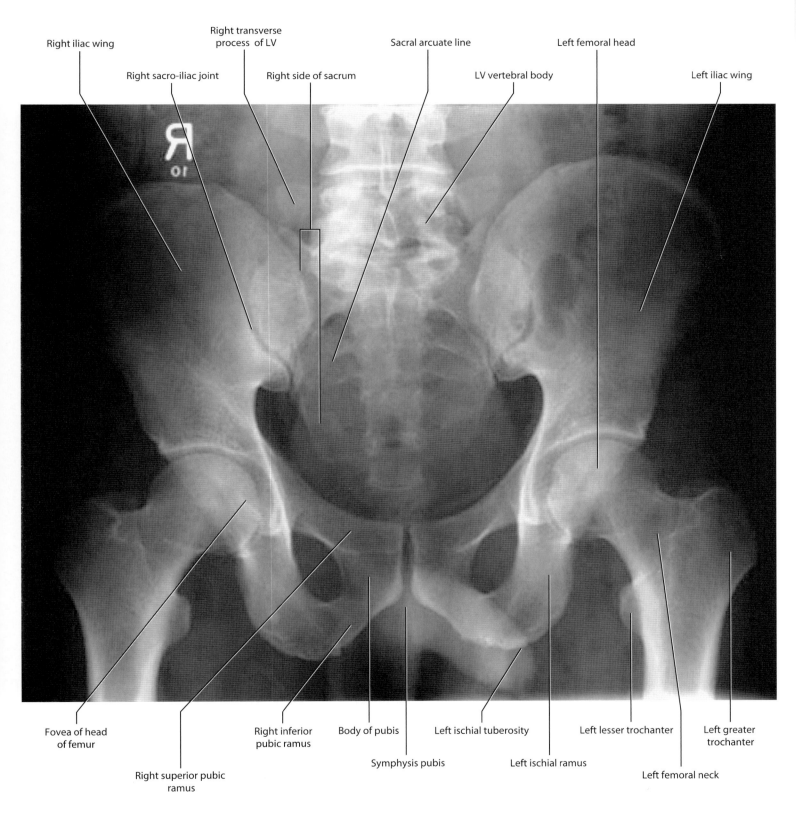

Right iliac wing

Right transverse process of LV

Sacral arcuate line

Left femoral head

Right sacro-iliac joint

Right side of sacrum

LV vertebral body

Left iliac wing

Fovea of head of femur

Right inferior pubic ramus

Body of pubis

Left ischial tuberosity

Left lesser trochanter

Left greater trochanter

Right superior pubic ramus

Symphysis pubis

Left ischial ramus

Left femoral neck

TRUNK Anterolateral abdominal wall and groin

Figure 35.12 Groin, male – plain film radiograph (anteroposterior view). Note that the shadow of the penis and testicles are visible inferior to the symphysis pubis. The left external inguinal ring is located just superior to the leader line for right superior pubic ramus. Under normal circumstances inguinal structures are not visible on plain radiographs

433

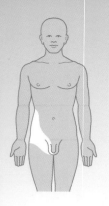

TRUNK

Anterolateral abdominal wall and groin

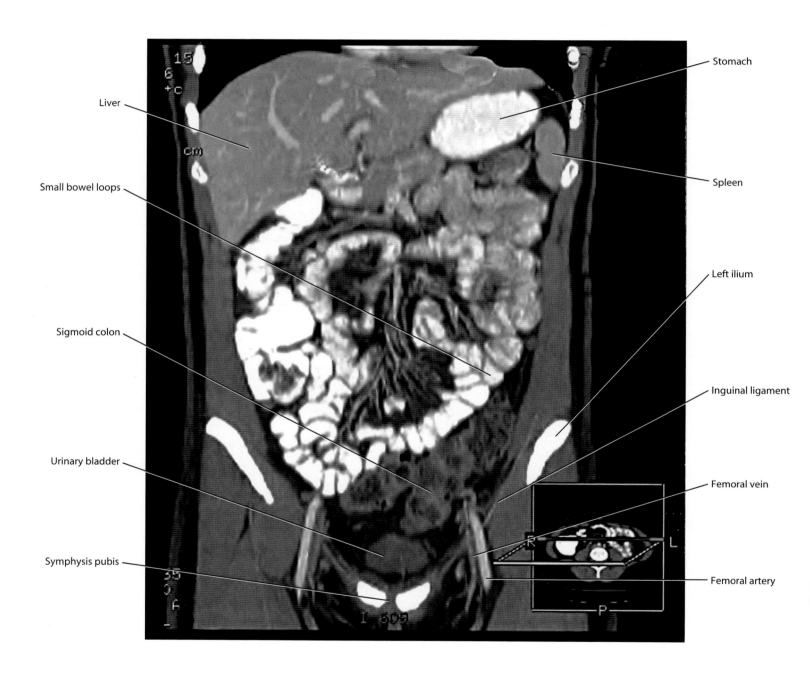

Liver

Small bowel loops

Sigmoid colon

Urinary bladder

Symphysis pubis

Stomach

Spleen

Left ilium

Inguinal ligament

Femoral vein

Femoral artery

Figure 35.13 Groin – CT scan (coronal view). Note the oblique course of the inguinal ligament from superior and lateral to inferior and medial. For the placement of femoral venous catheters it is important to note that the femoral vein is medial to the femoral artery

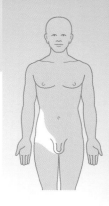

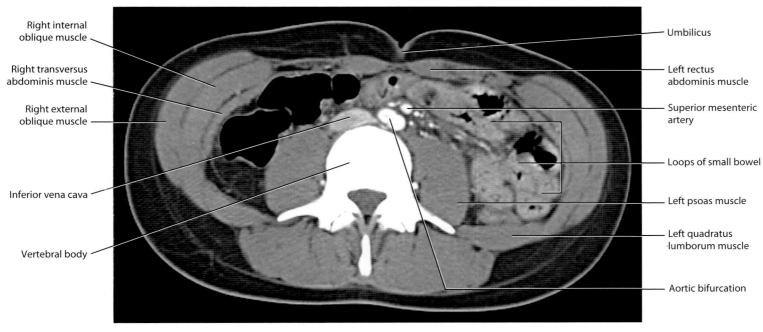

Right internal oblique muscle

Right transversus abdominis muscle

Right external oblique muscle

Inferior vena cava

Vertebral body

Umbilicus

Left rectus abdominis muscle

Superior mesenteric artery

Loops of small bowel

Left psoas muscle

Left quadratus lumborum muscle

Aortic bifurcation

Figure 35.14 Anterolateral abdominal wall – CT scan (axial view). Note the excellent visualization of the muscles of the anterolateral abdominal wall

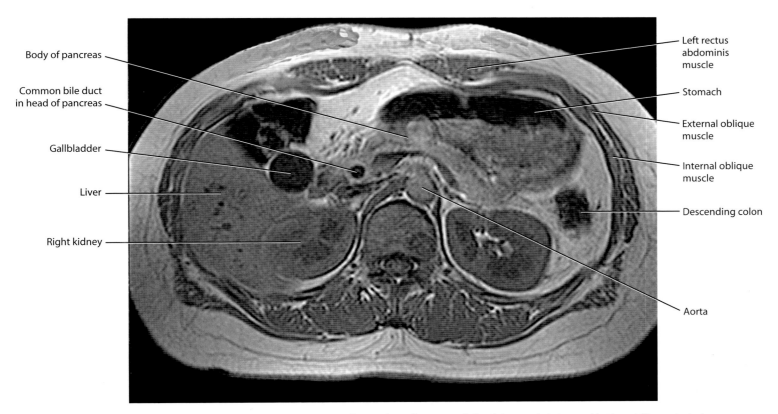

Body of pancreas

Common bile duct in head of pancreas

Gallbladder

Liver

Right kidney

Left rectus abdominis muscle

Stomach

External oblique muscle

Internal oblique muscle

Descending colon

Aorta

Figure 35.15 Anterolateral abdominal wall – MRI scan (axial view). Observe how the rectus abdominis muscle is located in the midline anteriorly

435

36

Pelvic girdle

The pelvic girdle is an attachment point for the vertebral column and lower limbs (Fig. 36.1). It is also involved in balance and weight transfer by transmitting the weight of the head and neck, trunk, and upper limbs to both lower limbs.

The left and right sides of the pelvic girdle are identical and are composed of two **hip bones**, which are formed from the fusion of the ilium, ischium, and pubis.

- The **ilium** forms the large superior part of the hip bone and has a body and an ala (wing). The superior part of the ala forms a crest (the **iliac crest**), which is palpable in most individuals.
- The **pubis** forms the anterior part of the pelvic girdle and has a body and superior and inferior rami. The two pubis bones are joined in the midline by the **pubic symphysis**, a joint at which movement is slight but nevertheless is of assistance during childbirth.
- The **ischium** forms the inferior part of the pelvic girdle and has a body and ramus, and a large **ischial tuberosity**, the 'sitting bone'.

The **sacrum** is in the midline of the posterior pelvic girdle. This triangular bone has multiple foramina for the sacral nerves to pass through. It unites the posterior pelvic girdle via the sacro-iliac joints.

At the inferior margin of the sacrum is the **coccyx**, which is made up of small, usually fused, bones.

The **sacrococcygeal joint** is a cartilaginous joint between the sacrum and coccyx. It is heavily reinforced by ligaments on its anterior, lateral, and posterior surfaces. The sacrum and coccyx stabilize the pelvis and provide attachment points for the ligaments and muscles of the pelvis, lower back (see Chapter 28), and thigh (see Chapters 40 and 42).

On the lateral surface of the pelvic girdle is the **acetabulum** – a cup-shaped depression where the head of the femur articulates with the pelvic girdle.

Two major ligaments join the sacrum to the ilium and ischium:

- the **sacrospinous ligament** extends from the sacrum to the ischial spine and forms the **lesser sciatic foramen**;
- the **sacrotuberous ligament** extends from the sacrum to the ischial tuberosity and forms the **greater sciatic foramen**.

Neurovascular structures from within the pelvic girdle pass through the greater and lesser sciatic foramina to the gluteal region, posterior thigh, and perineum:

- the piriformis muscle, sciatic nerve, inferior gluteal nerve and artery, internal pudendal nerve, artery, and vein, nerve to quadratus femoris, nerve to obturator internus, and posterior cutaneous nerve of thigh pass through the greater sciatic foramen;
- the tendon of obturator internus muscle, nerve to obturator internus, pudendal nerve, and internal pudendal artery pass through the lesser sciatic foramen.

The **obturator foramen** is inferior to the acetabulum (Fig. 36.1) and most of it is closed by a membrane of flat connective tissue, the **obturator membrane**.

MUSCLES

The pelvic girdle is lined by muscles that support the trunk and move the lower limbs. These muscles are described in Chapters 28, 32, 40, and 42. The pelvic girdle does not have any mobile joints, so there are no intrinsic muscles (muscles that move pelvic bones). However, several muscles span different parts of the pelvis and support the pelvic viscera (see Chapter 37) and perineum (see Chapter 38).

The muscles of the pelvis are described according to their location. The **obturator internus** muscle covers part of the lateral pelvic wall. It passes from the internal surface of the obturator membrane of the pelvis and its fibers converge to form a tendon that leaves the pelvis laterally through the lesser sciatic foramen and inserts onto the greater trochanter of the femur and assists with lateral rotation of the thigh.

The posterior pelvic wall is partly covered by the **piriformis** muscle. This muscle originates from the anterior surface of the sacrum, extends laterally through the greater sciatic foramen to insert onto the greater trochanter of the femur, and laterally rotates the femur. The nerves of the sacral plexus are medial to the origin of piriformis.

The **pelvic diaphragm** (pelvic floor) is formed from the levator ani and coccygeus muscles (see Chapter 38).

NERVES

The nerve supply to the pelvis is provided by voluntary (somatic) and involuntary (autonomic) nerves (Fig. 36.2). The somatic nerves are branches of the **sacral plexus** of nerves, which is formed from the joining of L4 and L5 lumbar spinal nerves (lumbosacral trunk) and sacral spinal nerves S1 to S4. Nerve fibers from this plexus intertwine in various combinations to form:

- The **superior gluteal nerve** (L4 to S1) exits the pelvis through the greater sciatic foramen to enter the gluteal region and innervate the gluteus medius and minimus muscles as well as the tensor fasciae latae muscle.

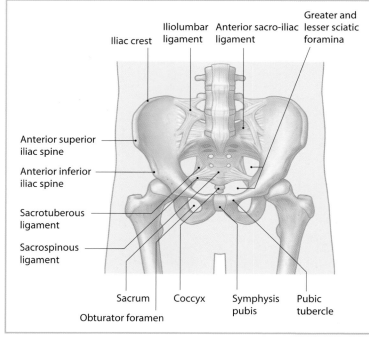

Iliolumbar ligament Anterior sacro-iliac ligament Greater and lesser sciatic foramina

Iliac crest

Anterior superior iliac spine

Anterior inferior iliac spine

Sacrotuberous ligament

Sacrospinous ligament

Sacrum Coccyx Symphysis pubis Pubic tubercle

Obturator foramen

Figure 36.1 Pelvis – anterior view

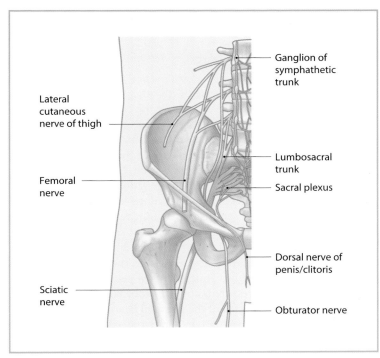

Figure 36.2 Nerves of the pelvis – anterior view

- The **inferior gluteal nerve** (L5 to S2) exits the pelvis through the greater sciatic foramen to innervate the gluteus maximus muscle.
- The **sciatic nerve** (L4 to S3) is the largest nerve in the body and leaves the pelvis through the greater sciatic foramen to innervate all structures of the posterior thigh, leg, ankle, and foot (except for a small area of skin on the anteromedial leg, supplied by the femoral nerve).
- The **nerve to obturator internus** (L5 to S2) leaves the pelvis medial to the sciatic nerve and enters the gluteal region to innervate the obturator internus and superior gemellus muscles.
- The **nerve to quadratus femoris** (L5 to S1) leaves the pelvis anterior to the sciatic nerve via the greater sciatic foramen. It supplies an articular branch to the hip joint and a muscular branch to the inferior gemellus muscle before terminating at the quadratus femoris muscle.
- The **pudendal nerve** (S2 to 4) leaves the pelvis through the greater sciatic foramen and is medial to the posterior cutaneous nerve of thigh in the gluteal region – from here, it turns medially and passes through the lesser sciatic notch to innervate structures of the ischiorectal fossa and perineum (see Chapter 38).

Several other nerves that originate from the sacral plexus do not leave the pelvis. These nerves are the **nerve to the piriformis** muscle, sacral branches to the levator ani muscles, coccygeal nerve, and inferior anal nerves.

The pelvic **splanchnic nerves** are autonomic (involuntary) parasympathetic nerves from sacral levels S2 to S4. The autonomic nerves of the pelvis are continuations of the autonomic plexuses of the abdomen. They are formed from nerve fibers that leave the sympathetic chain and form branching networks centered along the median plane of the abdominopelvic cavity. The **superior hypogastric plexus** is anterior to vertebra LV. It contains preganglionic and postganglionic sympathetic and parasympathetic nerve fibers, and innervates the lower gastrointestinal tract and pelvic viscera. It terminates inferiorly by sending out **left** and **right hypogastric nerves** to the inferior hypogastric plexus.

The **inferior hypogastric plexuses** are formed by the hypogastric nerves (from the superior hypogastric plexus), pelvic splanchnic nerves (from the sacral plexus of nerves), and sacral splanchnic nerves (from the sacrum). They are on the posterior pelvic wall on the left and right sides of the rectum and bladder and contain both sympathetic and parasympathetic ganglia, which send autonomic nerve fibers to the lower gastrointestinal tract (sigmoid colon, rectum, anus), the lower pelvic viscera, and the external genitalia. Disruption can cause erectile dysfunction in men.

ARTERIES

Blood is supplied to the pelvis primarily by the **internal iliac arteries** (Table 36.1), which are branches of the **common iliac artery**, and by other arteries (Table 36.2).

At the level of vertebra LIV, the aorta bifurcates into left and right common iliac arteries (Fig. 36.3). These vessels descend into the pelvis and further divide into the external and internal iliac arteries. As the ureter descends from the kidneys it crosses anterior to the origin of the internal iliac artery. Within the pelvis near the sacro-iliac joints, the internal iliac artery gives off anterior and posterior divisions (Table 36.2).

The anterior division of the internal iliac artery branches into the umbilical, obturator, inferior vesical, middle rectal, vaginal, uterine, internal pudendal, and inferior gluteal arteries. These vessels provide blood to the viscera of the pelvis (reproductive organs, bladder, and rectum).

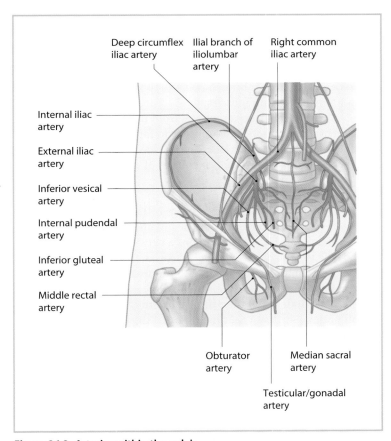

Figure 36.3 Arteries within the pelvis

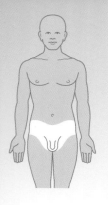
- The **umbilical artery** proceeds anteriorly from its origin in the posterior pelvis and branches to form the superior vesical artery, which supplies the bladder. During the prenatal period the umbilical artery carries deoxygenated blood from the fetus to the placenta. After birth, the distal part of the umbilical artery atrophies to form the medial umbilical ligaments (see Chapter 35).
- The **obturator artery** leaves the pelvis through the obturator foramen of the pelvis to supply the medial compartment of the thigh.
- The **inferior vesical artery** is present only in men. It provides blood to the bladder, prostate, ureter, seminal glands and ductus deferens (see Chapter 35). The vaginal artery is the female equivalent.
- The **middle rectal artery** supplies blood to the inferior rectum by anastomosing with the superior rectal artery (from the inferior mesenteric artery; see Chapter 34) and inferior rectal artery (from the pudendal artery; see Chapter 38). It also supplies the prostate (in men) and the vagina (in women).
- The **uterine artery** in women is homologous to the artery to the ductus deferens in men. It enters the broad ligament of uterus, then travels medially towards the uterus (see Chapter 37). This artery passes anterior to the ureter near the lateral part of the vagina and is of surgical significance during hysterectomy.
- The **internal pudendal artery** leaves the pelvis posteriorly with the internal pudendal nerve, then turns anteriorly to supply the perineal structures. The terminal branch is the **dorsal artery of penis/clitoris**.
- The **inferior gluteal artery** leaves the pelvis through the greater sciatic foramen to supply the gluteus muscles and posterior thigh.

The posterior division of the internal iliac artery branches into the superior gluteal, iliolumbar, lateral sacral, and ovarian arteries.

- The **superior gluteal artery** leaves the pelvis through the greater sciatic foramen and supplies the gluteal muscles.
- The **iliolumbar artery** runs toward the psoas major muscle and branches to form an **iliacus branch**, which supplies the iliacus muscle, and a **lumbar branch**, which supplies the psoas major and quadratus lumborum muscles.
- The **lateral sacral artery** originates from the posterior division of the internal iliac artery and branches to form several small spinal branches to the sacrum. These supply blood to the terminal branches (cauda equina) and meninges of the spinal cord.

VEINS AND LYMPHATICS

Primary venous drainage of the pelvis is by the **internal iliac veins**. Each of the named arteries has a concomitant vein that drains to the internal iliac vein. The pelvis contains a network of adjoining veins – the pelvic venous plexus. Venous plexuses also occur at the bladder, rectum, prostate, vagina, and uterus and drain to the internal iliac veins.

Lymphatic drainage of the pelvis is toward the **internal iliac lymph nodes**, which are near the origin of the first few arterial branches of the internal iliac lymph nodes. Lymph from the bladder, prostate, uterus, vagina, rectum, seminal glands, and part of the proximal male urethra flows toward these nodes.

Lymph from the gluteal region and posterior thigh flows along small, unnamed vessels toward the internal iliac nodes, and then to the **external iliac** and **common iliac nodes**.

Lymph from the posterior pelvic wall, prostate, vagina, and rectum drains to a second group of nodes, the **sacral nodes**, along the middle part of the anterior sacrum, and then toward the **common iliac nodes**.

■ CLINICAL CORRELATIONS
Pelvic fractures

A pelvic fracture may be associated with other serious injuries because it requires great force to fracture the pelvis. Most pelvic fractures occur as a result of motor vehicle accidents. The pelvic girdle can break at any point. Less serious injuries involve the pubic or ischial rami; more serious injuries involve the sacrum or sacroiliac joint – areas containing many blood vessels and nerves.

Patients usually complain of pain in the groin, buttocks, or hips. The most immediate concern is maintaining blood volume because of the likelihood of other serious injury. Intravenous fluids are administered to maintain volume and prevent shock. A trauma survey is carried out to assess the airway, breathing, and circulation. Once it has been verified that these are stable, the pelvis can be examined more thoroughly. Clinical signs of pelvic fracture include instability when light pressure is applied to the lateral margins of the pelvis, hematoma at the area of the inguinal ligament, tenderness or bleeding during rectal examination, and hypotension secondary to hypovolemia (decreased intravascular blood volume) caused by internal bleeding. Fracture is confirmed by radiography. This must be done with minimal movement of the patient because movement can worsen the injury.

Less serious fractures are treated conservatively, but more serious fractures may need surgical stabilization. The overall mortality rate for pelvic fracture is not low; prognosis improves after the first 24 hours.

Pressure ulcers

A pressure ulcer (decubitus ulcer, pressure sore, or bedsore) occurs when an area of soft tissue is compressed for a prolonged period of time. This can cause erythema (redness), blistering, ulceration, or a wound covered with darkened eschar (scab).

Pressure ulcers are common in elderly and debilitated patients. In the elderly, this may be partly because of the thinner skin, with decreased elasticity and vascularity. Patients who have inadequate nutrition, incontinence (loss of bladder or bowel control), inability to move or ambulate, and poor mental status (e.g. comatose) are at increased risk. Pressure ulcers typically develop in bedbound patients who stay in a supine position for long periods. The time it takes to develop a pressure ulcer varies. The most common sites are the posterior pelvis and sacral areas.

Pressure ulcers cause pain that worsens on movement. There is erythema over the affected area in early pressure ulcers. As the ulcer progresses the skin blisters and, if it is not treated, open sores develop. In some cases a black or dark eschar is visible over the sore. On removal of this scab the typical ulcer crater is visible. In advanced pressure ulcers, bone can be seen in the bed of the ulcer.

Treatment of ulcers aims to prevent progressions, by reducing pressure over the affected area using weight-distributing pads or air beds, combined with mobilization and movement of the patient. For less advanced ulcers, occlusive gas-permeable membrane-like dressings are applied and are changed every few days. This can help an ulcer heal quickly (days to weeks). More advanced ulcers contain larger amounts of necrotic tissue that has to be removed before wound healing can progress. Many advanced ulcers become infected and antibiotics may be needed. Advanced ulcers usually take weeks to months to heal.

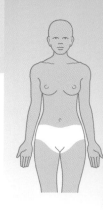

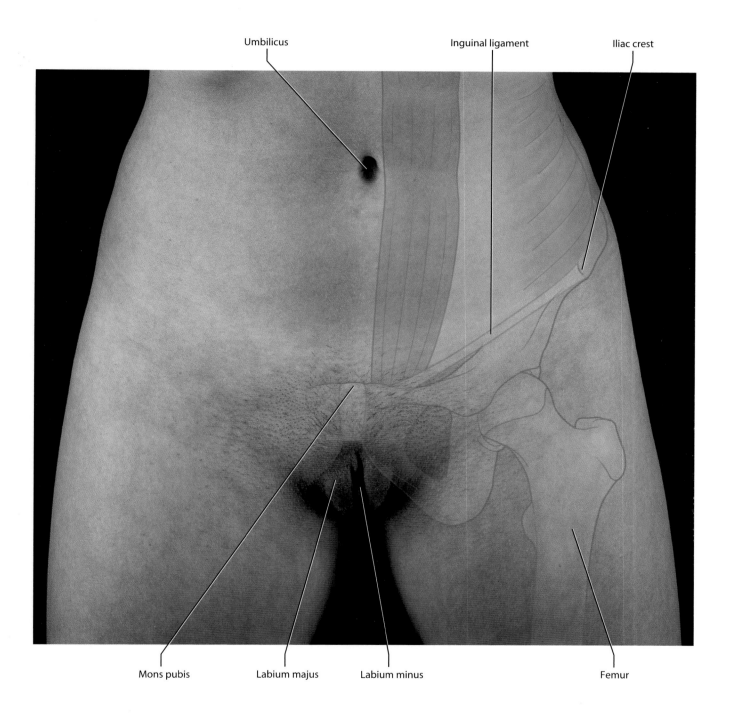

Umbilicus

Inguinal ligament

Iliac crest

Mons pubis

Labium majus

Labium minus

Femur

Figure 36.4 Pelvis – surface anatomy 1. Anterior view of the female pelvis. The pubic hair has been almost completely removed to show the labia majora and minora

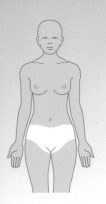

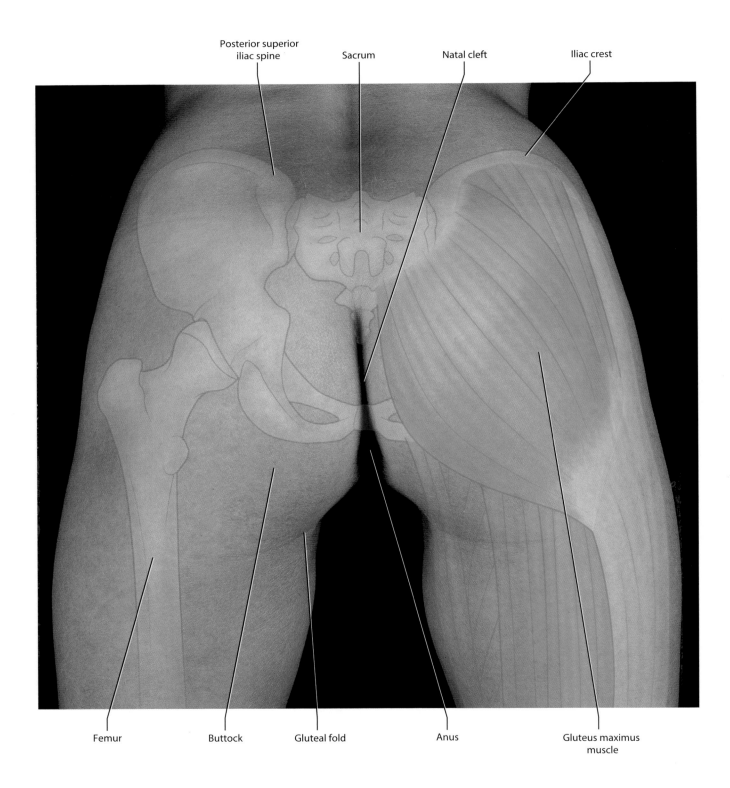

Posterior superior
iliac spine

Sacrum

Natal cleft

Iliac crest

Femur

Buttock

Gluteal fold

Anus

Gluteus maximus
muscle

Figure 36.5 Pelvis – surface anatomy 2. Posterior view of the female pelvis. Observe the posterior superior iliac spine and the location of the greater trochanter of the femur, which are anatomical landmarks in this region

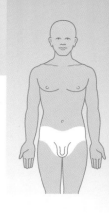

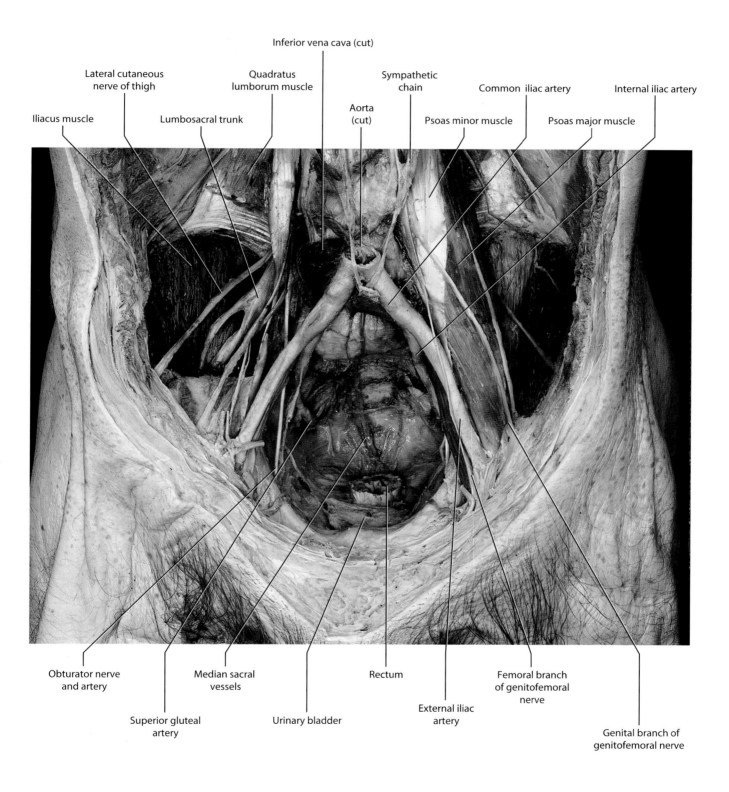

Inferior vena cava (cut)

Lateral cutaneous
nerve of thigh

Quadratus
lumborum muscle

Sympathetic
chain

Common iliac artery

Internal iliac artery

Iliacus muscle

Lumbosacral trunk

Aorta
(cut)

Psoas minor muscle

Psoas major muscle

Obturator nerve
and artery

Median sacral
vessels

Rectum

Femoral branch
of genitofemoral
nerve

Superior gluteal
artery

Urinary bladder

External iliac
artery

Genital branch of
genitofemoral nerve

Figure 36.6 Pelvis – superficial dissection. Anterior view looking into the dissected walls of a male pelvis. Observe the many nerves in this region and how they relate to the external and internal iliac arteries

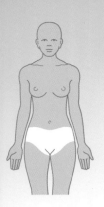

Pelvic girdle **TRUNK**

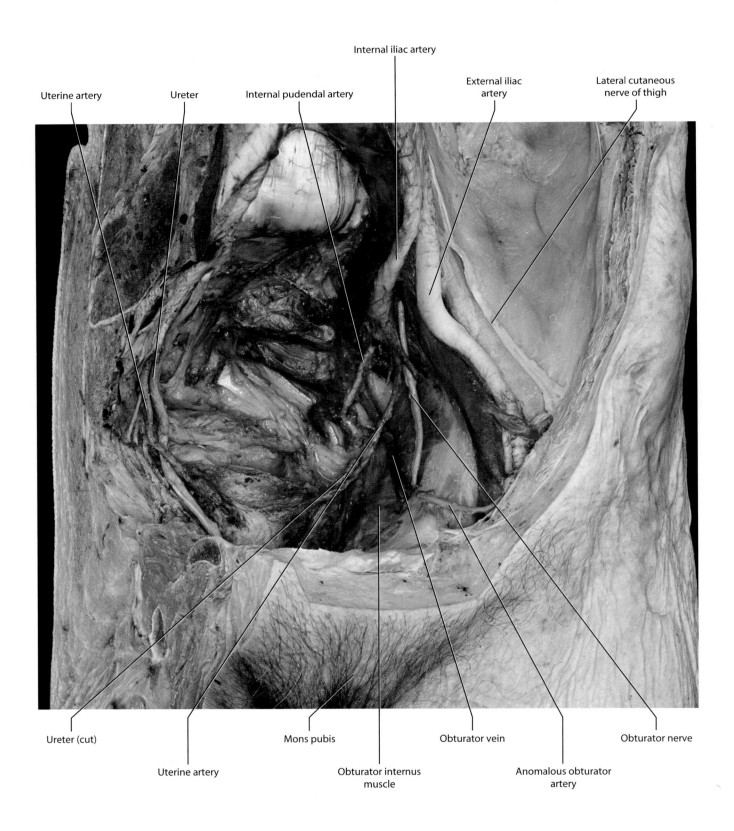

Internal iliac artery

Uterine artery   Ureter   Internal pudendal artery   External iliac artery   Lateral cutaneous nerve of thigh

Ureter (cut)   Mons pubis   Obturator vein   Obturator nerve

Uterine artery   Obturator internus muscle   Anomalous obturator artery

Figure 36.7 Pelvis – intermediate dissection. Anterolateral view looking into the left side of a female pelvis. Observe the external and internal iliac arteries on the internal wall of the pelvis

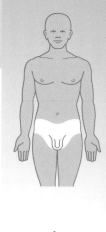

TABLE 36.1 BRANCHES OF THE ANTERIOR AND POSTERIOR DIVISIONS OF THE INTERNAL ILIAC ARTERIES

Artery	Origin	Course and distribution
Branches of the anterior division		
Obturator artery	Anterior division	Runs anterolaterally along the lateral pelvic wall and exits pelvis through obturator foramen to supply the medial thigh pelvic muscles, ilium, and head of femur
Umbilical artery	Anterior division	On anterior abdominal wall – closes and becomes the medial umbilical ligament. In pelvis – gives rise to superior vesical arteries to supply upper bladder. In males – can give rise to artery to ductus deferens
Superior vesical artery	Proximal patent portion of umbilical artery	Multiple branches that supply superior part of urinary bladder and pelvic part of ureter
Inferior vesical artery	Anterior division	Located retroperitoneally and passes to inferior aspect of male bladder
Artery to ductus deferens	Inferior or superior vesical artery	Runs retroperitoneally to supply ductus deferens
Prostatic arteries	Inferior vesical artery	Pass along posterolateral surface of prostate gland
Uterine artery	Anterior division	Runs in base of broad ligament of uterus superior to cardinal ligament and ureter and lateral to uterus. Supplies uterus, ligaments of uterus, uterine tube, and vagina
Vaginal artery	Uterine artery	Female homolog of the inferior vesical artery. Arises lateral to ureter and descends to lateral aspect of vagina, supplying the vagina and the inferior bladder and distal ureter
Middle rectal artery	Anterior division	Runs inferiorly in pelvis to lower rectum. Supplies lower rectum and the seminal vesicles
Internal pudendal artery	Anterior division	Exits pelvis through greater sciatic foramen and enters perineum through the lesser sciatic foramen. The main artery to the perineum (anal and urogenital triangles)
Inferior gluteal artery	Anterior division	Leaves the pelvis through the greater sciatic foramen and passes inferior to piriformis. Supplies pelvic diaphragm, piriformis, quadratus femoris, superior part of biceps femoris, gluteus maximus, and sciatic nerve
Branches of the posterior division Iliolumbar artery	Posterior division	Passes between the sacro-iliac joint and the common iliac vessels and deep to psoas major muscle, which it supplies along with the iliacus and quadratus lumborum muscles and the cauda equina
Lateral sacral artery	Posterior division	Runs medially along the piriformis and sends branches through the sacral foramina. Supplies piriformis, contents of the sacral canal, erector spinae, and overlying skin
Superior gluteal artery	Posterior division	Leaves the pelvis through the greater sciatic foramen by passing superior to piriformis. Supplies the piriformis, gluteus maximus, medius, and minimus, and tensor fasciae latae

TABLE 36.2 OTHER ARTERIES OF THE PELVIS

Artery	Origin	Course and distribution
Median sacral	Abdominal aorta	Runs anterior to the body of the sacrum; supplies lower lumbar vertebrae, sacrum, and coccyx
Superior rectal	Inferior mesenteric artery	Passes anterior to the left common iliac vessels. Enters pelvis through sigmoid mesocolon. Supplies rectum as far as the anal canal
Gonadal: ovarian (female), testicular (male)	Abdominal aorta, just below renal arteries	Ovarian artery descends retroperitoneally into pelvis, medial to the ureter, in suspensory ligament of ovary. Testicular artery passes through the inguinal canal to enter the scrotum and supply the testes
Internal iliac artery	Terminal branch of common iliac artery; at the level of the sacro-iliac joint passes inferoposteriorly on the posterior pelvic wall. Ureter lies antero-inferior to the artery	Major blood supply to pelvic viscera, musculoskeletal structures of the pelvis and perineum, and the gluteal region

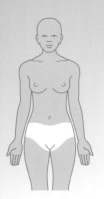

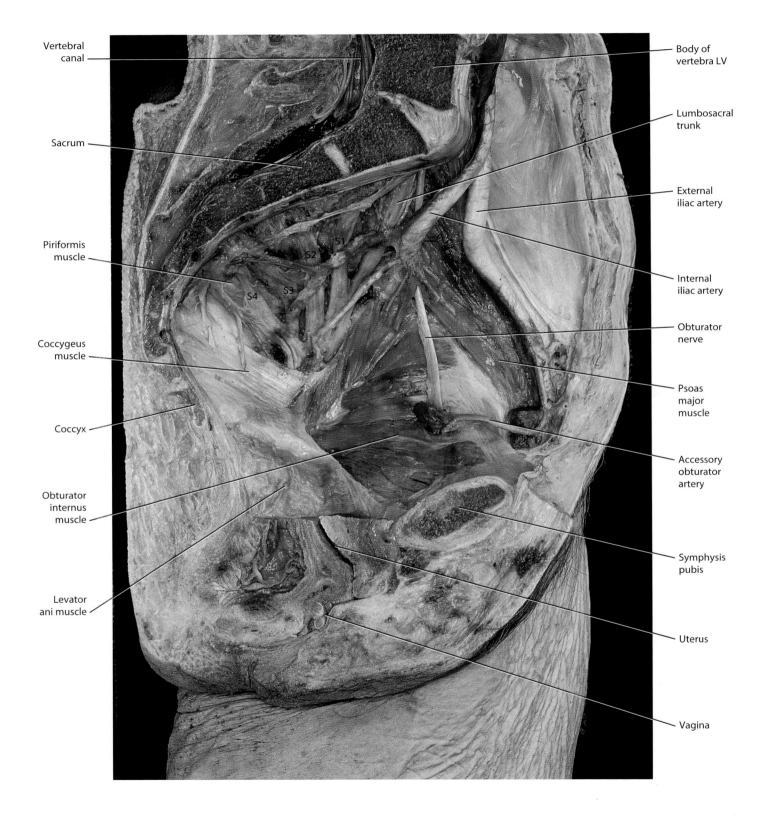

Vertebral canal

Sacrum

Piriformis muscle

Coccygeus muscle

Coccyx

Obturator internus muscle

Levator ani muscle

Body of vertebra LV

Lumbosacral trunk

External iliac artery

Internal iliac artery

Obturator nerve

Psoas major muscle

Accessory obturator artery

Symphysis pubis

Uterus

Vagina

S1
S2
S3
S4

Figure 36.8 Pelvis – sagittal section. Medial view looking into the left side of a female pelvis. The upper part of the uterus has been removed to show the levator ani and coccygeus muscles

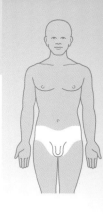

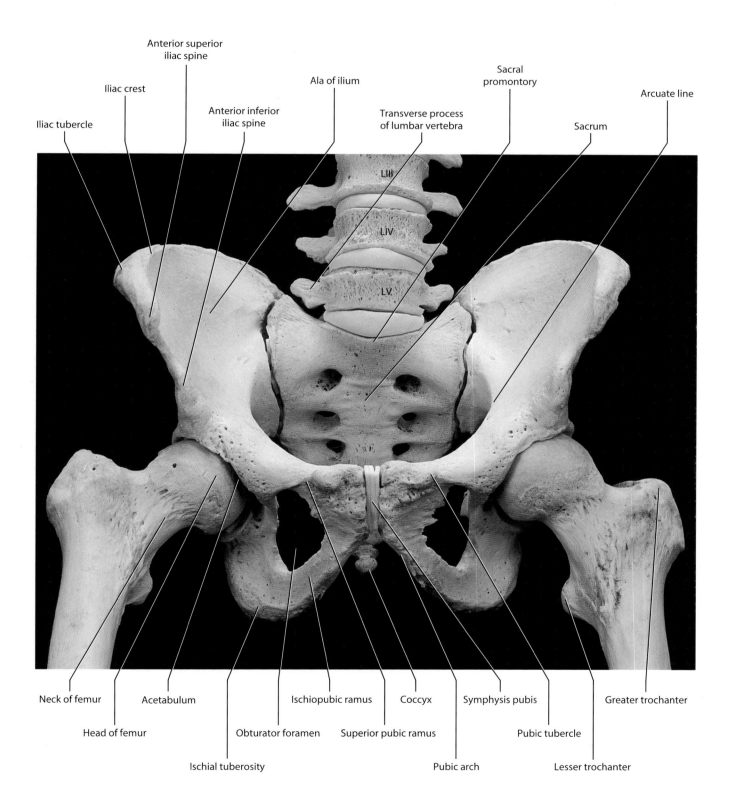

Iliac tubercle

Iliac crest

Anterior superior
iliac spine

Anterior inferior
iliac spine

Ala of ilium

Transverse process
of lumbar vertebra

Sacral
promontory

Sacrum

Arcuate line

LIII

LIV

LV

Neck of femur

Head of femur

Acetabulum

Ischial tuberosity

Obturator foramen

Ischiopubic ramus

Superior pubic ramus

Coccyx

Pubic arch

Symphysis pubis

Pubic tubercle

Lesser trochanter

Greater trochanter

Figure 36.9 Pelvis – osteology 1. Anterior view of the articulated pelvis. Observe how the sacrum and femur join the pelvis

445

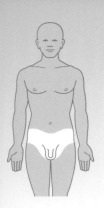

Pelvic girdle **TRUNK**

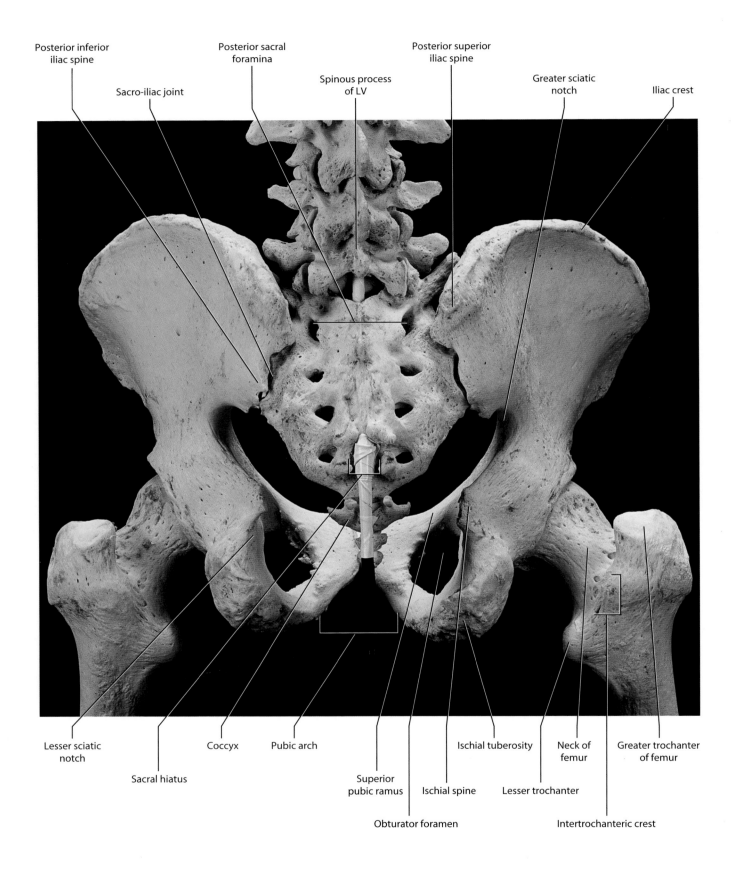

Posterior inferior
iliac spine

Posterior sacral
foramina

Posterior superior
iliac spine

Greater sciatic
notch

Iliac crest

Sacro-iliac joint

Spinous process
of LV

Lesser sciatic
notch

Coccyx

Pubic arch

Ischial tuberosity

Neck of
femur

Greater trochanter
of femur

Sacral hiatus

Superior
pubic ramus

Ischial spine

Lesser trochanter

Obturator foramen

Intertrochanteric crest

446   **Figure 36.10 Pelvis – osteology 2.** Posterior view of the articulated pelvis. Observe the sacro-iliac joints

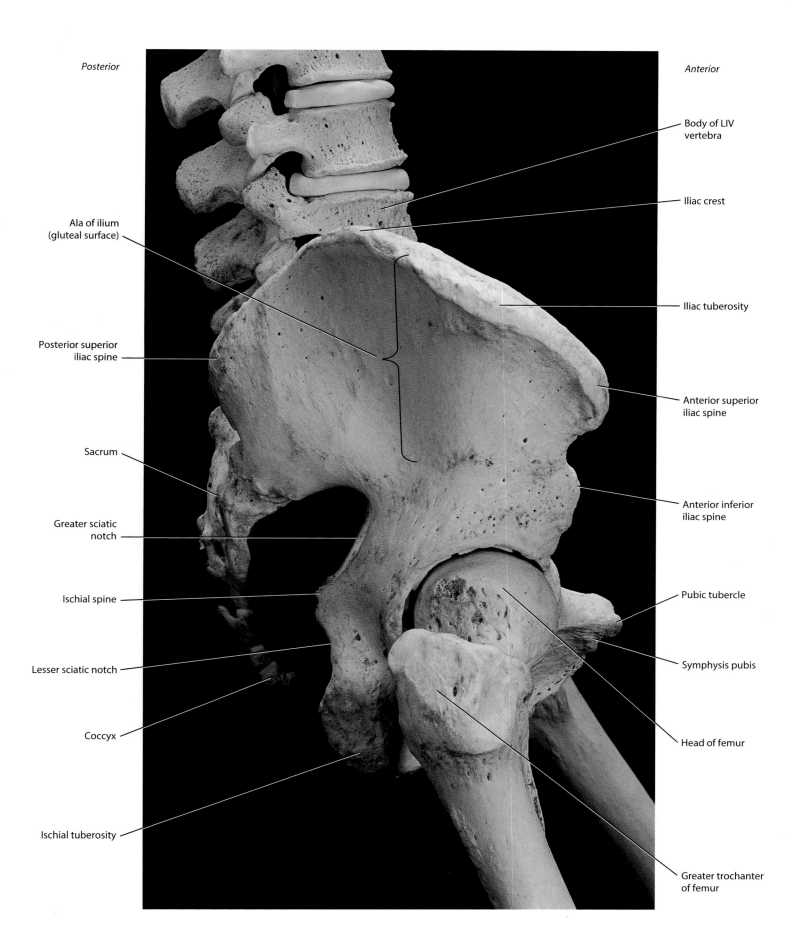

Posterior

Anterior

Body of LIV
vertebra

Iliac crest

Ala of ilium
(gluteal surface)

Iliac tuberosity

Posterior superior
iliac spine

Anterior superior
iliac spine

Sacrum

Anterior inferior
iliac spine

Greater sciatic
notch

Ischial spine

Pubic tubercle

Lesser sciatic notch

Symphysis pubis

Coccyx

Head of femur

Ischial tuberosity

Greater trochanter
of femur

Figure 36.11 Pelvis – osteology 3. Lateral view of the right side of the articulated pelvis. Observe how the head of the femur fits into the acetabulum

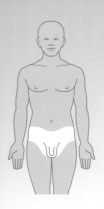

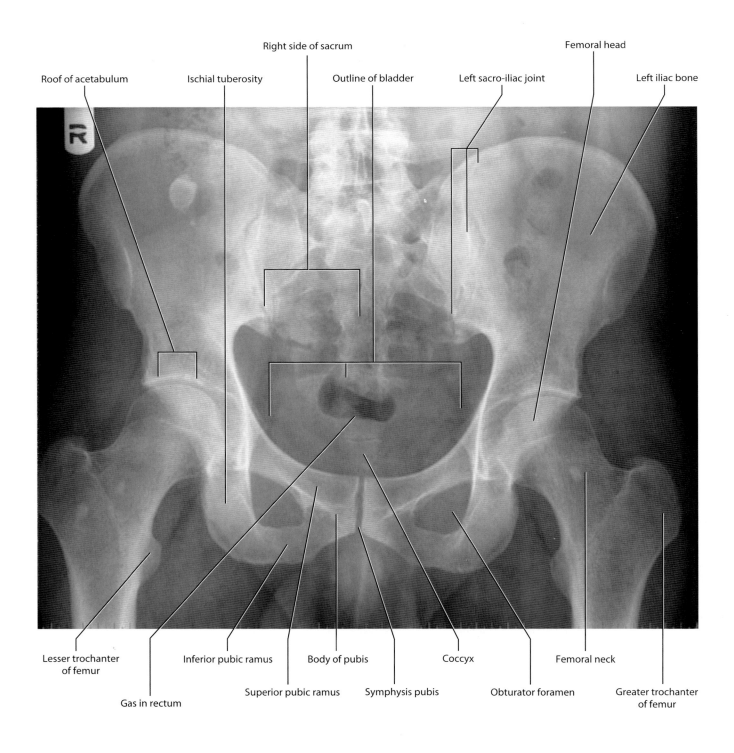

Roof of acetabulum

Ischial tuberosity

Right side of sacrum

Outline of bladder

Left sacro-iliac joint

Femoral head

Left iliac bone

Lesser trochanter of femur

Gas in rectum

Inferior pubic ramus

Superior pubic ramus

Body of pubis

Symphysis pubis

Coccyx

Obturator foramen

Femoral neck

Greater trochanter of femur

Figure 36.12 Pelvic girdle – plain film radiograph (anteroposterior view). The sacrum, iliac bones and ischial bones make up the pelvic girdle and act as a solid ring. If there is fracture of one side of the ring, there is almost always an associated fracture in the contralateral side. This is a normal radiograph

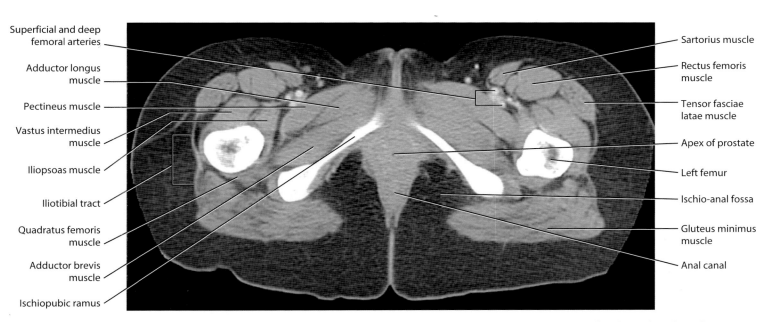

Superficial and deep femoral arteries

Adductor longus muscle

Pectineus muscle

Vastus intermedius muscle

Iliopsoas muscle

Iliotibial tract

Quadratus femoris muscle

Adductor brevis muscle

Ischiopubic ramus

Sartorius muscle

Rectus femoris muscle

Tensor fasciae latae muscle

Apex of prostate

Left femur

Ischio-anal fossa

Gluteus minimus muscle

Anal canal

Figure 36.13 Pelvic girdle – CT scan (axial view). In this scan of the lower pelvis note how the ischial and pubic bones are fused together along the ischiopubic ramus

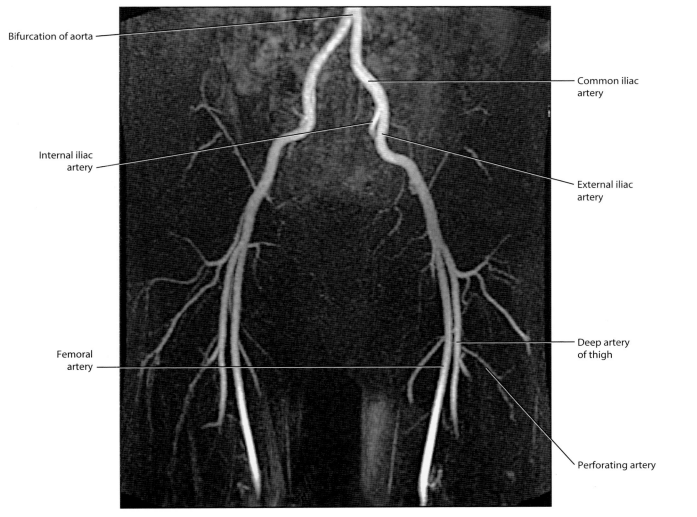

Bifurcation of aorta

Internal iliac artery

Femoral artery

Common iliac artery

External iliac artery

Deep artery of thigh

Perforating artery

Figure 36.14 Pelvic girdle – MRA scan (coronal view). The arteries of the pelvis and upper thigh are visible in this magnetic resonance angiogram (MRA). Observe the bifurcation of the common iliac arteries into internal and deep branches within the pelvis

TRUNK Pelvic girdle

449

The pelvic viscera include the urinary bladder, distal ureters, rectum, and reproductive organs (Table 37.1, Figs 37.1–37.4). Structural support for the pelvic viscera is provided by the bones and ligaments of the pelvis (see Chapter 36).

The urinary bladder, inferior part of the two ureters, and urethra are contained within the pelvis.

The **ureter** is a long retroperitoneal muscular tube that transports urine from the renal pelvis of the kidney to the urinary bladder. Descending from the posterior abdominal wall, they become pelvic structures when they cross the bifurcation of the common iliac artery. The ureter is:

- anterior to the internal iliac arteries within the pelvis;
- in men, posterior to ductus deferens, which crosses it superiorly near the bladder;
- in women, medial and inferior to the uterine artery, which crosses it anteriorly and superiorly in the base of the broad ligament.

The ureters are constricted at the uteropelvic junction, pelvic inlet, and bladder entrance.

The ureters are innervated by the autonomic nerve plexuses along their path to the bladder: renal, aortic, superior hypogastric, and inferior hypogastric plexuses. The blood supply to the pelvic part of the ureter is from adjacent branches of the common and internal

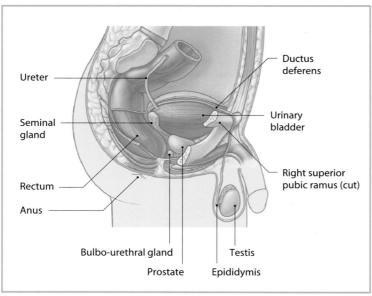

Figure 37.1 Male pelvic viscera

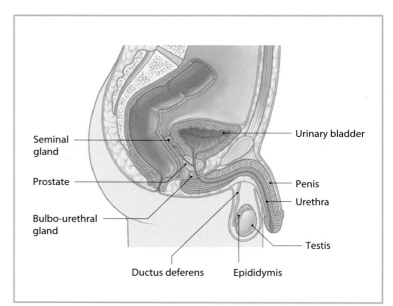

Figure 37.3 Male pelvic viscera – median sagittal section

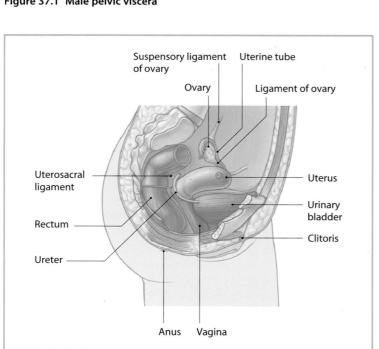

Figure 37.2 Female pelvic viscera

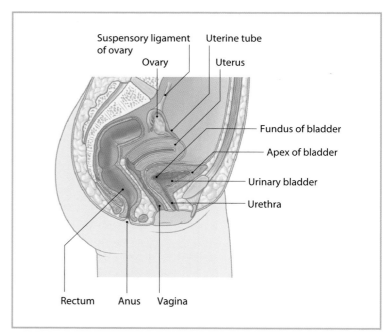

Figure 37.4 Female pelvic viscera – median sagittal section

iliac arteries. The main blood supply in females is from the uterine artery whereas in men blood is supplied by the inferior vesical artery. Venous drainage accompanies the arteries and empties toward the iliac veins. Lymphatic drainage is to the common iliac, external iliac, internal iliac, and lumbar lymph nodes.

The sac-like **urinary bladder** has strong muscular walls (the detrusor muscles). The **apex of bladder** is at the superior edge of the pubic symphysis and is attached to the umbilicus via the medial umbilical ligament. The base (**fundus of bladder**), created by the posterior wall of the bladder, is attached to the seminal vesicles and rectum in males and the uterus and vagina in females. The rest of the bladder between the apex and fundus is the **body of bladder**. The superior surface of the bladder is covered with peritoneum. Ureteral openings are at the posterior superior edge of the fundus of bladder and the urethral opening is at the midline inferior anterior part just below the apex of bladder.

The urinary bladder is a reservoir for urine transported from the kidneys via the ureters. When it is full, parasympathetic nerve fibers cause the **detrusor muscle** to contract and the **urethral sphincter** to relax. This can be suppressed voluntarily. Parasympathetic innervation is from **pelvic splanchnic nerves**. Sympathetic fibers are from the sympathetic trunk (levels T11 to L2). These nerves converge on the bladder to form the autonomic **vesical plexus**.

Blood supply to the bladder is from the **superior vesical artery** (a branch of the inferior mesenteric artery), and blood drains into the **internal iliac veins**. In addition, a smaller **vesical venous plexus** forms a network of small unnamed veins around the bladder. The vesical venous plexus also drains into the internal iliac veins.

Lymphatic drainage of the bladder is toward the superior surface of the bladder. From this point, lymph drains into the **external iliac nodes**. Lymph from the fundus of bladder drains into the **internal iliac nodes**.

The **urethra** exits the bladder via the **internal urethral orifice**. From here, urine flows to the **external urethral orifice**. In men, the urethra is 18–20 cm long, whereas in women it is only 4 cm. Innervation in men is from the **prostatic nerve plexus**; in women it is from the **pudendal nerve**. Blood supply in men is from **prostatic branches**, which are branches of the inferior vesical artery (a branch of the internal iliac artery) and **middle rectal arteries** (branches of the inferior mesenteric artery). In women, blood is supplied by the **internal pudendal** and **vaginal arteries**, which are both branches of the internal iliac artery.

The rectum is described as part of the gastrointestinal tract and is discussed in Chapter 34.

MALE PELVIC VISCERA
The male pelvic viscera (prostate, seminal glands, bladder, and rectum) have a role in sexual activity, reproduction, urination, and defecation (see Figs 37.1 and 37.3).

The **prostate** is a small, solid, ovoid gland (usually around 3 cm long) through which the first part of the urethra passes. It contains five lobes. Four are glandular and produce secretions that are added to the ejaculate during intercourse and orgasm (posterior, median, and paired lateral lobes). A fifth fibromuscular lobe is anterior to the urethra. Fluid, which is cloudy and milky in color, passes from the prostate to the urethra through several (usually 20–30) small **prostatic ducts**, and usually accounts for approximately 20% of the volume in semen. The prostate is surrounded by a thin capsule, a prostatic venous plexus, and pelvic fascia (false capsule). It is supported by the pubococcygeus muscle and the puboprostatic ligaments.

The prostate gland is inferior to the urinary bladder at the base of the penis within the pelvis (intrapelvic) and posteroinferior to the pubic symphysis. Because of its position between the bladder and rectum, the posterior part of the prostate can be partly examined by digital rectal examination to detect abnormalities, such as tumors.

Parasympathetic innervation to the prostate is from **pelvic splanchnic nerves** (S2 to S4); sympathetic innervation is through nerve fibers that originate in the **inferior hypogastric plexus**.

Blood supply to the prostate is provided by the **prostatic arteries** (small branches of the inferior vesical artery), the **middle rectal artery** and the **internal pudendal arteries** (branches of the internal iliac artery). Venous drainage is to the **prostatic venous plexus**, which drains toward the inferior **vesical venous plexus** and **internal iliac veins**. Lymphatic vessels from the prostate gland drain towards the **internal iliac** and **sacral nodes**.

The two **seminal glands** are small elongated organs between the rectum and bladder, and lateral to the ampulla of ductus deferens. They can be palpated through the anorectal canal. They produce a thick seminal fluid that passes into the **ejaculatory duct** (formed by the adjoining excretory ducts from the seminal glands and the ductus deferens) during ejaculation. Innervation is from the **inferior hypogastric plexus** (sympathetic) and **pelvic splanchnic nerves** (parasympathetic). Blood is supplied by the **inferior vesical** and **middle rectal arteries**, which are branches of the internal iliac artery. Venous drainage is to veins that correspond to the arteries and drain into the **internal iliac veins**. Lymph drains from the seminal glands toward the **internal iliac nodes**.

The **bulbo-urethral glands** are two small round glands (0.5–1 cm in diameter) in the **deep perineal pouch** embedded in the urethral sphincter muscle. Their ducts pass through the inferior fascia of the urogenital diaphragm and open into the proximal part of the spongy urethra just anterior to the prostate. The bulbo-urethral glands produce a mucus-like liquid, which is secreted directly into the spongy urethra during sexual arousal. Their neurovascular supply and lymphatic drainage are similar to those of the prostate.

The **ductus deferens** (vas deferens) is a thick-walled muscular tube through which sperm produced in the testis passes. It is an extension of the elongated **epididymis**. From its origin within the scrotum, the ductus deferens ascends in the spermatic cord, enters the inguinal canal at the superficial inguinal ring, then enters the abdominal cavity through the deep inguinal ring lateral to the inferior epigastric vessels (see Chapter 35). It remains extraperitoneal as it descends into the pelvis. When it enters the anterior pelvis the ductus deferens runs posteriorly along the superior surface of the urinary bladder, crosses the ureter near the ischial spine, and runs medially and downwards on the posterior surface of the bladder, terminating as it turns inferiorly to join the duct of the seminal glands at the ampulla of ductus deferens. These adjoining ducts form the ejaculatory ducts. Innervation is from the **inferior hypogastric plexus** of nerves. Blood supply to the pelvic part is from the **inferior vesical artery** and venous drainage follows the artery and is toward the **internal iliac vein**. Lymphatic drainage is along vessels that empty into the **external iliac nodes**.

FEMALE PELVIC VISCERA
The female pelvic viscera are the vagina (see Chapter 38), uterus, uterine tubes, and ovaries (see Figs 37.2 and 37.4).

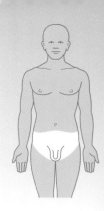

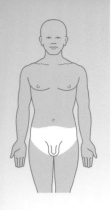

The **uterus** is a thick muscular organ (usually 6 × 5 × 2 cm) located centrally in the female pelvis partly superior to the urinary bladder. It has a body, fundus, isthmus, and cervix. The **body of uterus** forms the superior two-thirds, contains the uterine cavity, and includes the **uterine horns**, which is where the uterine tubes enter the uterus. A fertilized ovum travels from the ovary through the uterine tube to the uterus, and implants onto the internal uterine wall during embryogenesis. The **fundus of uterus** is the small midline part of the uterus superior to the uterine horns. Inferior to the fundus is the **isthmus of uterus**, which is a narrowed region that joins inferiorly to the **cervix of uterus**. The cervix is the cylindrical inferior third of the uterus and projects into the vagina (see Chapter 38). It is traversed by the cervical canal. The **internal os** and **external os** are the proximal and distal openings of the cervical canal. At childbirth, hormonal and autonomic stimulation relax and stretch the cervix of uterus and the fetus can then pass through the cervical canal and into the vagina.

The **round ligament of uterus** is a cord-like structure attached to the posterior part of the body of uterus and extending laterally toward the deep inguinal ring. It passes through the inguinal canal to insert into the fascia at the base of the labium majus. It is continuous with the **ligament of ovary**, a small ligament joining the ovary to the uterus and is anterior on the body of the uterus. The **broad ligament of uterus** is a folding of the peritoneum over the uterus and uterine tubes. This wide, drape-like ligament descends from the uterine tubes to the cervix and lateral pelvic wall and contains the uterine artery and vein.

Inferior support to the uterus is provided by the pelvic diaphragm (see Chapter 38) and transverse **cardinal ligaments**, which join the cervix to the lateral pelvic wall.

The uterus is innervated by the **uterovaginal plexus**. This contains sympathetic and parasympathetic fibers and is formed from the branching of nerve fibers from the inferior hypogastric plexus. There is additional parasympathetic innervation to the uterovaginal plexus from the pelvic splanchnic nerves (S2 to S4).

Blood supply to the uterus is provided by the **uterine arteries**, which are branches of the internal iliac arteries. These arteries run within the broad ligament and enter the uterus near the junction of the cervix and isthmus. Venous drainage is into the **uterine veins**, which empty into the **internal iliac veins**. The **uterine venous plexus** is a weblike arrangement of veins around the cervix that drains into the internal iliac veins.

Lymph from the uterus usually drains to the **lumbar lymph nodes**, but some also flows to the external iliac nodes and superficial inguinal nodes (through vessels along the round ligament of uterus).

The **uterine tubes** are approximately 10 cm long and extend laterally from the uterine cavity toward the ovaries. They open over each ovary at the **infundibulum**, which is a dilated horn-like expansion bordered by finger-like fimbriae. The infundibulum spreads over the surface of the ovary and directs the released ovum into the uterine tube and toward the uterus. Fertilization takes place in the **ampulla of uterine tube**. The narrowest part of the tube is called the **isthmus**. Innervation is provided by the **ovarian plexus** (formed from the uterine plexus and pelvic splanchnic nerves). Blood is supplied by the **uterine artery** (a branch of the internal iliac artery) and **ovarian artery** (a branch of the abdominal aorta). Lymphatic drainage is to the **lumbar lymph nodes**.

The **ovaries** are small oval organs suspended in the pelvis by ligaments. The **ligament of ovary** attaches to the medial side of the ovary and joins it to the uterus. The lateral side of the ovary is attached to the lateral pelvic wall by the **suspensory ligament of ovary**. The ovarian artery and vein pass through the suspensory ligament of ovary to supply the ovary. The **broad ligament of uterus** also supports the ovary.

The ovaries are innervated by the **ovarian plexus**, which receives sympathetic nerve fibers from the uterine plexus and parasympathetic nerve fibers from pelvic splanchnic nerves. Lymph drains from the ovary to the **lumbar lymph nodes**.

■ CLINICAL CORRELATIONS
Uterine leiomyoma

Uterine leiomyomas (fibroid tumors) are common benign tumors of the female reproductive tract. These single or multiple tumors occur within the smooth muscle of the uterus and vary in size from small pea-sized nodules to large tumors that fill the abdominal cavity. They are shiny, whitish, whorl-like, solid tumors.

Uterine leiomyomas may cause a variety of symptoms or be completely asymptomatic. Common symptoms are abnormal bleeding from the vagina, lower abdominal pain (sometimes reported as similar to menstrual cramp), and abnormal enlargement of the abdomen. Most women seek medical attention secondary to the abnormal vaginal bleeding, which can be profuse.

A careful abdominal and pelvic examination is needed to determine the size of the uterus, presence of uterine or abdominal tenderness, and extent of the bleeding. In a woman who has not been pregnant (nulliparous) the uterus is small (about the size of a walnut); in a woman who has had more than one child (multiparous) the uterus is larger (pear-sized). Abnormal masses palpated on examination warrant further study. Pelvic ultrasound is helpful in delineating the size and extent of leiomyomas. Radiographs can help rule out other causes. If there is excessive bleeding, blood counts are obtained to check for anemia.

Conservative options are medications or procedures to decrease the size of the tumor. Refractory uterine leiomyomas are referred for hysterectomy.

Prostate cancer

Prostate cancer is one of the most common cancers in men.

Its cause is unknown, but genetics and the environment do play a role. Although it mostly affects older men, it can also affect younger individuals.

Patients who have prostate cancer usually present with blood in the urine, pain on urination, slowing of the urinary stream, frequency of urination, inability to urinate, and/or impotence. A digital rectal examination (DRE) is carried out. Abnormalities in the shape or consistency of the prostate are referred to a specialist for biopsy. In addition, the blood is tested for prostatic-specific antigen (PSA). Abnormal PSA levels necessitate prostatic biopsy. The type and stage of cancer guide the choice of treatment option. Other tests such as radionuclide bone scans, magnetic resonance imaging (MRI), and computed tomography (CT) are carried out to search for metastasis. Prostate cancer can involve the posterior lobe; benign prostatic hypertrophy usually involves the medial lobe.

The treatment of prostate cancer depends on the cancer type, histologic grade, and presence or absence of metastasis. Common options are prostatectomy and radiation. If diagnosed early, prostate cancer is treatable and long-term survival is good.

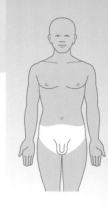

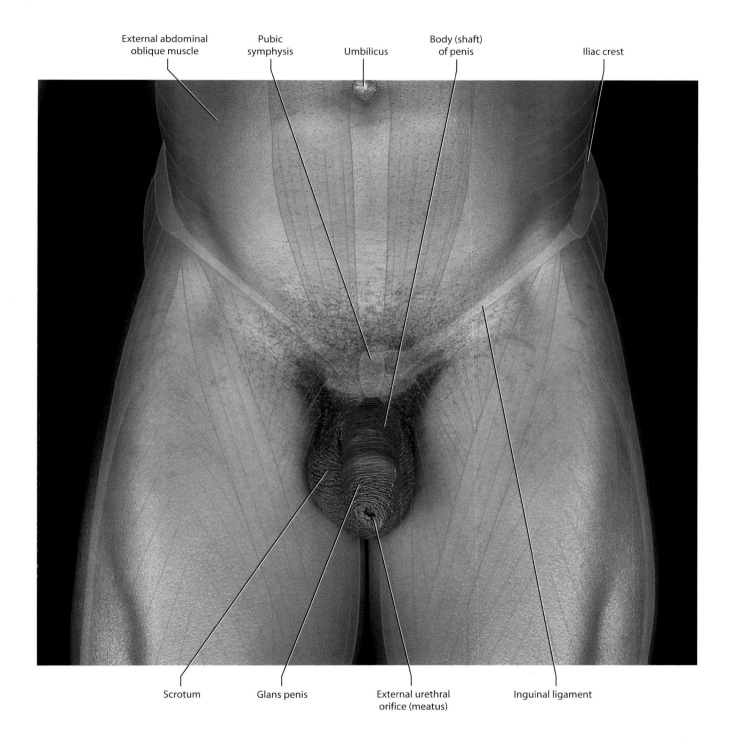

External abdominal oblique muscle

Pubic symphysis

Umbilicus

Body (shaft) of penis

Iliac crest

Scrotum

Glans penis

External urethral orifice (meatus)

Inguinal ligament

Figure 37.5 Pelvic viscera, male – surface anatomy. Surface landmarks of the male pelvic region in relation to the pelvic viscera. This man is uncircumcised

453

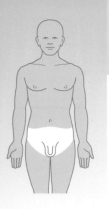

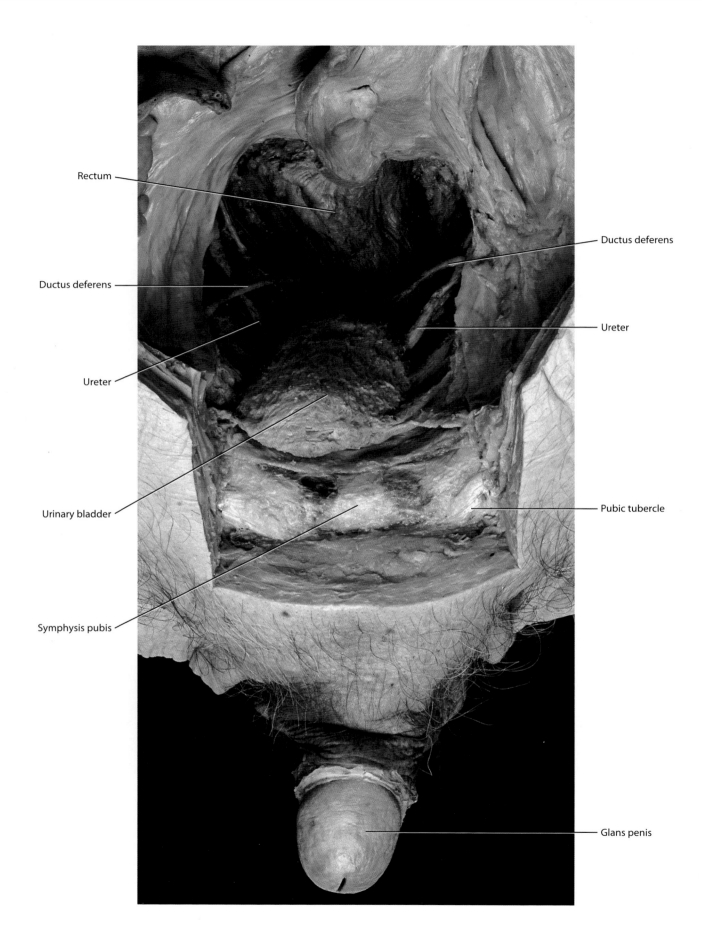

Rectum

Ductus deferens

Ductus deferens

Ureter

Ureter

Urinary bladder

Pubic tubercle

Symphysis pubis

Glans penis

Figure 37.6 Pelvic viscera, male – deep dissection 1. Anterior view looking into the male pelvis from above. The bladder, ureters, and seminal glands are visible in the pelvis anterior to the rectum

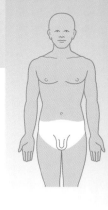

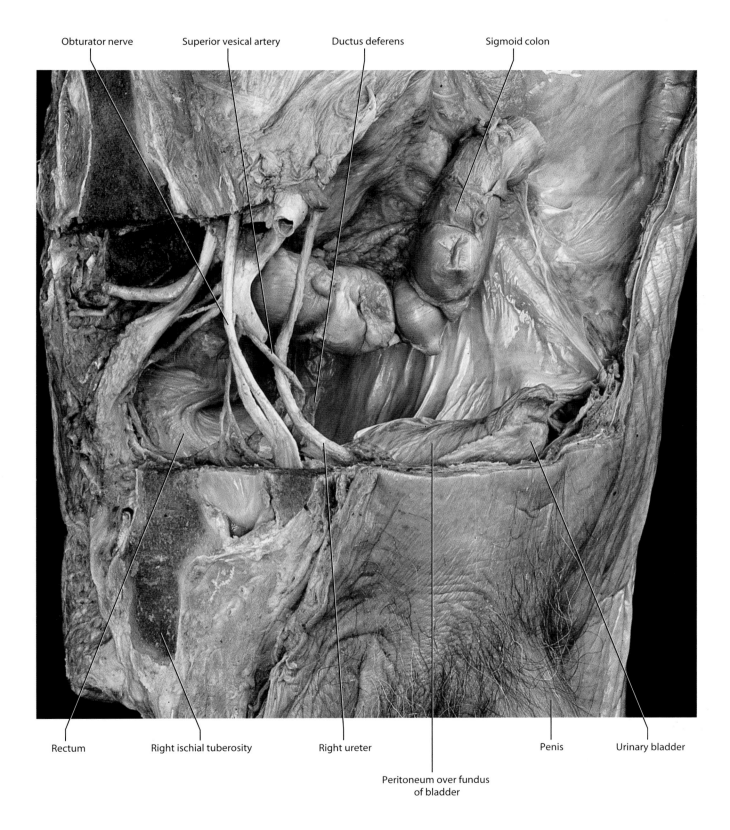

Obturator nerve   Superior vesical artery   Ductus deferens   Sigmoid colon

Rectum   Right ischial tuberosity   Right ureter   Penis   Urinary bladder

Peritoneum over fundus
of bladder

Figure 37.7 Pelvic viscera, male – deep dissection 2. Anterolateral view of a deep dissection of the right side of the male pelvis

455

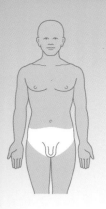

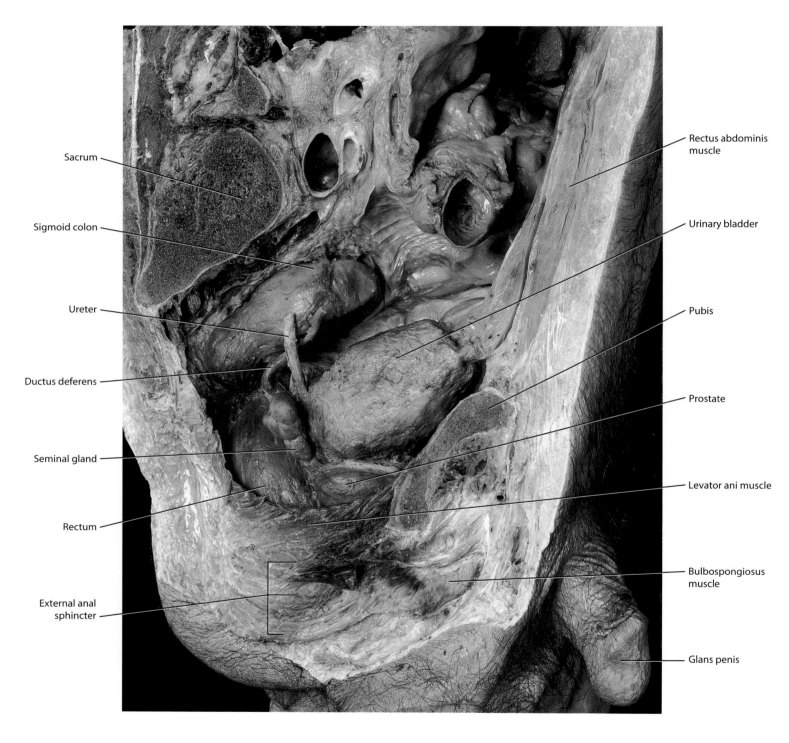

Sacrum

Sigmoid colon

Ureter

Ductus deferens

Seminal gland

Rectum

External anal
sphincter

Rectus abdominis
muscle

Urinary bladder

Pubis

Prostate

Levator ani muscle

Bulbospongiosus
muscle

Glans penis

Figure 37.8 Pelvic viscera, male – deep dissection 3. Lateral view of a deep dissection of the right side of the male pelvis

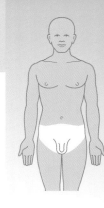

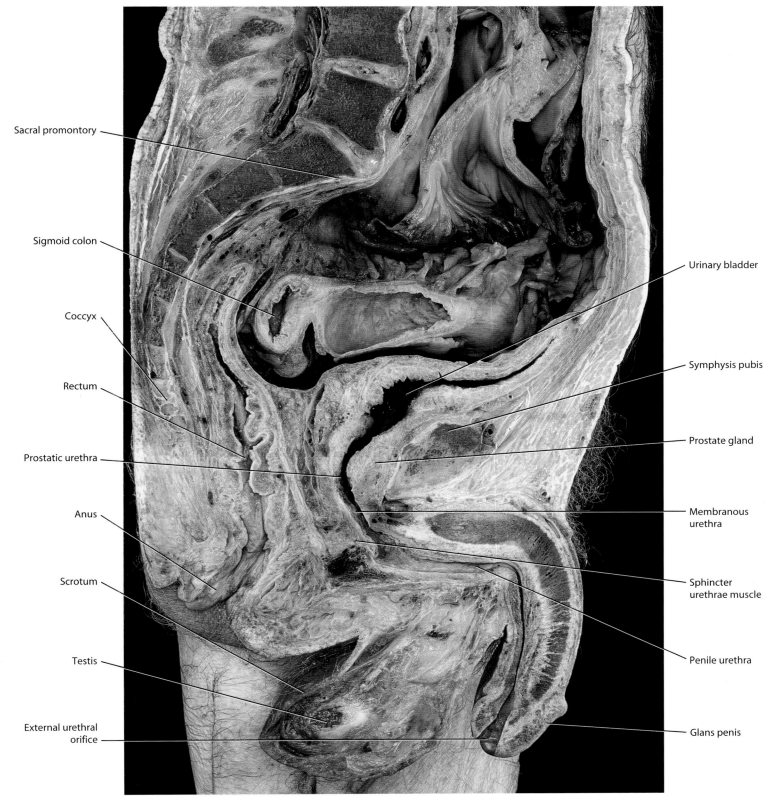

Sacral promontory

Sigmoid colon

Coccyx

Rectum

Prostatic urethra

Anus

Scrotum

Testis

External urethral orifice

Urinary bladder

Symphysis pubis

Prostate gland

Membranous urethra

Sphincter urethrae muscle

Penile urethra

Glans penis

Figure 37.9 Pelvic viscera, male – sagittal section 1. Median sagittal section. Observe the urinary bladder and its relationship to the prostate gland, seminal glands, and rectum

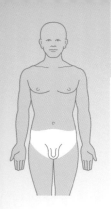

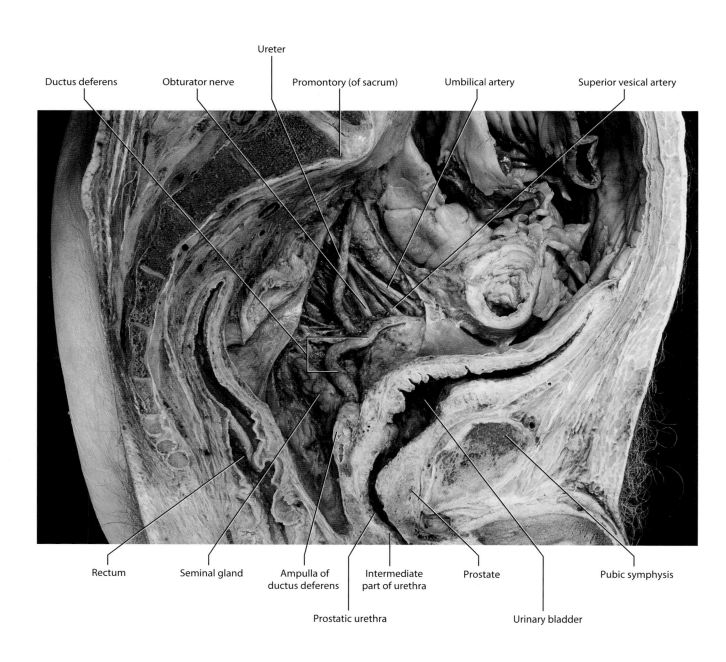

Ureter

Ductus deferens   Obturator nerve   Promontory (of sacrum)   Umbilical artery   Superior vesical artery

Rectum   Seminal gland   Ampulla of ductus deferens   Intermediate part of urethra   Prostate   Pubic symphysis

Prostatic urethra   Urinary bladder

    Figure 37.10 Pelvic viscera, male – sagittal section 2. Median sagittal section looking into the left side of the male pelvis

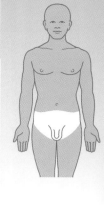

TABLE 37.1 NEUROVASCULAR SUPPLY OF THE PELVIC ORGANS

Organ	Blood supply	Venous drainage	Innervation
Pelvic organs common to male and female			
Ureter	Renal, gonadal, common iliac, uterine/inferior vesical, and middle rectal arteries	Parallel to the arteries	Sympathetic (T11 to L2) via renal, aortic and hypogastric plexuses. Parasympathetic – vagus [X] superior segment, sacral (S2 to S4) inferior segment, sensory nerves (T11 to L2)
Urinary bladder	Superior and inferior vesical arteries of anterior division of internal iliac artery	Internal iliac veins via vesical and prostatic venous plexuses	Sympathetics inhibit micturition and parasympathetics facilitate micturition. Pudendal nerve (somatic motor) causes voluntary relaxation of the external urethral sphincter
Male pelvic structures			
Seminal glands	Branches of inferior vesical and middle rectal arteries	Drain to internal iliac veins	Sympathetic: least splanchnic (T12). Parasympathetic: pelvic splanchnic nerves (S2 to S4)
Ductus deferens	Inferior epigastric artery, inferior vesical, and middle rectal arteries	Drain to internal iliac veins	Sympathetics: lesser splanchnic, least splanchnic (T12). Parasympathetics: pelvic splanchnic nerves (S2 to S4)
Prostate gland	Inferior vesical and middle rectal arteries	Prostatic venous plexus receives the deep dorsal vein of penis and vesical veins. It drains into the internal iliac veins	Sympathetic: lesser splanchnic (T11), least splanchnic (T12) and lumbar splanchnic (L1). Parasympathetic: pelvic splanchnic nerves (S2 to S4)
Female pelvic structures			
Ovary	Ovarian artery from abdominal aorta, which anastomoses with the uterine artery (a branch of the internal iliac artery)	Ovarian vein drains to inferior vena cava on the right and left renal vein on the left	Under hormonal control
Uterine tube	(See ovary)	(See ovary)	(See ovary)
Uterus	Branches of ovarian artery (from the aorta), uterine and vaginal arteries (from the internal iliac artery)	Ovarian vein (see ovary), uterine and vaginal veins (drain to the internal iliac veins)	Sympathetics: least splanchnic (T12), lumbar splanchnic (L1). Parasympathetics: pelvic splanchnic (S2 to S4). Sensory fibers travel with autonomics. Pain is felt in the lower back and perineum

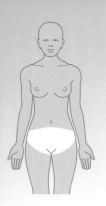

TRUNK

Pelvic viscera

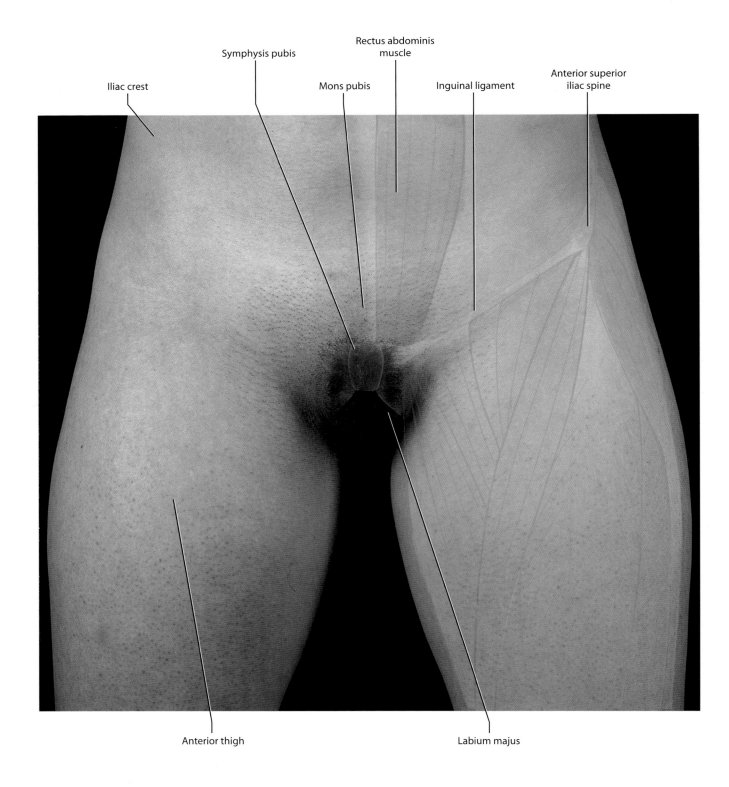

Iliac crest

Symphysis pubis

Rectus abdominis muscle

Mons pubis

Inguinal ligament

Anterior superior iliac spine

Anterior thigh

Labium majus

Figure 37.11 **Pelvic viscera, female – surface anatomy.** Surface landmarks of the female pelvic region in relation to the pelvic viscera

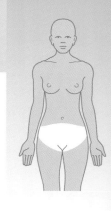

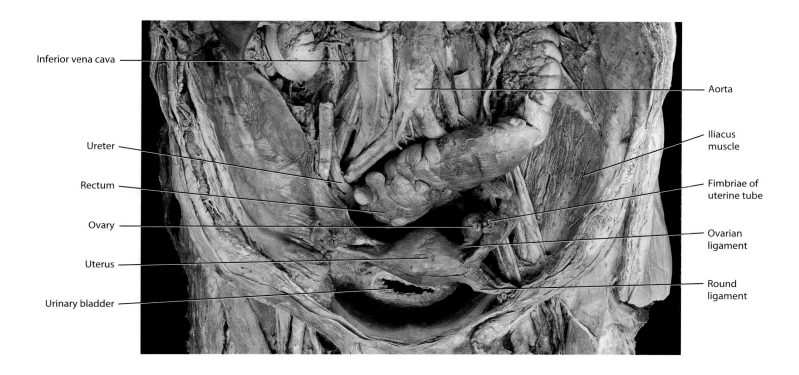

Inferior vena cava

Ureter

Rectum

Ovary

Uterus

Urinary bladder

Aorta

Iliacus muscle

Fimbriae of uterine tube

Ovarian ligament

Round ligament

Figure 37.12 Pelvic viscera, female – deep dissection 1. Anterior view looking into the female pelvis. Observe the relationship between the urinary bladder, uterus and rectum

461

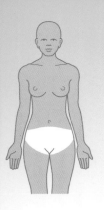

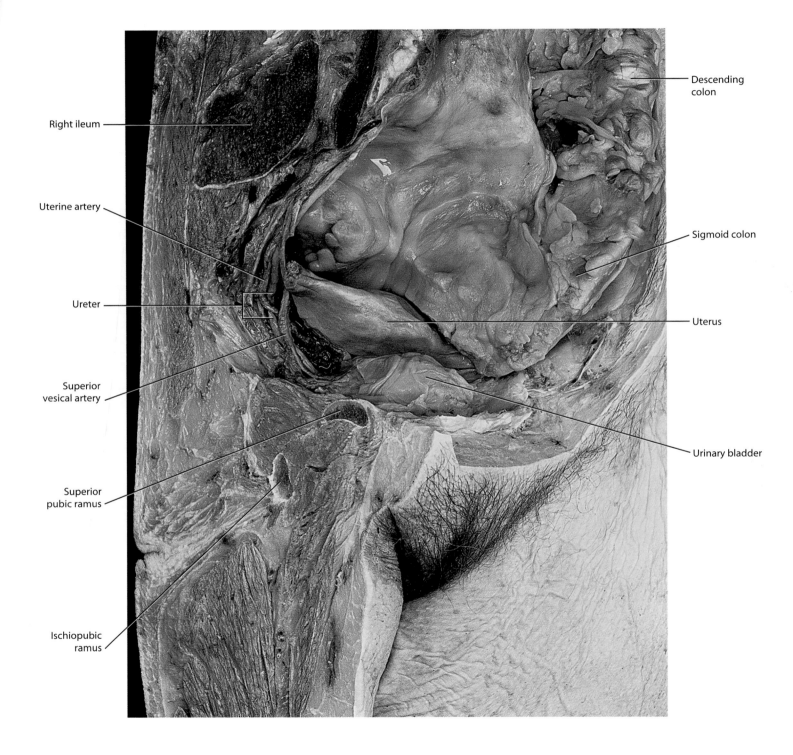

Right ileum

Uterine artery

Ureter

Superior
vesical artery

Superior
pubic ramus

Ischiopubic
ramus

Descending
colon

Sigmoid colon

Uterus

Urinary bladder

Figure 37.13 Pelvic viscera, female – deep dissection 2. Anterolateral view of a deep dissection of the right side of the female pelvis, just to the right of the midline

462

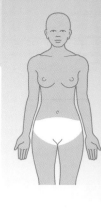

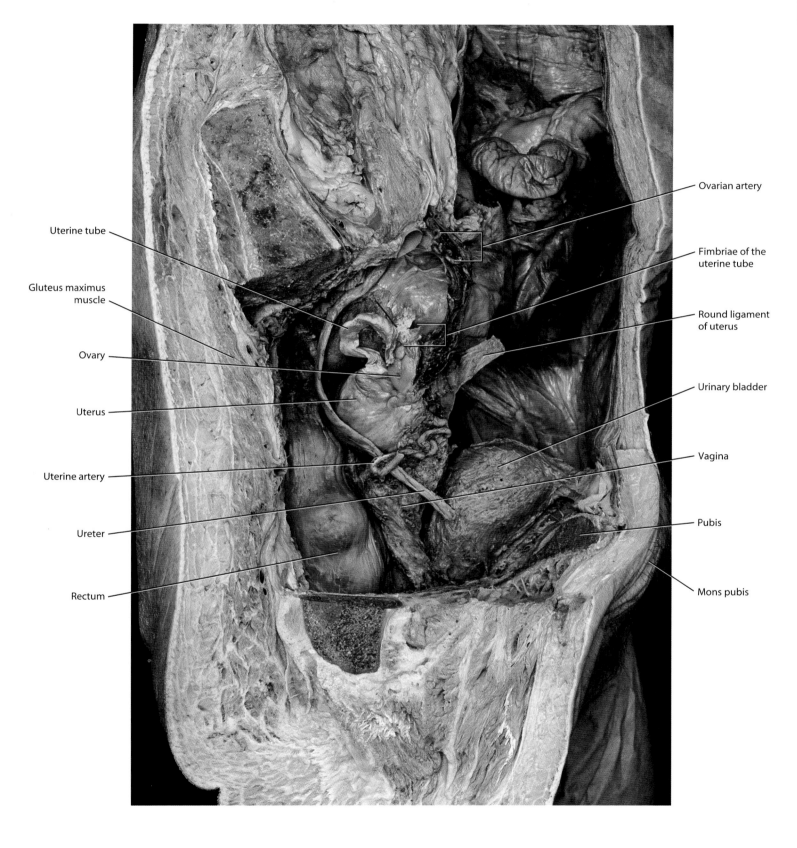

Uterine tube

Gluteus maximus muscle

Ovary

Uterus

Uterine artery

Ureter

Rectum

Ovarian artery

Fimbriae of the uterine tube

Round ligament of uterus

Urinary bladder

Vagina

Pubis

Mons pubis

Figure 37.14 Pelvic viscera, female – deep dissection 3. Lateral view of a deep dissection of the right side of the female pelvis

463

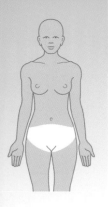

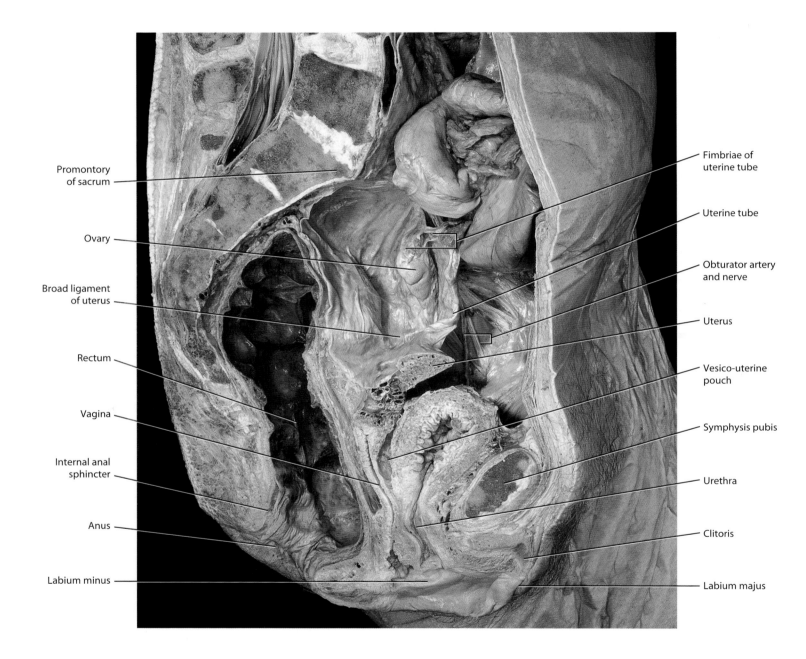

Promontory of sacrum

Ovary

Broad ligament of uterus

Rectum

Vagina

Internal anal sphincter

Anus

Labium minus

Fimbriae of uterine tube

Uterine tube

Obturator artery and nerve

Uterus

Vesico-uterine pouch

Symphysis pubis

Urethra

Clitoris

Labium majus

Figure 37.15 Pelvic viscera, female – sagittal section 1. Median sagittal section looking into the left side of a hemisected female pelvis. Observe the uterus and how it relates to the external genitalia and colon

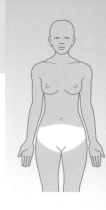

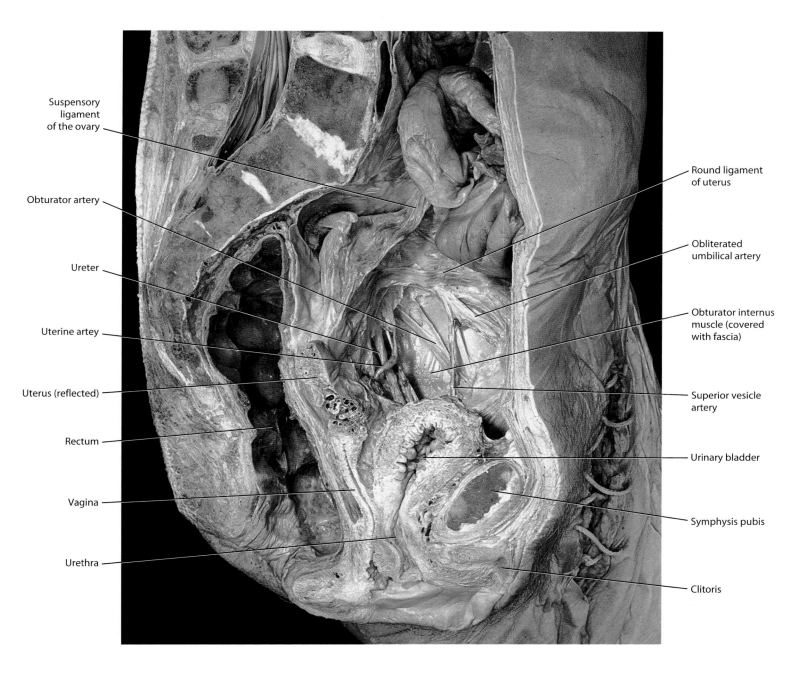

Suspensory
ligament
of the ovary

Obturator artery

Ureter

Uterine artey

Uterus (reflected)

Rectum

Vagina

Urethra

Round ligament
of uterus

Obliterated
umbilical artery

Obturator internus
muscle (covered
with fascia)

Superior vesicle
artery

Urinary bladder

Symphysis pubis

Clitoris

Figure 37.16 Pelvic viscera, female – sagittal section 2. Median sagittal view looking into the left side of the female pelvis. The uterus and ovarian tubes are visible. Also observe the location of the ovary

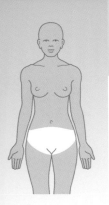

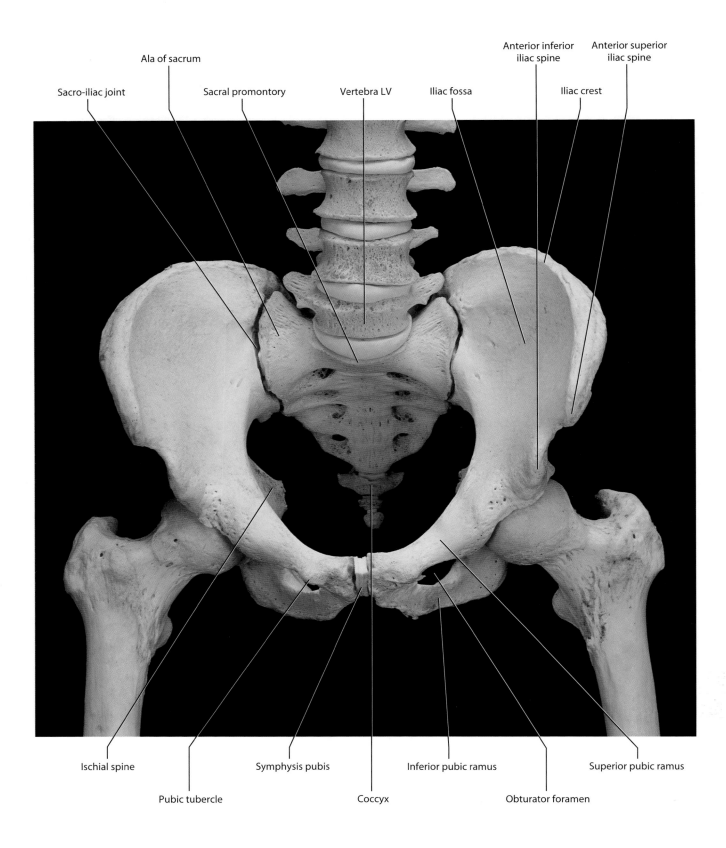

Ala of sacrum

Sacro-iliac joint

Sacral promontory

Vertebra LV

Iliac fossa

Anterior inferior iliac spine

Anterior superior iliac spine

Iliac crest

Ischial spine

Symphysis pubis

Inferior pubic ramus

Superior pubic ramus

Pubic tubercle

Coccyx

Obturator foramen

Figure 37.17 Pelvic viscera – osteology. Anterior view of the articulated pelvis

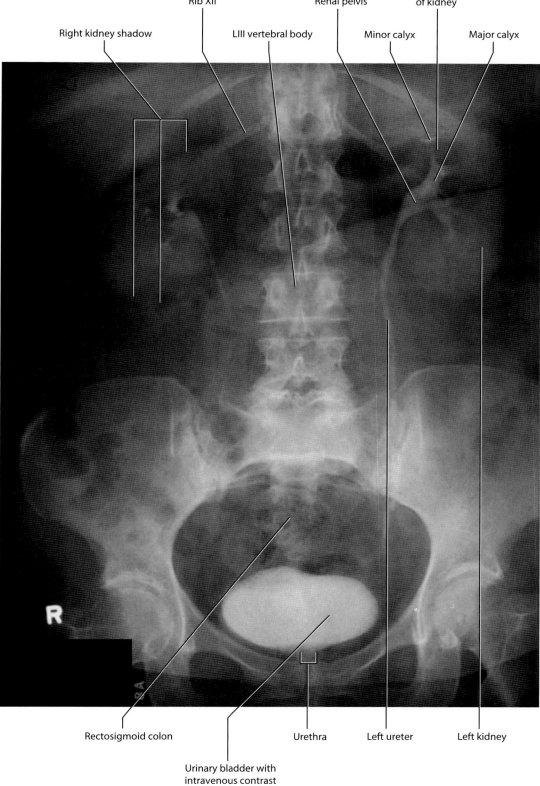

Figure 37.18 Pelvic viscera – intravenous pyelogram (anteroposterior view). In this view taken in the supine position 15 minutes after injection of dye, note the contrast in the collecting system of the kidneys, ureters, and bladder. The intravenous pyelogram is used to assess the urinary drainage of the kidneys and can show the presence of blockage, usually caused by calculi (stones), if present. This is a normal film

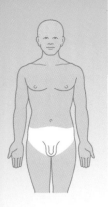

TRUNK

Pelvic viscera

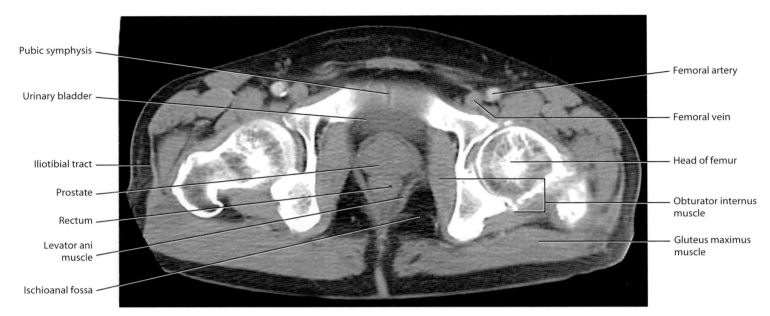

Pubic symphysis

Urinary bladder

Iliotibial tract

Prostate

Rectum

Levator ani muscle

Ischioanal fossa

Femoral artery

Femoral vein

Head of femur

Obturator internus muscle

Gluteus maximus muscle

Figure 37.19 Pelvic viscera, male – CT scan (axial view). The prostate gland is anterior to the rectum and posterior to the bladder in this axial view

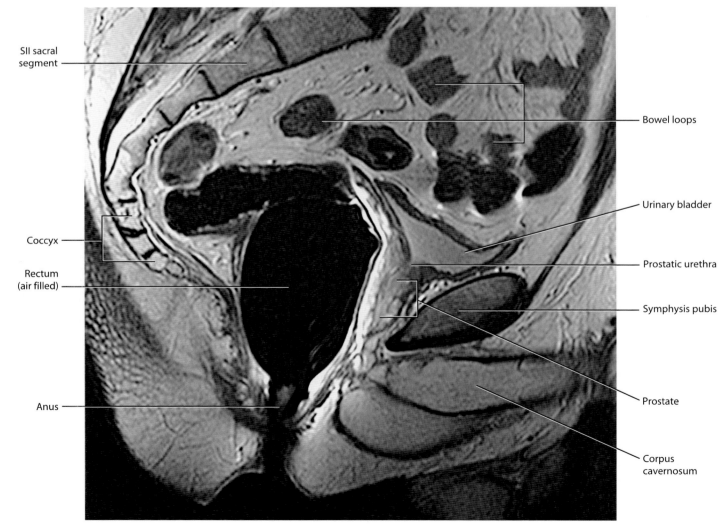

SII sacral segment

Coccyx

Rectum (air filled)

Anus

Bowel loops

Urinary bladder

Prostatic urethra

Symphysis pubis

Prostate

Corpus cavernosum

Figure 37.20 Pelvic viscera, male – MRI scan (sagittal view). In this scan, the rectum contains a medically placed probe that enables enhanced viewing of intrapelvic structures. The inverted pyramidal shape of the bladder is demonstrated. Observe how both the bladder and prostate are located behind the symphysis pubis

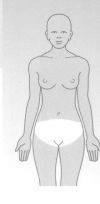

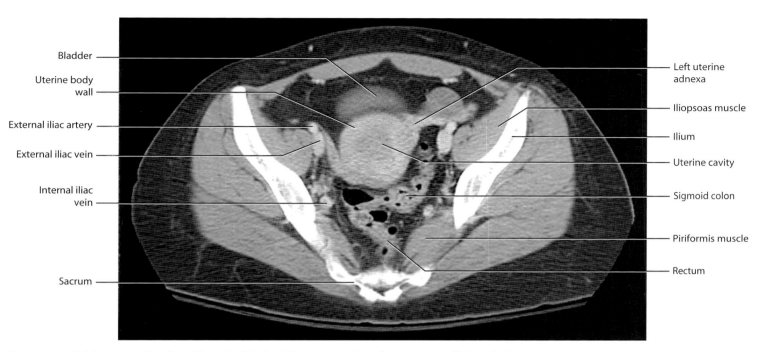

Bladder

Uterine body wall

External iliac artery

External iliac vein

Internal iliac vein

Sacrum

Left uterine adnexa

Iliopsoas muscle

Ilium

Uterine cavity

Sigmoid colon

Piriformis muscle

Rectum

Figure 37.21 Pelvic viscera, female – CT scan (axial view). Note the position of the uterus and bilateral adnexae (accessory reproductive organs) in this multiparous woman (a woman who has given birth to more than one child). Observe how the bladder is anterior to, and the rectum is posterior to, the uterus. Female reproductive organs are usually better visualized on MRI scans

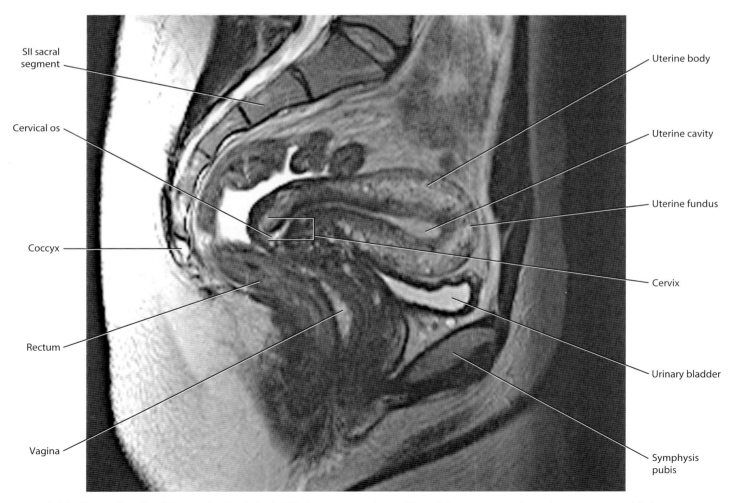

SII sacral segment

Cervical os

Coccyx

Rectum

Vagina

Uterine body

Uterine cavity

Uterine fundus

Cervix

Urinary bladder

Symphysis pubis

Figure 37.22 Pelvic viscera, female – MRI scan (sagittal view). This demonstrates the position of the uterus superior and posterior to the bladder

38 Perineum

The **perineum** is the area outlined by the diamond-shaped **pelvic outlet**. It contains the external genitalia and anus. The pelvic outlet is bounded:

- anteriorly by the pubic symphysis;
- posteriorly by the coccyx;
- laterally by the medial margins of the inferior pubic rami (anteriorly) and the sacrotuberous ligaments (posteriorly).

The perineum is further subdivided into **urogenital** and **anal triangles** by an imaginary line that joins the space between the anterior margins of the ischial tuberosities. Osseous support is provided by the pubic and ischial parts of the hip bones, the sacrum, and coccyx (see Chapter 36).

The floor of the perineum is formed by the skin and structures of the external genitalia, and the roof (the **pelvic diaphragm**) by a group of flat, sheet-like muscles (levator ani and coccygeus). These muscles extend across and cover the pelvic outlet to support the pelvic viscera (see Chapter 37). All the structures inferior or superficial to the pelvic diaphragm are constituents of the perineum (e.g. penis, vagina, and anus).

MUSCLES

The muscles of the perineum (Table 38.1) can be divided into three distinct groups: the pelvic diaphragm and supporting muscles, the urogenital diaphragm, and the superficial perineal muscles. These three layers of muscle are separated by several spaces containing fascia, fat, and loose connective tissue. These perirectal and perineal spaces are all adjoining, and infection in one area can quickly spread to another.

Pelvic diaphragm

The pelvic diaphragm is a collection of flat muscles that create a supportive basket-like floor for the pelvic viscera. These muscles are adjacent to each other and comprise the **levator ani** (**puborectalis**, **pubococcygeus**, and **iliococcygeus**) and **ischiococcygeus** muscles. The three levator ani muscles span the space between the body of the pubis, ischial spine, and coccyx. The **coccygeus** muscle attaches to the ischial spine and pelvic surface of the sacrospinous ligament, and to the coccyx and inferior sacrum. The coccygeus is superior and lateral to the levator ani muscles. These muscles support and elevate the pelvic floor when contracted.

The **piriformis** and **obturator internus** muscles provide additional support to the pelvic viscera. The piriformis muscle (see Chapter 42) is on the internal surface of the lateral sacrum and covers the opening in the pelvic outlet between the coccygeus muscle and the lateral wall of the pelvis. The obturator internus muscle is lateral to the levator ani muscles, spans the obturator foramen on the lateral wall of the pelvis, and leaves the pelvis through the lesser sciatic foramen to insert onto the femur.

Urogenital diaphragm

The **urogenital diaphragm** is composed of two muscles: the **deep transverse perineal** muscle and the **urethral sphincter**. These two muscles are superficial or inferior to the pelvic diaphragm. The deep transverse perineal muscles arise from the ischial tuberosities on the pelvic girdle and extend toward the midline, where they meet and help form the **perineal body**. Muscle fibers from the **external anal sphincter** and **puborectalis** (from the levator ani) also insert on this midline collection of muscle and soft tissue fibers. The perineal body is between the root of penis/vaginal fornix and the anus. Muscles of the superficial perineal group (superficial transverse perineal, bulbospongiosus, external anal sphincter) attach to it.

Just anterior to the deep transverse perineal muscles is the urethral sphincter muscle, which forms a circular ring around the urethra in both sexes; in women it also encircles the vagina. Small slips of muscle leave this ring laterally to insert onto the inferior pubic ramus. As a group, the urethral sphincter and deep transverse perineal muscles can be controlled voluntarily to delay micturition (urination). They are innervated by the **perineal branch** of the pudendal nerve.

Superficial perineal muscles

The superficial perineal muscles are the bulbospongiosus, ischiocavernosus, and superficial transverse perineal muscles, and the external anal sphincter (see Figs 38.1 and 38.3). These are superficial or inferior to the urogenital diaphragm. All are innervated by the pudendal nerve. The **bulbospongiosus** muscle originates from the perineal body and inserts into the corpus spongiosum of the penis where it maintains erection by preventing venous outflow. In women, the bulbospongiosus compresses the erectile tissue in the vestibule of the vagina and helps constrict the vaginal opening. This muscle also aids in expelling urine from the urethra in men and women.

The **ischiocavernosus** arises from the ischial tuberosity and inserts onto the corpus cavernosum of the penis or clitoris. It maintains erection in men and constricts the vagina and clitoris in women.

Like the other superficial perineal muscles, the **superficial transverse perineal muscle** arises from the ischium and inserts onto the perineal body. Its action stabilizes the perineal body.

The **external anal sphincter** is a circular muscle that surrounds the anus and provides voluntary control of defecation through the pudendal nerve.

MALE EXTERNAL GENITALIA

The **penis** is an elongated structure constructed of three tubular masses of erectile tissue (Fig. 38.1). It introduces sperm into the female genital tract during sexual intercourse and provides an exit point for urine through the **external urethral orifice**. The penis has a root, body, and head (glans penis).

The **root of penis** is the attachment point of the penis to the pelvis via the **urogenital diaphragm**. It is in the **superficial perineal pouch** and consists of three masses of erectile tissue: two lateral crura (legs) and the median **bulb of penis**. These structures are attached to the adjacent pubic arches and are covered superficially by the ischiocavernosus and bulbospongiosus muscles.

The three masses of erectile tissue – two **corpora cavernosa** and the **corpus spongiosum** (which contains the urethra) – continue into the **body of penis** (Fig. 38.2). The two corpora cavernosa expand and become firm during erection. Blood is supplied to the corpora cavernosa by the **dorsal artery of penis** (a branch of the

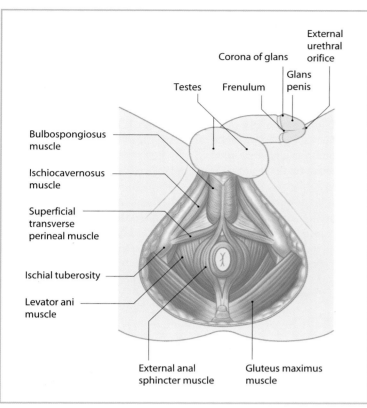

Figure 38.1 Male external genitalia

Labels in Figure 38.1:
Bulbospongiosus muscle; Ischiocavernosus muscle; Superficial transverse perineal muscle; Ischial tuberosity; Levator ani muscle; Testes; Frenulum; Corona of glans; Glans penis; External urethral orifice; External anal sphincter muscle; Gluteus maximus muscle

internal pudendal artery, which is a branch of the internal iliac artery). During sexual stimulation, contraction of the superficial perineal muscles maintains erection through autonomic innervation from the parasympathetic nervous system (the **pelvic splanchnic nerves**). This same process occurs in the clitoris of the female, although vascular enlargement of the clitoris is much less.

Distally, the corpus spongiosum becomes the **glans penis**. A midline slit near the tip of the glans penis is the external urethral orifice. The glans is covered by the **prepuce** (foreskin), which is a hood-like extension of the skin on the shaft of the penis.

The penis is innervated by the **pudendal nerve**, which carries parasympathetic nerve fibers from the pelvic splanchnic nerves, sympathetic fibers from the sympathetic trunk of the lower abdomen, and sensory fibers from spinal nerves S2 to S4.

Blood is supplied to the penis by the **internal pudendal artery**, which branches into the **artery of bulb of penis**, **dorsal artery of penis**, and **deep arteries of the penis**. Venous drainage from the corpora cavernosa, corpus spongiosum, and deep tissue is to the **deep dorsal vein of penis**, which empties into the **prostatic venous plexus**. Blood from the skin and superficial tissue of the penis flows along the **superficial dorsal vein** of penis to the **external pudendal vein**, which empties into the femoral vein in the groin. Lymph flows from the penis to the **superficial inguinal nodes** (see Chapter 32).

The **scrotum** is a fibromuscular sac that contains the testes and is described in Chapter 32.

FEMALE EXTERNAL GENITALIA

The female external genitalia (**vulva**) consist of the mons pubis, labia majora, labia minora, clitoris, and vestibule of the vagina (Fig. 38.3). The **vagina** is a distensible fibromuscular tube between

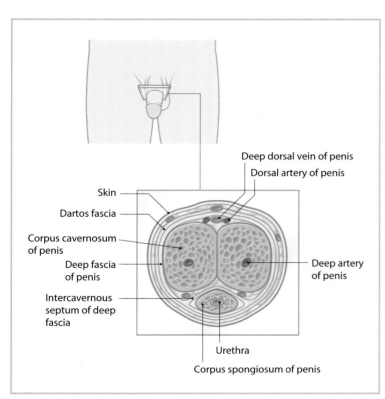

Figure 38.2 Cross section of the penis

Labels in Figure 38.2:
Skin; Dartos fascia; Corpus cavernosum of penis; Deep fascia of penis; Intercavernous septum of deep fascia; Deep dorsal vein of penis; Dorsal artery of penis; Deep artery of penis; Urethra; Corpus spongiosum of penis

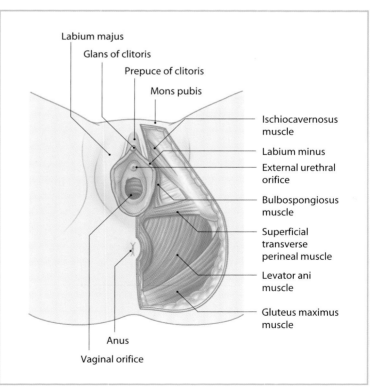

Figure 38.3 Female external genitalia (lithotomy position)

Labels in Figure 38.3:
Labium majus; Glans of clitoris; Prepuce of clitoris; Mons pubis; Ischiocavernosus muscle; Labium minus; External urethral orifice; Bulbospongiosus muscle; Superficial transverse perineal muscle; Levator ani muscle; Gluteus maximus muscle; Anus; Vaginal orifice

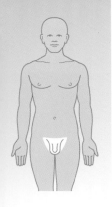
the uterus and perineum. It forms a recess around the uterine cervix and is subdivided into anterior, posterior, and lateral fornices. It is supported by the perineal body, urogenital diaphragm, levator ani muscles, and cardinal, uterosacral, and pubocervical ligaments. It is anterior to the perineal body, rectum, and recto-uterine pouch, and posterior to the urethra and bladder. It is the opening to the female pelvic viscera and is bounded by two sets of skin folds. The outer **labia majora** are longitudinal folds of hairbearing skin, sebaceous glands, and sweat glands. Superiorly, they meet at the **mons pubis**, which is a prominence of fatty tissue anterior to the pubic symphysis. Medial to the labia majora are the **labia minora**, the hairless folds of skin that surround the **vestibule** of the vagina.

Superiorly, the labia minora join at the **prepuce of clitoris**, which contains spongy erectile tissue that becomes engorged during sexual arousal. Just inferior to the prepuce formed by the labia minora is the **clitoris**. Resembling an upside down 'V', it contains two corpora cavernosa, two crura, and the **glans of clitoris**. Unlike the penis, the clitoris does not have any immediate connection with the urethra. Instead, the external urethral orifice is 2–3 cm inferior to the clitoris, within the vestibule of the vagina.

The vestibule of the vagina is the space between the labia minora and contains the **external urethral orifice**, **vaginal orifice**, and the openings of the ducts of the urethral glands. During sexual arousal the paired **greater vestibular glands** on either side of the vestibule secrete mucus into the vestibule through ducts that open into both sides of the vagina.

The vulva is innervated by the **ilio-inguinal, iliohypogastric**, and **pudendal nerves**, and the **posterior cutaneous nerve of thigh**. Blood is supplied by the **superficial external pudendal artery** (a branch of the femoral artery) and the **internal pudendal arteries** (branches of the internal iliac artery). Branches (**labial arteries**) from the internal pudendal artery supply the labia majora, labia minora, and vestibule of the vagina. **Clitoral branches** from the internal pudendal artery supply the clitoris and superior part of the vagina. Venous drainage is to the **internal pudendal vein** along vessels with the same name as the arteries. Lymphatic drainage of the vulva is to the **superficial inguinal nodes**.

■ CLINICAL CORRELATIONS
Hemorrhoids

Hemorrhoids are abnormal engorgements of the vascular cushions of the left lateral, right anterior, and right posterior areas external to the anal canal. These vascular cushions aid in anal continence and are supplied by the superior rectal and middle/inferior hemorrhoidal arteries. The cause of hemorrhoids is unknown, but chronic increased anal pressure secondary to chronic constipation, pregnancy, heredity, or other causes may lead to over-engorgement of the anal vascular cushions.

There are two types of hemorrhoids:

- external hemorrhoids are inferior to the pectinate (dentate) line within the anal canal – the skin inferior to this line is thin and richly innervated with pain fibers, whereas superior to this line the anal canal is lined by mucosa that produces pain only on extreme stretching;
- internal hemorrhoids are superior to the pectinate line and are usually asymptomatic until they bleed.

Patients with hemorrhoids commonly report blood in their stool. Other symptoms are anal itching, swelling, pain on wiping with toilet paper, mucus-like discharge, and a sense of a foreign body in the anal canal. Sometimes there is a long history of constipation or straining with defecation, and a diet lacking in fiber.

On examining the anal area for hemorrhoids patients are asked to strain (i.e. carry out a Valsalva maneuver) to see whether this causes the hemorrhoids to protrude (prolapse) from the anus. A hemorrhoid is visible as an outpouching of the anal tissue, usually in the shape of a teardrop or marble. The entire anal canal is examined by anoscopy to determine whether the hemorrhoids are internal or external. Severe internal hemorrhoids are referred for surgical treatment, but most hemorrhoids can be treated by simple measures, which include washing the anal area with warm water or taking a sitz bath several times a day, a high-fiber diet, stool softeners (as recommended by the clinician), and mild analgesics to minimize pain.

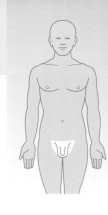

Body of penis

Pubic symphysis

Inguinal ligament

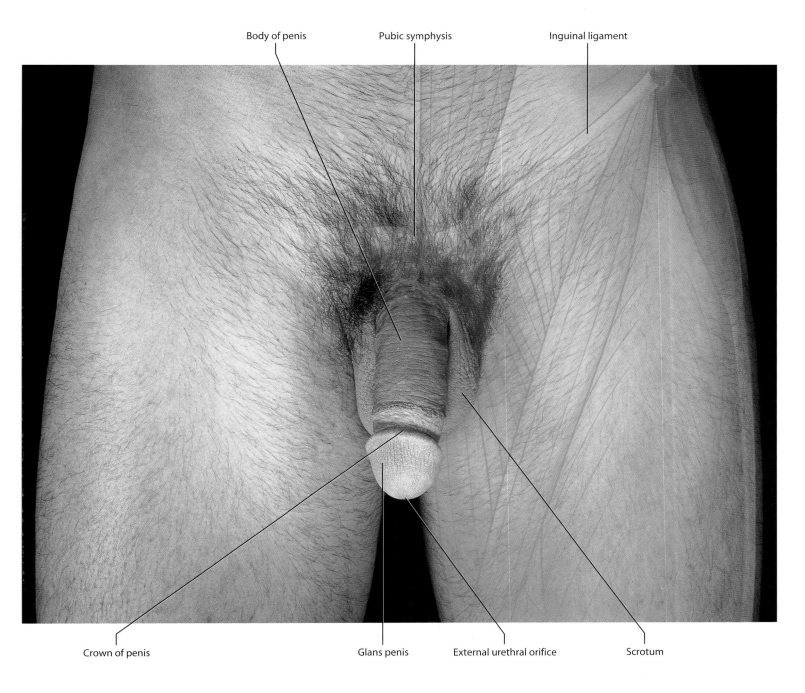

Crown of penis

Glans penis

External urethral orifice

Scrotum

Figure 38.4 Perineum, male – surface anatomy. Anterior view of the male external genitalia. This man is circumcised

473

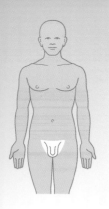

Perineum **TRUNK**

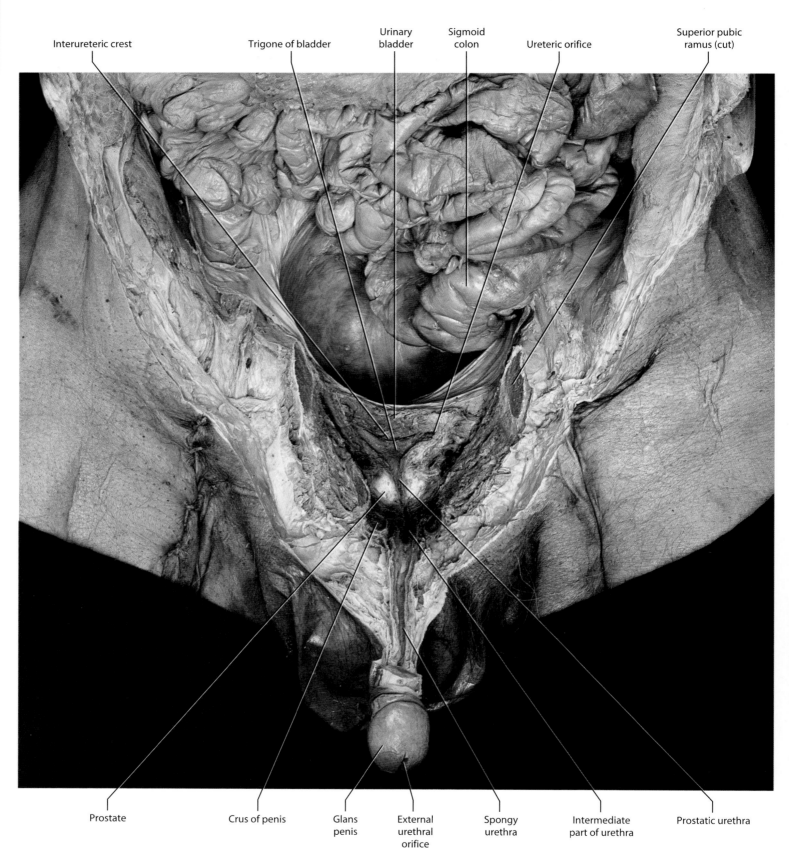

Interureteric crest

Trigone of bladder

Urinary
bladder

Sigmoid
colon

Ureteric orifice

Superior pubic
ramus (cut)

Prostate

Crus of penis

Glans
penis

External
urethral
orifice

Spongy
urethra

Intermediate
part of urethra

Prostatic urethra

474 **Figure 38.5 Genitalia, male – intermediate dissection.** Superoanterior view of an intermediate dissection of the male external genitalia and pelvic cavity

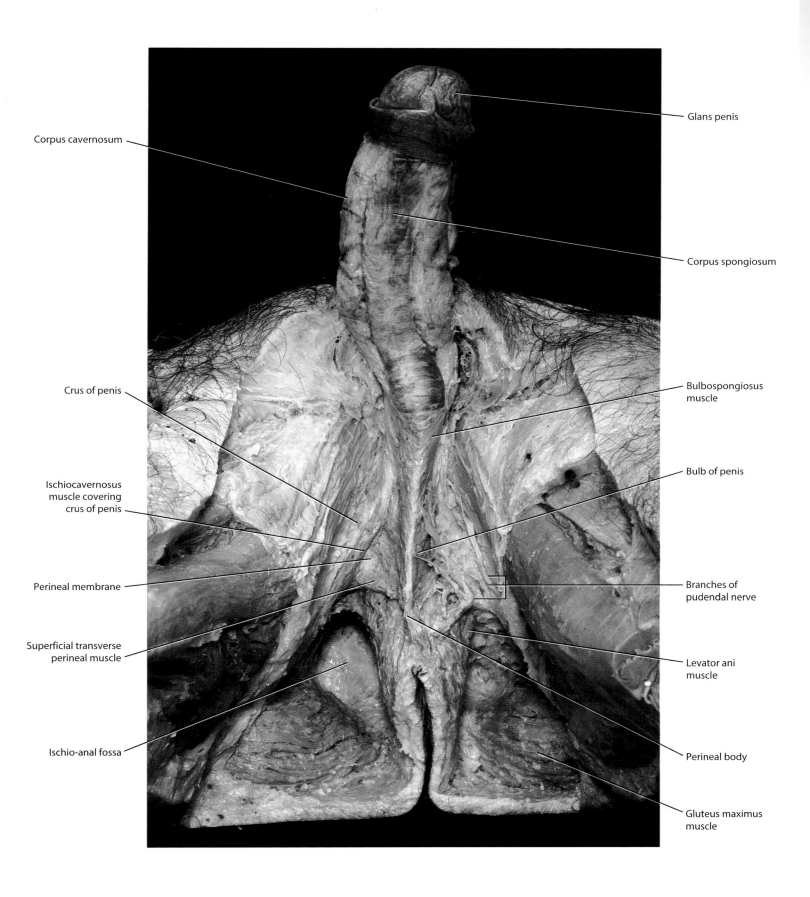

Glans penis

Corpus cavernosum

Corpus spongiosum

Crus of penis

Bulbospongiosus
muscle

Ischiocavernosus
muscle covering
crus of penis

Bulb of penis

Perineal membrane

Branches of
pudendal nerve

Superficial transverse
perineal muscle

Levator ani
muscle

Ischio-anal fossa

Perineal body

Gluteus maximus
muscle

Figure 38.6 Perineum, male – deep dissection. Inferior view of a deep dissection of the male perineum. The scrotum has been removed to reveal the root of the penis and the urogenital diaphragm

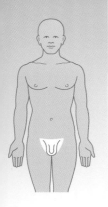

TABLE 38.1 MUSCLES OF THE PERINEUM

Muscle	Origin	Insertion	Action	Nerve supply	Blood supply
External anal sphincter Subcutaneous part	Encircles anal canal, no bony attachments	Coccyx	Forms voluntary anal sphincter with puborectalis muscle	Inferior anal nerve (branch of pudendal nerve)	Inferior rectal artery (branch of internal pudendal artery)
Superficial part	Perineal body	Coccyx	Forms voluntary anal sphincter with puborectalis muscle	Inferior anal nerve (branch of pudendal nerve)	Inferior rectal artery (branch of internal pudendal artery)
Deep part	Encircles anal canal, no bony attachments	Coccyx	" "	Inferior anal nerve (branch of pudendal nerve)	Inferior rectal artery (branch of internal pudendal artery)
Pelvic diaphragm Levator ani (pubococcygeus, puborectalis, and iliococcygeus)	Body of pubis, obturator fascia (tendinous arch of pelvic fascia), ischial spine	Perineal body, coccyx, anococcygeal body, prostate/vagina, rectum and anal canal	Forms floor of pelvic cavity; constricts lower end of rectum and vagina, supports pelvic viscera, muscle of forced defecation	Nerve to levator ani muscles (S4), inferior anal nerve, and coccygeal plexus	Muscular branches of internal pudendal, inferior rectal, and inferior gluteal arteries
Ischiococcygeus	Ischial spine and sacrospinous ligament	Coccyx and lower sacrum	Support for pelvic viscera, supports coccyx	Branches of S4 and S5	Muscular branches of internal pudendal and inferior rectal arteries
Pelvic walls Obturator internus	Pelvic aspect of ischium and ilium, obturator membrane	Greater trochanter of femur	Rotates thigh laterally, helps stabilize hip joint	Nerve to obturator internus	Obturator artery
Piriformis	Pelvic surface of sacrum, superior margin of greater sciatic notch, sacrotuberous ligament	Greater trochanter of femur	Rotates thigh laterally, abducts thigh, stabilizes hip joint	S1 and S2 (anterior rami)	Superior and inferior gluteal arteries
Ischiocavernosus	Ischial tuberosity	Crus of penis/clitoris	Assists in erection of penis/clitoris by compressing outflow of veins	Perineal branch of pudendal nerve	Perineal artery (branch of internal pudendal artery)
External urethral sphincter	Pubic arch	Surrounds urethra	Voluntary urethral sphincter	Perineal branch of pudendal nerve	Perineal artery (branch of internal pudendal artery)
Superficial transverse perineal muscle	Ischial tuberosity	Perineal body	Fixes perineal body	Perineal branch of pudendal nerve	Perineal artery (branch of internal pudendal artery)
Deep transverse perineal muscle	Ramus of ischium	Perineal body	Fixes perineal body	Perineal branch of pudendal nerve	Perineal artery (branch of internal pudendal artery)

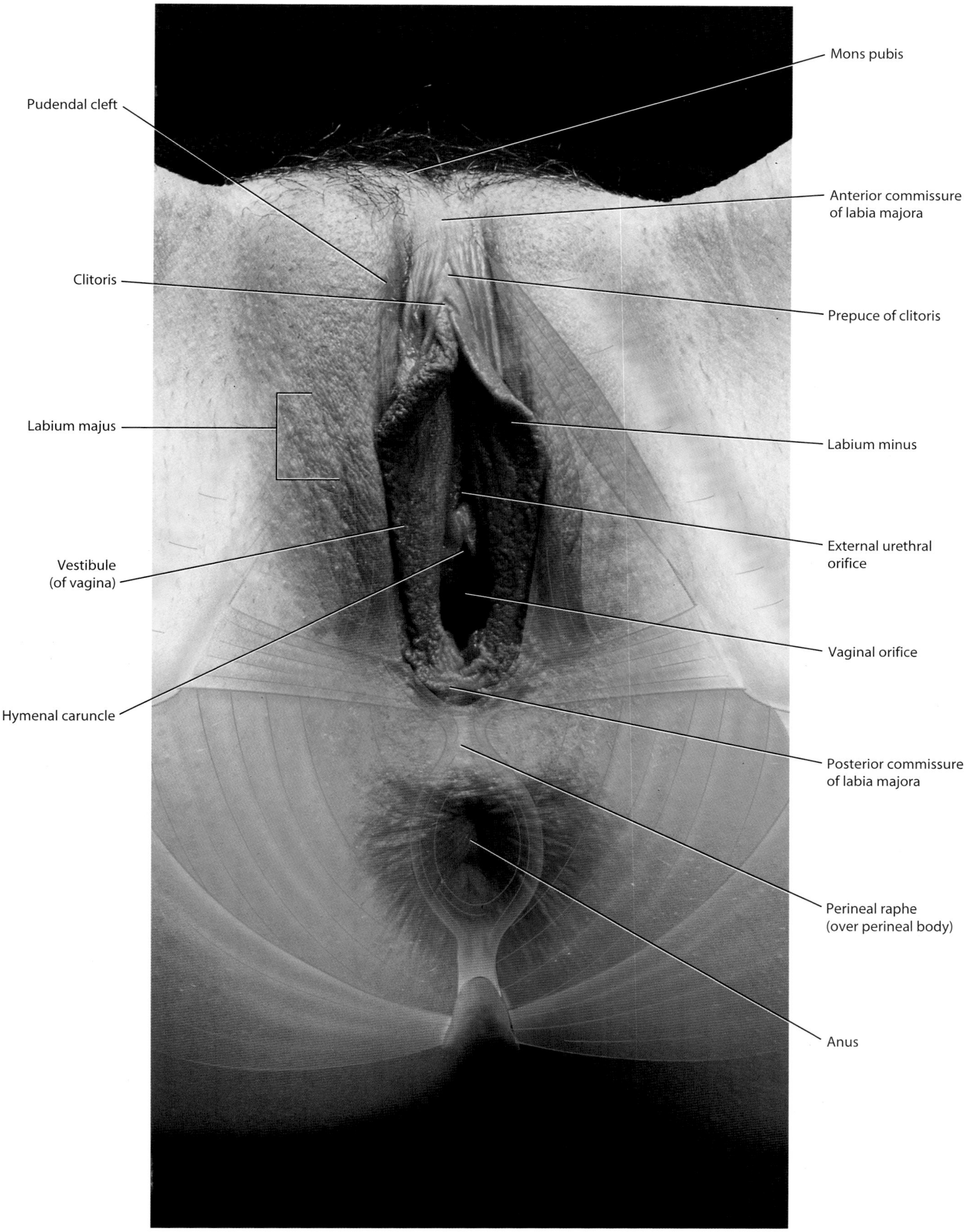

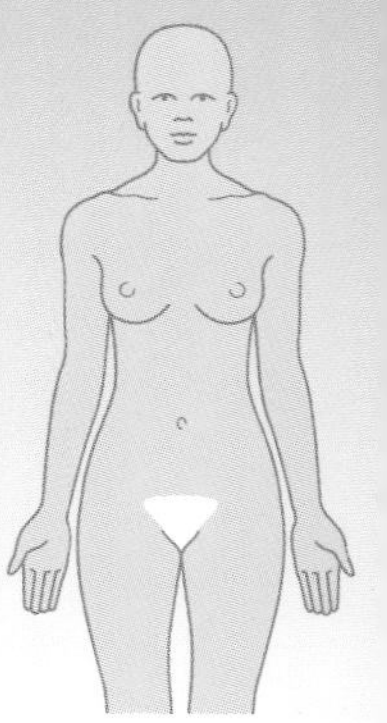

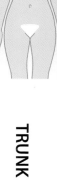

Mons pubis

Pudendal cleft

Anterior commissure
of labia majora

Clitoris

Prepuce of clitoris

Labium majus

Labium minus

External urethral
orifice

Vestibule
(of vagina)

Vaginal orifice

Hymenal caruncle

Posterior commissure
of labia majora

Perineal raphe
(over perineal body)

Anus

Figure 38.7 Perineum, female – surface anatomy. Inferior view of the female perineum of a woman who has given birth to more than one child

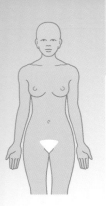

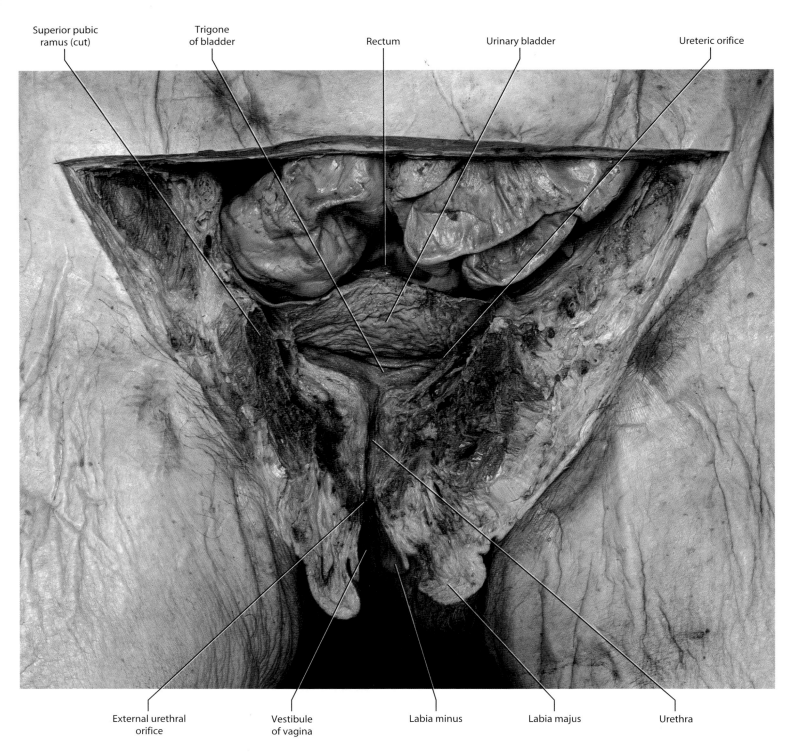

Superior pubic
ramus (cut)

Trigone
of bladder

Rectum

Urinary bladder

Ureteric orifice

External urethral
orifice

Vestibule
of vagina

Labia minus

Labia majus

Urethra

Figure 38.8 Genitalia, female – intermediate dissection. The female perineum viewed from an anterior perspective, showing the urinary bladder and vagina as they relate to the intestine

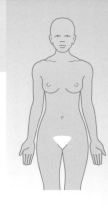

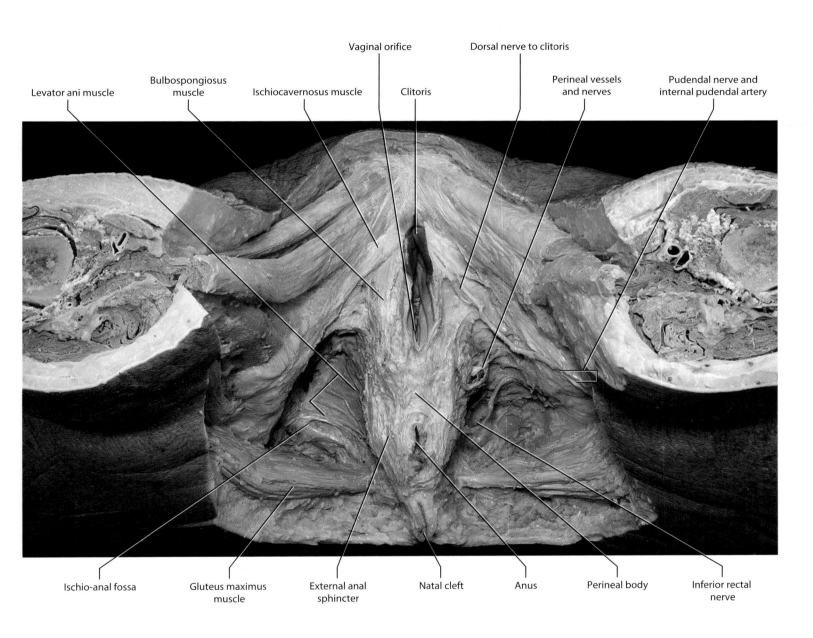

Vaginal orifice

Dorsal nerve to clitoris

Bulbospongiosus muscle

Perineal vessels and nerves

Pudendal nerve and internal pudendal artery

Levator ani muscle

Ischiocavernosus muscle

Clitoris

Ischio-anal fossa

Gluteus maximus muscle

External anal sphincter

Natal cleft

Anus

Perineal body

Inferior rectal nerve

Figure 38.9 Perineum, female – intermediate dissection 1. Inferior view. The labia minora and anus have been preserved as anatomical landmarks

479

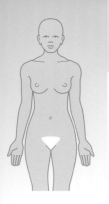

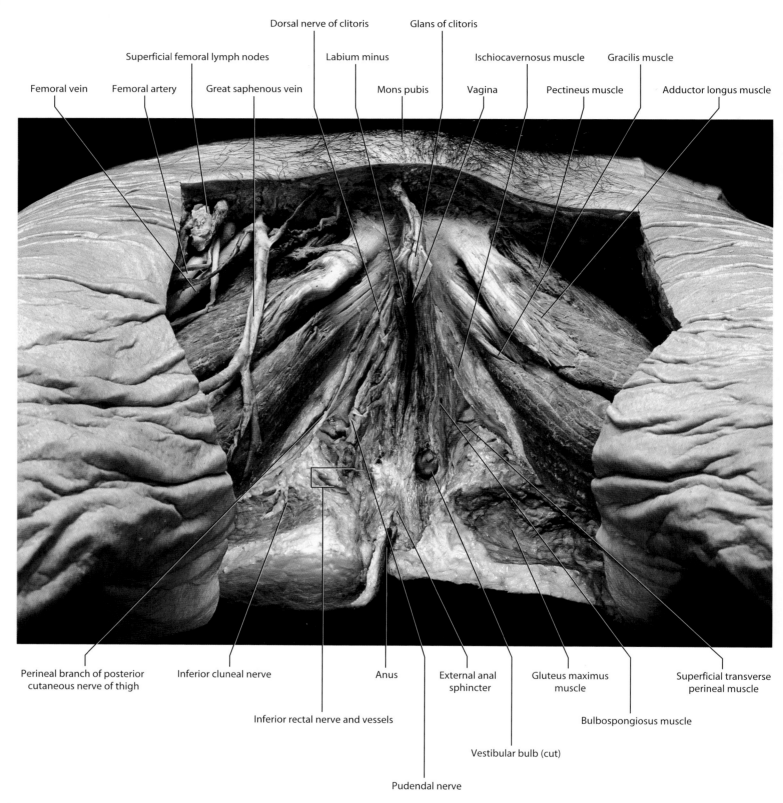

Dorsal nerve of clitoris

Glans of clitoris

Superficial femoral lymph nodes

Labium minus

Ischiocavernosus muscle

Gracilis muscle

Femoral vein

Femoral artery

Great saphenous vein

Mons pubis

Vagina

Pectineus muscle

Adductor longus muscle

Perineal branch of posterior cutaneous nerve of thigh

Inferior cluneal nerve

Anus

External anal sphincter

Gluteus maximus muscle

Superficial transverse perineal muscle

Inferior rectal nerve and vessels

Bulbospongiosus muscle

Vestibular bulb (cut)

Pudendal nerve

480   **Figure 38.10 Perineum, female – intermediate dissection 2.** Inferior view. The labia minora has been preserved as a landmark

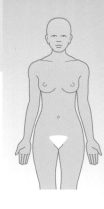

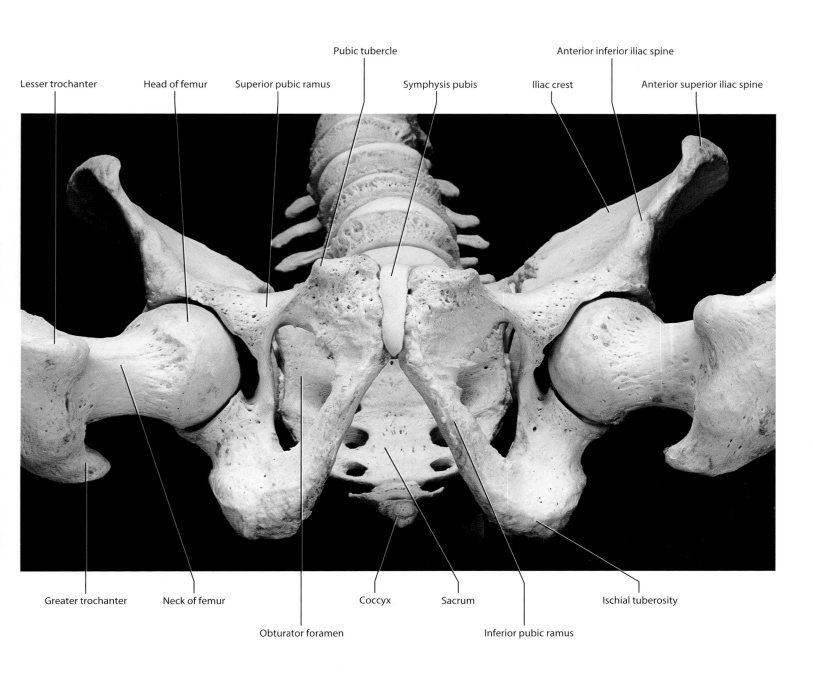

Lesser trochanter   Head of femur   Superior pubic ramus   Pubic tubercle   Symphysis pubis   Iliac crest   Anterior inferior iliac spine   Anterior superior iliac spine

Greater trochanter   Neck of femur   Obturator foramen   Coccyx   Sacrum   Inferior pubic ramus   Ischial tuberosity

Figure 38.11 Perineum – osteology. This is the view of the articulated pelvis as a clinician would encounter it during the pelvic examination of a woman

481

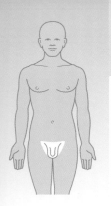

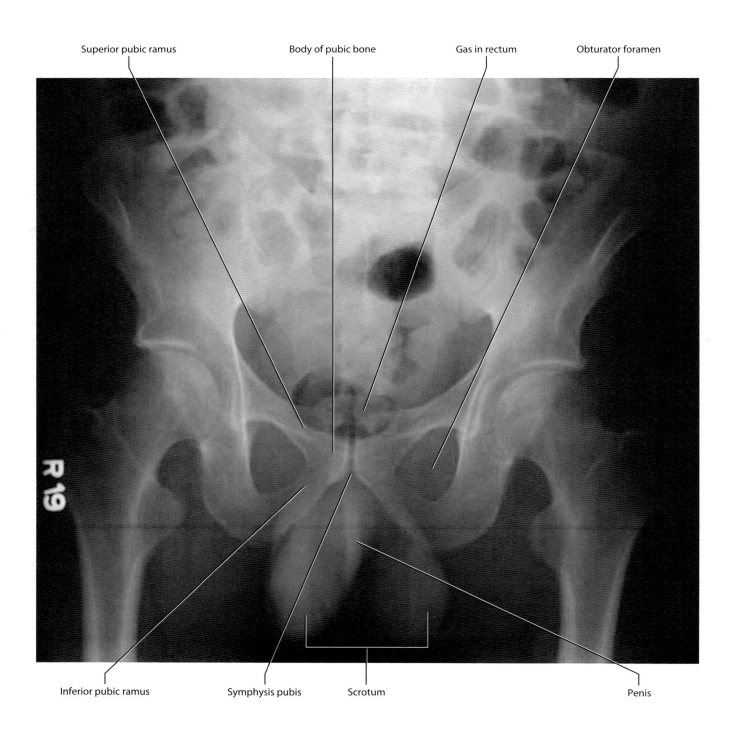

Superior pubic ramus   Body of pubic bone   Gas in rectum   Obturator foramen

Inferior pubic ramus   Symphysis pubis   Scrotum   Penis

Figure 38.12 Perineum, male – plain film radiograph (anteroposterior view). Observe the anatomical relationship of the male external genitalia with the pelvis

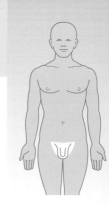

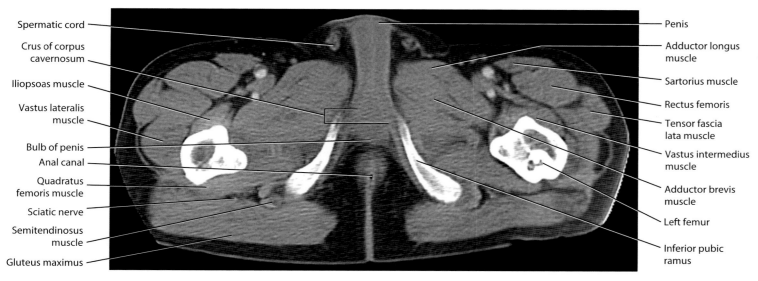

Spermatic cord

Crus of corpus cavernosum

Iliopsoas muscle

Vastus lateralis muscle

Bulb of penis

Anal canal

Quadratus femoris muscle

Sciatic nerve

Semitendinosus muscle

Gluteus maximus

Penis

Adductor longus muscle

Sartorius muscle

Rectus femoris

Tensor fascia lata muscle

Vastus intermedius muscle

Adductor brevis muscle

Left femur

Inferior pubic ramus

Figure 38.13 Perineum, male – CT scan (axial view). The penis and anal canal are visible in this view. Also observe the relationship of the spermatic cord to the penis

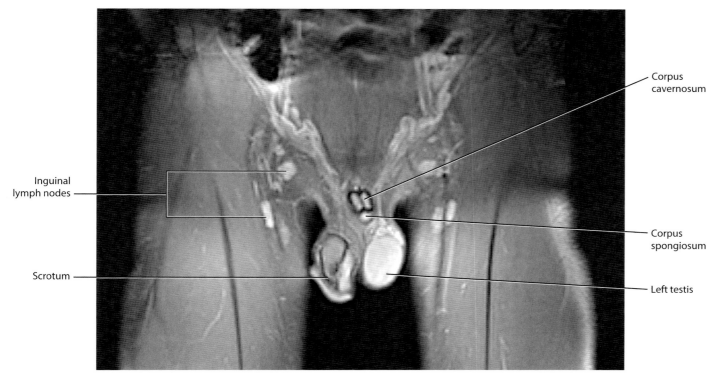

Inguinal lymph nodes

Scrotum

Corpus cavernosum

Corpus spongiosum

Left testis

Figure 38.14 Perineum, male – MRI scan (coronal view). Note the definition of the corpus spongiosum and cavernosum of the penis. Also, observe the distance between the penis and testes, which is essential for normal spermatogenesis

483

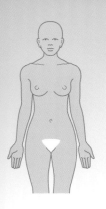

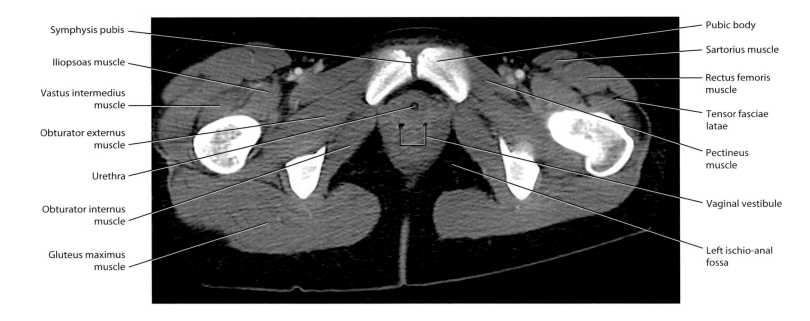

Symphysis pubis

Iliopsoas muscle

Vastus intermedius
muscle

Obturator externus
muscle

Urethra

Obturator internus
muscle

Gluteus maximus
muscle

Pubic body

Sartorius muscle

Rectus femoris
muscle

Tensor fasciae
latae

Pectineus
muscle

Vaginal vestibule

Left ischio-anal
fossa

Figure 38.15 Perineum, female – CT scan (axial view). This scan is at the level of the vaginal vestibule. Observe the urethra, which is located in the midline

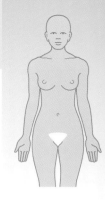

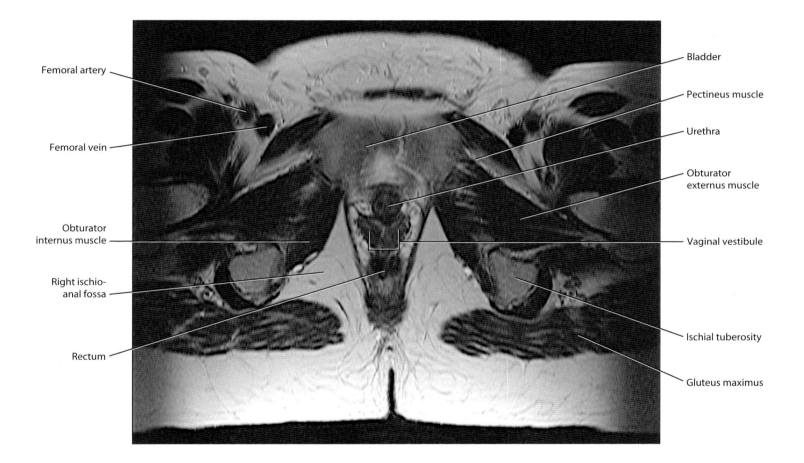

Femoral artery

Femoral vein

Obturator
internus muscle

Right ischio-
anal fossa

Rectum

Bladder

Pectineus muscle

Urethra

Obturator
externus muscle

Vaginal vestibule

Ischial tuberosity

Gluteus maximus

Figure 38.16 Perineum, female – MRI scan (axial view). Note the muscles of the pelvic floor and the proximity of the vaginal vestibule to the rectum

485

The basic structure of the lower limb is similar to that of the upper limb, but it is modified to support the weight of the body and for walking. The lower limb is divided into the thigh (between the hip and knee joints), gluteal area (region of the buttocks), leg (between the knee and ankle), and foot (from the heel to the toes).

The lower limb joins the **pelvic girdle** at the hip joint. This girdle is formed by the two hip bones (a fusion of ilium, ischium, and pubis bones), which join anteriorly at the pubic symphysis and, posteriorly, to the sacrum at the sacro-iliac joints.

The lower limb is supported by heavy bones that have pronounced areas for muscle and ligament attachment (Fig. 39.1). The **femur** articulates superiorly with the pelvis at the **hip joint** and inferiorly with the tibia at the **knee joint**. The **tibia** and **fibula** are the long bones of the leg. They articulate with each other proximally and distally at the **tibiofibular joint** and **tibiofibular syndesmosis**, respectively.

The distal ends of the tibia and fibula (**medial** and **lateral malleoli**) articulate with the **talus** (a tarsal bone) to form the ankle joint. The foot is made up of :
- seven **tarsal bones** – the talus, calcaneus, navicular, cuboid, medial cuneiform, intermediate cuneiform, and lateral cuneiform;
- five **metatarsals** (forefoot bones);
- five **digits**, each of which comprises three phalanges (proximal, middle, and distal) – except for the first digit (the great toe), which lacks the middle phalanx.

MUSCLES

The muscles of the lower limb are strong and the movements they produce are more coarse than those produced by the muscles of the upper limb. The deep fascia forms intermuscular septa, which divide the segments of the limb into unyielding compartments, each with its own group of muscles.

The thigh is divided into **anterior**, **medial**, and **posterior compartments**. The muscles in the anterior compartment of thigh are primarily extensors of the knee joint, whereas the medial thigh muscles are adductors of the hip joint. The posterior thigh muscles are extensors of the hip and flexors of the knee joint, and the gluteal muscles mainly rotate the thigh laterally.

The leg is similarly compartmentalized into three subdivisions (**anterior**, **lateral**, and **posterior compartments**) by intermuscular septa derived from the deep fascia of the leg. The anterior leg muscles are primarily dorsiflexors of the ankle and extensors of the toes. The lateral compartment contains two muscles, which plantarflex and evert the foot. The muscles of the posterior compartment of the leg are separated into a superficial and deep group by the **transverse fascia** of the leg. The superficial group, through its tendons, acts on the calcaneus to plantarflex the foot. The muscles of the deep group flex the toes and plantarflex the ankle.

The organization of the bones, muscles, and ligaments of the foot provides support and stability on varying surfaces. The sole of the foot is composed of four intricate layers of muscles and tendons.

NERVES

The nerves to the lower limb (Fig. 39.2) are derivatives of the **lumbar plexus** (L1 to L4) of nerves within the posterior abdominal wall and the **sacral plexus** (L4 to S4) in the posterior pelvis.

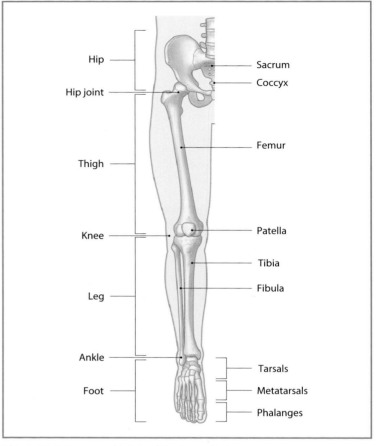

Figure 39.1 Bones and joints of the lower limb

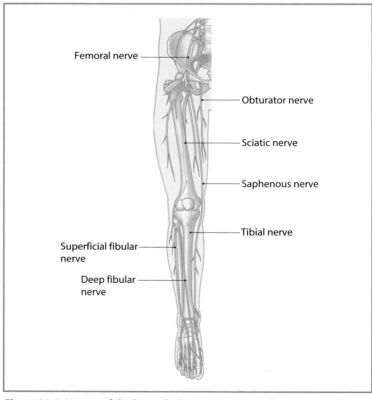

Figure 39.2 Nerves of the lower limb

The two main branches of the six branches of the lumbar plexus are the **femoral nerve**, which innervates the anterior thigh muscles, and the **obturator nerve**, which innervates the medial adductor muscles.

The largest branch of the nine branches of the sacral plexus is the **sciatic nerve** on the posterior surface of the buttock and lower limb. It descends through the posterior compartment of thigh, innervating the muscles in this compartment. Just before reaching the knee it divides into the **tibial** and **common fibular** nerves:

- the tibial nerve descends within the popliteal fossa (back of the knee) and innervates all muscles of the posterior leg – it then crosses the ankle posterior to the medial malleolus to enter the sole of the foot, where it divides into the **medial** and **lateral plantar nerves**, which innervate all muscles on the plantar surface of the foot;
- the common fibular nerve innervates all structures within the anterior and lateral compartments of leg, the superficial branch innervates the two lateral leg muscles and the **deep fibular nerve** branch innervates the four anterior leg muscles and the muscle on the dorsum of the foot.

Cutaneous innervation of the lower limb is shown in Figure 39.3.

ARTERIES

Blood is supplied to the lower limb by the **femoral artery**, which is a continuation of the external iliac artery (Fig. 39.4). The femoral artery begins at the inferior border of the inguinal ligament, then quickly branches to form the **deep artery of thigh**, which provides:

- **perforating arteries** to the posterior thigh;
- the **medial** and **lateral circumflex femoral arteries**, which encircle the upper part of the shaft of the femur and supply the femur, hip joint, and upper part of the thigh.

The femoral artery enters the **adductor canal** on the midanterior thigh and enters the posterior thigh through the **adductor hiatus** to become the **popliteal artery** (see Chapter 40). The popliteal artery descends through the popliteal fossa, giving off **genicular branches** to the knee joint. At the head of fibula, the popliteal artery divides into the **anterior** and **posterior tibial arteries**. The anterior tibial artery supplies the anterior and lateral compartments of the leg and terminates as the **dorsalis pedis artery** to the dorsum of the foot. The posterior tibial artery supplies the muscles in the posterior compartment of leg and crosses the ankle posterior to the medial malleolus, where it divides into the **medial** and **lateral plantar arteries**, which supply the sole of the foot.

VEINS AND LYMPHATICS

Deep venous drainage of the lower limb follows the arteries; the veins drain to the **femoral vein**. The superficial venous drainage originates from the **dorsal venous arch of foot**. Medially, this drains to the **great saphenous vein**, which ascends through the leg anterior to the medial malleolus (see Chapter 47). It continues along the medial leg and thigh before emptying into the femoral vein within the femoral triangle (see Chapter 40). The lateral side of the dorsal venous arch of foot gives rise to the **small saphenous vein**. This ascends into the calf posterior to the lateral malleolus and empties into the popliteal vein in the popliteal fossa (see Chapter 43).

Lymphatics superficial to the deep fascia of the lower limb drain into the **superficial inguinal nodes**, which are near the termination of the great saphenous vein in the femoral triangle. Lymph from the buttock, perineum, and lower abdomen also drains to these nodes. Deep lymphatic drainage of the lower limb follows the deep arteries and flows toward the **iliac** and **aortic lymph nodes** within the pelvis and lower posterior abdominal wall.

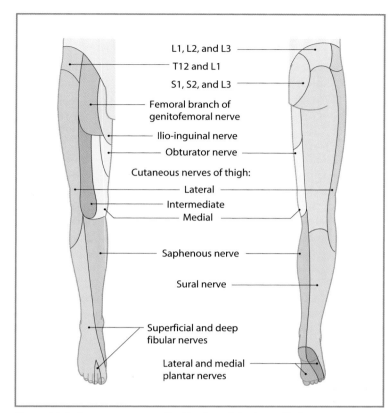

Figure 39.3 Cutaneous nerve distribution of the lower limb

L1, L2, and L3
T12 and L1
S1, S2, and L3
Femoral branch of genitofemoral nerve
Ilio-inguinal nerve
Obturator nerve
Cutaneous nerves of thigh:
Lateral
Intermediate
Medial
Saphenous nerve
Sural nerve
Superficial and deep fibular nerves
Lateral and medial plantar nerves

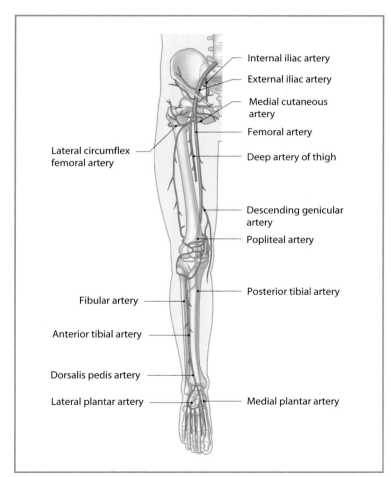

Figure 39.4 Arteries of the lower limb

Internal iliac artery
External iliac artery
Medial cutaneous artery
Femoral artery
Deep artery of thigh
Lateral circumflex femoral artery
Descending genicular artery
Popliteal artery
Posterior tibial artery
Fibular artery
Anterior tibial artery
Dorsalis pedis artery
Lateral plantar artery
Medial plantar artery

40 Anteromedial thigh

The thigh is the part of the lower limb between the hip and knee joints. The muscles of the thigh are divided into anterior, medial, and posterior groups. In addition, the psoas major and iliacus muscles enter the thigh from the posterior abdominal wall and iliac fossa (Fig. 40.1). These two muscles combine to form the iliopsoas muscle. The tensor fasciae latae muscle, innervated by the superior gluteal nerve, is discussed here because of its close proximity to the anteromedial thigh muscles.

The **femur** is the largest bone in the body and the only osseous support for the thigh. It is long and slender with a rounded **head** that articulates with the acetabulum of the pelvis. Inferiorly, it has two large prominences – the **medial** and **lateral condyles** – which articulate with the tibia and patella at the knee joint.

MUSCLES

The muscles of the thigh are enclosed within a strong fascial sleeve – the **fascia lata** (Fig. 40.2). Three intermuscular septa arising from the fascia lata divide the thigh into three compartments: anterior, medial, and posterior compartments.

The muscles of the **anterior compartment of thigh** (Table 40.1) are **sartorius** and **quadriceps femoris** with its four heads **rectus femoris**, **vastus medialis**, **vastus intermedius** (which includes the **articularis genu** – a distinct muscle considered to be part of the vastus intermedius muscle that pulls the synovial membrane of the knee superiorly during knee joint extension), and **vastus lateralis**. As a group, the anterior thigh muscles (Fig. 40.1) originate from either the anterior superior iliac spine of the pelvis or the shaft of the femur. The muscles insert onto the proximal tibia through tendinous attachments. These include the patellar tendon for the quadriceps femoris muscle and pes anserinus ('goose foot'), a three-pronged tendinous structure at the superior medial tibia with attachment for the sartorius, gracilis, and semitendinosus muscles. The anterior thigh muscles flex the thigh at the hip joint and extend the leg at the knee.

The muscles of the **medial compartment of thigh** (Table 40.2) are **pectineus**, **adductor longus**, **adductor brevis**, **adductor magnus**, **gracilis**, and **obturator externus**. The medial thigh muscles originate from the pubic rami and insert along the entire length of the posterior shaft of femur (Fig. 40.3). Collectively, these muscles are the adductors of the thigh, with the exception of obturator externus, which rotates the thigh laterally.

Two other muscles are related to the anteromedial thigh.

- The **tensor fasciae latae** is lateral to the superior part of the vastus medialis muscle and tightens the iliotibial tract, which helps to extend and stabilize the knee joint; it also aids in flexion and abduction of the hip joint.
- The **iliopsoas** muscle, formed from the union of the iliacus and psoas major muscles at the posterior abdominal wall, descends into the anteromedial thigh beneath the inguinal ligament to insert onto the lesser trochanter of the femur, and is the main flexor of the thigh at the hip joint.

The posterior thigh muscles are discussed in Chapter 42.

NERVES

The **femoral nerve** (L2 to L4) is the primary nerve to the anterior compartment of thigh. Originating in the posterior abdominal wall

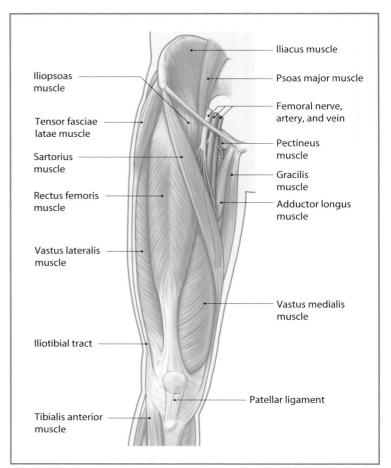

Figure 40.1 Muscles of the thigh – anterior view

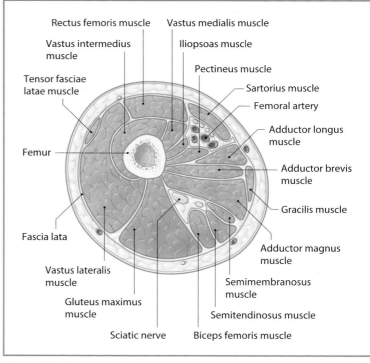

Figure 40.2 Cross-section of right thigh viewed from distal to proximal

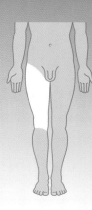

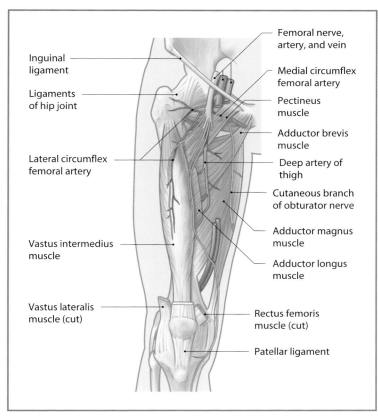

Figure 40.3 Deep muscles of the anterior thigh

as part of the lumbar plexus of nerves, the femoral nerve passes inferiorly and deep to the inguinal ligament in a groove formed by the psoas major and iliacus muscles to enter the anterior thigh. From the femoral nerve, muscular branches run to sartorius, pectineus, and each of the four heads of quadriceps femoris. The terminal branch of the femoral nerve is the **saphenous nerve**, which enters the adductor canal and descends toward the medial part of the leg, where it conveys sensation from the skin of the medial arch of the foot and the medial leg. Branches of the femoral nerve innervate the hip and knee joints.

The primary cutaneous nerves of the anteromedial thigh are the **anterior cutaneous branches** of the femoral nerve (L2, L3). Several of these branches descend over the quadriceps femoris to supply the skin of the distal three-quarters of the anterior thigh. The **medial femoral cutaneous nerve** supplies the skin of the distal two-thirds of the medial thigh, and the **lateral cutaneous nerve of thigh** (L2, L3), which is a direct branch of the lumbar plexus, supplies the skin over the tensor fasciae latae and vastus lateralis muscles of the lateral thigh.

The **obturator nerve** (L2 to L4) enters the medial thigh from the pelvis through the **obturator canal**. Superior to the adductor brevis muscle, the **obturator** nerve divides into **anterior** and **posterior branches**. The anterior branch innervates adductor longus, adductor brevis, and gracilis muscles before sending a cutaneous branch to the distal medial thigh and hip. The posterior branch of the obturator nerve supplies adductor magnus, obturator externus, and the adductor brevis muscles. This posterior branch pierces the adductor magnus muscle to end as an **articular branch** to the knee joint.

ARTERIES

The **femoral artery**, a continuation of the external iliac artery, begins at the lower border of the inguinal ligament, medial to the femoral nerve (see Fig. 40.3). After entering the thigh, it has three branches:

- the **superficial circumflex iliac artery** passes laterally toward the iliac crest;
- the **superficial external pudendal artery** runs medially to supply the external genitalia;
- the **superficial epigastric artery** reaches the umbilicus via the anterior abdominal wall.

The femoral artery descends inferiorly in the thigh. Its largest branch is the **deep artery of thigh**, which usually leaves the femoral artery a few centimeters inferior to the inguinal ligament. Two branches of the deep artery of thigh – the **medial** and **lateral circumflex femoral arteries** – wrap around the shaft of the femur to supply the immediate area and the hip joint. In addition, the deep artery of thigh branches to supply blood to the gluteal area, and, via perforating arterial branches, to the posterior thigh (see Chapter 42).

The **obturator artery** is a branch of the internal iliac artery that descends from within the pelvis medial to the psoas major muscle. It enters the thigh through the **obturator foramen** with the obturator nerve. After entering the medial thigh, the obturator artery divides into **anterior** and **posterior branches**. The anterior branch supplies the adductor muscles and the posterior branch gives off the **acetabular branch** to the hip joint.

VEINS AND LYMPHATICS

Superficial venous drainage of the anteromedial thigh is along small, unnamed veins that empty into the **great saphenous vein**, which in turn empties into the femoral vein within the femoral triangle. Deep venous drainage of the anteromedial thigh follows the course of the arteries and is toward the **femoral vein**.

Superficial lymphatic drainage, like superficial venous drainage, is through small lymphatic vessels that drain toward the **superficial inguinal nodes** within the femoral triangle at the groin. Deep lymphatic drainage is along lymphatic vessels that follow the large arteries and empty into the **iliac lymph nodes**.

FEMORAL TRIANGLE AND FEMORAL SHEATH

The **femoral triangle** (Fig. 40.4) is a subfascial area in the upper anterior thigh. It contains several neurovascular structures and has three boundaries – superior, medial, and lateral – formed by the inguinal ligament, adductor longus muscle, and sartorius muscle, respectively.

The muscular floor of the femoral triangle is formed (from lateral to medial) by the iliopsoas, pectineus, and adductor longus muscles. The femoral vein, artery, and nerve are within the triangle. In addition, the great saphenous vein empties into the femoral vein within the triangle.

The **femoral sheath** is a tube-like continuation of the **transversalis** and **iliac fasciae** of the abdominal wall and is medial to the femoral nerve. It extends into the anterior thigh inferior to the inguinal ligament and has three compartments – lateral, intermediate, and medial – for the femoral artery, femoral vein, and femoral canal (which contains lymph nodes and fat), respectively.

ADDUCTOR CANAL

The **adductor canal** is a passageway through the middle third of the thigh that allows the femoral vessels to pass through to the **adductor hiatus** of the posterior thigh. The saphenous nerve enters the canal

489

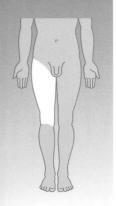
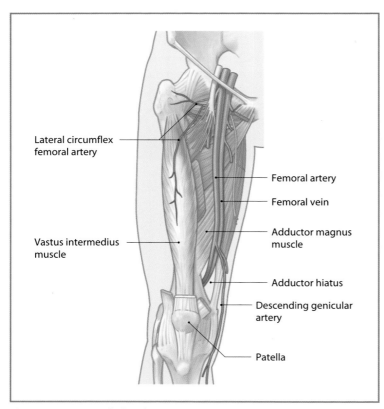

Figure 40.4 Femoral triangle

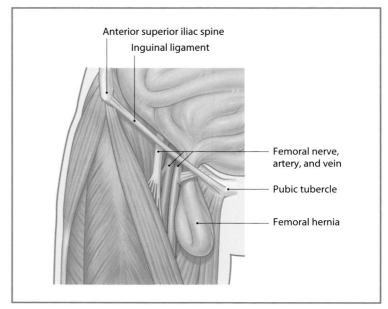

Figure 40.5 Femoral hernia

with the femoral vessels but pierces the medial fascial sleeve of the canal to become cutaneous opposite the knee joint.

■ CLINICAL CORRELATIONS
Femoral hernia
A femoral hernia occurs when part of the intra-abdominal contents (intestine or other) protrudes through the space inferior to the medial border of the inguinal ligament (Fig. 40.5). The hernia can be caused by any condition that chronically increases the intra-abdominal pressure or decreases the strength of the inferior abdominal and femoral tissues. Chronic constipation, prostate enlargement, vaginal delivery, cancer, smoking, and genetic defects are among the contributing factors. Femoral hernias are most common in women, but are much less common than inguinal hernias in both men and women (see Chapter 35).

A femoral hernia causes the sensation of a mass or bulge at or inferior to the groin crease on the superior anteromedial thigh. The mass may increase or decrease in size, depending on activity and abdominal straining from, for example, coughing or defecation. Medical advice is usually sought because of the discomfort that arises from having a mass in the groin.

The defect at the medial part of the inguinal ligament just medial to the femoral vein is usually small and there is a high risk that herniated abdominal contents will strangulate. Early referral to a surgeon for treatment is recommended. The management of femoral hernia is surgical and aimed at reducing the herniated abdominal contents back into the abdomen and closure of the defect at the medial inguinal ligament to prevent further hernia formation.

Chronic arterial occlusive disease of the femoral artery
Chronic arterial occlusive disease (CAOD) is caused by atherosclerosis, which is the result of repetitive injury of the endothelium. This injury is followed by a progressive build-up of lipid and the formation of plaque along the inner lumen of a blood vessel. This narrows the lumen of the vessel and, in some cases, complete obstruction can occur. Risk factors for CAOD include advanced age, smoking, hypertension, diabetes mellitus, hyperlipidemia, and family history. The most common location for CAOD in the lower limb is within the femoral artery as it passes through the adductor canal via the adductor hiatus. Patients with CAOD usually have shiny skin with very little hair and thick toenails on the affected limb.

Claudication, pain in a muscle group during activity, is common in the legs and is due to poor blood supply. It is brought on by exercise and alleviated with rest. Advanced arterial disease causes extreme burning pain in the legs and feet at night. Patients commonly awake in the night and place the involved limb in a dependent position to increase blood flow and cause the pain to subside. Occasionally painful ischemic ulcers develop on the foot inferior to the ankle malleoli.

Faint or nonpalpable popliteal or dorsalis pedis pulses, skin changes, and ischemic ulcers are observed on clinical examination. An ankle–brachial index (ABI, systolic blood pressure at the ankle/systolic blood pressure of the arm) is measured by many clinicians to determine the extent of arterial insufficiency: very low ABI values indicate advanced disease. Ultrasound and other modalities help in delineating the extent of disease. Patients with advanced arterial insufficiency are referred for vascular surgery, and may be treated by endarterectomy or a femoropopliteal bypass. Femoropopliteal bypass is a procedure in which a native vessel (saphenous vein) or synthetic arterial graft is attached to the femoral artery proximal to the stenosis and distally to the popliteal artery beyond the stenosis.

MNEMONICS	
Femoral triangle boundaries:	**So I May Always Love Sally** (**S**uperiorly – **I**nguinal ligament; **M**edially – **A**dductor longus; **L**aterally – **S**artorius)
Femoral triangle contents: (from lateral hip to medial navel)	**NAVEL** (**N**erve, **A**rtery, **V**ein, **E**mpty space, **L**ymph – nerve, artery, and vein all called femoral)

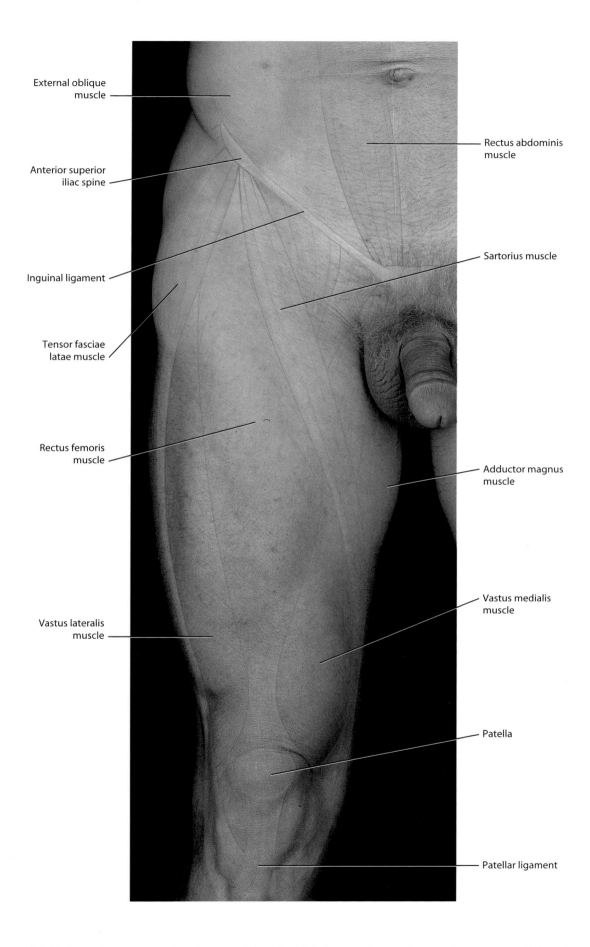

External oblique muscle

Anterior superior iliac spine

Inguinal ligament

Tensor fasciae latae muscle

Rectus femoris muscle

Vastus lateralis muscle

Rectus abdominis muscle

Sartorius muscle

Adductor magnus muscle

Vastus medialis muscle

Patella

Patellar ligament

Figure 40.6 Anteromedial thigh – surface anatomy. Anterior view of the right thigh. Observe the prominence of the vastus medialis and vastus lateralis muscles, which are members of the quadriceps femoris muscle group

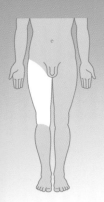

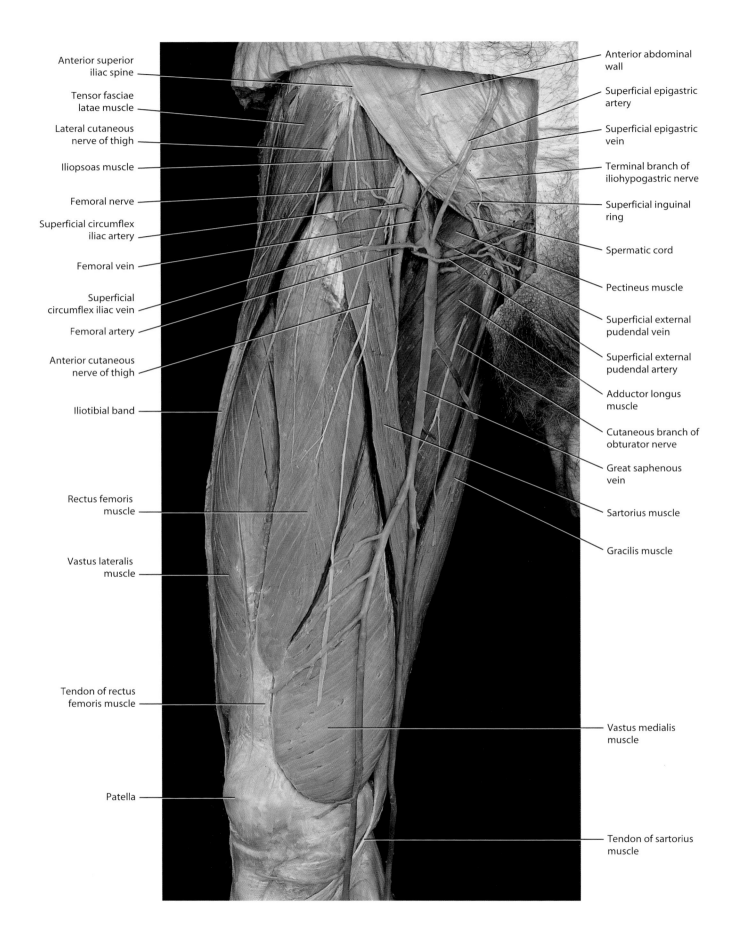

Anterior superior
iliac spine

Tensor fasciae
latae muscle

Lateral cutaneous
nerve of thigh

Iliopsoas muscle

Femoral nerve

Superficial circumflex
iliac artery

Femoral vein

Superficial
circumflex iliac vein

Femoral artery

Anterior cutaneous
nerve of thigh

Iliotibial band

Rectus femoris
muscle

Vastus lateralis
muscle

Tendon of rectus
femoris muscle

Patella

Anterior abdominal
wall

Superficial epigastric
artery

Superficial epigastric
vein

Terminal branch of
iliohypogastric nerve

Superficial inguinal
ring

Spermatic cord

Pectineus muscle

Superficial external
pudendal vein

Superficial external
pudendal artery

Adductor longus
muscle

Cutaneous branch of
obturator nerve

Great saphenous
vein

Sartorius muscle

Gracilis muscle

Vastus medialis
muscle

Tendon of sartorius
muscle

Figure 40.7 Anteromedial thigh – superficial dissection. Anterior view of the right thigh showing the greater saphenous vein, and the cutaneous nerves. Observe the muscle separation between the muscles of this compartment

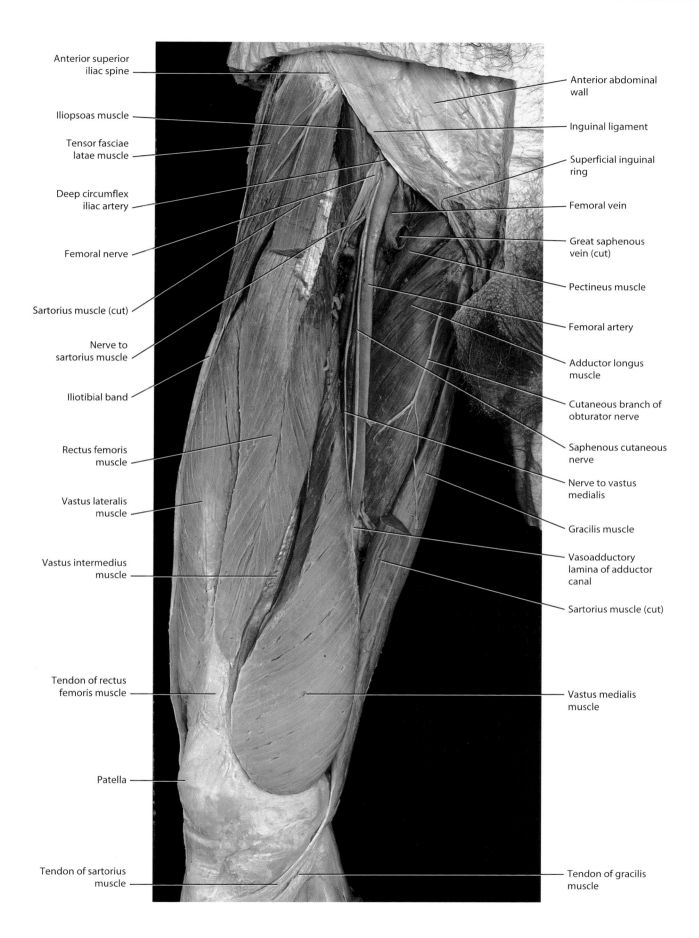

Anterior superior iliac spine

Iliopsoas muscle

Tensor fasciae latae muscle

Deep circumflex iliac artery

Femoral nerve

Sartorius muscle (cut)

Nerve to sartorius muscle

Iliotibial band

Rectus femoris muscle

Vastus lateralis muscle

Vastus intermedius muscle

Tendon of rectus femoris muscle

Patella

Tendon of sartorius muscle

Anterior abdominal wall

Inguinal ligament

Superficial inguinal ring

Femoral vein

Great saphenous vein (cut)

Pectineus muscle

Femoral artery

Adductor longus muscle

Cutaneous branch of obturator nerve

Saphenous cutaneous nerve

Nerve to vastus medialis

Gracilis muscle

Vasoadductory lamina of adductor canal

Sartorius muscle (cut)

Vastus medialis muscle

Tendon of gracilis muscle

LOWER LIMB Anteromedial thigh

Figure 40.8 Anteromedial thigh – intermediate dissection. Anterior view of the right thigh. The sartorius muscle has been cut and reflected to show the contents of the femoral triangle (femoral nerve, artery, and vein)

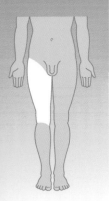

LOWER LIMB

Anteromedial thigh

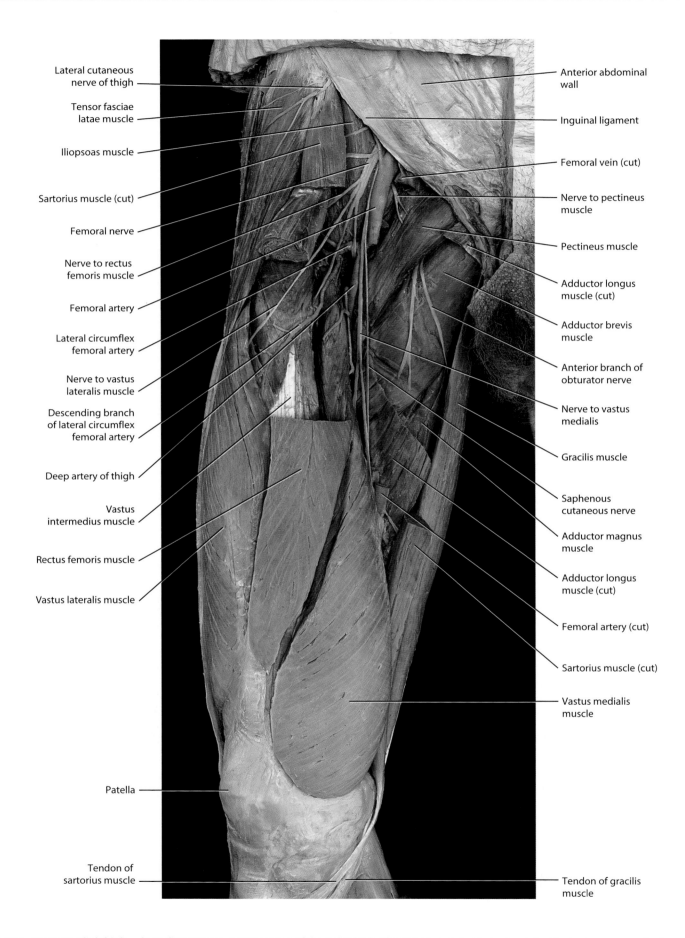

Lateral cutaneous nerve of thigh

Tensor fasciae latae muscle

Iliopsoas muscle

Sartorius muscle (cut)

Femoral nerve

Nerve to rectus femoris muscle

Femoral artery

Lateral circumflex femoral artery

Nerve to vastus lateralis muscle

Descending branch of lateral circumflex femoral artery

Deep artery of thigh

Vastus intermedius muscle

Rectus femoris muscle

Vastus lateralis muscle

Patella

Tendon of sartorius muscle

Anterior abdominal wall

Inguinal ligament

Femoral vein (cut)

Nerve to pectineus muscle

Pectineus muscle

Adductor longus muscle (cut)

Adductor brevis muscle

Anterior branch of obturator nerve

Nerve to vastus medialis

Gracilis muscle

Saphenous cutaneous nerve

Adductor magnus muscle

Adductor longus muscle (cut)

Femoral artery (cut)

Sartorius muscle (cut)

Vastus medialis muscle

Tendon of gracilis muscle

Figure 40.9 Anteromedial thigh – deep dissection 1. Anterior view of the right thigh. The sartorius, rectus femoris, and adductor longus muscles have been cut. Observe the deeper muscles not visible on superficial dissection (pectineus, adductor brevis, and adductor magnus), and the lateral circumflex femoral artery

494

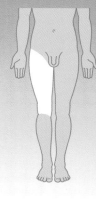

TABLE 40.1   ANTERIOR THIGH MUSCLES

Muscle	Origin	Insertion	Innervation	Action	Blood supply
Iliopsoas/ psoas major	Sides of vertebrae TXII to LV and transverse processes of LI to LV	Lesser trochanter of femur	Anterior rami of lumbar nerves (L1 to L3)	Flexes thigh at hip and stabilizes the hip	Lumbar branches of iliolumbar artery
Iliacus	Iliac crest, iliac fossa, ala of sacrum, and anterior sacro-iliac ligaments	Tendon of psoas major and body of femur, inferior to lesser trochanter	Femoral nerve (L2, L3)	Flexes thigh at hip and stabilizes the hip	Iliac branches of iliolumbar artery
Tensor fasciae latae	Anterior superior iliac spine and anterior part of external lip of iliac crest	Iliotibial tract that attaches to lateral condyle of tibia	Superior gluteal nerve (L4, L5)	Abducts, medially rotates and flexes the thigh, stabilizes trunk on thigh	Superior gluteal arteries, lateral circumflex femoral artery
Sartorius	Anterior superior iliac spine and superior part of notch inferior to it	Superior part of medial surface of tibia	Femoral nerve (L2, L3)	Abducts, medially rotates and flexes the thigh	Femoral artery
Quadriceps femoris, rectus femoris	Anterior inferior iliac spine and groove superior to acetabulum	Base of patella via patellar ligament	Femoral nerve (L2 to L4)	Extends the leg at the knee joint and flexes the thigh at the hip joint	Lateral circumflex femoral artery, deep femoral artery
Vastus lateralis	Greater trochanter and lateral lip of linea aspera of femur	Base of patella via patellar ligament	Femoral nerve (L2 to L4)	Extends the leg at the knee joint	Lateral circumflex femoral artery, deep femoral artery
Vastus medialis	Intertrochanteric line and medial lip of linea aspera of femur	Base of patella via patellar ligament	Femoral nerve (L2 to L4)	Extends the leg at the knee joint	Femoral artery, deep femoral artery
Vastus intermedius	Anterior and lateral surfaces of body of femur	Base of patella via patellar ligament	Femoral nerve (L2 to L4)	Extends the leg at the knee joint	Lateral circumflex femoral artery, deep femoral artery

TABLE 40.2   MEDIAL THIGH MUSCLES

Muscle	Origin	Insertion	Innervation	Action	Blood supply
Pectineus	Pecten pubis	Pectineal line of femur	Femoral nerve (L2, L3) and sometimes obturator nerve	Adducts and flexes thigh	Medial circumflex femoral artery, obturator artery
Adductor longus	Body of pubis, inferior to pubic crest	Middle third of linea aspera of femur	Obturator nerve (anterior division) (L2 to L4)	Adducts thigh	Medial circumflex femoral artery, obturator artery
Adductor brevis	Body and inferior pubic ramus	Pectineal line and proximal part of linea aspera of femur	Obturator nerve (L2 to L4)	Adducts and flexes thigh	Medial circumflex femoral artery, obturator artery
Adductor magnus	Inferior pubic ramus, ramus of ischium, and ischial tuberosity	Gluteal tuberosity, linea aspera, supracondylar line, and adductor tubercle	Adductor part: obturator nerve (L2 to L4) hamstring part: tibial nerve (L4)	Adducts and flexes thigh (adductor part) Extends thigh (hamstring part)	Deep femoral artery, popliteal artery, obturator artery
Gracilis	Body of pubis and inferior pubic ramus	Superior part of medial surface of tibia	Obturator nerve (L2, L3)	Adducts thigh, flexes and medially rotates the leg	Deep femoral artery, medial circumflex femoral artery
Obturator externus	Margins of obturator foramen and obturator membrane	Trochanteric fossa of femur	Obturator nerve (L2, L3)	Laterally rotates the thigh and stabilizes head of femur in acetabulum	Medial circumflex femoral artery, obturator artery

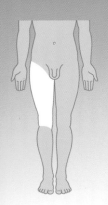

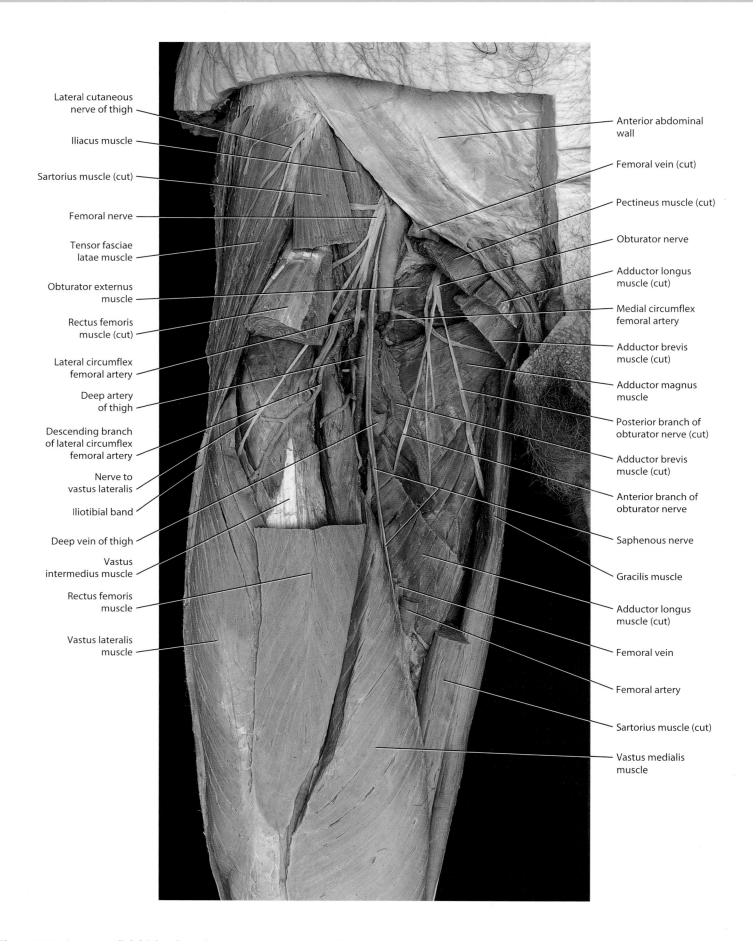

Lateral cutaneous nerve of thigh

Iliacus muscle

Sartorius muscle (cut)

Femoral nerve

Tensor fasciae latae muscle

Obturator externus muscle

Rectus femoris muscle (cut)

Lateral circumflex femoral artery

Deep artery of thigh

Descending branch of lateral circumflex femoral artery

Nerve to vastus lateralis

Iliotibial band

Deep vein of thigh

Vastus intermedius muscle

Rectus femoris muscle

Vastus lateralis muscle

Anterior abdominal wall

Femoral vein (cut)

Pectineus muscle (cut)

Obturator nerve

Adductor longus muscle (cut)

Medial circumflex femoral artery

Adductor brevis muscle (cut)

Adductor magnus muscle

Posterior branch of obturator nerve (cut)

Adductor brevis muscle (cut)

Anterior branch of obturator nerve

Saphenous nerve

Gracilis muscle

Adductor longus muscle (cut)

Femoral vein

Femoral artery

Sartorius muscle (cut)

Vastus medialis muscle

Figure 40.10 Anteromedial thigh – deep dissection 2. Anterior view of the right thigh. The sartorius, rectus femoris, adductor longus, and adductor brevis muscles have been cut to show the deepest structures of the anteromedial thigh. Observe the adductor magnus muscle and the anterior and posterior divisions of the obturator nerve

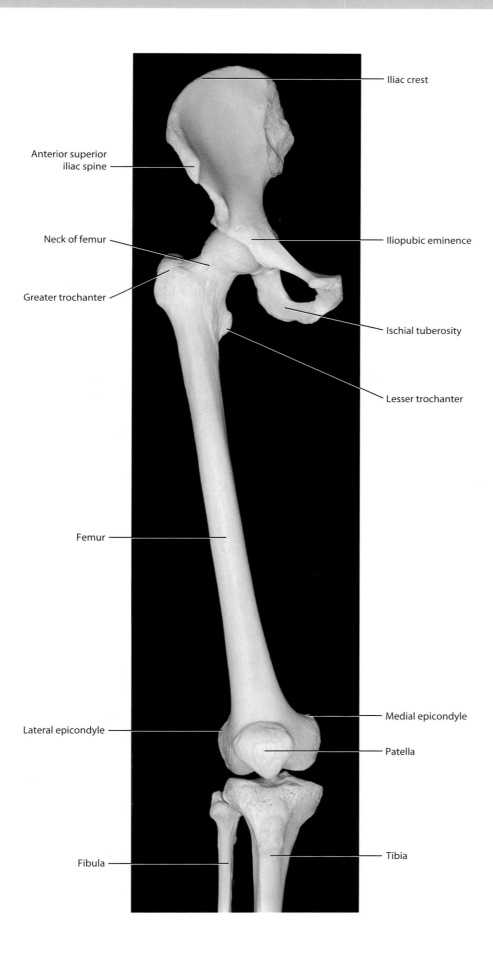

Iliac crest

Anterior superior
iliac spine

Iliopubic eminence

Neck of femur

Greater trochanter

Ischial tuberosity

Lesser trochanter

Femur

Medial epicondyle

Lateral epicondyle

Patella

Fibula

Tibia

Figure 40.11 Anteromedial thigh – osteology. Anterior view of the articulated bones of the right lower limb. Observe the shape of the femur, which is the largest bone in the body

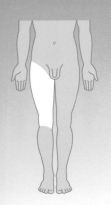

LOWER LIMB

Anteromedial thigh

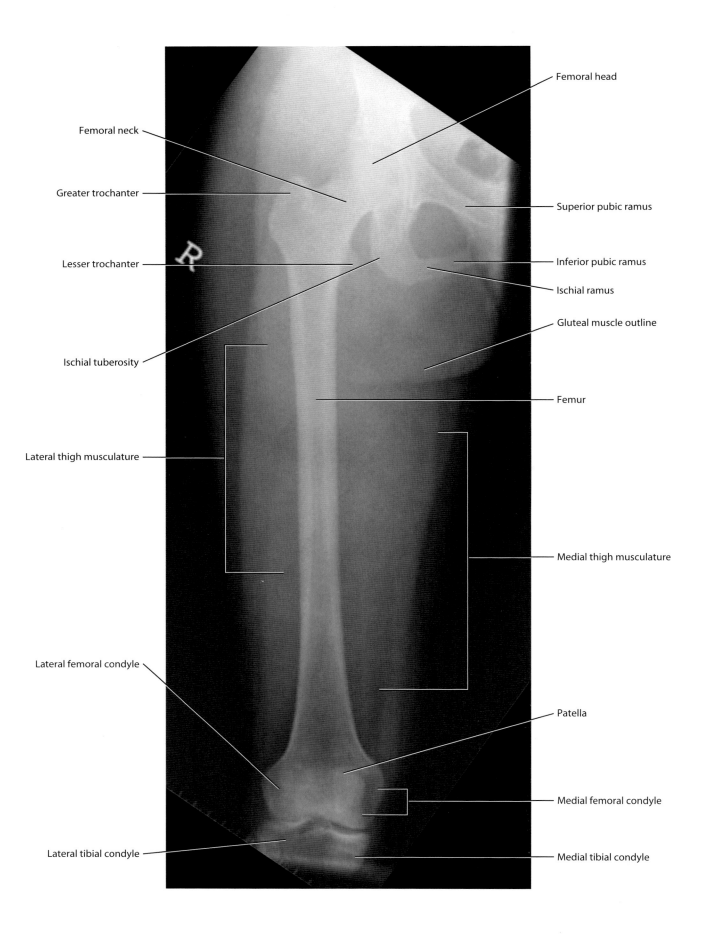

Femoral neck

Greater trochanter

Lesser trochanter

Ischial tuberosity

Lateral thigh musculature

Lateral femoral condyle

Lateral tibial condyle

Femoral head

Superior pubic ramus

Inferior pubic ramus

Ischial ramus

Gluteal muscle outline

Femur

Medial thigh musculature

Patella

Medial femoral condyle

Medial tibial condyle

Figure 40.12 Anteromedial thigh – plain film radiograph (anteroposterior view). Radiographs of the long bones should include superior and inferior joints, as does this one. An orthogonal (lateral) view is also required for full evaluation. Observe the position of the femur as it relates to the soft tissues of the gluteal region and thigh

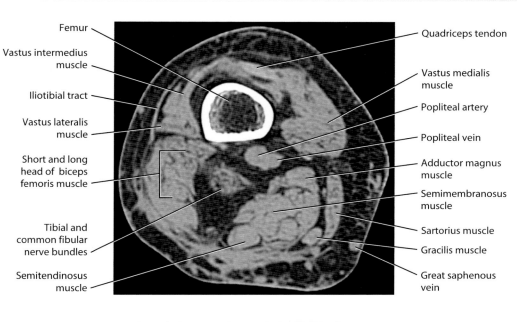

Femur

Vastus intermedius muscle

Iliotibial tract

Vastus lateralis muscle

Short and long head of biceps femoris muscle

Tibial and common fibular nerve bundles

Semitendinosus muscle

Quadriceps tendon

Vastus medialis muscle

Popliteal artery

Popliteal vein

Adductor magnus muscle

Semimembranosus muscle

Sartorius muscle

Gracilis muscle

Great saphenous vein

Figure 40.13 Anteromedial thigh – CT scan (axial view, from distal to proximal). In this scan of the lower thigh, muscles are well delineated by the fat that surrounds them. Observe the location of the sartorius muscle which indicates the level at which this scan was taken

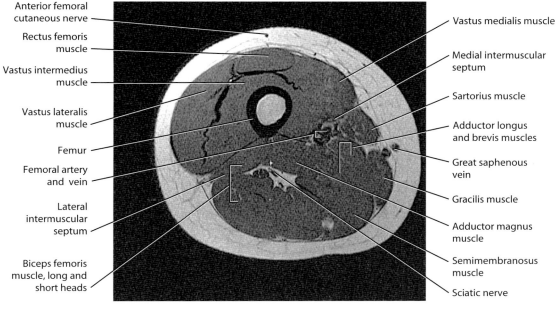

Anterior femoral cutaneous nerve

Rectus femoris muscle

Vastus intermedius muscle

Vastus lateralis muscle

Femur

Femoral artery and vein

Lateral intermuscular septum

Biceps femoris muscle, long and short heads

Vastus medialis muscle

Medial intermuscular septum

Sartorius muscle

Adductor longus and brevis muscles

Great saphenous vein

Gracilis muscle

Adductor magnus muscle

Semimembranosus muscle

Sciatic nerve

Figure 40.14 Anteromedial thigh – MRI scan (axial view, from distal to proximal). In this scan of the mid thigh, note the excellent muscle delineation due to the clear visualization of the medial and lateral intermuscular septa. Vessels and nerves are also better visualized on MRI than on CT scans. There is clear separation between the muscles of the anterior (quadriceps) and posterior (hamstrings) compartments of the thigh

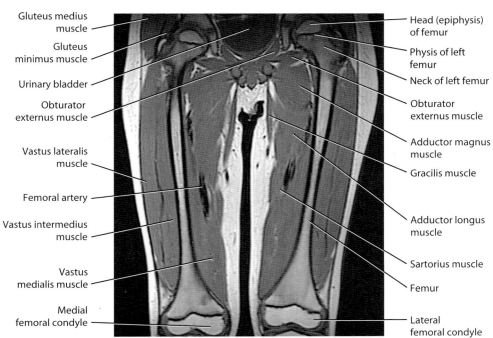

Gluteus medius muscle

Gluteus minimus muscle

Urinary bladder

Obturator externus muscle

Vastus lateralis muscle

Femoral artery

Vastus intermedius muscle

Vastus medialis muscle

Medial femoral condyle

Head (epiphysis) of femur

Physis of left femur

Neck of left femur

Obturator externus muscle

Adductor magnus muscle

Gracilis muscle

Adductor longus muscle

Sartorius muscle

Femur

Lateral femoral condyle

Figure 40.15 Anteromedial thigh – MRI scan (coronal view). The muscle bundles and vessels are well visualized. Note the locations of the adductor longus and adductor magnus muscles

LOWER LIMB Anteromedial thigh

499

The hip joint is the ball-and-socket synovial joint that connects the lower limb to the pelvis (Fig. 41.1). It is formed by the **head** of the femur and the **acetabular fossa** of the hip bone, and is a multiaxial joint that allows multiple movements (flexion, extension, abduction, adduction, lateral and medial rotation, and circumduction). The hip joint is supported by the muscles and ligaments in the hip area (Table 41.1).

The **acetabulum** is a cup-shaped fossa on the lateral pelvis. Parts of the ilium, ischium, and pubis bones contribute to it. The **acetabular labrum** is a fibrocartilage lip that attaches to the edges of the acetabulum to make the fossa deeper. This provides a deeper socket for the head of the femur and helps prevent easy dislocation of the hip. The anterior rim of the acetabular labrum is partly deficient at the **acetabular notch** and is bridged by the **transverse acetabular ligament**.

The femoral head has a central depression (**fovea for ligament of head**) for the attachment of the vascular intracapsular **ligament of head of femur**. The artery to the head of the femur and accompanying veins and nerves run with the intracapsular ligament and nourish and innervate the head of the femur.

Surrounding the hip joint is a very strong joint capsule. It completely encloses the hip joint, but is thin anteriorly at the location of the tendon of the iliopsoas muscle. Proximally, the joint capsule is attached to the acetabular labrum and the edge of the acetabular notch. Distally, it is attached to the femur along the intertrochanteric line and to the neck of femur approximately 1 cm superior to the intertrochanteric crest.

The fibrous joint capsule is reinforced anteriorly by the strong Y-shaped **iliofemoral ligament**, which joins the anterior superior iliac spine and acetabular margin of the pelvis proximally to the intertrochanteric line of the femur distally. The iliofemoral ligament tightens when standing and contributes to maintenance of posture and limitation of joint hyperextension.

The **pubofemoral ligament** is on the inferior and anterior surfaces of the joint. It originates from the inferior half of the acetabular margin and inserts laterally onto the inferior fibers of the iliofemoral ligament. The pubofemoral ligament tightens during extension and abduction, thus preventing overabduction of the joint.

The **ischiofemoral ligament**, the thinnest of the three hip joint ligaments, is on the posterior surface of the joint capsule (Fig. 41.2). It originates on the inferior part of the acetabulum and inserts laterally onto the superior surface of the neck of femur just medial to the greater trochanter. The ischiofemoral ligament helps prevent hyperextension of the hip joint.

MUSCLES

The muscles of the hip and thigh traverse the hip joint and provide support. From the anterior side, the anteromedial thigh muscles pass from the pelvis to the femur and move and support the joint (see Chapter 40). Posteriorly, the hip joint is supported by the muscles of the gluteal region and posterior thigh (see Chapter 42).

NERVES

Innervation to the hip joint is from small branches of the nerves that pass nearby. The **femoral nerve** (L2 to L4) innervates the hip joint as it passes over it anteriorly (see Figs 40.1 and 40.3). The posterior side of the hip joint is innervated by the **nerve to the quadratus femoris** (L4 to S1) as it crosses to innervate the quadratus femoris and inferior gemellus muscles. As the **sciatic**

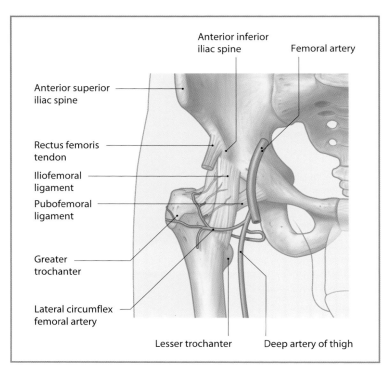

Figure 41.1 Hip joint (anterior view)

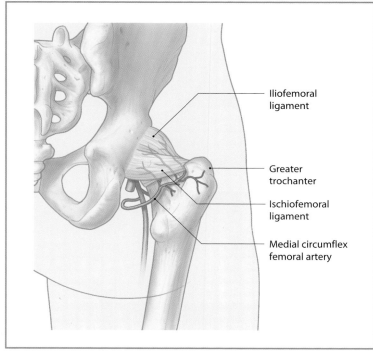

Figure 41.2 Main ligaments of the hip joint (posterior view)

nerve descends through the gluteal region and posterior thigh it sends out small articular branches to supply the hip joint (see Fig. 39.2). The anterior division of the **obturator nerve** and **superior gluteal nerve** also provide innervation to the hip joint.

ARTERIES

Blood is supplied to the hip joint by the rich anastomoses of arteries that surround it. Anteriorly, branches of the **deep artery of**

thigh bring blood to the area, and posteriorly, the **inferior gluteal artery** and the **medial** and **lateral circumflex femoral arteries** form a branching array of vessels to the area (Figs 41.1 and 41.2). The deep branch of the **superior gluteal artery** and the posterior branch of the **obturator artery** also contribute to these anastomoses.

The artery of the ligament of head of femur (a branch of the obturator artery) is a small artery that runs from the acetabulum of the pelvis along the intracapsular ligament of the head. It enters the fovea for the ligament of head of femur to supply the femoral head. This artery is important in children because it is a major source of blood for growth and development of the head of femur.

VEINS AND LYMPHATICS

Venous drainage of the hip joint follows the arterial blood supply. Anteriorly, blood flows to the **femoral vein** (see Figs 40.1 and 40.3). Posteriorly, the series of veins that follows the branching of the inferior gluteal artery and medial circumflex femoral artery drains blood toward the **internal iliac vein**.

Lymphatic vessels follow the veins so lymph from the anterior hip joint drains to the **inguinal nodes** and lymph from the posterior hip joint drains to the **internal iliac nodes**.

■ CLINICAL CORRELATIONS

Hip dislocation

Dislocation of the hip joint (Fig. 41.3) occurs when the head of femur leaves the acetabulum. This injury requires a great amount of force because the hip joint is supported by some of the largest muscles and ligaments in the body. Motor vehicle accidents, pedestrians struck by a vehicle, and other similar accidents are the most common causes.

Most hip dislocations are posterior and they most frequently occur in motor vehicle accidents. As the vehicle crashes, the seated occupant's knees strike the dashboard, causing a tremendous posterior stress on the femur that results in dislocation and/or fracture. Patients complain of extreme pain and cannot walk.

On examination, the injured limb is flexed, adducted, internally rotated, and shortened. There may be a vascular deficit manifest by decreased or absent femoral or dorsalis pedis pulses. The sciatic and femoral nerves should be tested carefully for injury.

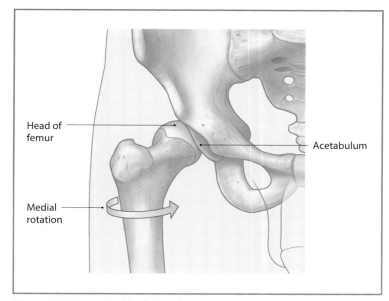

Figure 41.3 Posterior hip dislocation

Dislocation of the hip joint is diagnosed by physical examination and plain radiographs. The deformity is usually obvious on anteroposterior and lateral views of the pelvis.

Hip dislocation is an orthopedic emergency. Reduction should be carried out immediately to restore blood flow and neural stability. Prolongation of reduction, or delay in returning the femoral head to its socket, increases the risk of avascular necrosis of the head of femur, joint instability, arthritis, and chronic pain. Treatment is carried out by a clinician with specialized training who administers pain and sedative medications and then performs maneuvers to reduce the dislocation. Because of the tremendous energy required to cause a hip dislocation, careful clinical examination of the entire patient is warranted because most patients with hip dislocation have other serious injuries. Many patients with hip dislocation also have a fracture of the femur. A fracture–dislocation of the hip joint presents a challenge: patients require emergency treatment that should be carried out only by closed reduction under general anesthesia or open reduction (surgery) in the operating room by an orthopedic surgeon.

TABLE 41.1 LIGAMENTS OF THE HIP JOINT			
Ligament	Attachment	Movement limited	Comments
Joint capsule	Superiorly, attached to bony rim of acetabulum; inferiorly, in front attached to intertrochanteric line, in back just short of intertrochanteric crest	Containment of synovial fluid within joint space	Very strong, being thicker anteriorly; strengthened by: • reflected head of rectus femoris • gluteus minimus
Iliofemoral	Anterior inferior iliac spine and acetabular margin proximally to the intertrochanteric line distally	Prevents overextension when standing; (superior fibers limit adduction, inferior fibers limit abduction)	Strong, Y-shaped anterior ligament
Pubofemoral	Pubic part of acetabular margin of anterior intertrochanteric fossa	Tightens during extension and abduction, prevents overabduction	Reinforces joint capsule inferiorly and anteriorly
Ischiofemoral	Ischial part of acetabular margin to medial base of greater trochanter	Tightens during extension; spiral arrangement prevents hyperextension	Reinforces joint capsule posteriorly; shows a superolateral spiral with poor definition
Ligament of head of femur	Margins of the acetabular notch to fovea of head of femur	Tightens in adduction of the femur	Intracapsular but extrasynovial
Transverse acetabular	Connects the inferior ends of the acetabular labrum	Creates a foramen with the notch	Articular vessels and nerves enter the fossa under its deep border

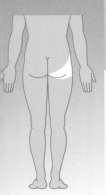

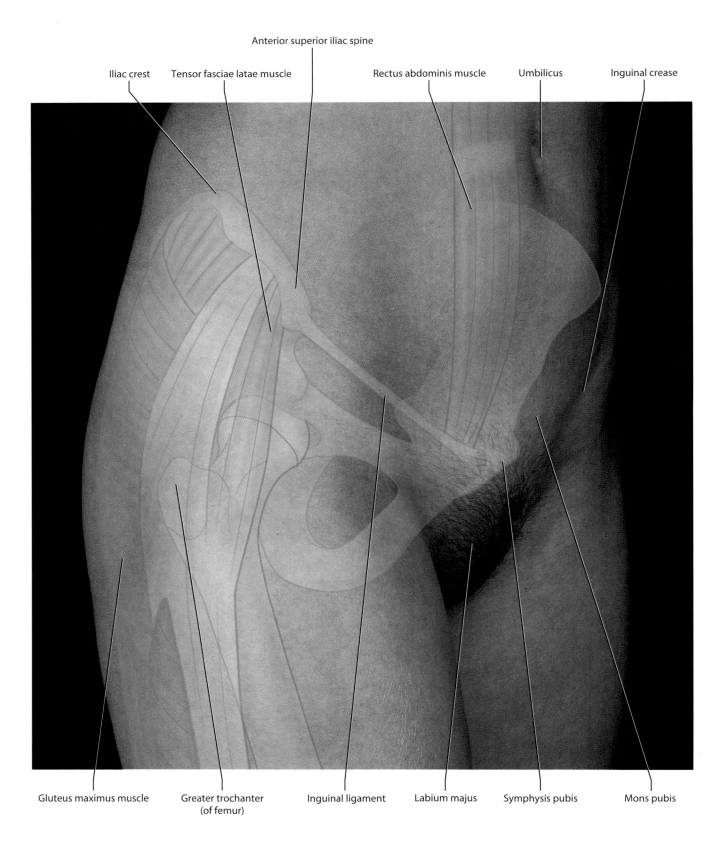

Anterior superior iliac spine

Iliac crest   Tensor fasciae latae muscle   Rectus abdominis muscle   Umbilicus   Inguinal crease

Gluteus maximus muscle   Greater trochanter   Inguinal ligament   Labium majus   Symphysis pubis   Mons pubis
(of femur)

Figure 41.4 Hip joint – surface anatomy 1. Anterolateral view of the right hip joint region. Observe the major surface landmarks for this region – the iliac crest and greater trochanter of the femur. The small 'dent' on the lateral buttock is immediately posterior to the greater trochanter of the femur

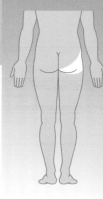

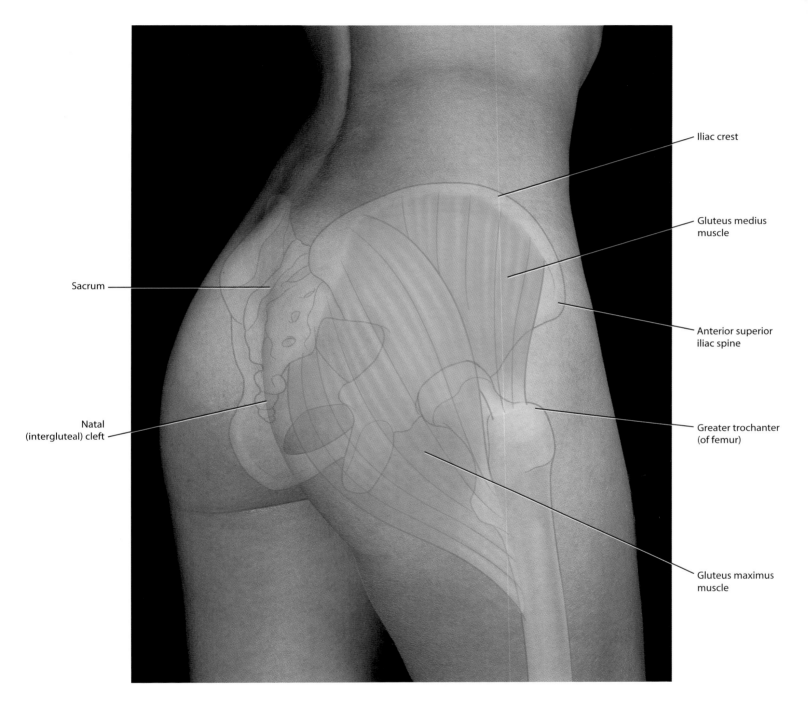

Iliac crest

Gluteus medius
muscle

Sacrum

Anterior superior
iliac spine

Natal
(intergluteal) cleft

Greater trochanter
(of femur)

Gluteus maximus
muscle

Figure 41.5 Hip joint – surface anatomy 2. Posterolateral view of the right hip. Observe the prominence of the greater trochanter of the femur

503

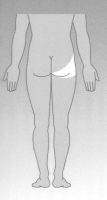

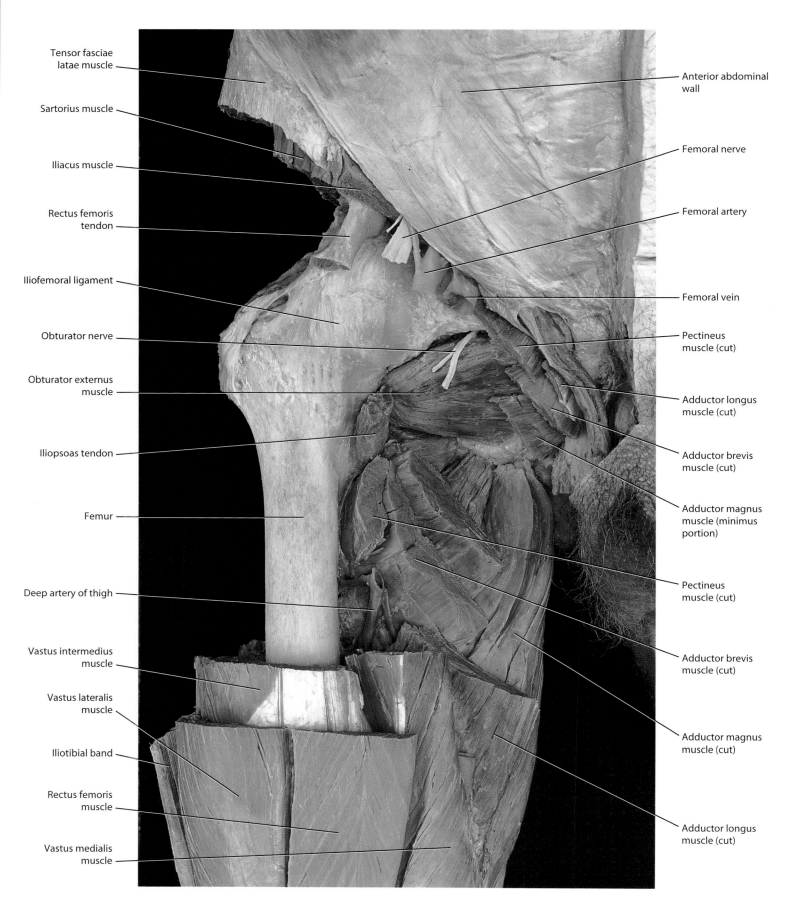

Tensor fasciae latae muscle

Sartorius muscle

Iliacus muscle

Rectus femoris tendon

Iliofemoral ligament

Obturator nerve

Obturator externus muscle

Iliopsoas tendon

Femur

Deep artery of thigh

Vastus intermedius muscle

Vastus lateralis muscle

Iliotibial band

Rectus femoris muscle

Vastus medialis muscle

Anterior abdominal wall

Femoral nerve

Femoral artery

Femoral vein

Pectineus muscle (cut)

Adductor longus muscle (cut)

Adductor brevis muscle (cut)

Adductor magnus muscle (minimus portion)

Pectineus muscle (cut)

Adductor brevis muscle (cut)

Adductor magnus muscle (cut)

Adductor longus muscle (cut)

Figure 41.6 Hip joint – deep dissection 1. Unique dissection of the right hip from an anterior viewpoint to expose the anterior wall of the joint capsule and its reinforcement by the iliofemoral ligament, and the muscles inferior and medial to the joint

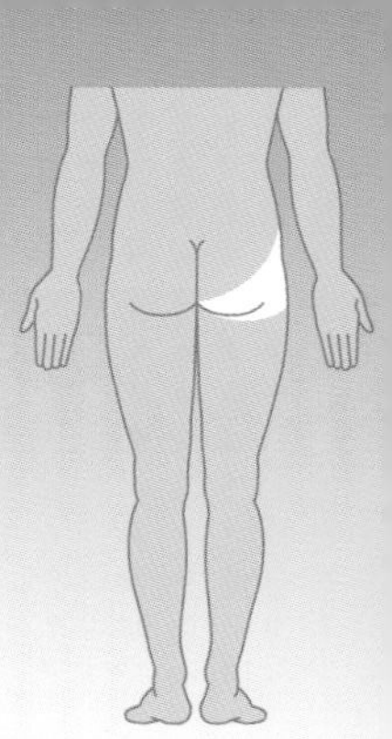

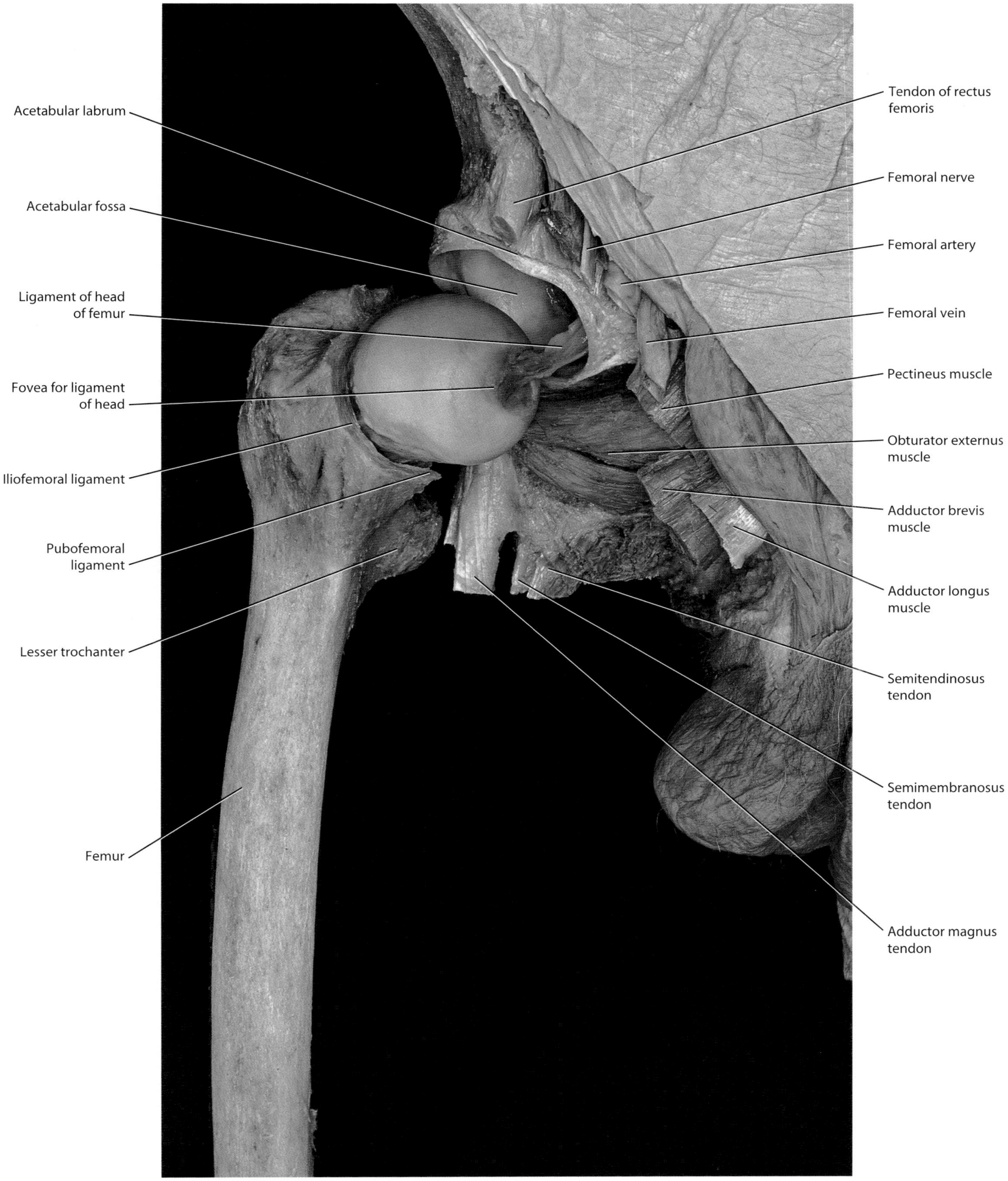

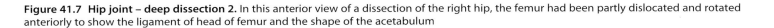

Acetabular labrum

Acetabular fossa

Ligament of head of femur

Fovea for ligament of head

Iliofemoral ligament

Pubofemoral ligament

Lesser trochanter

Femur

Tendon of rectus femoris

Femoral nerve

Femoral artery

Femoral vein

Pectineus muscle

Obturator externus muscle

Adductor brevis muscle

Adductor longus muscle

Semitendinosus tendon

Semimembranosus tendon

Adductor magnus tendon

Figure 41.7 Hip joint – deep dissection 2. In this anterior view of a dissection of the right hip, the femur had been partly dislocated and rotated anteriorly to show the ligament of head of femur and the shape of the acetabulum

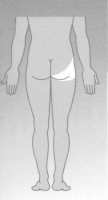

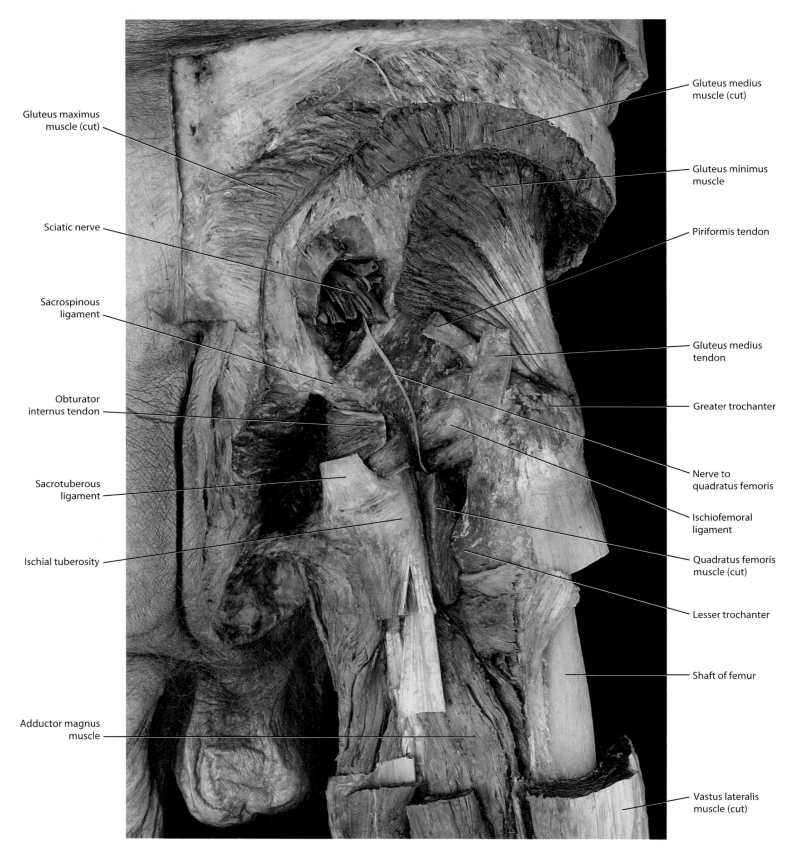

Gluteus maximus
muscle (cut)

Sciatic nerve

Sacrospinous
ligament

Obturator
internus tendon

Sacrotuberous
ligament

Ischial tuberosity

Adductor magnus
muscle

Gluteus medius
muscle (cut)

Gluteus minimus
muscle

Piriformis tendon

Gluteus medius
tendon

Greater trochanter

Nerve to
quadratus femoris

Ischiofemoral
ligament

Quadratus femoris
muscle (cut)

Lesser trochanter

Shaft of femur

Vastus lateralis
muscle (cut)

Figure 41.8 Hip joint – deep dissection 3. Posterior view of the dissected right hip of an elderly man. Many of the overlying muscles have been removed to show the joint. Observe the gluteus minimus muscle attachment onto the lateral femur. The vastus lateralis muscle, which almost appears to be the same color as the femur, has been cut to show the shaft of femur. The sciatic nerve, also cut, is visible in the superior part of the dissection entering the gluteal region from the pelvis

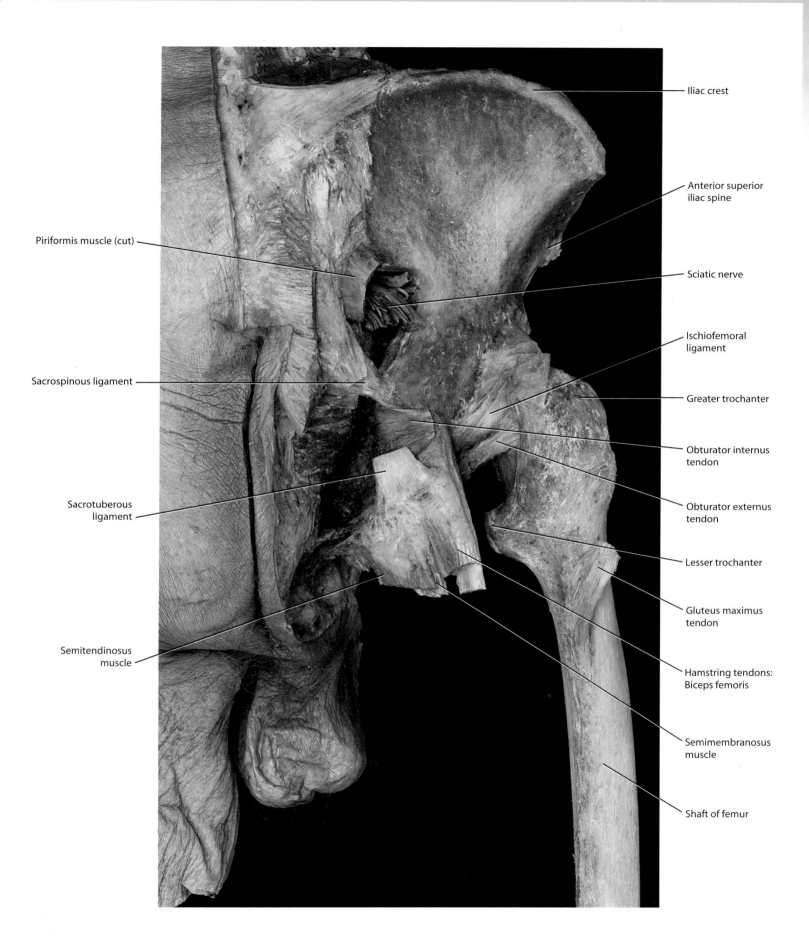

Iliac crest

Anterior superior
iliac spine

Sciatic nerve

Ischiofemoral
ligament

Greater trochanter

Obturator internus
tendon

Obturator externus
tendon

Lesser trochanter

Gluteus maximus
tendon

Hamstring tendons:
Biceps femoris

Semimembranosus
muscle

Shaft of femur

Piriformis muscle (cut)

Sacrospinous ligament

Sacrotuberous
ligament

Semitendinosus
muscle

LOWER LIMB   Hip joint

Figure 41.9 Hip joint – deep dissection 4. Posterior view of the dissected right hip of an elderly man. Many of the overlying muscles have been removed. Observe the ischiofemoral ligament superior to the obturator externus tendon

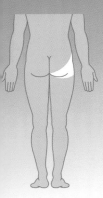

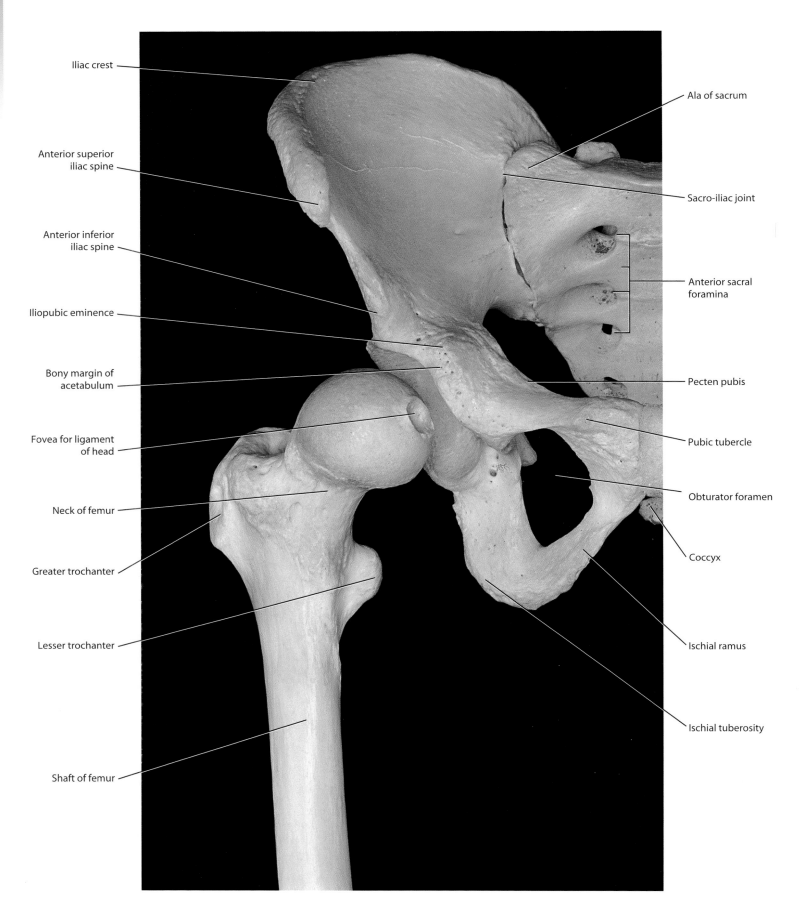

Iliac crest

Anterior superior
iliac spine

Anterior inferior
iliac spine

Iliopubic eminence

Bony margin of
acetabulum

Fovea for ligament
of head

Neck of femur

Greater trochanter

Lesser trochanter

Shaft of femur

Ala of sacrum

Sacro-iliac joint

Anterior sacral
foramina

Pecten pubis

Pubic tubercle

Obturator foramen

Coccyx

Ischial ramus

Ischial tuberosity

Figure 41.10 Hip joint – osteology 1. Anterior view of the right hip joint. The femur has been partly dislocated and rotated laterally so that the fovea for the ligament of head of femur is visible

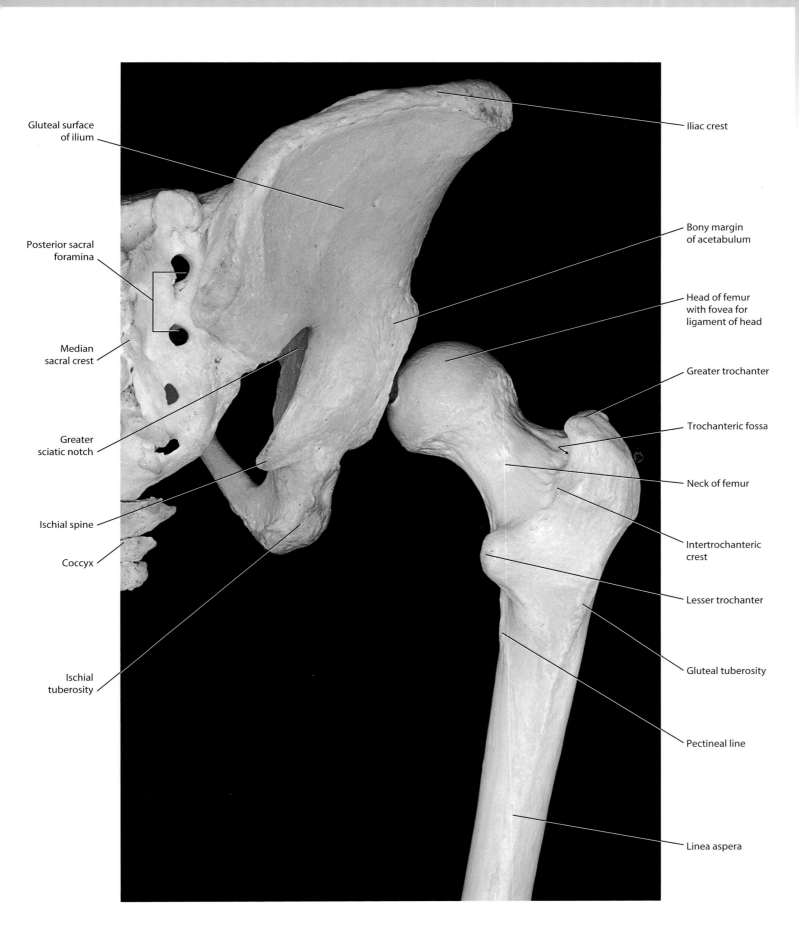

Gluteal surface of ilium

Posterior sacral foramina

Median sacral crest

Greater sciatic notch

Ischial spine

Coccyx

Ischial tuberosity

Iliac crest

Bony margin of acetabulum

Head of femur with fovea for ligament of head

Greater trochanter

Trochanteric fossa

Neck of femur

Intertrochanteric crest

Lesser trochanter

Gluteal tuberosity

Pectineal line

Linea aspera

Figure 41.11 Hip joint – osteology 2. Posterior view of the right hip joint. The femur has been partly dislocated so that its posterior surface can be completely visualized

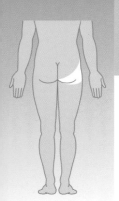

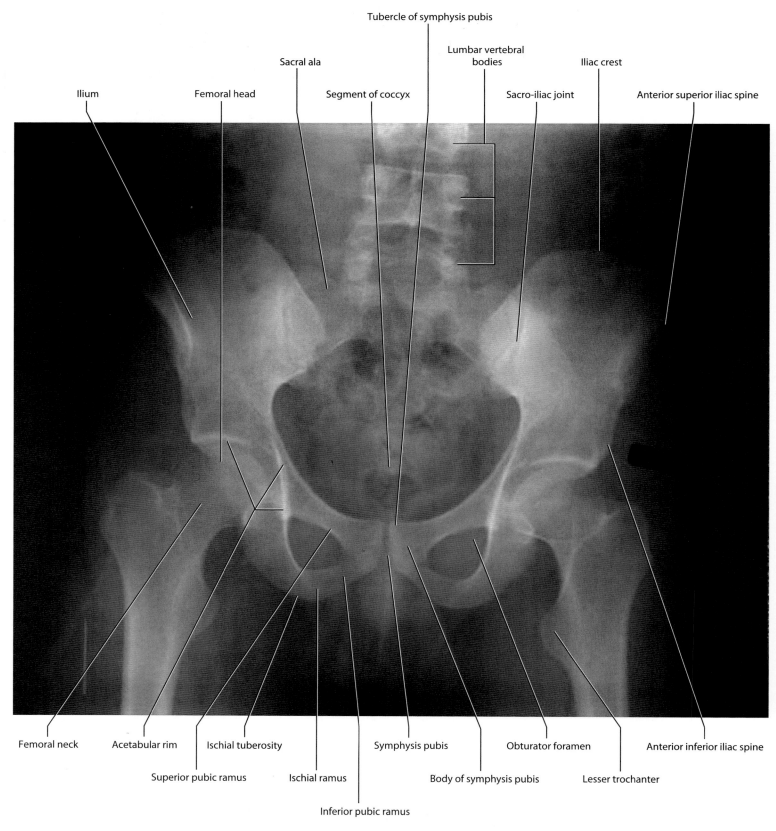

Tubercle of symphysis pubis

Lumbar vertebral bodies

Sacral ala

Iliac crest

Segment of coccyx

Sacro-iliac joint

Ilium

Femoral head

Anterior superior iliac spine

Femoral neck

Acetabular rim

Ischial tuberosity

Symphysis pubis

Obturator foramen

Anterior inferior iliac spine

Superior pubic ramus

Ischial ramus

Body of symphysis pubis

Lesser trochanter

Inferior pubic ramus

Figure 41.12 Hip joint – plain film radiograph (anteroposterior view). The head of the femur is seen articulating with the acetabulum of the pelvis in this normal radiograph. A thorough anteroposterior clinical evaluation of the hips should show the lower lumbar spine and proximal femora. In addition, when evaluating a joint for injury it is helpful to have a corresponding radiograph of the opposite joint for comparison

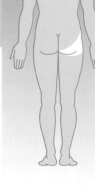

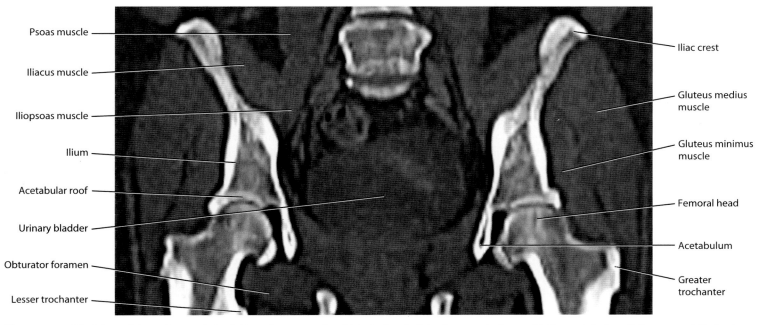

Psoas muscle

Iliacus muscle

Iliopsoas muscle

Ilium

Acetabular roof

Urinary bladder

Obturator foramen

Lesser trochanter

Iliac crest

Gluteus medius muscle

Gluteus minimus muscle

Femoral head

Acetabulum

Greater trochanter

Figure 41.13 Hip joint – CT scan (coronal view). Note the manner in which the head of the femur articulates with the acetabulum. If there are subtle fractures of the acetabulum or neck of femur, a coronal CT scan will demonstrate this

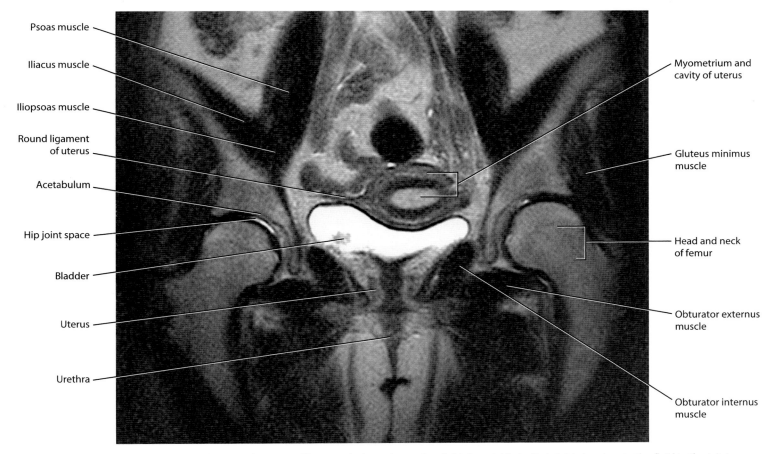

Psoas muscle

Iliacus muscle

Iliopsoas muscle

Round ligament of uterus

Acetabulum

Hip joint space

Bladder

Uterus

Urethra

Myometrium and cavity of uterus

Gluteus minimus muscle

Head and neck of femur

Obturator externus muscle

Obturator internus muscle

Figure 41.14 Hip joint – MRI scan (coronal view). This scan utilizes a technique that makes fluid detectable by its bright signal: note the fluid in the joint space of the right hip. A large amount of fluid in the joint space is abnormal and may be an indicator of injury or infection

Gluteal region and posterior thigh

The gluteal region (buttock) extends from the upper border of the posterior iliac crest to the inferior border of the gluteus maximus muscle. The posterior thigh extends from the inferior edge of the gluteus maximus muscle down to the upper border of the popliteal fossa. Support for the gluteal region and posterior thigh is from the pelvic girdle and femur. These bones provide attachment for the muscles and ligaments of the region. Enclosing the tissues of the gluteal region and posterior thigh are the **gluteal aponeurosis** and **fascia lata**. These are heavy, thickened fasciae that form an enveloping sleeve over the muscles of the gluteal region and thigh.

The parts of the pelvic girdle (hip bones, sacrum, and coccyx) are bound together by dense ligaments. The sacrotuberous and sacrospinous ligaments convert the sciatic notches of the hip bones into greater and lesser sciatic foramina (see Chapter 36).

MUSCLES

The muscles of the gluteal region (Fig. 42.1) include three large gluteal muscles and the deeper group of smaller muscles. The **gluteus maximus** is a large fan-like muscle and a strong extensor of the thigh that acts during jumping or running. The **gluteus medius** and **gluteus muscles minimus** stabilize the pelvis during standing or

walking. Overall, these muscles extend and abduct the thigh at the hip joint.

The deeper group (Fig. 42.2) of five muscles (from superior to inferior) comprises **piriformis, gemellus superior, obturator internus, gemellus inferior,** and **quadratus femoris.** These muscles originate from the lateral pelvis and insert onto the greater trochanter of the femur. As a group, the deep muscles externally rotate the thigh at the hip joint (Table 42.1).

The posterior thigh has three (hamstring) muscles that originate from the ischial tuberosity of the pelvis and insert onto the proximal tibia or fibula. These muscles, which are the **semitendinosus, semimembranosus,** and **biceps femoris,** span the hip and knee joints and are therefore two-joint muscles, extend the thigh and flex the leg (Table 42.2).

NERVES

The skin of the gluteal region is innervated by the **superior, medial,** and **inferior clunial nerves.** The superior clunial (L1 to L3) and medial clunial (S1 to S3) nerves (constituents of the lumbosacral plexus of nerves; see Chapters 32 and 36) exit the pelvis through the posterior sacral foramina to enter the gluteal region.

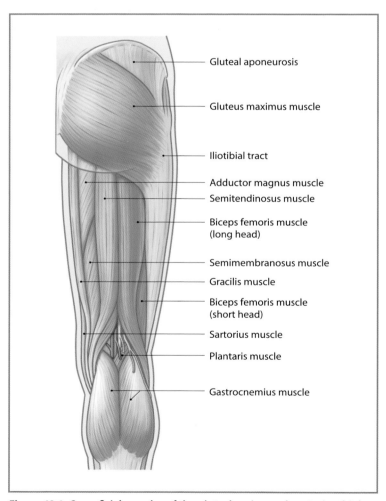

Figure 42.1 Superficial muscles of the gluteal region and posterior thigh

Labels:
- Gluteal aponeurosis
- Gluteus maximus muscle
- Iliotibial tract
- Adductor magnus muscle
- Semitendinosus muscle
- Biceps femoris muscle (long head)
- Semimembranosus muscle
- Gracilis muscle
- Biceps femoris muscle (short head)
- Sartorius muscle
- Plantaris muscle
- Gastrocnemius muscle

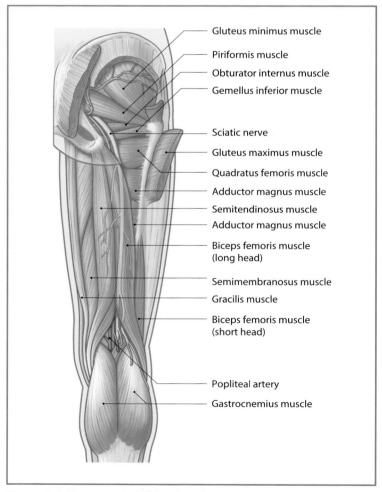

Figure 42.2 Deep muscles of the gluteal region and posterior thigh

Labels:
- Gluteus minimus muscle
- Piriformis muscle
- Obturator internus muscle
- Gemellus inferior muscle
- Sciatic nerve
- Gluteus maximus muscle
- Quadratus femoris muscle
- Adductor magnus muscle
- Semitendinosus muscle
- Adductor magnus muscle
- Biceps femoris muscle (long head)
- Semimembranosus muscle
- Gracilis muscle
- Biceps femoris muscle (short head)
- Popliteal artery
- Gastrocnemius muscle

The inferior clunial nerves are branches of the posterior cutaneous nerve of thigh and curve around the inferior border of gluteus maximus to innervate the skin of this region. The skin over the posterior aspect of the thigh and calf is supplied by the **posterior cutaneous nerve of thigh** (S1 to S3), which leaves the pelvis through the greater sciatic foramen inferior to the piriformis muscle. From here, it descends within the gluteal region and emerges onto the posterior thigh at the inferior border of the gluteus maximus muscle. The posterior cutaneous nerve of thigh is the largest single cutaneous nerve of the body.

The muscles of the gluteal region and posterior thigh are innervated by branches of the sacral plexus of nerves. The gluteal muscles are innervated by the **superior** (L4 to S1) and **inferior** (L5 to S2) **gluteal nerves**, which originate in the pelvis and pass through the greater sciatic foramen, to enter the gluteal region. These nerves can be identified in the gluteal region along the superior and inferior borders of the piriformis muscle.

The five deeper muscles of the gluteal region (see above) are innervated by three other branches of the sacral plexus: the **nerve to piriformis** (S1, S2), **nerve to obturator internus** (L5 to S2), and **nerve to quadratus femoris** (L4 to S1).

The **sciatic nerve** is the largest nerve in the body. It is also a constituent of the sacral plexus of nerves and exits the pelvis through the greater sciatic foramen. In the gluteal region the sciatic nerve emerges inferior to the piriformis muscle to descend in the thigh and innervate the posterior thigh muscles, the hip and knee joints, and part of the skin of the anal region. It terminates midway down the posterior thigh by splitting into the **tibial nerve** medially and the **common fibular nerve** laterally.

ARTERIES

The blood supply to the gluteal region is from branches of the **internal iliac artery** within the pelvis. The largest branch is the **superior gluteal artery**, which enters the gluteal region from the pelvis along the superior border of the piriformis muscle. Here the superior gluteal artery divides into a **superficial branch**, which supplies the gluteus maximus muscle, and a **deep branch**, which runs between the gluteus medius and minimus muscles, supplying them and the tensor fasciae latae muscle (see Chapter 40).

The **inferior gluteal artery**, which is also a branch of the internal iliac artery, enters the gluteal region from the pelvis but is inferior to the piriformis muscle. It supplies gluteus maximus, obturator internus, quadratus femoris, and the superior parts of the posterior thigh muscles (hamstrings).

The **internal pudendal artery**, a branch of the internal iliac artery, enters the gluteal region from the pelvis with the pudendal nerve, then turns back and re-enters the pelvis through the lesser sciatic foramen to supply the external genitalia and pelvic muscles.

The **deep artery of thigh**, which is the largest branch of the femoral artery, originates in the upper thigh and descends through the anterior thigh, branching to form three major perforating muscular branches to the posterior thigh muscles. It ends in the inferior third of the thigh as the fourth perforating artery, which pierces and supplies the adductor magnus and lower parts of the hamstring muscles.

VEINS

Venous drainage from the gluteal region is by the **superior** and **inferior gluteal veins**, which follow the course of the same arteries. These veins drain primarily to the pelvis, but also communicate with the femoral veins, so providing an alternative route of venous drainage from the lower limb. The **internal pudendal veins**, next to the internal pudendal arteries, drain blood from the external genitalia and empty into the **internal iliac veins**.

Venous drainage from the large veins of the posterior thigh follows the course of the **deep artery of thigh** and empties into the **femoral vein**.

Deep lymphatic drainage of the gluteal region follows the vessels named above and empties into the **iliac lymph nodes**. Superficial lymphatic drainage follows the superficial unnamed vessels of the skin and subcutaneous tissues to the **superficial inguinal nodes**, which then drain to the **iliac lymph nodes**.

■ CLINICAL CORRELATIONS
Fracture of neck of femur

The neck of the femur is strong if bone density is normal, and usually only major trauma will cause fracture. People with decreased bone density (e.g. osteoporosis) are at risk of fracture after mild trauma, such as a ground-level fall (falling to the ground from a standing position). A patient with a fracture of neck of femur is most commonly an elderly patient with osteoporosis who sustains a ground-level fall while carrying out a nonstrenuous activity (e.g. standing, walking).

On examination, the injured limb is shortened, abducted, and externally rotated (opposite of posterior femoral dislocation, see Chapter 41). There is usually pain and inability to walk, and sometimes weakness. The distal pulses are examined carefully and neural testing is carried out on the distal injured limb to check for any neurovascular injury. Anteroposterior and lateral radiographs usually show the deformity. The fractured limb should be kept immobile because movement can worsen vascular and neural damage. Urgent consultation with an orthopedic surgeon is needed because these injuries are commonly treated surgically.

Fracture of the shaft of femur

Fracture of the shaft of femur is usually caused by a high-velocity injury, such as a motor vehicle accident. Patients with a femoral shaft fracture cannot walk and complain of deformity to their injured thigh and extreme pain.

On examination, the injured limb is unstable and can rotate to either side (left or right) without concomitant movement of the hip joint. Plain radiographs of the femur reveal the fracture, which is described – according to its appearance – as transverse, spiral, comminuted (broken into many pieces), and/or open (with skin laceration by the fractured bone). Shock and hemorrhage into the thigh from injured blood vessels or muscular damage and resultant bleeding can be significant because the thigh can hold a large proportion of the total blood volume. It is therefore important to administer intravenous fluids and/or blood to maintain blood pressure and blood volume. Stabilization of the fracture is usually surgical and is carried out by placement of an intramedullary rod (i.e. specialized titanium or other rod placed within the shaft of the fractured bone and screwed in place) by an orthopedic surgeon.

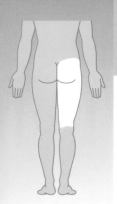

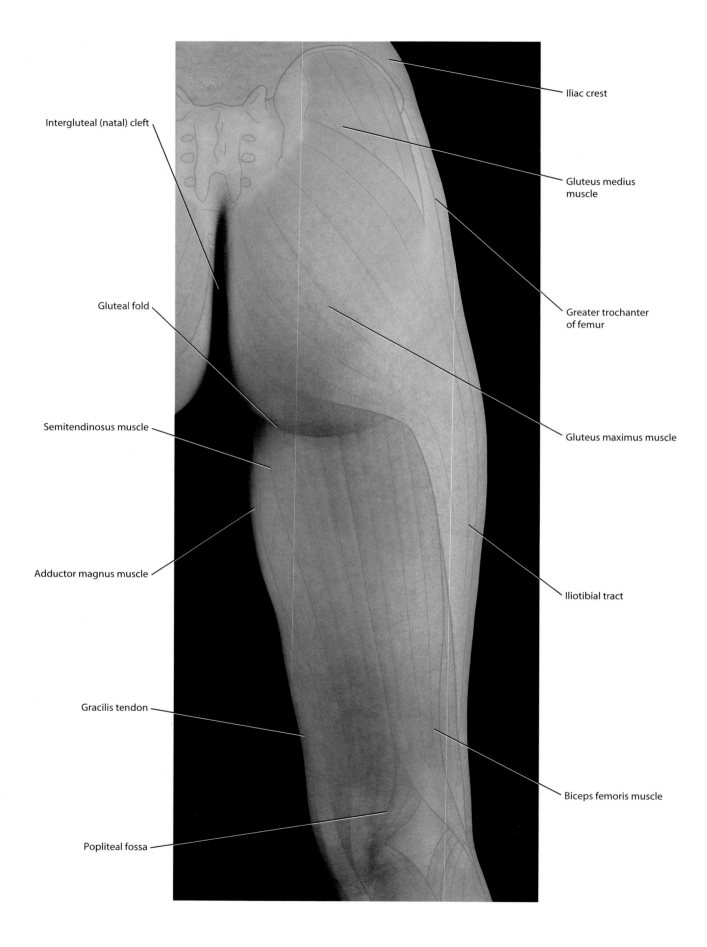

Intergluteal (natal) cleft

Gluteal fold

Semitendinosus muscle

Adductor magnus muscle

Gracilis tendon

Popliteal fossa

Iliac crest

Gluteus medius muscle

Greater trochanter of femur

Gluteus maximus muscle

Iliotibial tract

Biceps femoris muscle

Figure 42.3 Gluteal region and posterior thigh – surface anatomy. Posterior view of the left gluteal region and posterior thigh of a young woman. Observe the crease at the inferior part of the buttock. The midline separation between the buttocks is the intergluteal (natal) cleft

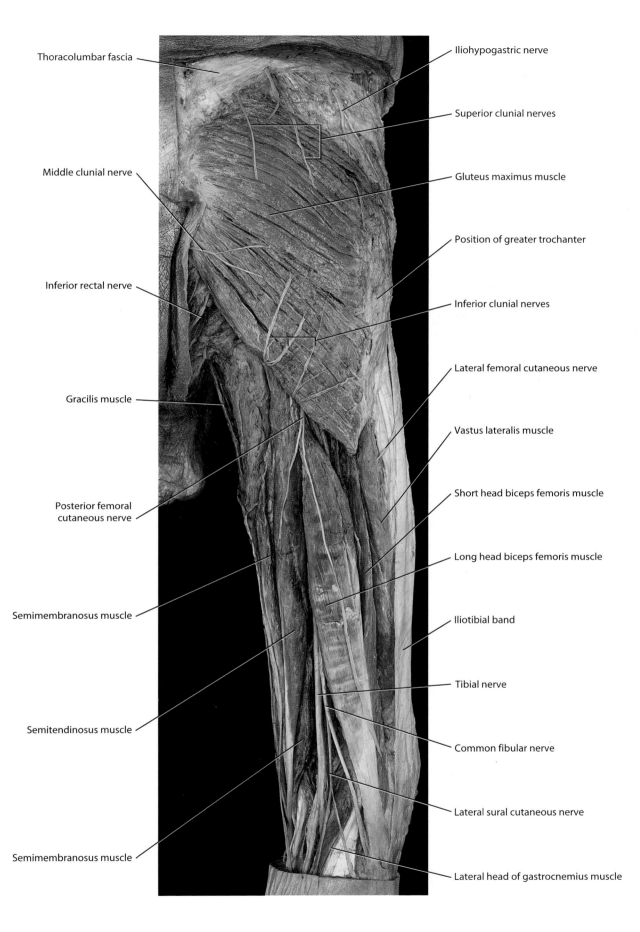

Thoracolumbar fascia

Middle clunial nerve

Inferior rectal nerve

Gracilis muscle

Posterior femoral cutaneous nerve

Semimembranosus muscle

Semitendinosus muscle

Semimembranosus muscle

Iliohypogastric nerve

Superior clunial nerves

Gluteus maximus muscle

Position of greater trochanter

Inferior clunial nerves

Lateral femoral cutaneous nerve

Vastus lateralis muscle

Short head biceps femoris muscle

Long head biceps femoris muscle

Iliotibial band

Tibial nerve

Common fibular nerve

Lateral sural cutaneous nerve

Lateral head of gastrocnemius muscle

LOWER LIMB Gluteal region and posterior thigh

Figure 42.4 Gluteal region and posterior thigh – superficial dissection 1. Posterior view of the right thigh. Observe the hamstring muscles (semitendinosus, semimembranosus, and biceps femoris), the position of the clunial nerves around the gluteus maximus muscle, and the posterior cutaneous nerve of thigh running down the biceps femoris muscle

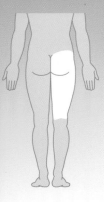

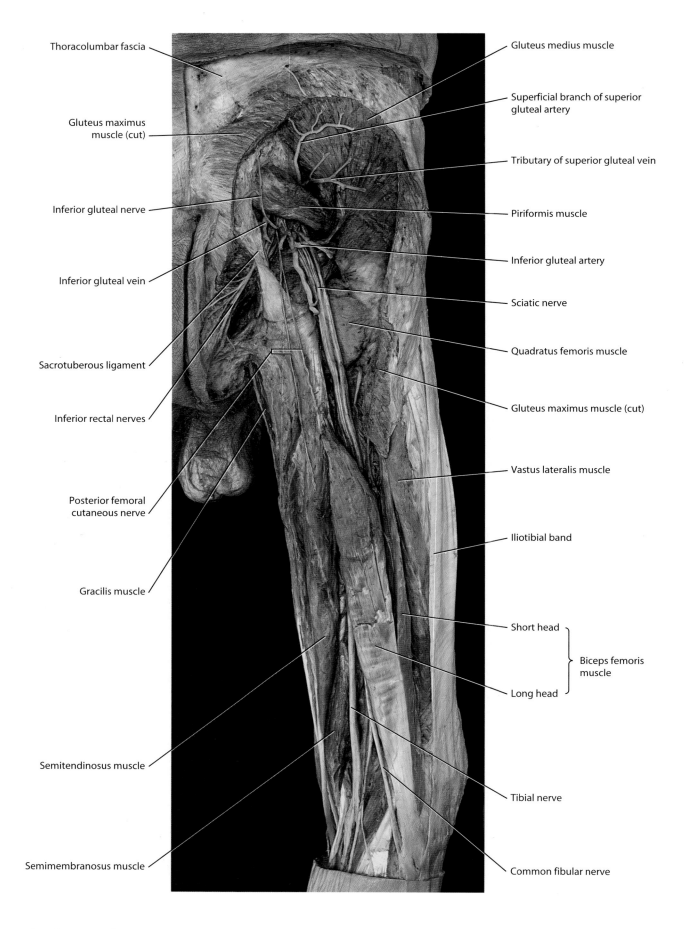

Thoracolumbar fascia

Gluteus maximus muscle (cut)

Inferior gluteal nerve

Inferior gluteal vein

Sacrotuberous ligament

Inferior rectal nerves

Posterior femoral cutaneous nerve

Gracilis muscle

Semitendinosus muscle

Semimembranosus muscle

Gluteus medius muscle

Superficial branch of superior gluteal artery

Tributary of superior gluteal vein

Piriformis muscle

Inferior gluteal artery

Sciatic nerve

Quadratus femoris muscle

Gluteus maximus muscle (cut)

Vastus lateralis muscle

Iliotibial band

Short head

Long head

Biceps femoris muscle

Tibial nerve

Common fibular nerve

Figure 42.5 Gluteal region and posterior thigh – intermediate dissection. Posterior view of the right thigh. The gluteus maximus muscle has been removed to show the gluteus medius and piriformis muscles, and the sacrotuberous ligament. Also note the superficial branch of the superior gluteal artery on the gluteus medius

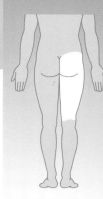

TABLE 42.1 MUSCLES OF THE GLUTEAL REGION

Muscle	Origin	Insertion	Innervation	Action	Blood supply
Gluteus maximus	Posterior gluteal line of ilium, dorsal sacrum, sacrotuberous ligament	Iliotibial tract of fascia lata, gluteal tuberosity of femur	Inferior gluteal nerve (L5 to S2)	Extends thigh, assists in adducting and lateral rotation	Superior and inferior gluteal arteries, first perforating branch of deep femoral artery
Gluteus medius	Lateral surface of ilium between anterior and posterior gluteal lines	Lateral surface of greater trochanter of femur	Superior gluteal nerve (L4 to S1)	Abducts thigh, rotates thigh medially	Deep branch of superior gluteal artery
Gluteus minimus	Lateral surface of ilium between anterior and inferior gluteal lines	Anterior border of greater trochanter of femur	Superior gluteal nerve (L4 to S1)	Abducts thigh, rotates thigh medially	Deep branch of superior gluteal artery
Piriformis	Anterior surface of sacrum and sacrotuberous ligament	Superior border of greater trochanter of femur	Anterior rami of S1 and S2	Laterally rotates thigh, abducts thigh when limb is flexed	Superior and inferior gluteal arteries, internal pudendal artery
Obturator internus	Pelvic surface of obturator membrane and margins of obturator foramen	Medial surface of greater trochanter of femur	Nerve to obturator internus (L5 to S2)	Laterally rotates thigh, abducts thigh when limb is flexed	Internal pudendal and superior gluteal arteries
Gemellus superior	Outer surface of ischial spine	Medial surface of greater trochanter of femur	Nerve to obturator internus (L5 to S2)	Laterally rotates thigh	Inferior gluteal artery
Gemellus inferior	Upper margin of ischial tuberosity	Medial surface of greater trochanter of femur	Nerve to quadratus femoris (L4 to S1)	Laterally rotates thigh	Inferior gluteal artery
Quadratus femoris	Lateral margin of ischial tuberosity	Quadrate tubercle on intertrochanteric crest of femur	Nerve to quadratus femoris (L4 to S1)	Laterally rotates thigh, adducts thigh	Medial circumflex femoral artery

TABLE 42.2 POSTERIOR THIGH MUSCLES

Muscle	Origin	Insertion	Innervation	Action	Blood supply
Semitendinosus	Upper and medial ischial tuberosity	Superior part of medial surface of tibia	Tibial division of sciatic nerve (L5 to S2)	Flexes leg, extends thigh	Perforating branch of deep artery of thigh, superior muscular branches of popliteal artery
Semimembranosus	Upper and lateral ischial tuberosity	Posterior part of medial condyle of tibia	Tibial division of sciatic nerve (L5 to S2)	Flexes leg, extends thigh	Perforating branch of deep artery of thigh, superior muscular branches of popliteal artery
Biceps femoris	Long head – ischial tuberosity Short head – lateral lip of linea aspera, lateral supracondylar line of femur	Head of fibula, lateral condyle of tibia	Long head – tibial division of sciatic nerve (L5 to S2) Short head – common fibular division of sciatic nerve (L5 to S2)	Flexes and laterally rotates leg, extends the thigh	Perforating branch of deep artery of thigh, superior muscular branches of popliteal artery

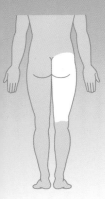

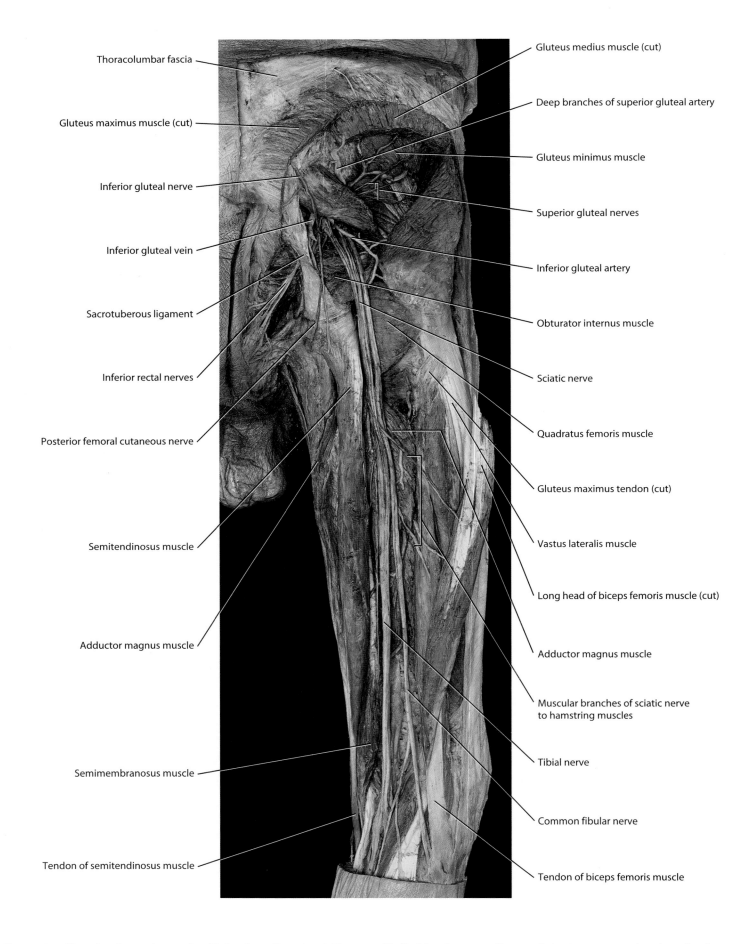

Thoracolumbar fascia

Gluteus maximus muscle (cut)

Inferior gluteal nerve

Inferior gluteal vein

Sacrotuberous ligament

Inferior rectal nerves

Posterior femoral cutaneous nerve

Semitendinosus muscle

Adductor magnus muscle

Semimembranosus muscle

Tendon of semitendinosus muscle

Gluteus medius muscle (cut)

Deep branches of superior gluteal artery

Gluteus minimus muscle

Superior gluteal nerves

Inferior gluteal artery

Obturator internus muscle

Sciatic nerve

Quadratus femoris muscle

Gluteus maximus tendon (cut)

Vastus lateralis muscle

Long head of biceps femoris muscle (cut)

Adductor magnus muscle

Muscular branches of sciatic nerve
to hamstring muscles

Tibial nerve

Common fibular nerve

Tendon of biceps femoris muscle

Figure 42.6 Gluteal region and posterior thigh – deep dissection 1. The central half of the gluteus medius muscle has been removed to show the gluteus minimus muscle and the deep branches of the superior gluteal artery. Also exposed is the sciatic nerve and all its branches to the hamstring muscles

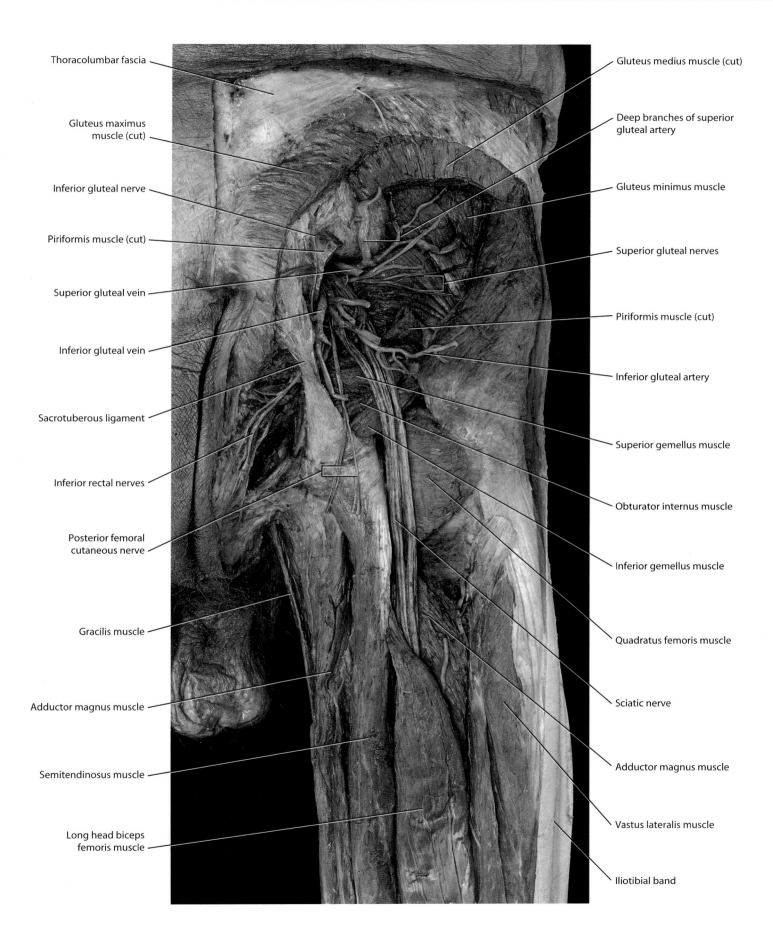

Thoracolumbar fascia

Gluteus maximus muscle (cut)

Inferior gluteal nerve

Piriformis muscle (cut)

Superior gluteal vein

Inferior gluteal vein

Sacrotuberous ligament

Inferior rectal nerves

Posterior femoral cutaneous nerve

Gracilis muscle

Adductor magnus muscle

Semitendinosus muscle

Long head biceps femoris muscle

Gluteus medius muscle (cut)

Deep branches of superior gluteal artery

Gluteus minimus muscle

Superior gluteal nerves

Piriformis muscle (cut)

Inferior gluteal artery

Superior gemellus muscle

Obturator internus muscle

Inferior gemellus muscle

Quadratus femoris muscle

Sciatic nerve

Adductor magnus muscle

Vastus lateralis muscle

Iliotibial band

LOWER LIMB Gluteal region and posterior thigh

Figure 42.7 Gluteal region and posterior thigh – deep dissection 2. This is a close-up view of Figure 42.6 with the piriformis muscle removed. The obturator internus and gemelli muscles are evident beneath the sciatic nerve. The superior and inferior gluteal arteries can also be seen

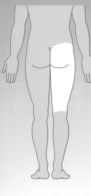

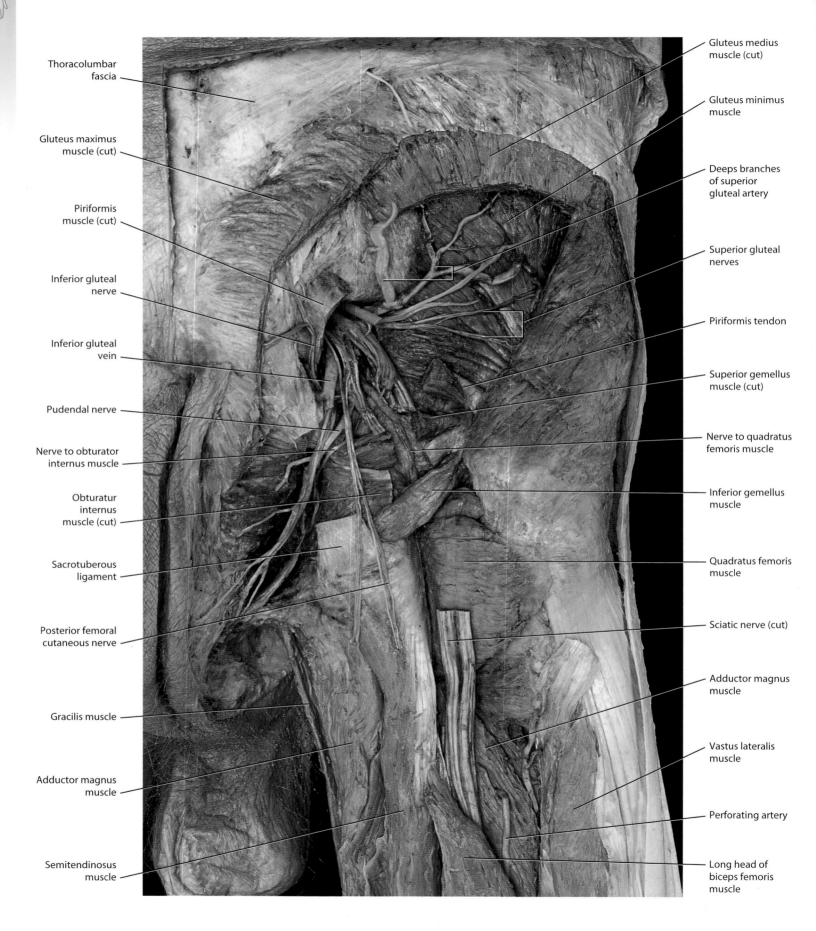

Thoracolumbar fascia

Gluteus maximus muscle (cut)

Piriformis muscle (cut)

Inferior gluteal nerve

Inferior gluteal vein

Pudendal nerve

Nerve to obturator internus muscle

Obturatur internus muscle (cut)

Sacrotuberous ligament

Posterior femoral cutaneous nerve

Gracilis muscle

Adductor magnus muscle

Semitendinosus muscle

Gluteus medius muscle (cut)

Gluteus minimus muscle

Deeps branches of superior gluteal artery

Superior gluteal nerves

Piriformis tendon

Superior gemellus muscle (cut)

Nerve to quadratus femoris muscle

Inferior gemellus muscle

Quadratus femoris muscle

Sciatic nerve (cut)

Adductor magnus muscle

Vastus lateralis muscle

Perforating artery

Long head of biceps femoris muscle

Figure 42.8 Gluteal region and posterior thigh – deep dissection 3. Close-up posterior view of the right gluteal region. The gluteus maximus and medius muscles have been partly cut and removed. The superior and inferior gemellus muscles and the obturator internus muscle have been partly cut to show the nerve to quadratus femoris muscle. The sciatic nerve has also been cut to show this

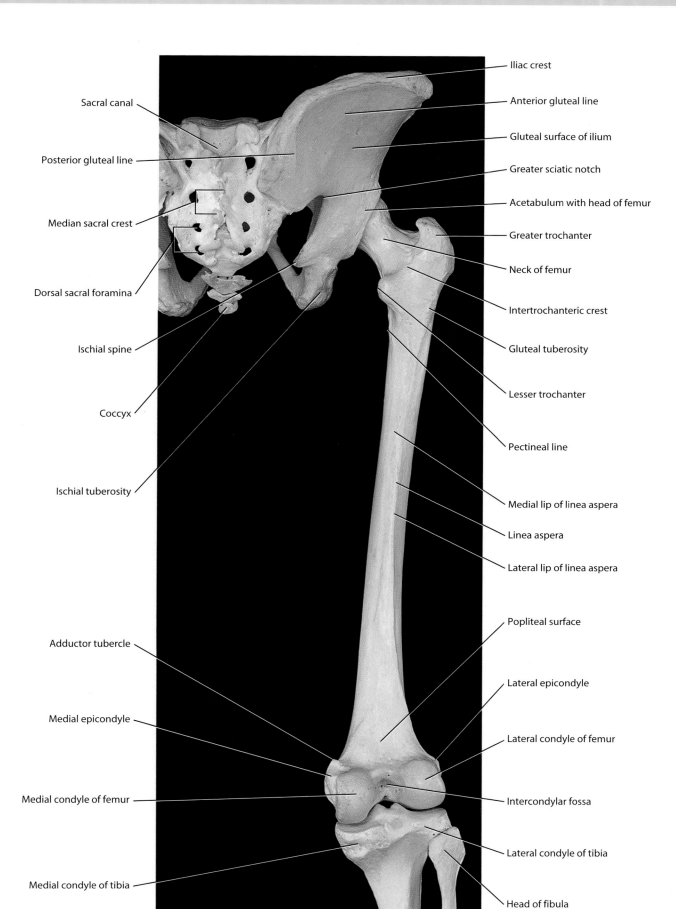

Iliac crest

Anterior gluteal line

Gluteal surface of ilium

Greater sciatic notch

Acetabulum with head of femur

Greater trochanter

Neck of femur

Intertrochanteric crest

Gluteal tuberosity

Lesser trochanter

Pectineal line

Medial lip of linea aspera

Linea aspera

Lateral lip of linea aspera

Popliteal surface

Lateral epicondyle

Lateral condyle of femur

Intercondylar fossa

Lateral condyle of tibia

Head of fibula

Sacral canal

Posterior gluteal line

Median sacral crest

Dorsal sacral foramina

Ischial spine

Coccyx

Ischial tuberosity

Adductor tubercle

Medial epicondyle

Medial condyle of femur

Medial condyle of tibia

LOWER LIMB Gluteal region and posterior thigh

Figure 42.9 Gluteal region and posterior thigh – osteology. Posterior view of the bones that support the gluteal region and posterior thigh

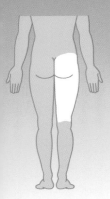

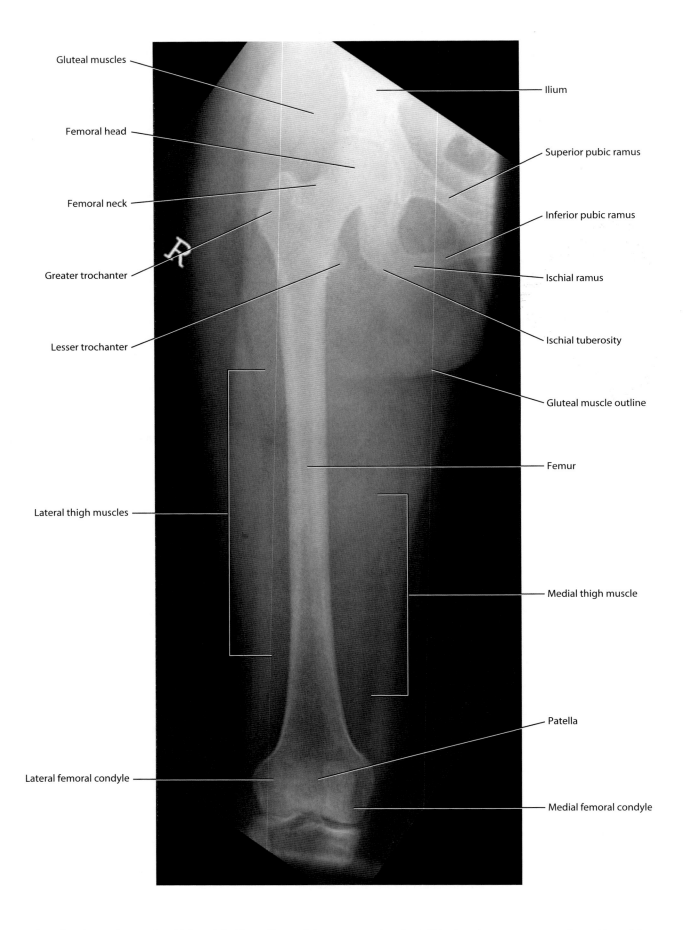

Gluteal muscles

Femoral head

Femoral neck

Greater trochanter

Lesser trochanter

Lateral thigh muscles

Lateral femoral condyle

Ilium

Superior pubic ramus

Inferior pubic ramus

Ischial ramus

Ischial tuberosity

Gluteal muscle outline

Femur

Medial thigh muscle

Patella

Medial femoral condyle

Figure 42.10 Gluteal region and posterior thigh – plain film radiograph (anteroposterior view). This view demonstrates superimposition of the osseous and soft tissues from anterior to posterior. Osseous structures are also superimposed. Note the location of the inferior gluteal crease (gluteal muscle outline), which is an anatomic surface landmark that separates the gluteal region from the posterior thigh

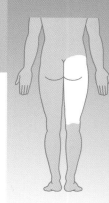

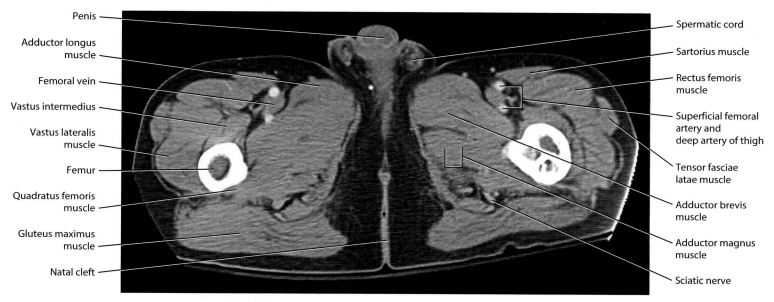

Penis

Adductor longus muscle

Femoral vein

Vastus intermedius

Vastus lateralis muscle

Femur

Quadratus femoris muscle

Gluteus maximus muscle

Natal cleft

Spermatic cord

Sartorius muscle

Rectus femoris muscle

Superficial femoral artery and deep artery of thigh

Tensor fasciae latae muscle

Adductor brevis muscle

Adductor magnus muscle

Sciatic nerve

Figure 42.11 Gluteal region – CT scan (axial view). In this scan of the upper thigh, the superficial and deep branches of the femoral artery are clearly visible within the anterior compartment. The sciatic nerve is also visible in the gluteal region

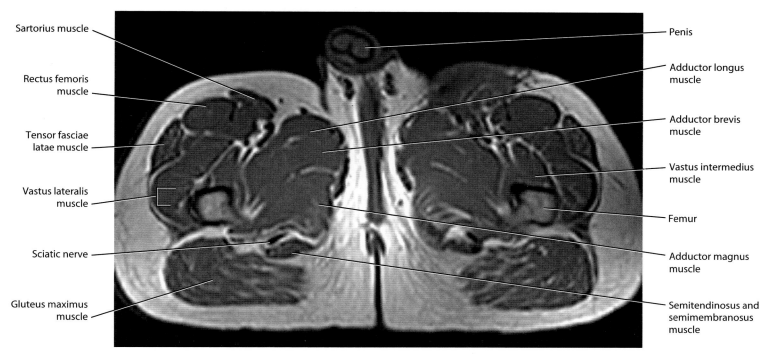

Sartorius muscle

Rectus femoris muscle

Tensor fasciae latae muscle

Vastus lateralis muscle

Sciatic nerve

Gluteus maximus muscle

Penis

Adductor longus muscle

Adductor brevis muscle

Vastus intermedius muscle

Femur

Adductor magnus muscle

Semitendinosus and semimembranosus muscle

Figure 42.12 Gluteal region – MRI scan (axial view). In this scan of the lower pelvis the muscles are well visualized. Note the reduction in the signal intensity of the normally bright fat in the anterior left thigh (related to prior surgery). The sciatic nerve appears black, and the gluteus maximus has a marbled appearance due to the presence of fat between the muscle fibers

43 Knee joint and popliteal fossa

The knee joint is a synovial hinge-type joint between the femur and tibia; its range of movement is limited primarily to flexion and extension, but with some rotation. The superior part of the knee joint is formed by the **condyles** of the femur. These enlarged bony prominences transfer weight to the flattened superior surfaces of the tibia and the **medial** and **lateral condyles**.

The **patella** is a large sesamoid bone that supports and protects the anterior knee joint through its attachments to the **quadriceps femoris tendon** and **patellar ligament**.

MUSCLES

The knee joint is supported anteriorly by the aponeurotic expansion of the quadriceps femoris muscle. This large tendon emerges from the inferior quadriceps femoris muscle and attaches to the superior aspect of the patella. At the inferior patella, the patellar ligament (Fig. 43.1) emerges inferiorly to insert onto the tibial tuberosity. With this design, the quadriceps femoris muscle is the primary extensor for the knee joint and supports the anterior knee via its tendon and the patella. The lateral portion of the knee is supported by the iliotibial tract and the tendon of the biceps femoris muscle, while the medial side of the knee is supported by the muscle tendons of the pes anserinus.

The hamstring muscles and posterior leg muscles support the posterior knee joint (Fig. 43.2). Medially the semimembranosus, semitendinosus, gracilis, and sartorius muscles and tendons, which originate in the upper thigh, insert onto points along the proximal medial tibia. The lateral part of the posterior knee joint is supported by biceps femoris, which originates in the thigh and inserts onto the head of the fibula (see Chapter 42).

NERVES

The knee joint is innervated by several nerves that pass the joint, including articular branches from the **tibial** and **common fibular nerves** and articular branches from the **femoral nerve**. The posterior division of the **obturator nerve** also supplies the knee after supplying the adductor magnus muscle.

Cutaneous innervation to the anterior skin of the knee joint is conveyed by anterior cutaneous branches of the femoral nerve. Posterior cutaneous innervation is conveyed by medial sural cutaneous branches of the tibial nerve (see Chapters 40 and 42).

ARTERIES

Blood supply to the knee is from the genicular anastomoses, which consist of ten arteries:

- the **descending genicular artery** and the **descending branch of the lateral circumflex femoral artery** (both of which are branches of the femoral artery) descend and supply the knee;
- five branches from the popliteal artery provide blood to the posterior side – the **superior medial genicular, superior lateral genicular, middle genicular, inferior medial genicular**, and **inferior lateral genicular arteries**;
- the remaining three vessels arise from the anterior tibial artery of the leg (see Chapter 44) – the **posterior tibial recurrent artery, circumflex fibular artery**, and **anterior tibial recurrent artery**.

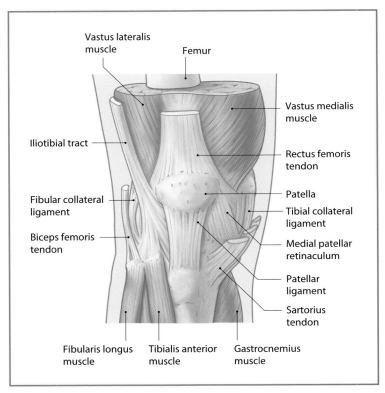

Figure 43.1 Knee joint – superficial anterior view

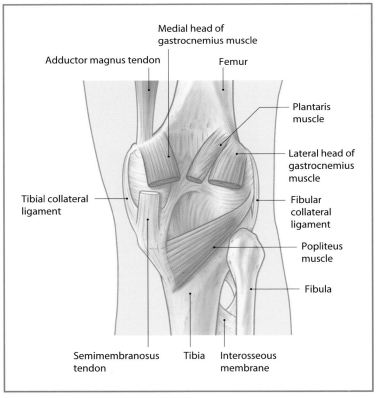

Figure 43.2 Knee joint – posterior view

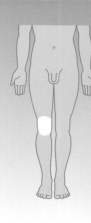

VEINS AND LYMPHATICS

Venous drainage of the superficial structures at the knee joint is to the **great saphenous vein** and other unnamed superficial veins at the knee. Deep venous drainage of the knee joint follows the arteries that comprise the genicular anastomoses named above.

Lymphatic drainage of the superficial structures of the knee (skin and soft tissue) follows the great saphenous vein and ends in the **inguinal lymph nodes**. Deep lymphatic drainage of the knee is to the **popliteal nodes**, which eventually drain toward the inguinal and **gluteal nodes**.

LIGAMENTS AND MENISCI

The knee has a strong fibrous joint capsule that completely surrounds the joint and is strengthened by five intrinsic ligaments (Table 43.1):

- the patellar ligament anteriorly;
- the **oblique popliteal** and **arcuate popliteal ligaments** posteriorly;
- the **tibial** (medial) and **fibular** (lateral) **collateral ligaments**.

Deep to this joint capsule, but superficial to the synovial cavity, the **anterior** and **posterior cruciate ligaments** ascend from the anterior and posterior areas of the tibia to attach to the inner sides of the femoral condyles. They prevent anterior and posterior displacement of the tibia relative to the femur.

The **medial** and **lateral menisci** of the knee joint are crescent-shaped plates of fibrocartilage that deepen the articulating surfaces of the knee and act as shock absorbers.

POPLITEAL FOSSA

Posterior to the knee joint, the muscles of the lower thigh and upper leg create a diamond-shaped region, the **popliteal fossa** (Fig. 43.3). The semimembranosus and semitendinosus muscles form the upper medial border, and the upper lateral border is formed by the biceps femoris muscle. The medial and lateral heads of the gastrocnemius muscle form the lower borders. The roof of the popliteal fossa is formed from the skin and fascia overlying the region, and the floor by the **popliteal surface** of the femur, the oblique popliteal ligament, and the fascia enclosing the popliteus muscle. From superficial to deep, the structures in the popliteal fossa are:

- skin;
- subcutaneous tissue and cutaneous nerves – the posterior cutaneous nerve of thigh and sural nerve;
- the small saphenous vein, which empties into popliteal vein;
- the tibial and common fibular nerves;
- the popliteal vein;
- the popliteal artery with genicular branches;
- the popliteus muscle with the arcuate popliteal ligament;
- the joint capsule with the oblique popliteal ligament.

■ CLINICAL CORRELATIONS
Knee injuries

The knee is a large joint with very little external supportive tissue, which predisposes it to injury. The main support is from the ligaments within and around the joint, with the muscles from the thigh and leg that cross the joint adding stability.

An anterior cruciate ligament injury (Fig. 43.4) usually results from a strenuous activity that involves running at high speed and then stopping suddenly to change direction – typically a sport that places great stress on the knee joint (e.g. football, skiing, tennis). Commonly, patients report hearing or feeling a 'popping' sound within the knee followed by pain and swelling. Inability to walk on the injured limb encourages patients to seek medical advice.

On examination the knee is swollen and tender to palpation. It has a decreased range of movement secondary to pain immediately after the injury. A Lachman test can be carried out by placing the patient in the supine position with the knee bent in 20–30° of flexion. The examiner grasps the lower thigh in one hand and upper leg in the other and attempts to move the tibia anteriorly

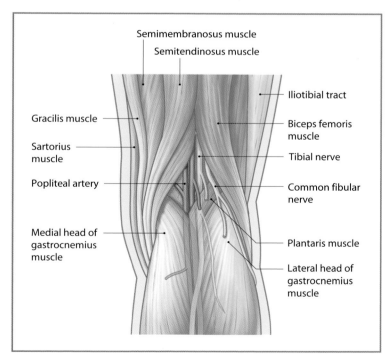

Figure 43.3 Popliteal fossa

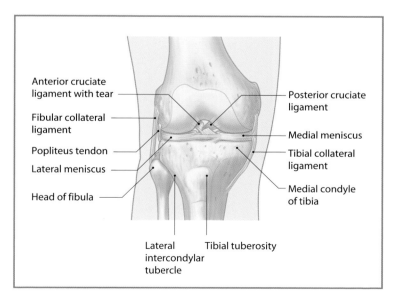

Figure 43.4 Injury to the anterior cruciate ligament

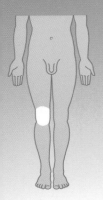

and posteriorly while maintaining the position of the femur. Laxity during this maneuver is highly suggestive of an anterior cruciate ligament injury and indicates a positive test result. Radiographs do not usually reveal fracture. Depending on the severity of the knee injury, other ligaments and/or menisci may be damaged. Initial conservative treatment is the RICE regimen:

- **R**est the injured joint;
- apply **I**ce-packs/cool packs as needed;
- place a **C**ompressive dressing (ACE – elastic – bandage);
- **E**levate the injured joint.

Crutches are also recommended to minimize weightbearing and facilitate healing. Aggressive orthopedic surgical management involves reconstruction of the anterior cruciate ligament.

Posterior cruciate ligament injury (Fig. 43.5) occurs in a similar fashion to anterior cruciate ligament injury. The patient's complaints, diagnostic work-up, and nonsurgical treatment are similar. When surgical repair is required it is important to distinguish between anterior and posterior cruciate ligament injuries because the surgical approaches differ.

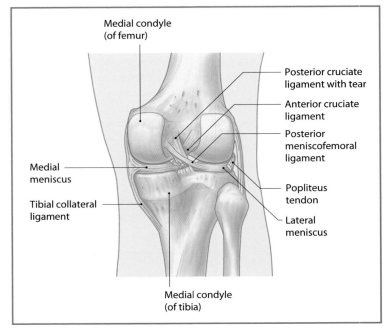

Figure 43.5 Injury to the posterior cruciate ligament

MNEMONIC	
Path and insertions of cruciate ligaments:	**PAMs ApPLes** (**P**osterior [passes] **A**nteriorly [and inserts] **M**edially; **A**nterior [passes] **P**osteriorly [and inserts] **L**aterally)

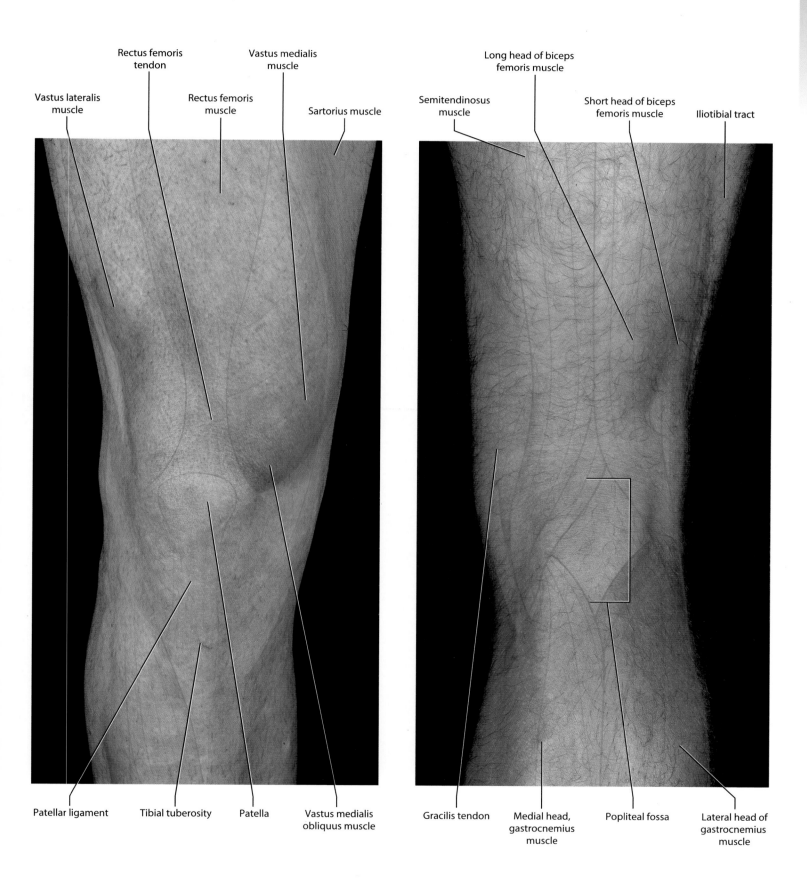

Vastus lateralis muscle

Rectus femoris tendon

Rectus femoris muscle

Vastus medialis muscle

Sartorius muscle

Long head of biceps femoris muscle

Semitendinosus muscle

Short head of biceps femoris muscle

Iliotibial tract

Patellar ligament

Tibial tuberosity

Patella

Vastus medialis obliquus muscle

Gracilis tendon

Medial head, gastrocnemius muscle

Popliteal fossa

Lateral head of gastrocnemius muscle

**Figure 43.6 Knee joint – surface anatomy. **Anterior view of the right knee. With the knee in extension, note the muscle bulge, which is the vastus medialis obliquus muscle

**Figure 43.7 Popliteal fossa – surface anatomy. **Posterior view of the popliteal fossa. The rough outline of its diamond shape can be discerned from the hamstrings superiorly and the calf muscles inferiorly

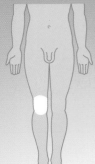

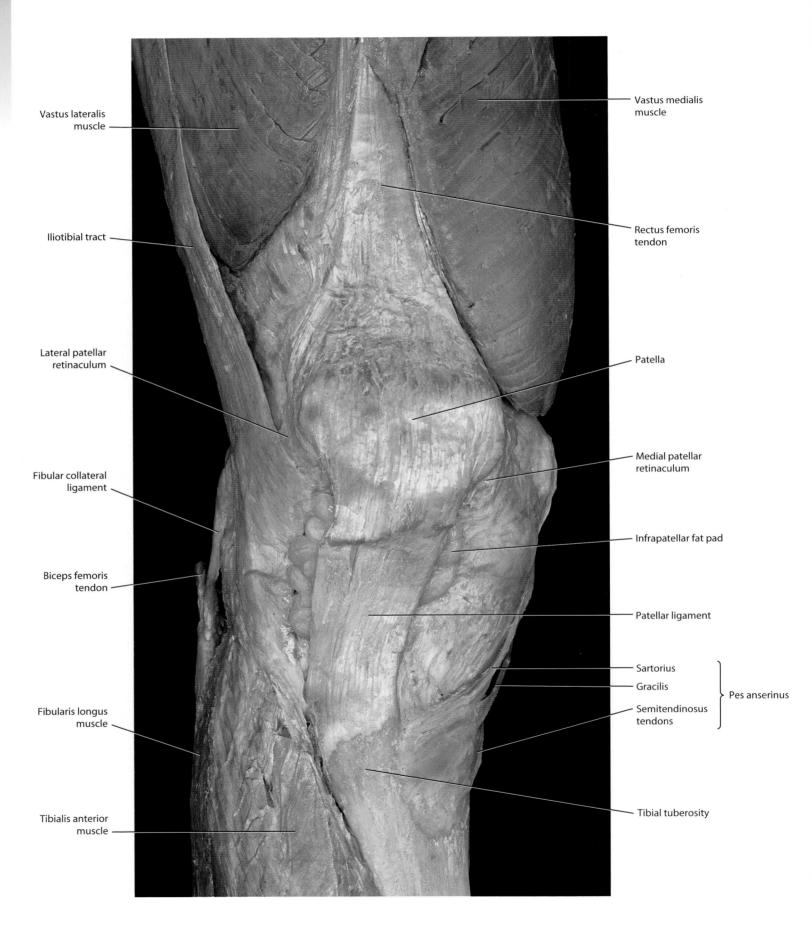

Vastus lateralis muscle

Iliotibial tract

Lateral patellar retinaculum

Fibular collateral ligament

Biceps femoris tendon

Fibularis longus muscle

Tibialis anterior muscle

Vastus medialis muscle

Rectus femoris tendon

Patella

Medial patellar retinaculum

Infrapatellar fat pad

Patellar ligament

Sartorius

Gracilis

Semitendinosus tendons

Pes anserinus

Tibial tuberosity

Figure 43.8 Knee joint – superficial dissection. Anterior view of the dissected right knee. Observe the patella and how it joins the quadriceps femoris tendon superiorly and the patellar ligament inferiorly, and the infrapatellar fat pad beneath the patellar ligament

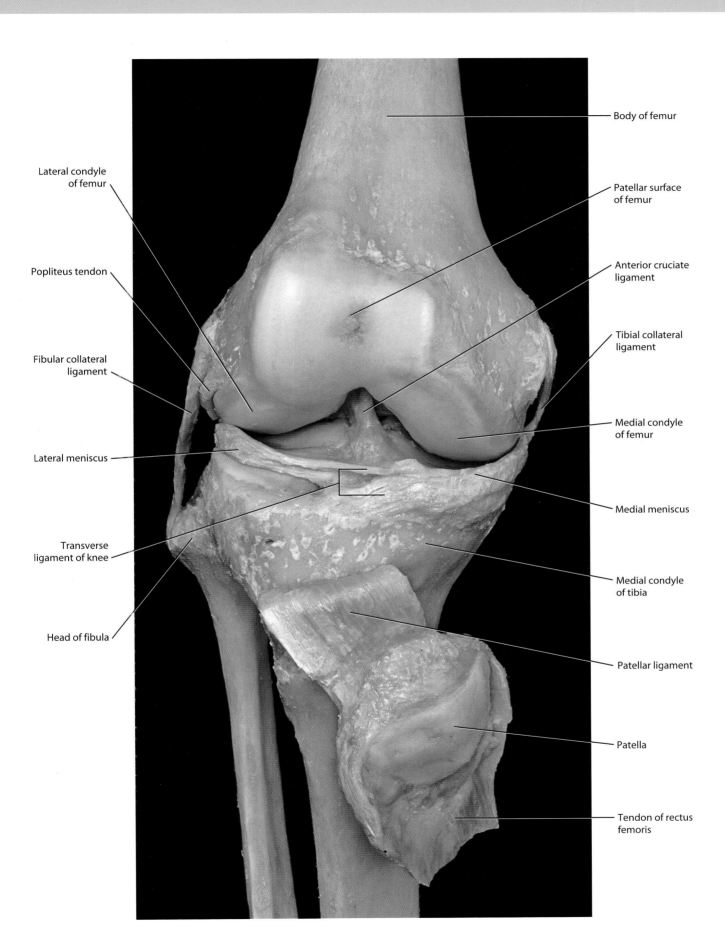

Body of femur

Lateral condyle
of femur

Popliteus tendon

Fibular collateral
ligament

Lateral meniscus

Transverse
ligament of knee

Head of fibula

Patellar surface
of femur

Anterior cruciate
ligament

Tibial collateral
ligament

Medial condyle
of femur

Medial meniscus

Medial condyle
of tibia

Patellar ligament

Patella

Tendon of rectus
femoris

Figure 43.9 Knee joint – deep dissection 1. This anterior view of a right knee dissection shows the cut quadriceps femoris tendon with the patella reflected downward to show the anterior cruciate ligament

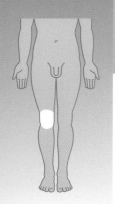

TABLE 43.1 LIGAMENTS AND MENISCI OF THE KNEE JOINT

Ligament	Attachment	Movement limited	Comments
Joint capsule	Superiorly, just proximal to articular margins of condyles of femur; inferiorly, to articular margin of tibia	Containment of synovial fluid within joint space	Strengthened by: • fibers from fascia lata and iliotibial tract • tendons of the vasti, hamstrings, and sartorius muscles
Patellar	Apex of patella to tuberosity of tibia	Helps hold patella in place	Serves as part of tendon of quadriceps femoris muscle
Oblique popliteal	Lateral femur, over condyles to posterior head of tibia	Limits extension, strengthens the fibrous joint capsule posteriorly	An expansion of the tendon of semimembranosus muscle
Arcuate popliteal	Lateral condyle of femur to styloid process of fibula	May limit medial rotation of leg	Passes superiomedially over the tendon of popliteus muscle
Tibial collateral	Medial epicondyle of femur to medial condyle and shaft of tibia	Limits extension, hyperflexion, and lateral flexion	Deeper fibers are firmly attached to medial meniscus
Fibular collateral	Lateral epicondyle of femur to lateral surface of head of fibula	Limits hyperextension (is relaxed in flexion)	Separated from lateral meniscus by tendon of popliteus
Anterior cruciate	Anterior part of intercondylar area of tibia; extends superiorly, posteriorly, and laterally to posterior part of medial side of lateral condyle of femur	Limits extension, lateral rotation, and posterior slipping of tibia on femur	Slack when the knee is flexed, and taut when it is fully extended
Posterior cruciate	Posterior part of intercondylar area of tibia; extends superiorly and medially to anterior part of lateral surface of medial condyle of femur	Taut in full flexion and lateral rotation, limits posterior slipping of tibia on femur	In the weightbearing flexed knee, it stabilizes the femur
Medial meniscus	Anterior end attaches to anterior intercondylar area of tibia; posterior end attaches to posterior intercondylar area	Deepens the medial condyle of tibia	Crescent-shaped and firmly adherent to the deep surface of tibial collateral ligament
Lateral meniscus	More freely movable, through the posterior meniscofemoral ligament, it is attached to the medial condyle of the femur	Deepens the lateral condyle of tibia	Nearly circular, separated from the fibular collateral ligament
Transverse	Joins the anterior edges of the two menisci	Allows menisci to move together during movements of femur on tibia	A slender fibrous band
Coronary	Attaches menisci margins to the tibial condyles	Helps hold the menisci in place	

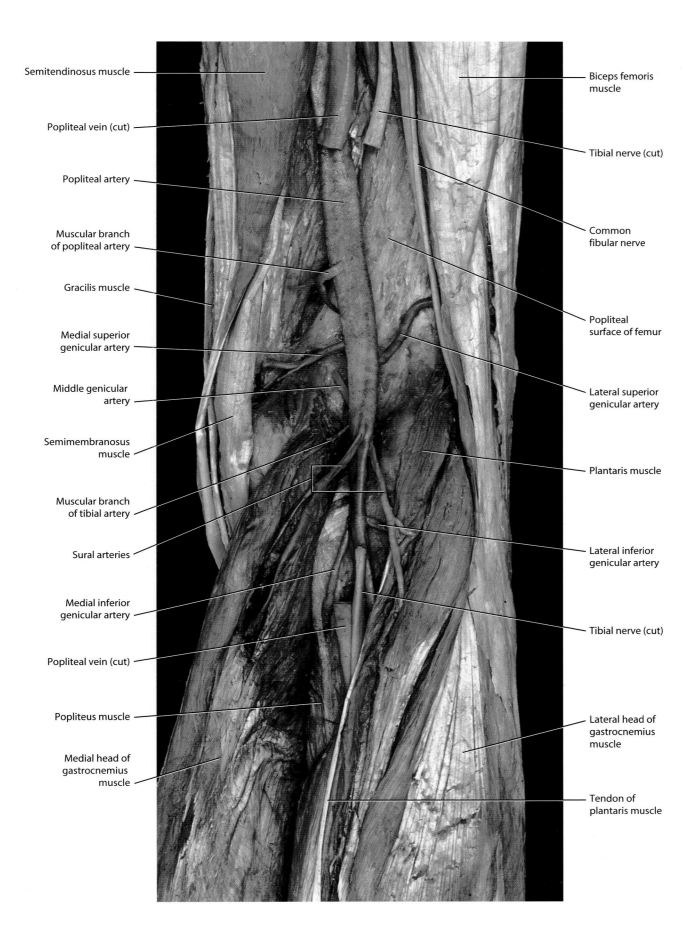

Semitendinosus muscle

Popliteal vein (cut)

Popliteal artery

Muscular branch of popliteal artery

Gracilis muscle

Medial superior genicular artery

Middle genicular artery

Semimembranosus muscle

Muscular branch of tibial artery

Sural arteries

Medial inferior genicular artery

Popliteal vein (cut)

Popliteus muscle

Medial head of gastrocnemius muscle

Biceps femoris muscle

Tibial nerve (cut)

Common fibular nerve

Popliteal surface of femur

Lateral superior genicular artery

Plantaris muscle

Lateral inferior genicular artery

Tibial nerve (cut)

Lateral head of gastrocnemius muscle

Tendon of plantaris muscle

LOWER LIMB Knee joint and popliteal fossa

Figure 43.10 Popliteal fossa – superficial dissection. Posterior view of the right knee showing the popliteal fossa. Observe all five genicular branches plus the sural arteries (which supply the heads of the gastrocnemius) arising from the popliteal artery, which lies against the inferior part of the femur

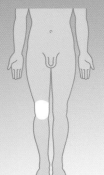

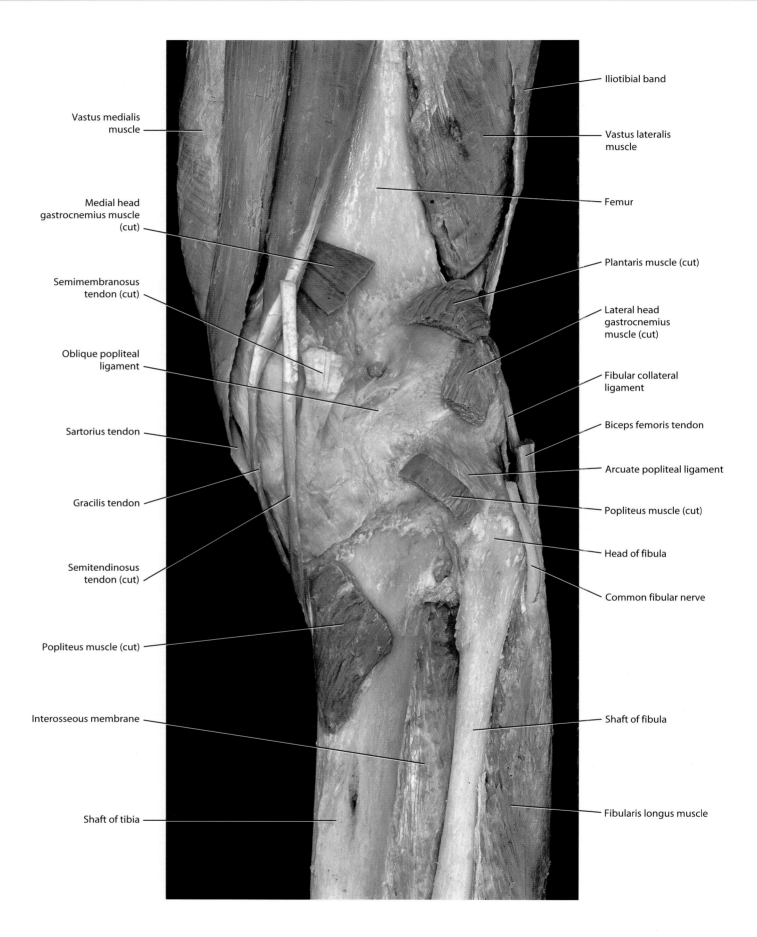

Vastus medialis muscle

Medial head gastrocnemius muscle (cut)

Semimembranosus tendon (cut)

Oblique popliteal ligament

Sartorius tendon

Gracilis tendon

Semitendinosus tendon (cut)

Popliteus muscle (cut)

Interosseous membrane

Shaft of tibia

Iliotibial band

Vastus lateralis muscle

Femur

Plantaris muscle (cut)

Lateral head gastrocnemius muscle (cut)

Fibular collateral ligament

Biceps femoris tendon

Arcuate popliteal ligament

Popliteus muscle (cut)

Head of fibula

Common fibular nerve

Shaft of fibula

Fibularis longus muscle

Figure 43.11 Knee joint – deep dissection 2. Posterior view of the right knee. Most of the muscles have been cut and removed to show the joint capsule and relationships of the femur, tibia, and fibula to the musculature. The pes anserinus muscles (sartorius, gracilis, and semitendinosus) have been displaced posteriorly

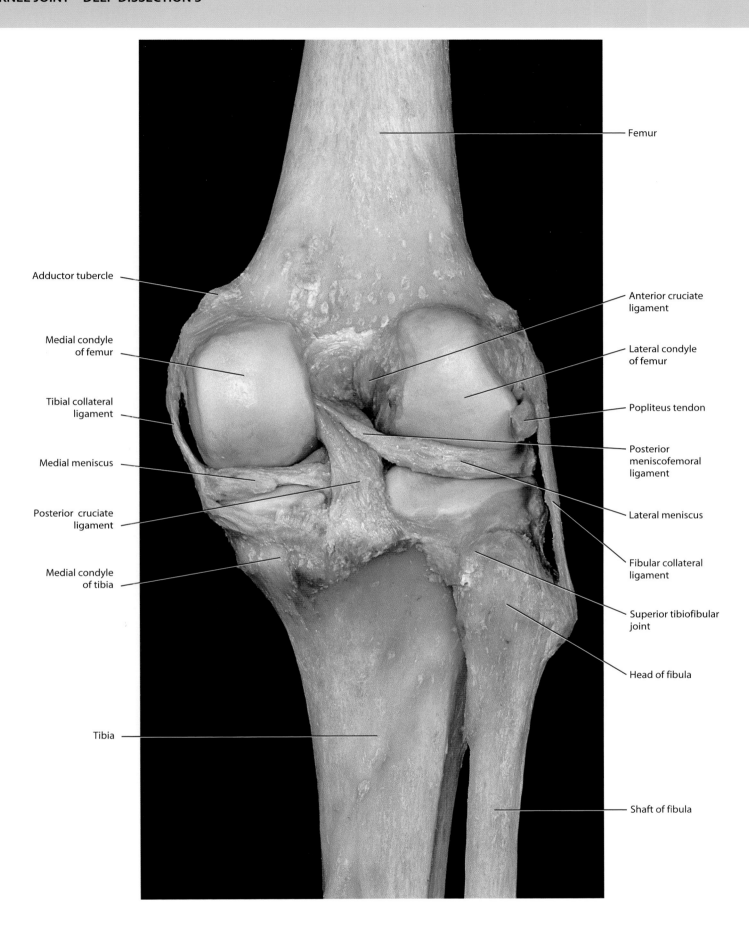

Femur

Adductor tubercle

Anterior cruciate ligament

Medial condyle of femur

Lateral condyle of femur

Tibial collateral ligament

Popliteus tendon

Medial meniscus

Posterior meniscofemoral ligament

Posterior cruciate ligament

Lateral meniscus

Medial condyle of tibia

Fibular collateral ligament

Superior tibiofibular joint

Tibia

Head of fibula

Shaft of fibula

Figure 43.12 Knee joint – deep dissection 3. Posterior view of the knee ligaments of the right knee. Observe the posterior cruciate ligament and the medial and lateral menisci

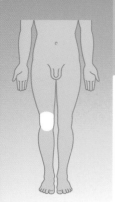

LOWER LIMB

Knee joint and popliteal fossa

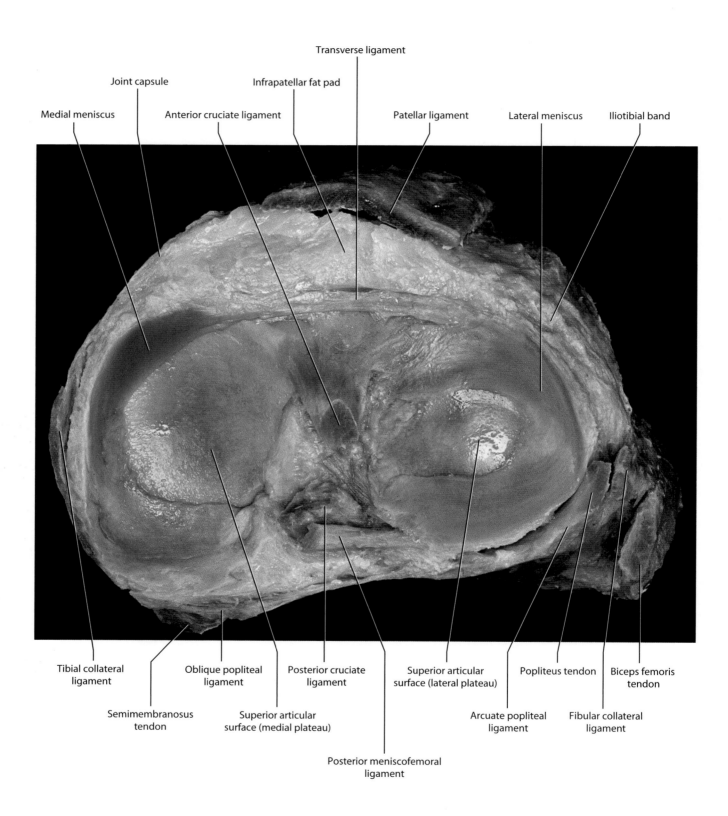

Transverse ligament

Joint capsule

Infrapatellar fat pad

Medial meniscus

Anterior cruciate ligament

Patellar ligament

Lateral meniscus

Iliotibial band

Tibial collateral ligament

Oblique popliteal ligament

Posterior cruciate ligament

Superior articular surface (lateral plateau)

Popliteus tendon

Biceps femoris tendon

Semimembranosus tendon

Superior articular surface (medial plateau)

Arcuate popliteal ligament

Fibular collateral ligament

Posterior meniscofemoral ligament

Figure 43.13 Knee joint – deep dissection 4. Superior view as if looking down at the lower half of one's own right knee joint, showing the menisci on the tibial plateaus

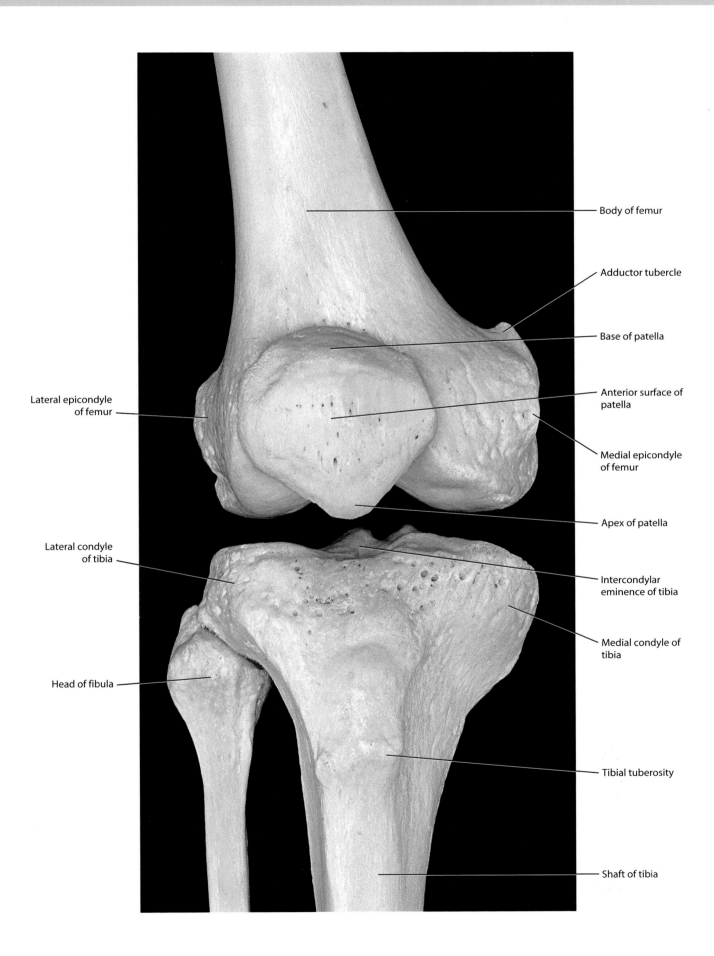

Figure 43.14 Knee joint – osteology 1. Anterior view of the bones of the right knee. The joint has been opened slightly to show the intercondylar eminence of the tibia

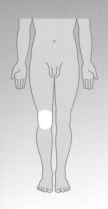

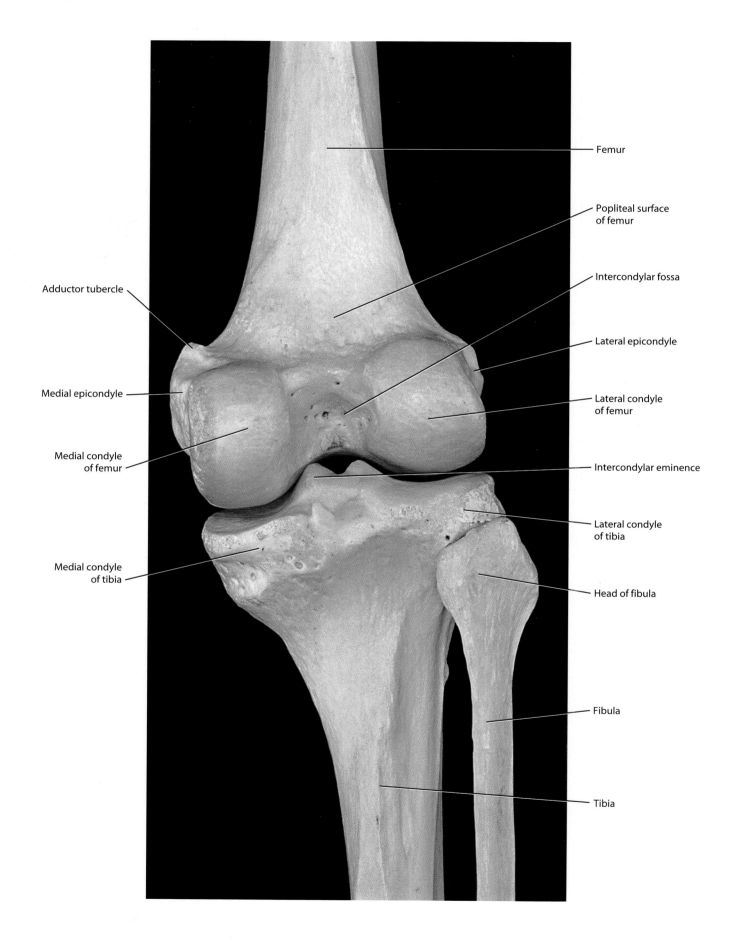

Adductor tubercle

Medial epicondyle

Medial condyle
of femur

Medial condyle
of tibia

Femur

Popliteal surface
of femur

Intercondylar fossa

Lateral epicondyle

Lateral condyle
of femur

Intercondylar eminence

Lateral condyle
of tibia

Head of fibula

Fibula

Tibia

Figure 43.15 Knee joint – osteology 2. Posterior view of the bones of the right knee. The condyles of the femur sit on the condyles of the tibia

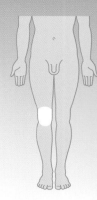

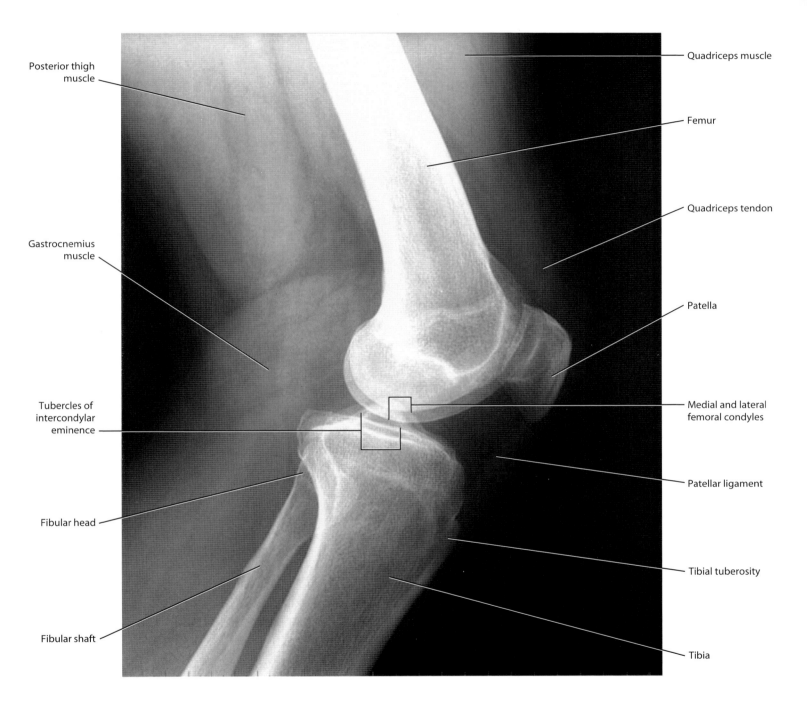

Posterior thigh muscle

Gastrocnemius muscle

Tubercles of intercondylar eminence

Fibular head

Fibular shaft

Quadriceps muscle

Femur

Quadriceps tendon

Patella

Medial and lateral femoral condyles

Patellar ligament

Tibial tuberosity

Tibia

Figure 43.16 Knee joint – plain film radiograph (lateral view). This view is routinely taken in slight flexion for better evaluation of the patellofemoral joint. Observe how the patella is normally located anterior to the distal femur when the knee is in slight flexion

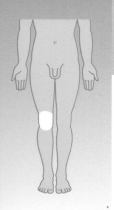

Knee joint and popliteal fossa

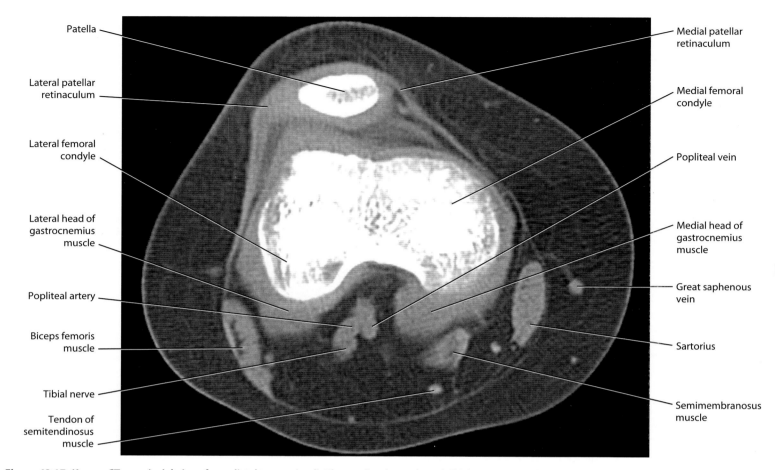

Patella

Lateral patellar retinaculum

Lateral femoral condyle

Lateral head of gastrocnemius muscle

Popliteal artery

Biceps femoris muscle

Tibial nerve

Tendon of semitendinosus muscle

Medial patellar retinaculum

Medial femoral condyle

Popliteal vein

Medial head of gastrocnemius muscle

Great saphenous vein

Sartorius

Semimembranosus muscle

Figure 43.17 Knee – CT scan (axial view, from distal to proximal). The popliteal vessels and tibial nerve are well visualized in the popliteal fossa. The retropatellar region located between the patella and the femur is also well delineated. Fat appears bright in this scan

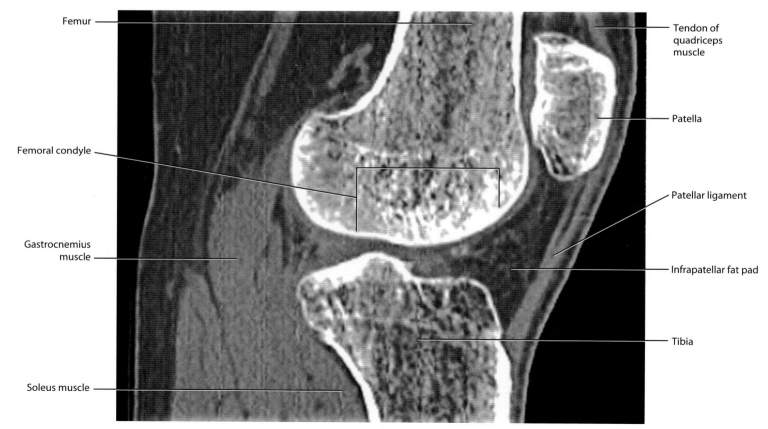

Femur

Femoral condyle

Gastrocnemius muscle

Soleus muscle

Tendon of quadriceps muscle

Patella

Patellar ligament

Infrapatellar fat pad

Tibia

Figure 43.18 Knee – CT scan (sagittal view). This scan is slightly off midline. Note the location of the patella with respect to the femur when the knee is in full extension

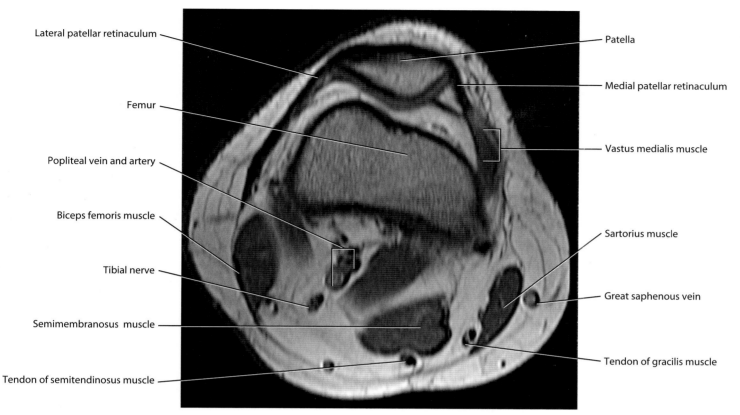

Lateral patellar retinaculum

Femur

Popliteal vein and artery

Biceps femoris muscle

Tibial nerve

Semimembranosus muscle

Tendon of semitendinosus muscle

Patella

Medial patellar retinaculum

Vastus medialis muscle

Sartorius muscle

Great saphenous vein

Tendon of gracilis muscle

Figure 43.19 Knee – MRI scan (axial view, from distal to proximal). The tendons appear black due their dense fibrous nature. The retropatellar fat is well visualized

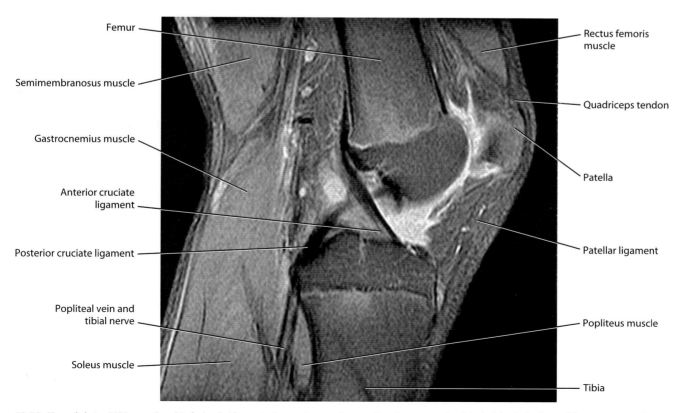

Femur

Semimembranosus muscle

Gastrocnemius muscle

Anterior cruciate ligament

Posterior cruciate ligament

Popliteal vein and tibial nerve

Soleus muscle

Rectus femoris muscle

Quadriceps tendon

Patella

Patellar ligament

Popliteus muscle

Tibia

Figure 43.20 Knee joint – MRI scan (sagittal view). The anterior and posterior cruciate ligaments are black due their dense fibrous nature; this makes the integrity of these ligaments easy to assess on MRI

The anterolateral leg is between the knee and the ankle (Fig. 44.1). The two bones of the leg are:

- the **tibia** (the shin bone), which is a large, weightbearing bone that contributes to the medial part of the ankle;
- the **fibula**, a smaller bone, which is primarily for muscle attachment, but also contributes to the lateral part of the ankle.

The tibia is flattened superiorly, with medial and lateral **superior articular surfaces** (commonly called 'plateaus') separated by the **intercondylar eminence**. The roughened areas below the medial and lateral facets are the **medial** and **lateral condyles**, respectively. The **tibial tuberosity** is a bony prominence on the anterior proximal tibia where the patellar ligament attaches. The tibia descends as a triangular shaft toward the ankle and becomes the **medial malleolus**.

The fibula is on the lateral aspect of the leg and is a slender bone, with a proximal **head** that articulates with the lateral condyle of the tibia. The distal **lateral malleolus** of the fibula makes up the lateral ankle. Together, the tibia and fibula transfer the weight of the body onto the talus bone of the foot.

MUSCLES

The muscles of the anterolateral leg are divided into an anterior group of four muscles and a lateral group of two muscles (Table 44.1, Fig. 44.2). These muscle groups are separated by the thick intermuscular **crural fascia**: the **anterior intermuscular septum of leg** separates the anterior and lateral muscle groups and the **posterior intermuscular septum of leg** separates the lateral group of muscles from the posterior leg muscles (see Chapter 45).

The tibialis anterior, extensor hallucis longus, extensor digitorum longus, and fibularis tertius muscles are the **anterior leg muscles**. They:

- originate from the tibia and fibula and insert onto the dorsal metatarsals and distal phalanges of the foot;
- dorsiflex the ankle and extend the toes.

The fibularis longus and fibularis brevis muscles comprise the **lateral group of muscles**. These two muscles:

- originate from the lateral surface of the tibia and insert on the bases of metatarsals I and V;
- evert the foot and weakly plantarflex the ankle.

NERVES

The anterolateral leg is innervated by the **common fibular nerve** (L4 to L5, S1 to S2 nerve roots), which is the lateral branch of the sciatic nerve. Just after the common fibular nerve separates from the tibial nerve in the popliteal fossa, it gives off a small cutaneous branch – the **lateral sural cutaneous nerve**. This nerve, in turn, gives off a fibular communicating branch, which joins the **medial sural cutaneous nerve** (from the tibial nerve) to form the **sural nerve**. The sural nerve conveys sensation from the skin of the posterolateral leg and foot.

The common fibular nerve descends through the popliteal fossa and enters the leg by wrapping around the neck of the fibula. At this point, it divides into the **superficial** and **deep fibular nerves**. The superficial fibular nerve descends in the lateral leg to innervate the

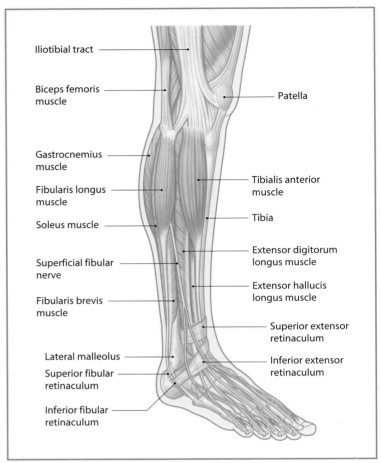

Figure 44.1 Muscles of the anterolateral leg

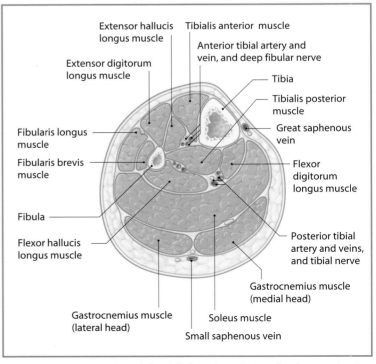

Figure 44.2 Cross-section of the right leg viewed from distal to proximal

fibularis longus and fibularis brevis muscles, and to convey sensation from the skin of the lateral leg and foot.

The deep fibular nerve descends down the leg and innervates the anterior muscles of the leg. It enters the foot between the extensor digitorum longus and extensor hallucis longus muscles and conveys sensation from the small patch of skin of the dorsal webspace between toes I and II.

ARTERIES

Blood is supplied to the anterior leg by the **anterior tibial artery**, which is a branch of the popliteal artery.

The anterior tibial artery starts on the posterior superior side of the leg and passes through a high opening in the **interosseous membrane** to enter the anterior compartment of the leg. It descends inferiorly on the interosseous membrane in the anterior leg between the tendons of the tibialis anterior and extensor hallucis longus muscles. As it enters the foot it becomes the **dorsalis pedis artery**.

Additional branches of the anterior tibial artery include:

- the **anterior tibial recurrent artery**, which branches off soon after entering the anterior compartment and anastomoses with the **genicular branches** of the popliteal artery;
- an **anterior medial malleolar artery**, which branches off at the far inferior end and anastomoses with the **medial malleolar branch** of the posterior tibial artery;
- an **anterior lateral malleolar artery**, which anastomoses with the **perforating branch** of the fibular artery.

The blood supply to the two fibularis muscles in the lateral leg is mainly from the **fibular artery** (a lateral branch of the posterior tibial artery). The fibularis longus muscle also receives blood from the anterior tibial artery.

VEINS AND LYMPHATICS

Superficial venous drainage of the dorsum of the foot is to the **dorsal venous arch of foot**. Blood from the medial end of the dorsal venous arch enters the **great saphenous vein**, which ascends the leg anterior to the medial malleolus, passes through the medial leg and thigh, and drains into the **femoral vein** at the femoral triangle (see Chapter 40).

The **small saphenous vein** begins at the lateral end of the dorsal venous arch. It ascends with the sural nerve posterior to the lateral malleolus and drains the superficial tissues of the foot and lower leg before emptying into the **popliteal vein** at the popliteal fossa (see Chapter 43).

Deep venous drainage of the anterolateral leg is through venae comitantes (accompanying veins) that follow the anterior and posterior tibial arteries and their branches. These deep veins contribute to the formation of the popliteal vein.

Large lymph vessels of the leg follow the major arteries and the great and small saphenous veins and drain directly to the **inguinal nodes**. Smaller and more superficial lymphatic vessels from the medial leg drain to the inguinal nodes. Lymph from the lateral leg drains to the **popliteal nodes** behind the knee and then to the inguinal nodes.

■ CLINICAL CORRELATIONS

Compartment syndrome

Compartment syndrome is abnormally increased pressure within a specific anatomical region of the leg. This increased pressure results in decreased arterial flow, ischemia, and nerve damage. Common causes are trauma, deep vein thrombosis, and external pressure from a cast or other dressing. The four compartments in the leg are:

- the anterior compartment – containing the tibialis anterior, extensor hallucis longus, and extensor digitorum longus muscles, and the deep fibular nerve;
- the lateral compartment – containing the fibularis longus and brevis muscles and the superficial fibular nerve;
- the superficial posterior compartment – containing the gastrocnemius and soleus muscles and the sural nerve;
- the deep posterior compartment – containing the flexor digitorum longus, flexor hallucis longus, and tibialis posterior muscles, and the tibial nerve.

Because of the tight fascia surrounding it, the risk for compartment syndrome developing in the anterior compartment of the leg is high.

Compartment syndrome causes extreme pain, which is made much worse by small movements and palpation during the physical examination (the pain can sometimes seem out of all proportion to the examination).

Signs on examination are weak dorsiflexion of the great toe and decreased sensation at the first webspace of the toes due to compression of the deep fibular nerve. The diagnosis is confirmed by direct measurement of the pressure within the compartment. Normal compartment pressure is less than 10 mmHg. Abnormal pressure is defined as pressure that will cause ischemia and death of tissue if not decreased; this is usually above 40 mmHg.

Untreated compartment syndrome results in cyanosis, loss of peripheral pulses, paresthesia, and paralysis of the involved limb. The treatment is fasciotomy (surgical opening of the fascial compartment) and debridement of any necrotic tissue. After surgery, the wound is left open for several days until the swelling of the compartment has decreased and the wound can be closed or other treatment can be carried out as necessary.

Tibia fracture

The tibia is superficial in the anterolateral leg and is easily palpated. Direct impact to the tibia can cause open or closed fractures of the tibial shaft. Fractures of the tibial plateau usually result from axial loading (compression). Patients with a tibial fracture usually cannot walk because of pain and instability in the leg. A splint should be applied to the area until further medical attention is available. In the hospital, clinical examination and radiographs will determine the type of fracture. Transverse fractures of the tibia can be treated intraoperatively with intramedullary rod placement. Open, comminuted fractures are treated with external fixation. In young patients or patients with a spiral fracture of the tibia, cast placement may be the definitive treatment.

MNEMONICS

Nerves of the leg and their functions: **FED** (**F**ibular nerve **E**verts and **D**orsiflexes the foot)

　　　　　　　　　　　　　　　　　　　　　　TIP (**T**ibial nerve **I**nverts and **P**lantarflexes the foot)

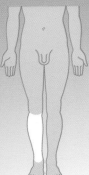

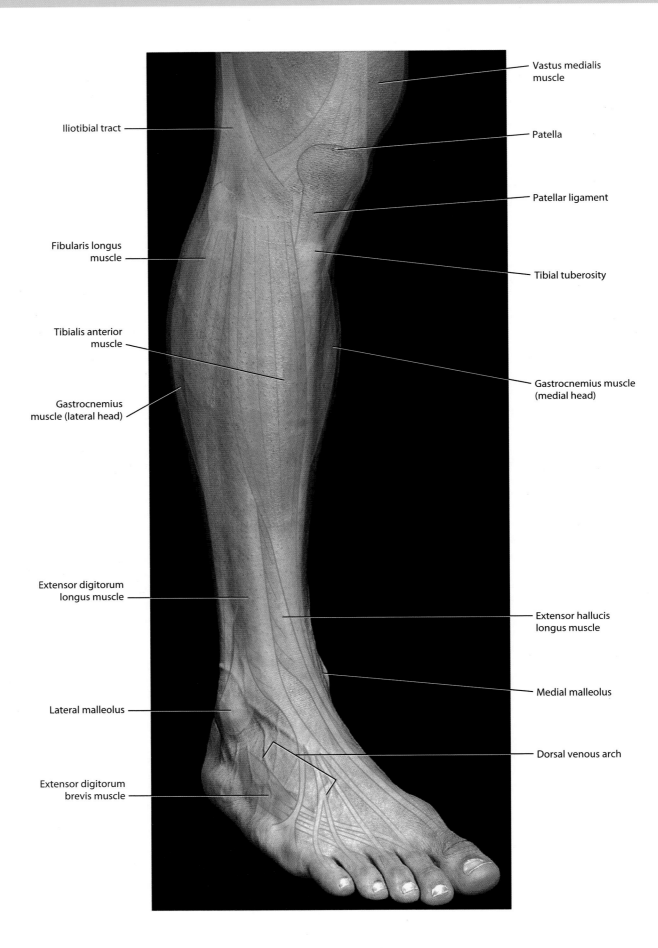

Iliotibial tract

Fibularis longus
muscle

Tibialis anterior
muscle

Gastrocnemius
muscle (lateral head)

Extensor digitorum
longus muscle

Lateral malleolus

Extensor digitorum
brevis muscle

Vastus medialis
muscle

Patella

Patellar ligament

Tibial tuberosity

Gastrocnemius muscle
(medial head)

Extensor hallucis
longus muscle

Medial malleolus

Dorsal venous arch

Figure 44.3 Anterolateral leg – surface anatomy. Anterolateral view of the right leg of a young man. Note the veins on the dorsum of the foot, which will form the saphenous system of superficial venous drainage

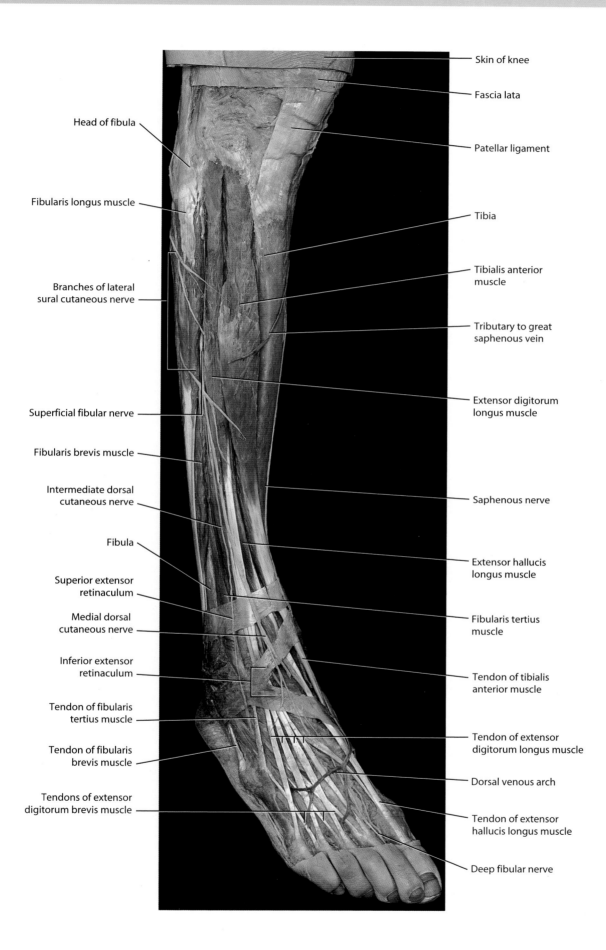

Skin of knee

Fascia lata

Patellar ligament

Head of fibula

Fibularis longus muscle

Tibia

Branches of lateral sural cutaneous nerve

Tibialis anterior muscle

Tributary to great saphenous vein

Extensor digitorum longus muscle

Superficial fibular nerve

Fibularis brevis muscle

Intermediate dorsal cutaneous nerve

Saphenous nerve

Fibula

Extensor hallucis longus muscle

Superior extensor retinaculum

Medial dorsal cutaneous nerve

Fibularis tertius muscle

Inferior extensor retinaculum

Tendon of tibialis anterior muscle

Tendon of fibularis tertius muscle

Tendon of extensor digitorum longus muscle

Tendon of fibularis brevis muscle

Dorsal venous arch

Tendons of extensor digitorum brevis muscle

Tendon of extensor hallucis longus muscle

Deep fibular nerve

Figure 44.4 Anterolateral leg –superficial dissection. Superficial dissection of the right anterolateral leg. All six muscles can be seen; their tendons are prevented from 'bowstringing' by the extensor retinacula. Observe the tibialis anterior muscle, which is lateral to the tibia in this view

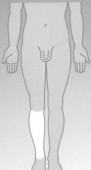

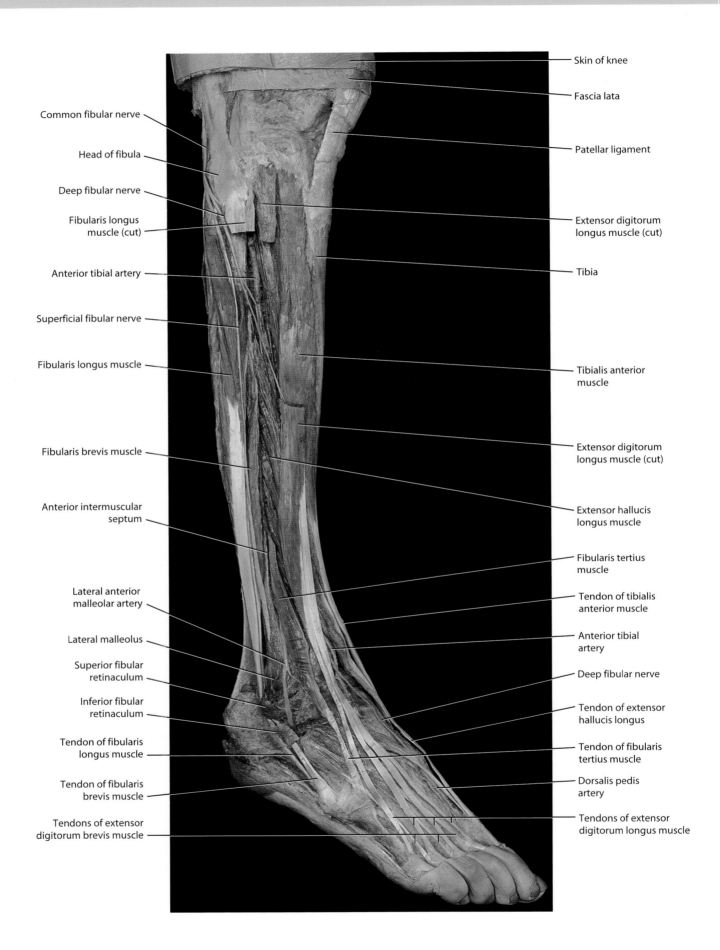

Skin of knee

Fascia lata

Common fibular nerve

Head of fibula

Patellar ligament

Deep fibular nerve

Fibularis longus muscle (cut)

Extensor digitorum longus muscle (cut)

Anterior tibial artery

Tibia

Superficial fibular nerve

Fibularis longus muscle

Tibialis anterior muscle

Fibularis brevis muscle

Extensor digitorum longus muscle (cut)

Anterior intermuscular septum

Extensor hallucis longus muscle

Fibularis tertius muscle

Lateral anterior malleolar artery

Tendon of tibialis anterior muscle

Lateral malleolus

Anterior tibial artery

Superior fibular retinaculum

Deep fibular nerve

Inferior fibular retinaculum

Tendon of extensor hallucis longus

Tendon of fibularis longus muscle

Tendon of fibularis tertius muscle

Tendon of fibularis brevis muscle

Dorsalis pedis artery

Tendons of extensor digitorum brevis muscle

Tendons of extensor digitorum longus muscle

Figure 44.5 Anterolateral leg – intermediate dissection. A dissection of the right anterolateral leg. The extensor digitorum longus and fibularis longus muscles have been cut to show the superficial and deep fibular nerves and the anterior tibial artery

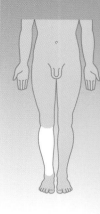

TABLE 44.1 MUSCLES OF THE ANTEROLATERAL LEG

Muscle	Origin	Insertion	Innervation	Action	Blood supply
Anterior muscles					
Tibialis anterior	Lateral condyle and proximal half of lateral tibia	Medial plantar surfaces of medial cuneiform and base of metatarsal I	Deep fibular nerve (L4, L5)	Dorsiflexes ankle and inverts foot	Anterior tibial artery
Extensor hallucis longus	Middle half of anterior surface of fibula and interosseous membrane	Base of distal phalanx of great toe (toe I)	Deep fibular nerve (L5, S1)	Extends toe I and dorsiflexes ankle	Anterior tibial artery
Extensor digitorum longus	Lateral condyle of tibia and proximal three-quarters of anterior surface of interosseous membrane	Middle and distal phalanges of toes II to V	Deep fibular nerve (L5, S1)	Extends toes II to V and dorsiflexes ankle	Anterior tibial artery
Fibularis tertius	Distal third of anterior surface of fibula and interosseous membrane	Dorsum of base of metatarsal V	Deep fibular nerve (L5, S1)	Dorsiflexes ankle and aids in eversion of foot	Anterior tibial artery
Lateral muscles					
Fibularis longus	Head and proximal two-thirds of lateral fibula	Plantar base of metatarsal I and medial cuneiform	Superficial fibular nerve (L5 to S2)	Everts foot and weakly plantarflexes ankle	Anterior tibial artery, fibular artery
Fibularis brevis	Distal two-thirds of lateral surface of fibula	Dorsal surface of tuberosity on base of metatarsal V	Superficial fibular nerve (L5 to S2)	Everts foot and weakly plantarflexes ankle	Fibular artery

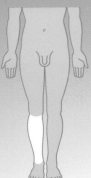

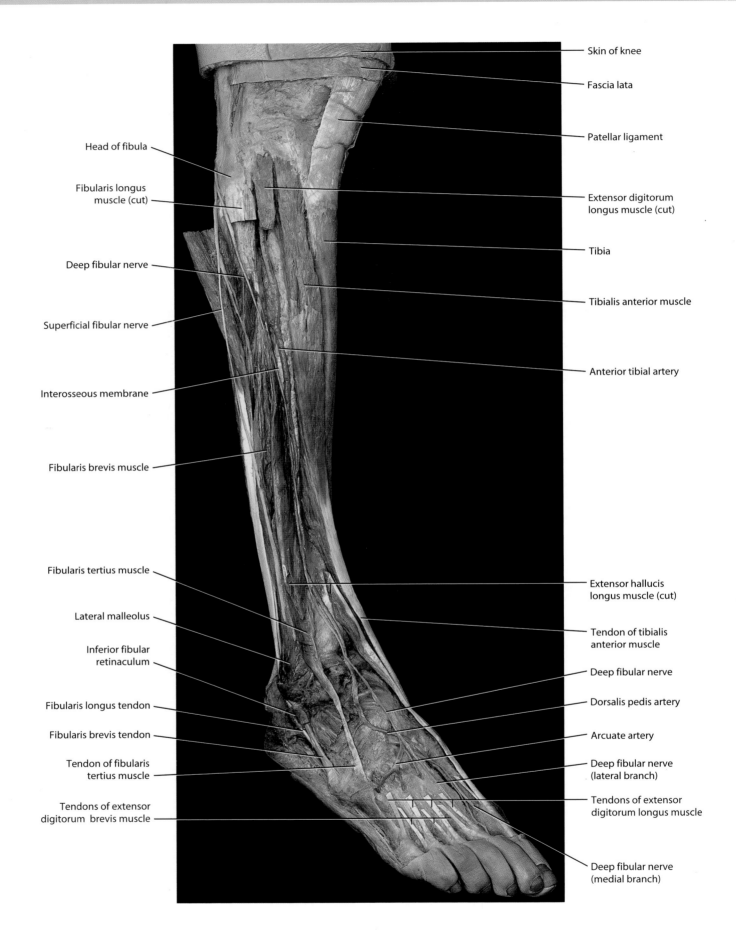

Head of fibula

Fibularis longus
muscle (cut)

Deep fibular nerve

Superficial fibular nerve

Interosseous membrane

Fibularis brevis muscle

Fibularis tertius muscle

Lateral malleolus

Inferior fibular
retinaculum

Fibularis longus tendon

Fibularis brevis tendon

Tendon of fibularis
tertius muscle

Tendons of extensor
digitorum brevis muscle

Skin of knee

Fascia lata

Patellar ligament

Extensor digitorum
longus muscle (cut)

Tibia

Tibialis anterior muscle

Anterior tibial artery

Extensor hallucis
longus muscle (cut)

Tendon of tibialis
anterior muscle

Deep fibular nerve

Dorsalis pedis artery

Arcuate artery

Deep fibular nerve
(lateral branch)

Tendons of extensor
digitorum longus muscle

Deep fibular nerve
(medial branch)

Figure 44.6 Anterolateral leg – deep dissection. This is a continuation of the dissection shown in Figure 44.5 of the right anterolateral leg. The extensor digitorum muscle and tendons have been removed to show the entire length of the anterior tibial artery, the dorsalis pedis artery, and superficial and deep fibular nerves. The deep fibular nerve is on the interosseous membrane

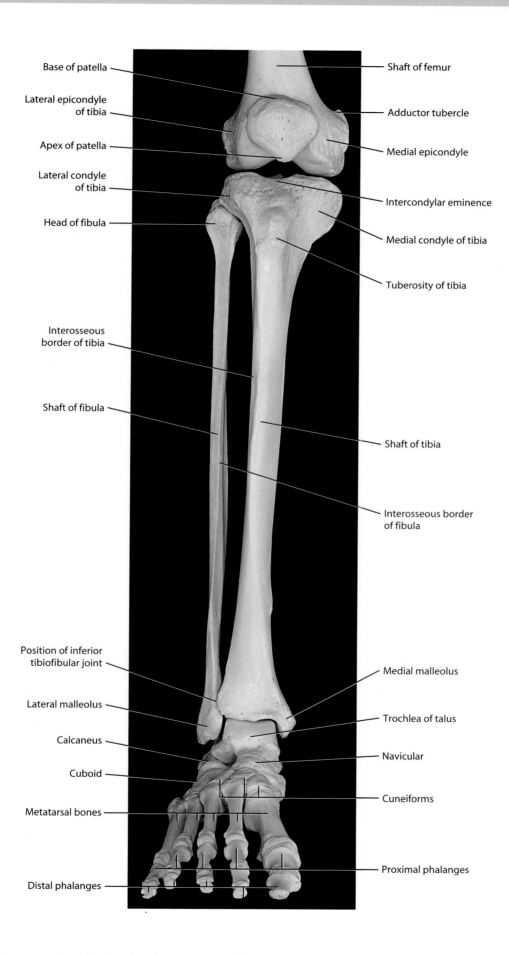

Base of patella

Lateral epicondyle of tibia

Apex of patella

Lateral condyle of tibia

Head of fibula

Interosseous border of tibia

Shaft of fibula

Position of inferior tibiofibular joint

Lateral malleolus

Calcaneus

Cuboid

Metatarsal bones

Distal phalanges

Shaft of femur

Adductor tubercle

Medial epicondyle

Intercondylar eminence

Medial condyle of tibia

Tuberosity of tibia

Shaft of tibia

Interosseous border of fibula

Medial malleolus

Trochlea of talus

Navicular

Cuneiforms

Proximal phalanges

Figure 44.7 Anterolateral leg – osteology. Anterior view showing the parallel arrangement of the tibia and fibula; they are united by an interosseous membrane to become one unit functionally

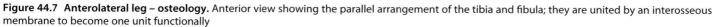

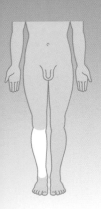

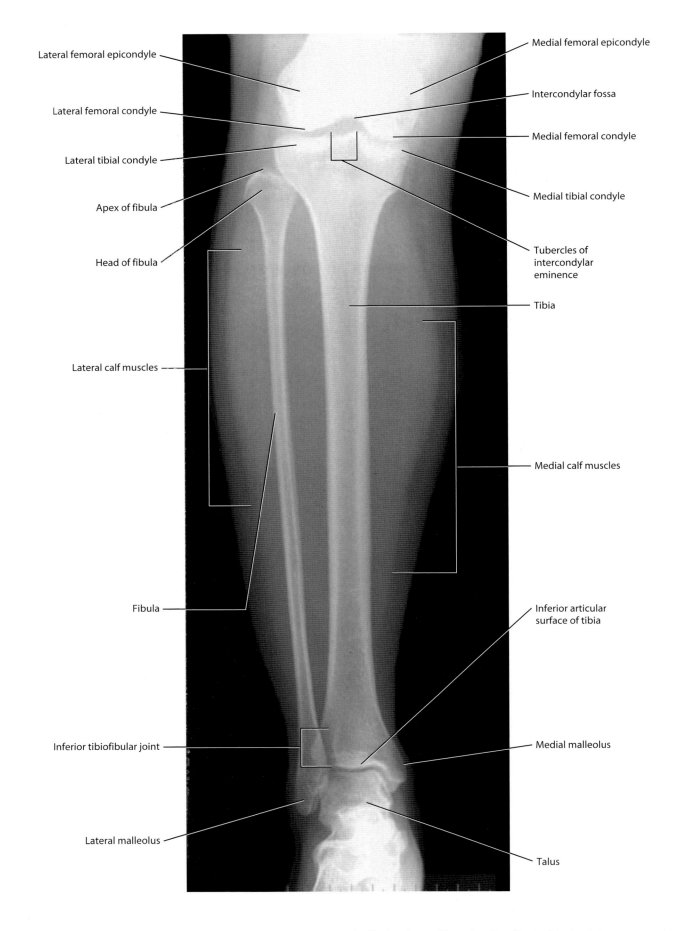

Lateral femoral epicondyle

Lateral femoral condyle

Lateral tibial condyle

Apex of fibula

Head of fibula

Lateral calf muscles

Fibula

Inferior tibiofibular joint

Lateral malleolus

Medial femoral epicondyle

Intercondylar fossa

Medial femoral condyle

Medial tibial condyle

Tubercles of intercondylar eminence

Tibia

Medial calf muscles

Inferior articular surface of tibia

Medial malleolus

Talus

Figure 44.8 Anterolateral leg – plain film radiograph (anteroposterior view). The fibula is located lateral to the tibia. In this view it is easy to see how weight is transferred from the femur to the tibia and then from the tibia to the talus. In plain film radiographs, soft tissue detail is not well delineated but the margin between muscle and cutaneous fat is visualized

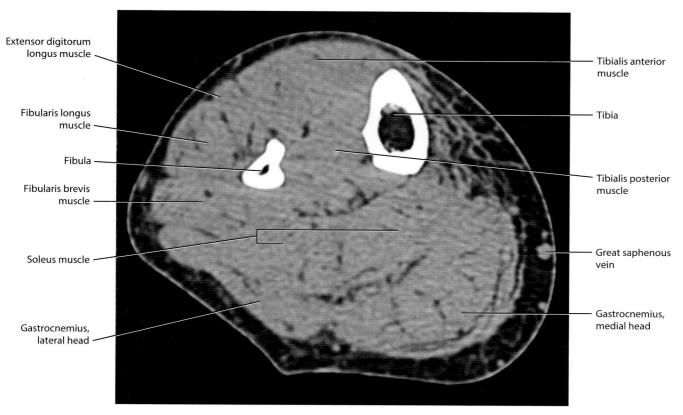

Extensor digitorum longus muscle

Fibularis longus muscle

Fibula

Fibularis brevis muscle

Soleus muscle

Gastrocnemius, lateral head

Tibialis anterior muscle

Tibia

Tibialis posterior muscle

Great saphenous vein

Gastrocnemius, medial head

Figure 44.9 Anterolateral leg – CT scan (axial view, from distal to proximal). Intermuscular definition is dependent on the amount of intermuscular fat. Note the position of the great saphenous vein

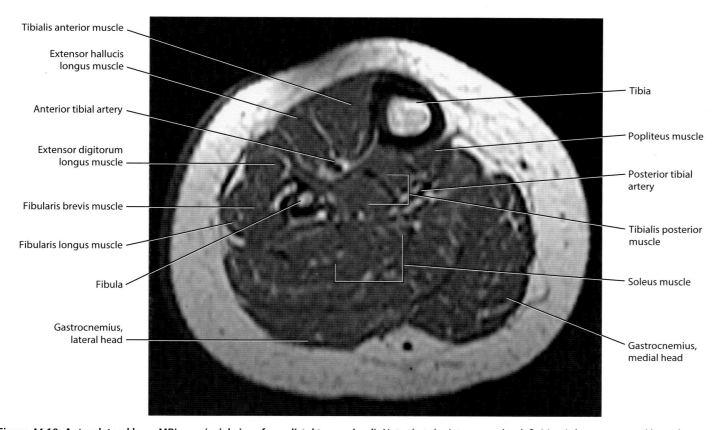

Tibialis anterior muscle

Extensor hallucis longus muscle

Anterior tibial artery

Extensor digitorum longus muscle

Fibularis brevis muscle

Fibularis longus muscle

Fibula

Gastrocnemius, lateral head

Tibia

Popliteus muscle

Posterior tibial artery

Tibialis posterior muscle

Soleus muscle

Gastrocnemius, medial head

Figure 44.10 Anterolateral leg – MRI scan (axial view, from distal to proximal). Note that the intermuscular definition is better assessed here than on CT scans due to the bright appearance of fat. Vessels are well visualized in black. Note the position of the tibialis anterior muscle

Posterior leg

The posterior leg (the calf) is between the knee and the ankle and contains superficial muscles that flex the ankle and deep muscles that flex the toes (Table 45.1). The bones of the leg, tibia, and fibula (see Chapter 44) provide support and muscle attachment for the posterior leg.

MUSCLES

The muscles of the posterior compartment of the leg are divided into superficial and deep groups by a thickened layer of deep fascia. The three **superficial muscles** plantarflex the ankle and are the **gastrocnemius, soleus,** and **plantaris** muscles (Fig. 45.1). They have a general origin from the femoral condyles and the superior part of the tibia and fibula. All three muscle tendons fuse inferiorly to the calcaneus through the large calcaneal tendon (Achilles' tendon).

The four **deep muscles** of the posterior leg are the **popliteus, flexor hallucis longus, flexor digitorum longus,** and **tibialis posterior** muscles (Fig. 45.2). With the exception of the popliteus muscle, they have a general origin from the posterior tibia and fibula and plantarflex the foot and toes. The popliteus muscle originates from the lateral condyle of the femur, inserts onto the posterior aspect of the superior tibia, and medially rotates the leg, so unlocking and flexing the hyperextended knee.

NERVES

The **tibial nerve** (L4 to S3) originates in the thigh as a division of the sciatic nerve and descends into the leg through the popliteal fossa. At this point it gives off the **medial sural cutaneous nerve,** which unites with the **lateral sural cutaneous nerve** (from the fibular nerve) to form the **sural nerve** (see Chapter 44). The sural nerve conveys sensation from the skin of the posterolateral leg and foot.

From the popliteal fossa, the tibial nerve enters the posterior compartment of the leg and innervates all superficial and deep posterior leg muscles. It continues distally and is located between the flexor digitorum longus and flexor hallucis longus tendons at the level of the medial malleolus of the ankle. On entering the foot, it divides into the **medial** and **lateral plantar nerves.**

ARTERIES

Branches of the **popliteal artery** supply the posterior leg.

The popliteal artery descends through the popliteal fossa of the knee and at the distal border of the popliteus muscle gives off the **anterior tibial artery,** which travels forward between the leg bones to the anterior compartment of leg. Before the anterior tibial artery pierces the interosseous membrane it usually gives off the **posterior tibial recurrent artery** medially and a small **circumflex fibular artery** laterally. Both these branches anastomose with the **inferior lateral genicular artery.**

The posterior branch of the popliteal artery – the **posterior tibial artery** – gives off muscular branches to the soleus and flexor digitorum longus muscles. Its largest branch is the **fibular artery,** which gives muscular branches to soleus, flexor hallucis longus, and tibialis posterior muscles, as well as to the two lateral fibularis muscles. At its distal end, the posterior tibial artery gives off a posterior **medial malleolar artery** (which anastomoses with the

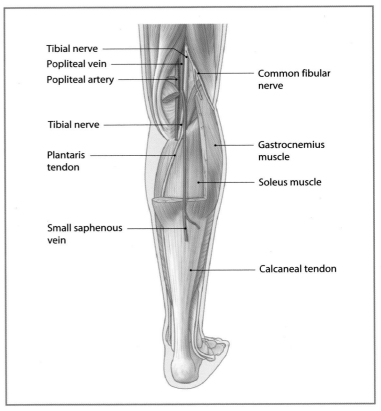

Figure 45.1 Superficial muscles of the posterior leg

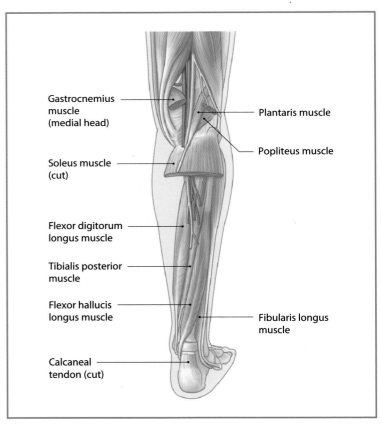

Figure 45.2 Deep muscles of the posterior leg

anterior medial malleolar artery) and a medial **calcaneal branch** (which travels to the medial and posterior heel).

As the posterior tibial artery descends in the deep leg it is accompanied by the tibial nerve and the posterior tibial vein. They pass posterior to the medial malleolus between the tendons of the flexor digitorum longus and flexor hallucis longus muscles. The posterior tibial artery divides into **medial** and **lateral plantar arteries** before entering the plantar surface of the foot.

VEINS AND LYMPHATICS

Superficial venous drainage of the posterior leg is through the **small saphenous vein**, which originates at the lateral end of the **dorsal venous arch of foot**. It ascends posteriorly to the lateral malleolus, along the back of the leg, and pierces the fascial roof of the popliteal fossa to enter the **popliteal vein**. Tributaries of the small saphenous vein communicate with the **great saphenous vein** and the deep veins that accompany the posterior tibial and fibular arteries. Contracting the muscles of the leg applies pressure to the deep veins and facilitates blood return to the heart.

Lymphatic vessels of the posterior leg follow the above-named vessels and drain into the **popliteal nodes**.

■ CLINICAL CORRELATIONS

Calcaneal tendon rupture

Calcaneal tendon rupture usually occurs during strenuous physical activity. A snapping sensation in the posterior ankle region is usually reported. An inability to walk because the foot cannot be plantarflexed is accompanied by severe calf pain (Fig. 45.3). The diagnosis is confirmed by Thompson's test (squeezing the gastrocnemius muscle). A positive Thompson's test results in plantarflexion of the foot. Calcaneal tendon rupture results in a negative Thompson's test. Treatment of calcaneal tendon rupture is either by nonsurgical casting or surgical repair of the tendon.

Atherosclerotic disease of the leg

Chronic arterial occlusive disease is caused by atherosclerosis and affects many arteries. In the thigh and leg, the superficial arteries risk becoming stenosed (narrowed) because of their smaller size. Sometimes this causes aching and cramping pain in the calves during exertion (walking or running), which is relieved by resting for a few minutes (intermittent claudication). This pain is reproducible, in that patients will say that walking a specific distance will cause the pain. Resting for a few minutes will relieve the pain and walking again will reactivate it. If a patient does not seek treatment at this stage, atherosclerotic changes in the vessels will continue until ischemic rest pain develops. This is a severe burning pain that usually occurs in the feet at night. Many patients try to alleviate the pain by hanging the affected foot over the side of the bed in a dependent position. The resulting vascular insufficiency can cause painful ulcers to develop on the foot (Fig. 45.4). Patients who do not seek medical treatment for ischemic rest pain are likely to need amputation at a later time.

A diagnosis of arterial occlusive disease of the lower limb can be confirmed by Doppler analysis, plethysmography, and Doppler ultrasound.

Treatment of arterial occlusive disease is initially medical and involves stopping smoking, weight reduction, exercise, and antiplatelet medication to prevent vascular complications. Most patients treated medically do not require amputation, but severe

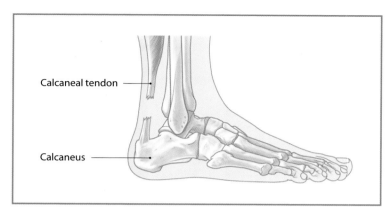

Figure 45.3 Rupture of the calcaneal tendon

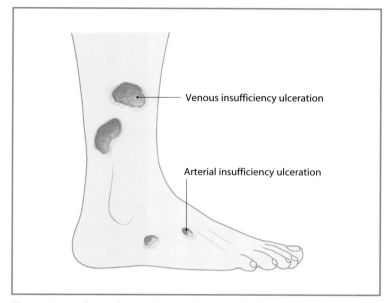

Figure 45.4 Atherosclerotic disease of the leg

symptoms and findings consistent with irreversible limb-threatening ischemia (cyanosis and tissue necrosis) will necessitate amputation.

Varicose veins

Varicose veins are enlarged superficial veins that usually occur in the lower limb. They result from incompetent valves within the veins and occur in around 10% of the population. Symptoms are pain, achiness, and heaviness of the affected leg, which is worsened by prolonged standing. Elastic stockings and avoiding prolonged standing can help alleviate some of the symptoms. Definitive treatment is sclerotherapy (injecting a sclerosing agent into the involved vein to cause it to shrink and close) or surgery. There are two types of surgery – vein stripping (removal of the involved veins) or proximal ligation of the great saphenous vein at the point where it enters the femoral vein in the groin.

MNEMONIC	
Origins of deep posterior leg muscles: (medial to lateral)	**Down The Hatch** (Flexor **D**igitorum longus, **T**ibialis posterior, flexor **H**allucis longus)

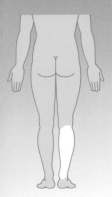

LOWER LIMB

Posterior leg

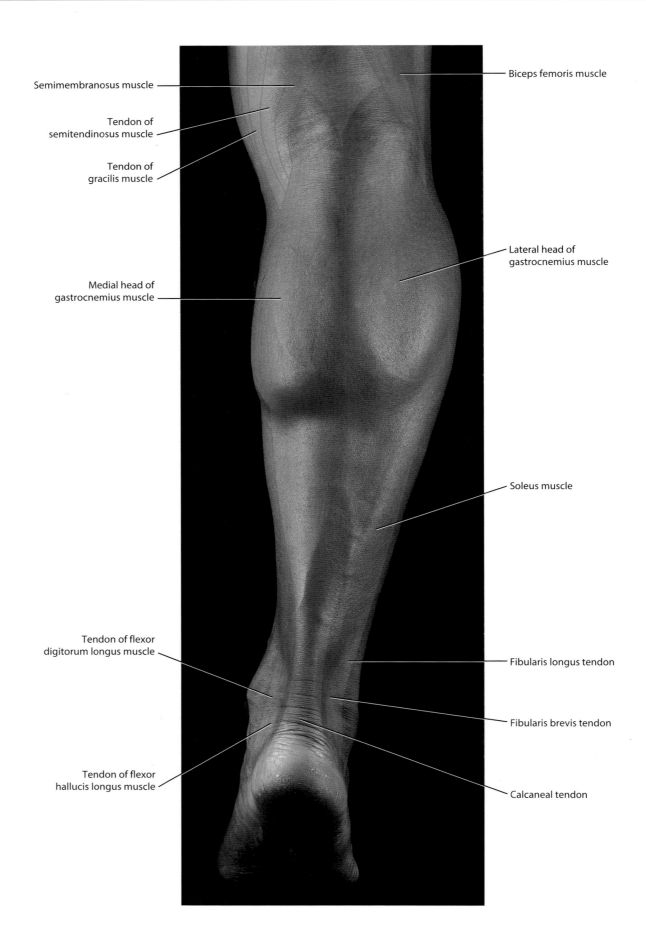

Semimembranosus muscle

Tendon of
semitendinosus muscle

Tendon of
gracilis muscle

Medial head of
gastrocnemius muscle

Tendon of flexor
digitorum longus muscle

Tendon of flexor
hallucis longus muscle

Biceps femoris muscle

Lateral head of
gastrocnemius muscle

Soleus muscle

Fibularis longus tendon

Fibularis brevis tendon

Calcaneal tendon

Figure 45.5 Posterior leg – surface anatomy. The heel is slightly raised by plantarflexion of the ankle. This enhances the heads of gastrocnemius and the calcaneal tendon

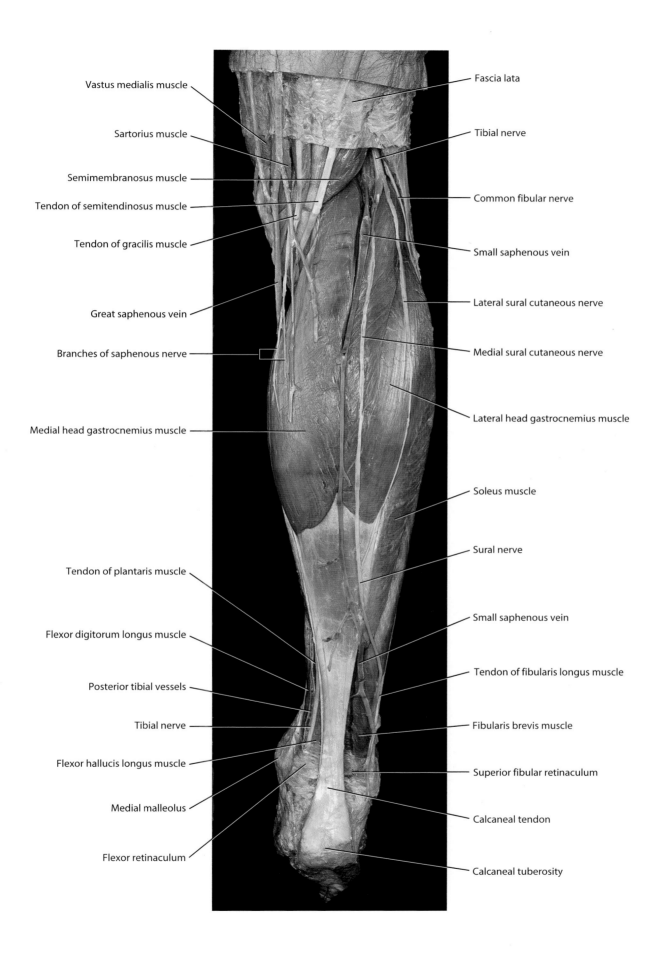

Vastus medialis muscle

Sartorius muscle

Semimembranosus muscle

Tendon of semitendinosus muscle

Tendon of gracilis muscle

Great saphenous vein

Branches of saphenous nerve

Medial head gastrocnemius muscle

Tendon of plantaris muscle

Flexor digitorum longus muscle

Posterior tibial vessels

Tibial nerve

Flexor hallucis longus muscle

Medial malleolus

Flexor retinaculum

Fascia lata

Tibial nerve

Common fibular nerve

Small saphenous vein

Lateral sural cutaneous nerve

Medial sural cutaneous nerve

Lateral head gastrocnemius muscle

Soleus muscle

Sural nerve

Small saphenous vein

Tendon of fibularis longus muscle

Fibularis brevis muscle

Superior fibular retinaculum

Calcaneal tendon

Calcaneal tuberosity

Figure 45.6 Posterior leg – superficial dissection. Observe the small saphenous vein along the midline of the posterior leg

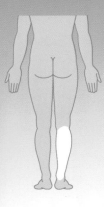

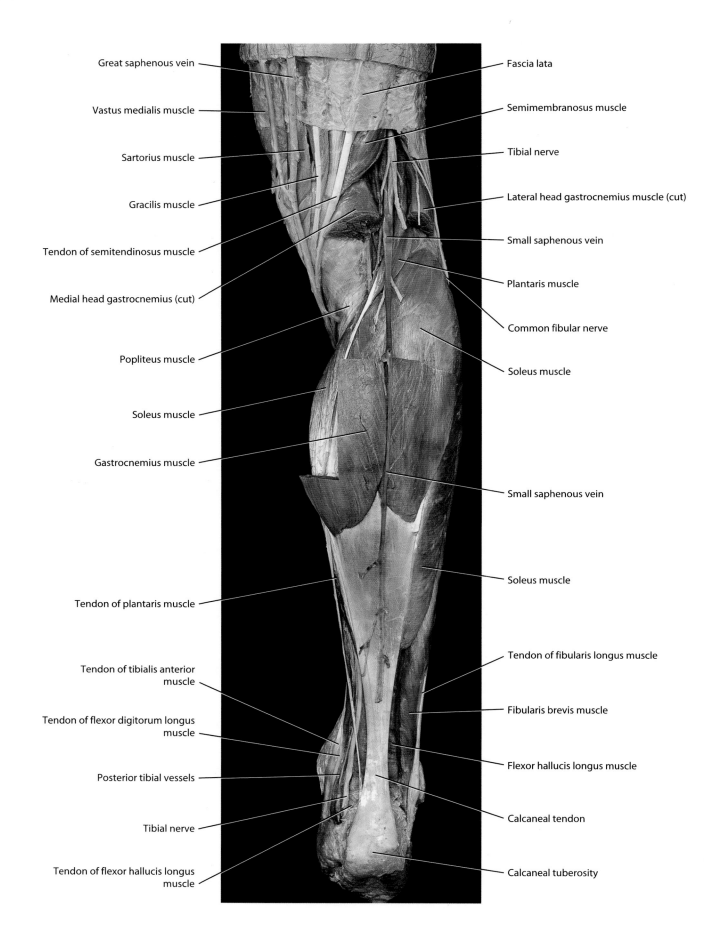

Great saphenous vein

Vastus medialis muscle

Sartorius muscle

Gracilis muscle

Tendon of semitendinosus muscle

Medial head gastrocnemius (cut)

Popliteus muscle

Soleus muscle

Gastrocnemius muscle

Tendon of plantaris muscle

Tendon of tibialis anterior muscle

Tendon of flexor digitorum longus muscle

Posterior tibial vessels

Tibial nerve

Tendon of flexor hallucis longus muscle

Fascia lata

Semimembranosus muscle

Tibial nerve

Lateral head gastrocnemius muscle (cut)

Small saphenous vein

Plantaris muscle

Common fibular nerve

Soleus muscle

Small saphenous vein

Soleus muscle

Tendon of fibularis longus muscle

Fibularis brevis muscle

Flexor hallucis longus muscle

Calcaneal tendon

Calcaneal tuberosity

Figure 45.7 Posterior leg – intermediate dissection. The gastrocnemius muscle has been partly removed to show some of the deeper structures – soleus muscle, popliteal artery, tendon of plantaris muscle

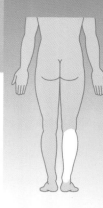

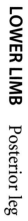

		TABLE 45.1 MUSCLES OF THE POSTERIOR LEG			
Muscle	**Origin**	**Insertion**	**Innervation**	**Action**	**Blood supply**
Superficial muscles					
Gastrocnemius	Lateral head – lateral aspect of lateral condyle of femur. Medial head – popliteal surface and medial condyle of femur	Posterior aspect of calcaneus via the calcaneal tendon	Tibial nerve (S1, S2)	Plantarflexes the ankle joint, assists in flexion of the knee joint	Popliteal artery
Soleus	Posterior aspect of head of fibula, proximal fourth of posterior surface of fibula, soleal line of tibia	Posterior aspect of calcaneus via the calcaneal tendon	Tibial nerve (S1, S2)	Plantarflexes the ankle and stabilizes the leg over the foot	Posterior tibia artery, fibular artery, popliteal artery
Plantaris	Popliteal surface of femur	Calcaneal tendon	Tibial nerve (L5, S1)	Weakly assists gastrocnemius	Popliteal artery
Deep muscles					
Popliteus	Lateral aspect of lateral condyle of femur and lateral meniscus	Posterior tibia above soleal line	Tibial nerve (L4 to S1)	Medially rotates the knee	Popliteal artery
Flexor hallucis longus	Distal two-thirds of posterior fibula and inferior part of interosseous membrane	Base of distal phalanx of great toe (toe I)	Tibial nerve (L5 to S2)	Flexes toe I, plantarflexes the ankle	Fibular artery
Flexor digitorum longus	Medial part of posterior tibia inferior to soleal line	Plantar bases of distal phalanges of lateral four toes	Tibial nerve (L5, S1)	Flexes lateral four toes, plantarflexes ankle	Posterior tibial artery
Tibialis posterior	Lateral part of posterior tibia, interosseous membrane, proximal half of posterior fibula	Tuberosity of navicular bone, all cuneiforms, cuboid and bases of metatarsals II to IV	Tibial nerve (L5, S1)	Plantarflexes the ankle and inverts the foot	Fibular artery

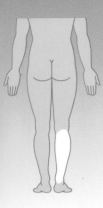

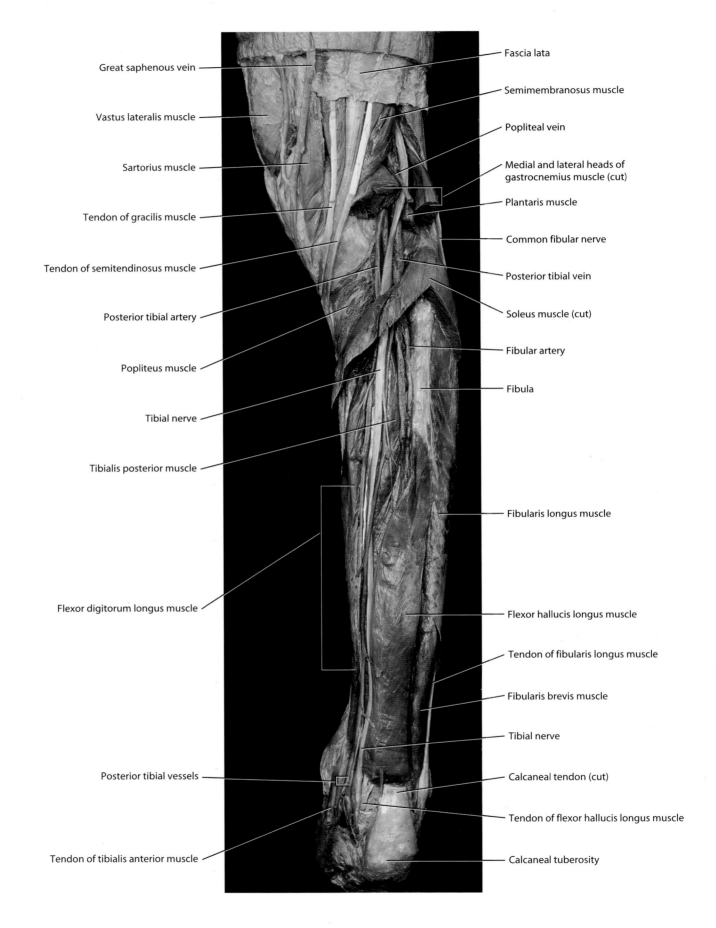

Great saphenous vein

Vastus lateralis muscle

Sartorius muscle

Tendon of gracilis muscle

Tendon of semitendinosus muscle

Posterior tibial artery

Popliteus muscle

Tibial nerve

Tibialis posterior muscle

Flexor digitorum longus muscle

Posterior tibial vessels

Tendon of tibialis anterior muscle

Fascia lata

Semimembranosus muscle

Popliteal vein

Medial and lateral heads of gastrocnemius muscle (cut)

Plantaris muscle

Common fibular nerve

Posterior tibial vein

Soleus muscle (cut)

Fibular artery

Fibula

Fibularis longus muscle

Flexor hallucis longus muscle

Tendon of fibularis longus muscle

Fibularis brevis muscle

Tibial nerve

Calcaneal tendon (cut)

Tendon of flexor hallucis longus muscle

Calcaneal tuberosity

Figure 45.8 Posterior leg – deep dissection. The gastrocnemius, and soleus muscles have been almost completely removed. The popliteus muscle can therefore be seen more clearly and the other deep muscles (flexor digitorum longus, tibialis posterior, and flexor hallucis longus) can be seen in their entirety. The tibial nerve is seen passing from the knee to the ankle

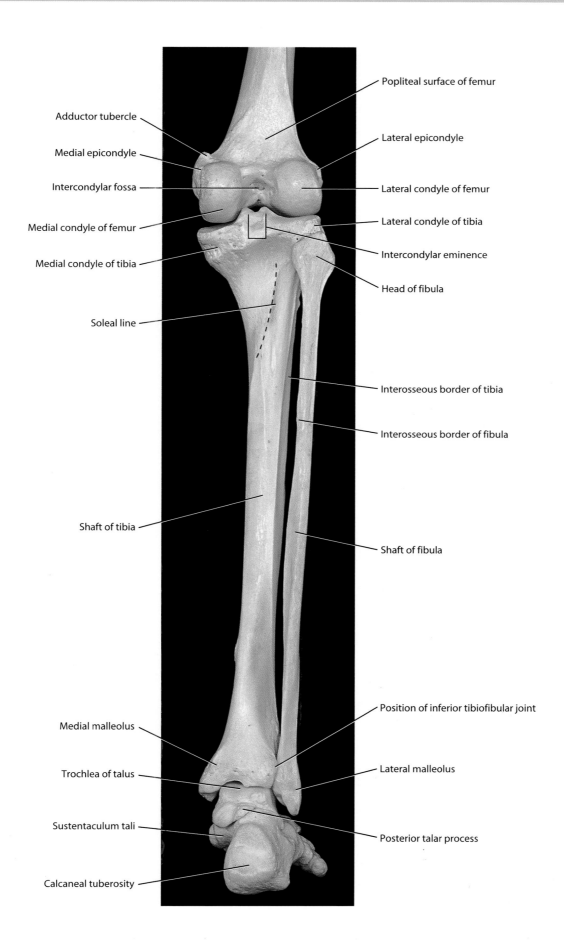

Adductor tubercle

Medial epicondyle

Intercondylar fossa

Medial condyle of femur

Medial condyle of tibia

Soleal line

Shaft of tibia

Medial malleolus

Trochlea of talus

Sustentaculum tali

Calcaneal tuberosity

Popliteal surface of femur

Lateral epicondyle

Lateral condyle of femur

Lateral condyle of tibia

Intercondylar eminence

Head of fibula

Interosseous border of tibia

Interosseous border of fibula

Shaft of fibula

Position of inferior tibiofibular joint

Lateral malleolus

Posterior talar process

LOWER LIMB   Posterior leg

Figure 45.9 Posterior leg – osteology. Posterior view of the articulated leg bones. Note the soleal line (dotted) and the shallow popliteal depression just above it

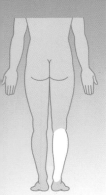

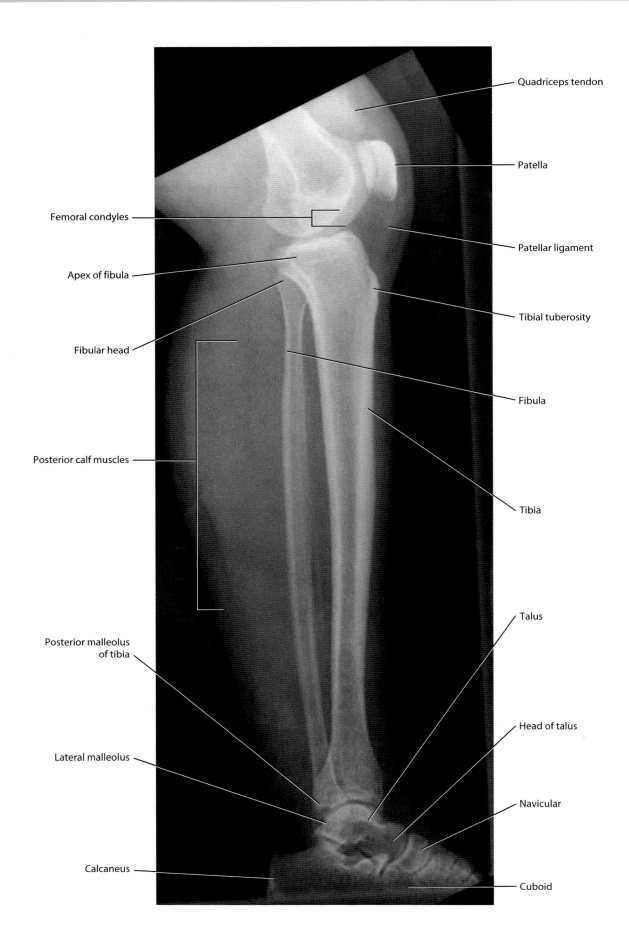

Quadriceps tendon

Patella

Femoral condyles

Patellar ligament

Apex of fibula

Tibial tuberosity

Fibular head

Fibula

Posterior calf muscles

Tibia

Talus

Posterior malleolus
of tibia

Head of talus

Lateral malleolus

Navicular

Calcaneus

Cuboid

Figure 45.10 Posterior leg – plain film radiograph (lateral view). Note that the majority of the muscle bulk is posterior. From a lateral perspective it is easy to see that the tibia is located more anteriorly than the fibula

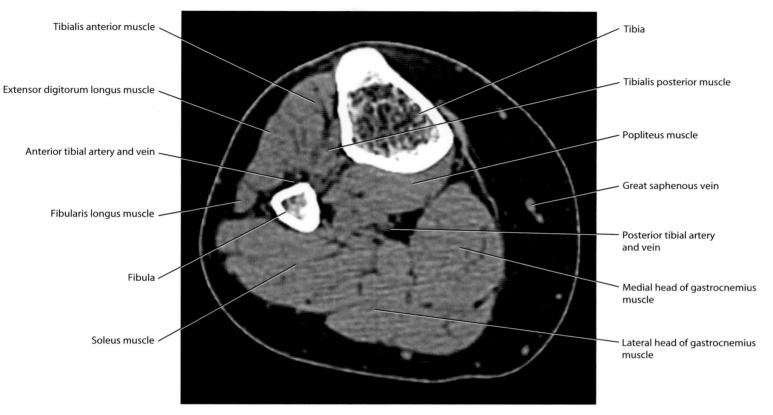

Tibialis anterior muscle

Extensor digitorum longus muscle

Anterior tibial artery and vein

Fibularis longus muscle

Fibula

Soleus muscle

Tibia

Tibialis posterior muscle

Popliteus muscle

Great saphenous vein

Posterior tibial artery and vein

Medial head of gastrocnemius muscle

Lateral head of gastrocnemius muscle

Figure 45.11 Posterior leg – CT scan (axial view, from distal to proximal). This scan is at the level of the tibial tubercle. Observe the location of the posterior tibial artery and vein deep within the leg. Also note the great saphenous vein within the subcutaneous tissue of the medial leg

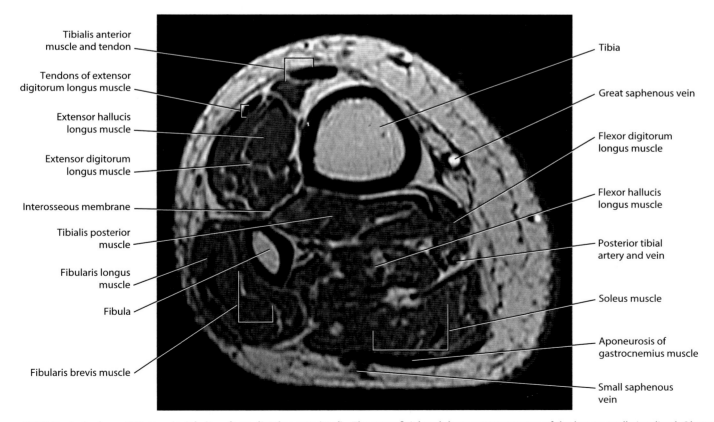

Tibialis anterior muscle and tendon

Tendons of extensor digitorum longus muscle

Extensor hallucis longus muscle

Extensor digitorum longus muscle

Interosseous membrane

Tibialis posterior muscle

Fibularis longus muscle

Fibula

Fibularis brevis muscle

Tibia

Great saphenous vein

Flexor digitorum longus muscle

Flexor hallucis longus muscle

Posterior tibial artery and vein

Soleus muscle

Aponeurosis of gastrocnemius muscle

Small saphenous vein

Figure 45.12 Posterior leg – MRI scan (axial view, from distal to proximal). The superficial and deep compartments of the leg are well visualized. Observe the location of the tibialis posterior muscle. The tendons appear black because of their dense fibrous nature

559

46 Ankle and foot joints

The **ankle joint** is a freely moving hinge joint between the leg and the foot. It is formed by the lower ends of the tibia and fibula and the **trochlea** of the talus. The tibia and the fibula form a socket that is wider anteriorly than posteriorly, and the talus moves in the socket during dorsiflexion and plantarflexion of the ankle. The joint capsule of the ankle is thickened on each side by ligaments (Figs 46.1 and 46.2).

The foot consists of individual bones supported by ligaments and muscles (Fig. 46.3). All joints between the bones in the foot are synovial. Together, the bones and joints create an arch that supports the body's weight, serves as a shock absorber, and acts as a lever to propel the body forward.

The most important joints in the foot are the **subtalar**, **talocalcaneonavicular**, and **calcaneocuboid joints**. The last two form the **transverse tarsal joint**. The subtalar joint is where the talus rests on the calcaneus and where most of the inversion and eversion movements of the foot occur. It has a joint capsule reinforced by ligaments. The remaining joints are listed in Table 46.1.

LIGAMENTS AND FASCIA

Because of the angle at the junction of the leg and foot, the tendons of the extrinsic foot muscles need to be bound down by fascial bands (retinacula). On the lateral side of the ankle, the fibularis muscle tendons are kept in place by the **superior fibular retinaculum**, which joins the lateral malleolus to the calcaneus. The **inferior fibular retinaculum** between the dorsum of the foot and the lateral aspect of the calcaneus prevents displacement of these tendons.

On the medial side of the ankle, the **flexor retinaculum** (between the medial malleolus and the calcaneus, plantar aponeurosis, and adjacent bony prominences of the foot) helps maintain the position of the flexor tendons from the posterior leg.

On the front of the ankle, two extensor retinacula prevent the extensor muscle tendons from bowing during extension (dorsiflexion) of the foot and toes. A **superior extensor retinaculum** is attached to the anterior borders of the fibula and tibia. A Y-shaped **inferior extensor retinaculum** has its lateral base on the upper calcaneus, and its arms are attached to the medial malleolus and the medial side of the plantar aponeurosis.

The fibrous joint capsule of the ankle joint is thin anteriorly and posteriorly, but supported on each side by strong collateral ligaments. It is reinforced medially by the strong **medial (deltoid) ligament**, which contains superficial and deep fibers that arise from the medial malleolus and insert onto the talus, navicular, and calcaneus bones of the foot. The main function of the medial ligament is to prevent eversion of the foot.

The **lateral ligament** is composed of three separate bands that arise from the lateral malleolus and insert onto the neck of the talus (**anterior talofibular ligament**), the calcaneus (**calcaneofibular ligament**), and the lateral tubercle of the talus (**posterior talofibular ligament**). The lateral ligament is weaker than the medial ligament and prevents inversion of the foot.

The foot has numerous dorsal and plantar ligaments (Figs 46.3 and 46.4), but three ligaments maintain the important **longitudinal arch of foot**:

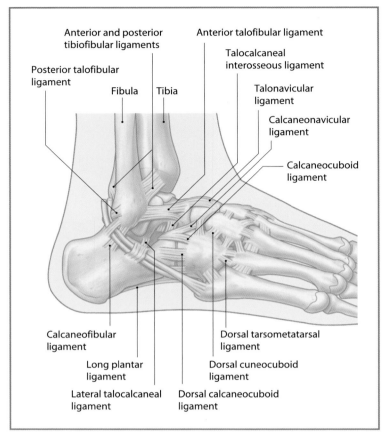

Figure 46.1 Lateral view of ankle ligaments

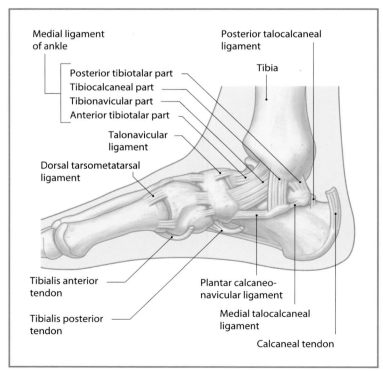

Figure 46.2 Medial view of ankle ligaments

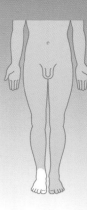

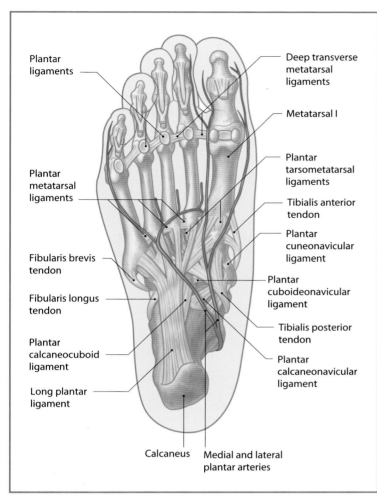

Figure 46.3 Plantar surface showing ligaments and arterial supply

Labels (clockwise from top left):
Plantar ligaments
Plantar metatarsal ligaments
Fibularis brevis tendon
Fibularis longus tendon
Plantar calcaneocuboid ligament
Long plantar ligament
Calcaneus
Medial and lateral plantar arteries
Plantar calcaneonavicular ligament
Tibialis posterior tendon
Plantar cuboideonavicular ligament
Plantar cuneonavicular ligament
Tibialis anterior tendon
Plantar tarsometatarsal ligaments
Metatarsal I
Deep transverse metatarsal ligaments

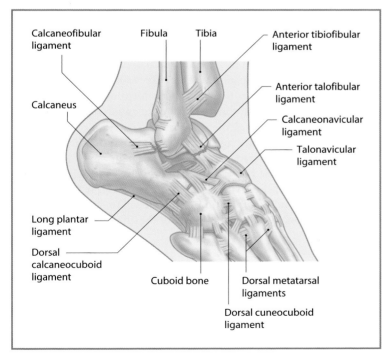

Figure 46.4 Dorsal ligaments of the foot

Labels:
Calcaneofibular ligament
Calcaneus
Long plantar ligament
Dorsal calcaneocuboid ligament
Cuboid bone
Fibula
Tibia
Dorsal metatarsal ligaments
Dorsal cuneocuboid ligament
Anterior tibiofibular ligament
Anterior talofibular ligament
Calcaneonavicular ligament
Talonavicular ligament

- the **plantar calcaneonavicular ligament** (spring ligament) connects the sustentaculum tali of the calcaneus to the navicular bone and strengthens the longitudinal arch of the foot;
- the **long plantar ligament** extends from the calcaneus to the tuberosity of the cuboid bone – some fibers extend to the bases of the metatarsals, forming a tunnel for the tendon of the fibularis longus muscle;
- the **plantar calcaneocuboid ligament** (short plantar ligament) is deep to the long plantar ligament and extends from the calcaneus to the inferior surface of the cuboid.

STRUCTURES AROUND THE ANKLE JOINT

The ankle joint has no intrinsic muscles. Instead, muscle tendons from the three compartments of the leg extend across the ankle to the foot. These structures provide additional support to the ankle joint and facilitate movement.

On the medial side of the ankle joint, just posterior to the medial malleolus, are (from anterior to posterior):

- the tendons of tibialis posterior and flexor digitorum longus muscles;
- the posterior tibial vein and artery, and tibial nerve;
- the tendon of flexor hallucis longus muscle;
- the calcaneal tendon, which is the most posterior structure at the ankle.

The main structures on the anterior surface of the ankle between the malleoli are (from medial to lateral):

- the tendon of the tibialis anterior muscle;
- the dorsalis pedis artery;
- the deep fibular nerve;
- the extensor hallucis longus muscle;
- the extensor digitorum longus muscle.

The cutaneous nerves at the ankle are the sural, superficial fibular, and saphenous nerves and cutaneous branches of the tibial nerve.

DEEP FOOT MUSCLES

Four dorsal and three plantar interosseous muscles (interossei) are the deepest muscles of the foot and all are innervated by the **lateral plantar nerve** (see Chapter 47):

- the **dorsal interossei** abduct the toes, help flex the metatarsophalangeal joints, and extend the interphalangeal joints of the toes;
- the **plantar interossei** adduct the toes and assist the dorsal interossei with flexing the metatarsophalangeal joints and extending the interphalangeal joints (see Table 46.1).

NERVES

The ankle and foot joints are innervated by branches of the **tibial** and **deep fibular nerves** as they pass each joint. Injury to these nerves, for example with ankle sprain, can cause problems with joint proprioception (see below). The cutaneous nerves that pass the ankle are the **saphenous**, **superficial fibular**, **deep fibular**, and **sural nerves**. In addition, the **medial** and **lateral plantar nerves** from the tibial nerve convey sensation from the plantar surface of the foot. **Calcaneal branches** from the tibial and sural nerves innervate the heel.

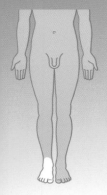
ARTERIES

Blood is supplied to the ankle and the foot by three arteries that descend from the leg:

- the **anterior tibial artery** gives off medial and lateral malleolar arteries to the ankle before becoming the **dorsalis pedis artery**, which supplies the foot;
- the **posterior tibial artery** supplies the ankle and then descends posteriorly to the medial malleolus, where it divides into the **medial** and **lateral plantar arteries** of the foot;
- the **fibular artery** (a branch of the posterior tibial artery), gives off a **lateral malleolar branch** to the ankle.

VEINS AND LYMPHATICS

Venous drainage of the deep structures of the foot and ankle follows the major arteries listed above. The skin and superficial tissues drain to the great and small saphenous veins.

The lymphatics of the foot and ankle also follow the major arteries and drain superiorly. The medial foot drains to the medial superficial lymphatic vessels, which accompany the great saphenous vein to the groin. The lateral foot drains to the lateral superficial lymphatic vessels, which follow the small saphenous vein and drain toward the **popliteal nodes**.

ARCHES OF THE FOOT

The two major arches of the foot are the transverse and longitudinal arches.

The **transverse arch of foot** between the medial and lateral foot is formed by the navicular, three cuneiform bones (medial, intermediate and lateral), and cuboid bones, and by the bases of each metatarsal bone.

The **longitudinal arch of foot** has two parts:

- the **medial part** is composed of the calcaneus, talus, navicular, cuneiforms, and metatarsals I, II and III;
- the **lateral part**, which is flatter than the medial part, is on the lateral side of the foot and comprises the calcaneus and cuboid, and the lateral two metatarsals.

The integrity of these bony arches is maintained by the supporting ligaments and the plantar aponeurosis (see Chapter 47). The arches provide the foot with resilience, so minimizing degeneration of the joints of the ankle, foot, and lower limb.

■ CLINICAL CORRELATIONS

Lateral ankle sprain

Injuries caused by rolling the ankle inward (inversion) cause a lateral ankle sprain. A sprain is defined as a torn ligament. In lateral ankle sprains the most commonly injured ligament is the anterior talofibular ligament. Patients usually report carrying out some kind of ambulatory activity (walking, running, playing sport) during which they accidentally roll their ankle inward and experience pain and swelling. Typical findings on physical examination are edema of the lateral ankle and pain over the injured ligament. Point tenderness and bone deformity suggest a fracture and radiographs should be obtained. Treatment involves support bandages, casting or crutches, and avoiding strenuous activity until healing occurs. Pain killers can be used. Ligament injuries usually take at least six months to heal. Medial ankle

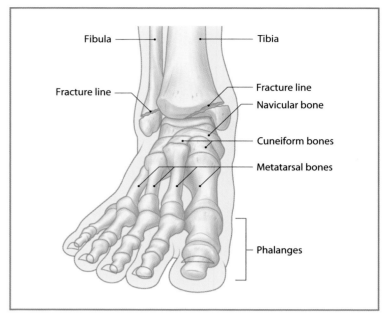

Figure 46.5 Ankle fracture (dorsal view)

sprains are rare because of the high strength of the deltoid ligament.

Ankle fracture

An ankle fracture occurs when the force applied to the ankle exceeds the strength of its bones. The medial and lateral malleoli are the weakest points and account for most ankle fractures (Fig. 46.5); the talus and calcaneus are strong bones and usually do not break with nonmajor ankle trauma. Symptoms are pain, swelling, and inability to bear weight on the affected limb. On examination, there is point tenderness on the bone and bone deformity. Radiographs are carried out to confirm and delineate the diagnosis. Treatment depends on the severity and type of the fracture. Unstable ankle fractures, such as bimalleolar fractures (fracture of the medial and lateral malleoli), are repaired surgically.

Ingrown toenail (onychocryptosis)

Overgrowth of the toenail into the soft tissues at the medial or lateral nail margin can cause pain. This may result from poor foot care, badly fitting shoes, or hereditary placement of the nailbed on the toe, and causes pain at the margins of the involved toe (usually the great toe). Without treatment, persistent irritation can lead to breakdown of the skin and infection. On examination, the toe is swollen, erythematous (red), and tender. The pain can be out of proportion, and a very small amount of pressure can elicit a great deal of pain. Treatment involves soaks, antibiotics (if indicated to treat infection), and manipulation of the toenail to facilitate normal growth. Occasionally, surgical removal of the affected part of the nail is necessary.

MNEMONIC	
Structures traveling behind medial malleolus (anterior to posterior)	**Tom, Dick and Harry** (**T**ibialis posterior, flexor **D**igitorum longus, flexor **H**allucis longus)
	('and' = space with neurovascular structures: **VAN** – posteriortibial **V**ein and **A**rtery, tibial **N**erve)

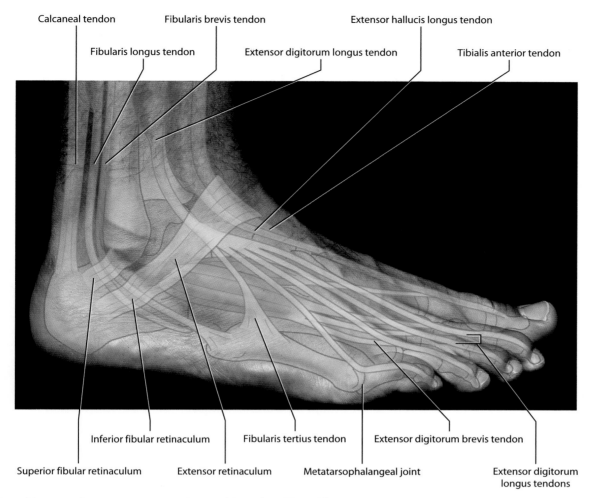

Calcaneal tendon

Fibularis longus tendon

Fibularis brevis tendon

Extensor digitorum longus tendon

Extensor hallucis longus tendon

Tibialis anterior tendon

Superior fibular retinaculum

Inferior fibular retinaculum

Extensor retinaculum

Fibularis tertius tendon

Metatarsophalangeal joint

Extensor digitorum brevis tendon

Extensor digitorum longus tendons

Figure 46.6 Ankle and foot – surface anatomy 1. Lateral view of the right ankle and foot

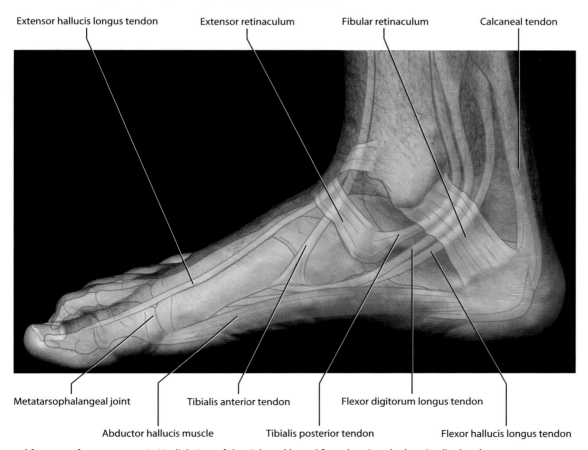

Extensor hallucis longus tendon

Extensor retinaculum

Fibular retinaculum

Calcaneal tendon

Metatarsophalangeal joint

Abductor hallucis muscle

Tibialis anterior tendon

Tibialis posterior tendon

Flexor digitorum longus tendon

Flexor hallucis longus tendon

Figure 46.7 Ankle and foot – surface anatomy 2. Medial view of the right ankle and foot showing the longitudinal arch

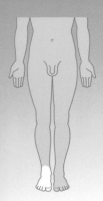

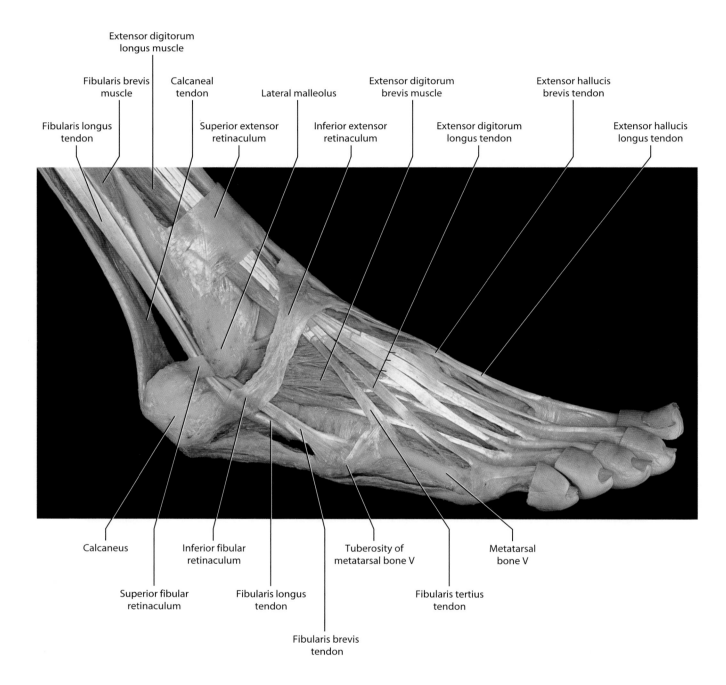

Extensor digitorum
longus muscle

Fibularis brevis
muscle

Calcaneal
tendon

Lateral malleolus

Extensor digitorum
brevis muscle

Extensor hallucis
brevis tendon

Fibularis longus
tendon

Superior extensor
retinaculum

Inferior extensor
retinaculum

Extensor digitorum
longus tendon

Extensor hallucis
longus tendon

Calcaneus

Inferior fibular
retinaculum

Tuberosity of
metatarsal bone V

Metatarsal
bone V

Superior fibular
retinaculum

Fibularis longus
tendon

Fibularis tertius
tendon

Fibularis brevis
tendon

Figure 46.8 Ankle and foot – superficial dissection 1. Lateral view of a right ankle and foot. Note the long extensor tendons covering the only intrinsic muscle of the dorsum (extensor digitorum brevis muscle). Observe how the tendons passing from the leg to the foot are kept in place by the extensor retinacula around the ankle

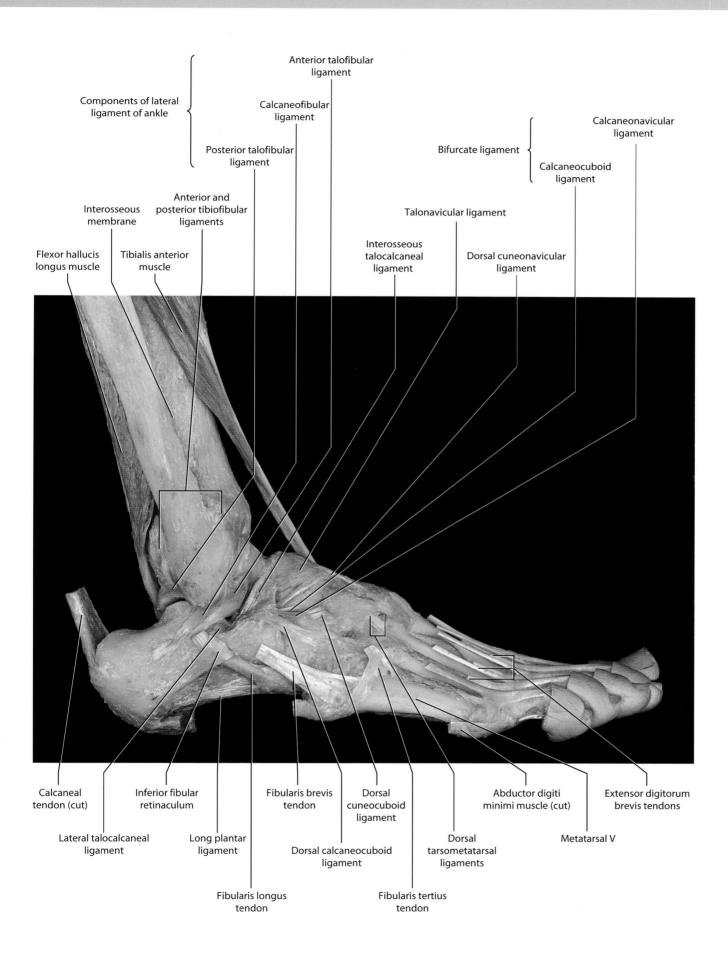

Components of lateral ligament of ankle

Anterior talofibular ligament

Calcaneofibular ligament

Posterior talofibular ligament

Anterior and posterior tibiofibular ligaments

Interosseous membrane

Flexor hallucis longus muscle

Tibialis anterior muscle

Calcaneonavicular ligament

Bifurcate ligament

Calcaneocuboid ligament

Talonavicular ligament

Interosseous talocalcaneal ligament

Dorsal cuneonavicular ligament

Calcaneal tendon (cut)

Inferior fibular retinaculum

Fibularis brevis tendon

Dorsal cuneocuboid ligament

Abductor digiti minimi muscle (cut)

Extensor digitorum brevis tendons

Lateral talocalcaneal ligament

Long plantar ligament

Dorsal calcaneocuboid ligament

Dorsal tarsometatarsal ligaments

Metatarsal V

Fibularis longus tendon

Fibularis tertius tendon

Figure 46.9 Ankle and foot – deep dissection 1. Lateral view of a right ankle and foot. Observe the ligaments and tendons that support the foot and particularly the three ligaments that form the lateral ligament of the ankle

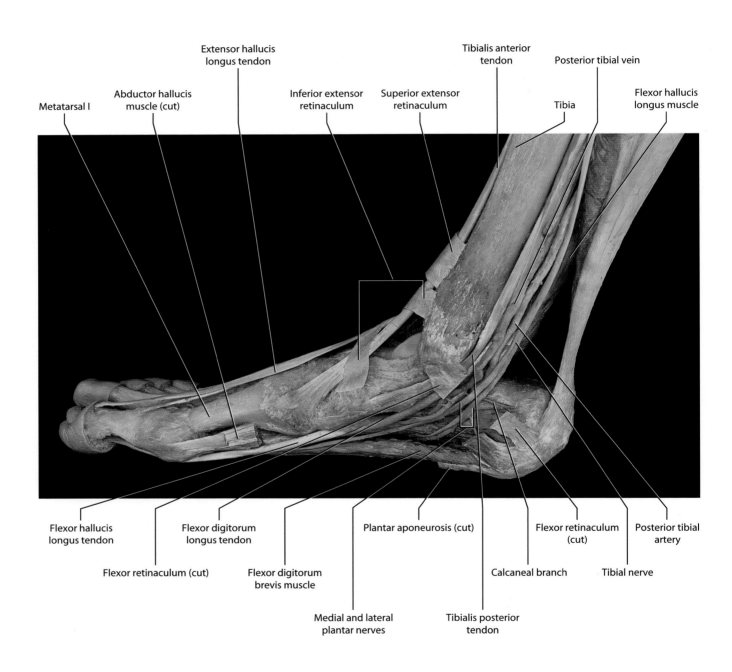

Metatarsal I

Abductor hallucis
muscle (cut)

Extensor hallucis
longus tendon

Inferior extensor
retinaculum

Superior extensor
retinaculum

Tibialis anterior
tendon

Tibia

Posterior tibial vein

Flexor hallucis
longus muscle

Flexor hallucis
longus tendon

Flexor retinaculum (cut)

Flexor digitorum
longus tendon

Flexor digitorum
brevis muscle

Medial and lateral
plantar nerves

Plantar aponeurosis (cut)

Tibialis posterior
tendon

Calcaneal branch

Flexor retinaculum
(cut)

Tibial nerve

Posterior tibial
artery

Figure 46.10 Ankle and foot – superficial dissection 2. Medial view of a right foot and ankle dissection. This shows the tendons of the deep posterior leg muscles with their nerves and vessels reaching the plantar surface by passing posterior to the medial malleolus. The tibialis anterior, tibialis posterior, and calcaneal tendons are visible

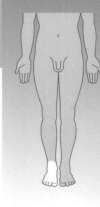

TABLE 46.1 JOINTS OF THE ANKLE AND FOOT

Joint	Type	Articular surface	Ligaments	Function/description
Inferior tibiofibular	Fibrous union (syndesmosis)	Concave facet of tibia and convex facet of fibula	Anterior tibiofibular Posterior tibiofibular	Runs inferiorly and laterally Thicker and broader, runs in same direction as anterior tibiofibular Strong principal connector
Ankle (talocrural)	Hinge-type synovial joint	Talus and distal tibia (tibiotalar) and talus and fibula (talofibular)	Medial – anterior tibiotalar – tibionavicular – tibiocalcaneal – posterior tibiotalar Lateral – anterior talofibular – calcaneofibular – posterior talofibular	Fan-shaped 'deltoid' ligament: – controls plantarflexion – controls abduction (eversion) – controls abduction (eversion) – controls dorsiflexion Weaker and more prone to injury – controls plantarflexion (1° stabilizer) – controls adduction (inversion) – controls dorsiflexion
Subtalar (talocalcaneal)	Plane-type synovial joint	Inferior surface of body of talus with superior surface of calcaneus	Four talocalcaneal – interosseous – lateral – posterior – medial	Two thick bands in sinus tarsi Parallel and deep to calcaneofibular Short band (lateral talus → medial calcaneus) Medial talus → posterior sustentaculum tali
Talocalcaneonavicular (medial half of transverse tarsal joint)	Ball and socket-type synovial joint	Head of talus with medial calcaneus and posterior navicular bone	Plantar calcaneonavicular Bifurcate Dorsal talonavicular	Forms inferior–medial socket Calcaneocuboid and calcaneonavicular parts Reinforces dorsally
Calcaneocuboid (lateral half of transverse tarsal joint)	Plane-type synovial joint	Anterior end of calcaneus with posterior surface of cuboid	Dorsal calcaneocuboid Long plantar Plantar calcaneocuboid	Relatively thin broad band Calcaneal tubercles to cuboidal ridge Deep to long plantar
Tarsometatarsal	Plane-type synovial joint	Anterior tarsal bones with bases of metatarsal bones	Dorsal and plantar tarsometatarsal, and cuneometatarsal interosseous	1st joint – metatarsal I with medial cuneiform 2nd joint – metatarsal II with all three cuneiforms 3rd joint – metatarsal III with lateral cuneiform 4th joint – metatarsal IV with medial cuboid 5th joint – metatarsal V with lateral cuboid
Metatarsophalangeal	Condylar-type synovial joint	Heads of metatarsal bones with bases of proximal phalanges	Collateral Plantar Deep transverse metatarsal	Supporting capsule on each side A dense fibrocartilaginous plate Interconnectors
Interphalangeal	Hinge-type synovial joint	Head of one phalanx with base of one distal to it	Collateral Plantar	Five proximal interphalangeal joints Four distal interphalangeal joints

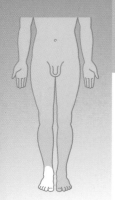

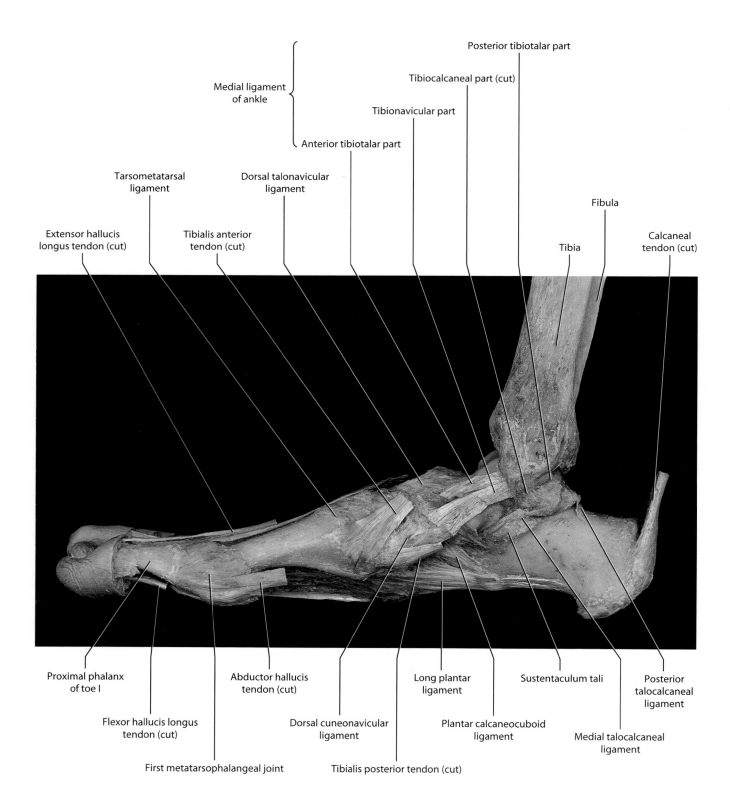

Posterior tibiotalar part

Tibiocalcaneal part (cut)

Medial ligament
of ankle

Tibionavicular part

Anterior tibiotalar part

Tarsometatarsal
ligament

Dorsal talonavicular
ligament

Fibula

Extensor hallucis
longus tendon (cut)

Tibialis anterior
tendon (cut)

Tibia

Calcaneal
tendon (cut)

Proximal phalanx
of toe I

Abductor hallucis
tendon (cut)

Long plantar
ligament

Sustentaculum tali

Posterior
talocalcaneal
ligament

Flexor hallucis longus
tendon (cut)

Dorsal cuneonavicular
ligament

Plantar calcaneocuboid
ligament

Medial talocalcaneal
ligament

First metatarsophalangeal joint

Tibialis posterior tendon (cut)

Figure 46.11 Ankle and foot – deep dissection 2. Medial view of a deep dissection of the right ankle and foot. This shows the parts of the medial ligament of the ankle

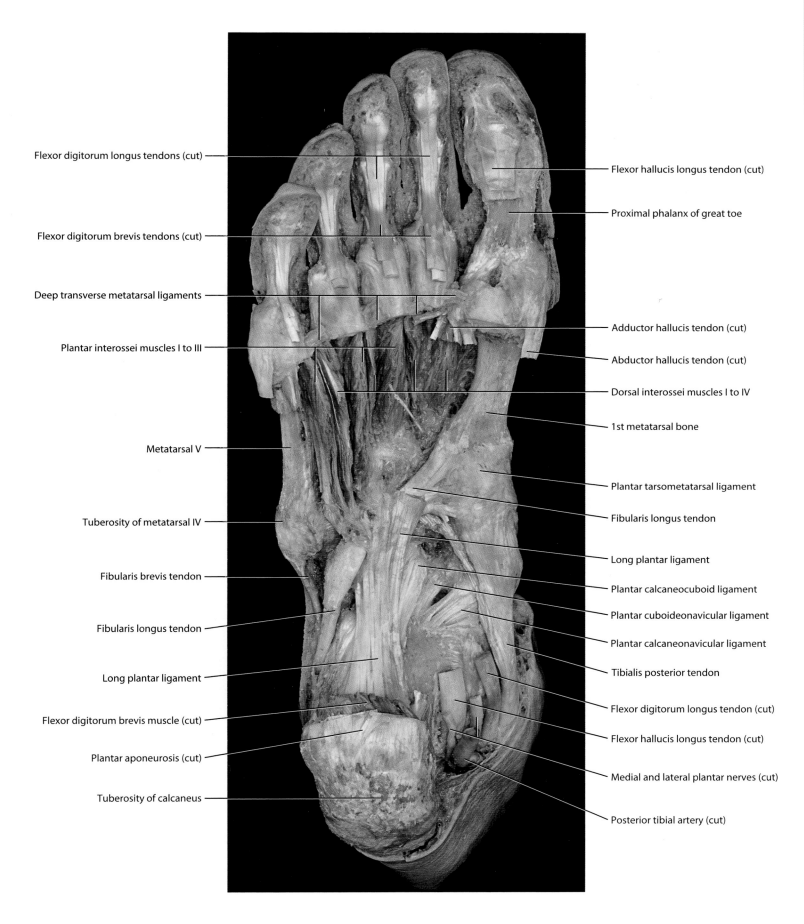

Flexor digitorum longus tendons (cut)

Flexor digitorum brevis tendons (cut)

Deep transverse metatarsal ligaments

Plantar interossei muscles I to III

Metatarsal V

Tuberosity of metatarsal IV

Fibularis brevis tendon

Fibularis longus tendon

Long plantar ligament

Flexor digitorum brevis muscle (cut)

Plantar aponeurosis (cut)

Tuberosity of calcaneus

Flexor hallucis longus tendon (cut)

Proximal phalanx of great toe

Adductor hallucis tendon (cut)

Abductor hallucis tendon (cut)

Dorsal interossei muscles I to IV

1st metatarsal bone

Plantar tarsometatarsal ligament

Fibularis longus tendon

Long plantar ligament

Plantar calcaneocuboid ligament

Plantar cuboideonavicular ligament

Plantar calcaneonavicular ligament

Tibialis posterior tendon

Flexor digitorum longus tendon (cut)

Flexor hallucis longus tendon (cut)

Medial and lateral plantar nerves (cut)

Posterior tibial artery (cut)

Figure 46.12 Foot – deep dissection 3. Plantar view of the right foot. Observe the ligaments that maintain the longitudinal arch in the hindfoot and all seven interossei in the forefoot

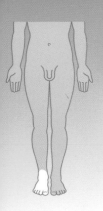

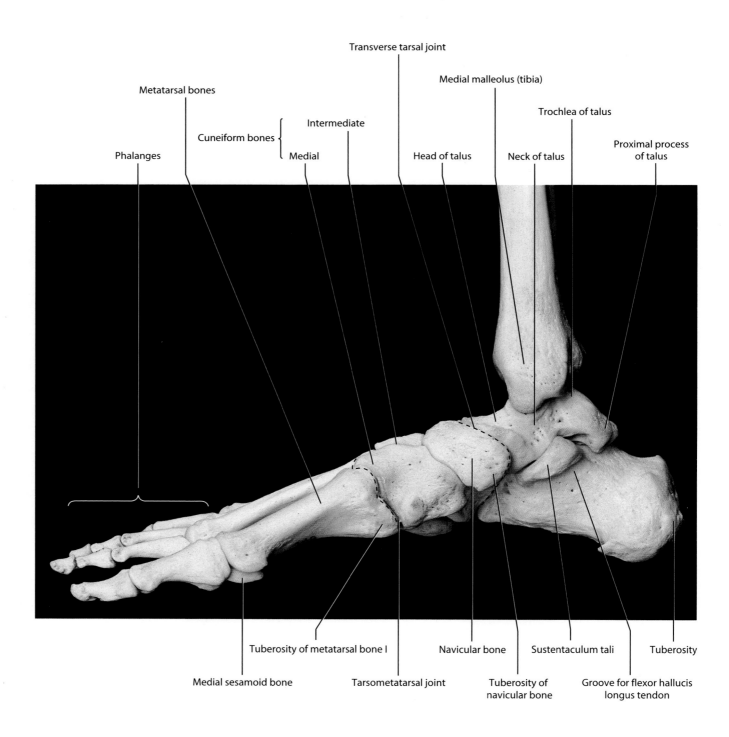

Transverse tarsal joint

Metatarsal bones

Medial malleolus (tibia)

Intermediate

Cuneiform bones

Trochlea of talus

Phalanges

Medial

Head of talus

Neck of talus

Proximal process of talus

Tuberosity of metatarsal bone I

Navicular bone

Sustentaculum tali

Tuberosity

Medial sesamoid bone

Tarsometatarsal joint

Tuberosity of navicular bone

Groove for flexor hallucis longus tendon

Figure 46.13 Ankle and foot joints – osteology 1. Medial view of the articulated bones of the right ankle and foot

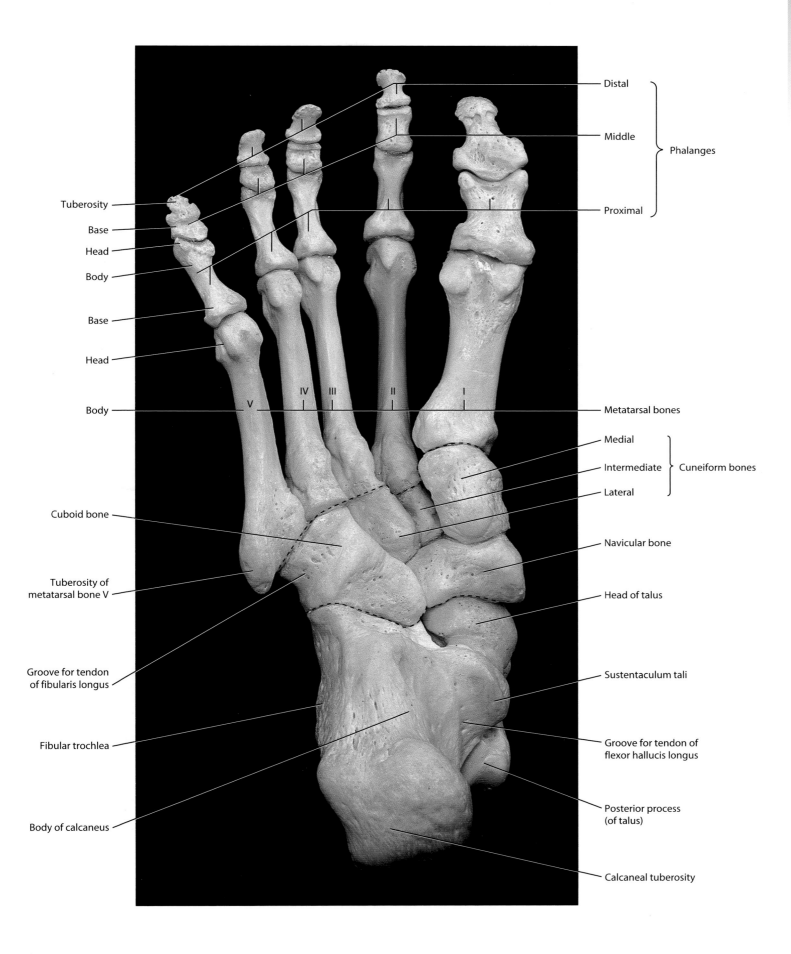

Distal

Middle — Phalanges

Proximal

Tuberosity

Base

Head

Body

Base

Head

Body

IV   III   II   I

V   Metatarsal bones

Medial

Intermediate   Cuneiform bones

Lateral

Cuboid bone

Navicular bone

Head of talus

Tuberosity of
metatarsal bone V

Sustentaculum tali

Groove for tendon
of fibularis longus

Fibular trochlea

Groove for tendon of
flexor hallucis longus

Body of calcaneus

Posterior process
(of talus)

Calcaneal tuberosity

Figure 46.14 Ankle and foot joints – osteology 2. Inferior view of the articulated bones of the right foot

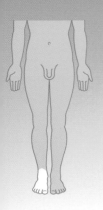

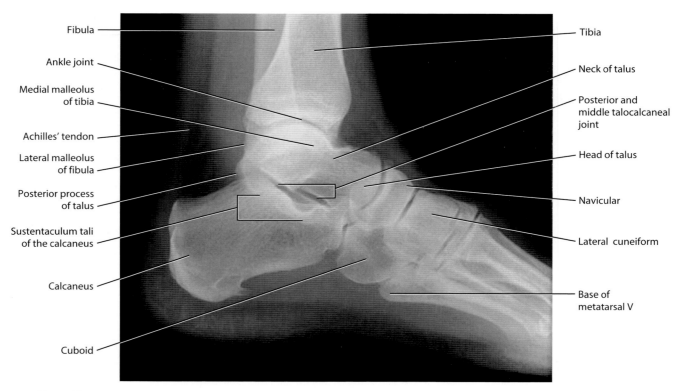

Figure 46.15 Ankle and foot – plain film radiograph (lateral view). The talus and calcaneus are readily evaluated. The ankle joint and posterior and middle talocalcaneal joints are well visualized on lateral views

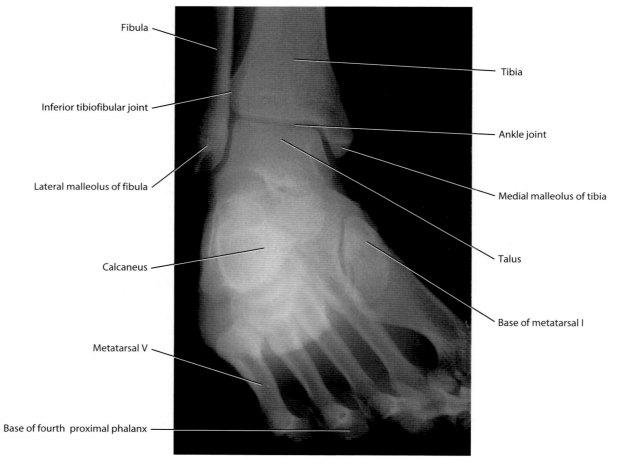

Figure 46.16 Ankle and foot joints – plain film radiograph (oblique view). This view, also known as a mortise view, is used to evaluate the integrity of the ankle mortise and its supporting ligaments. The joint spaces between the lateral and medial malleoli and the talus should be equal

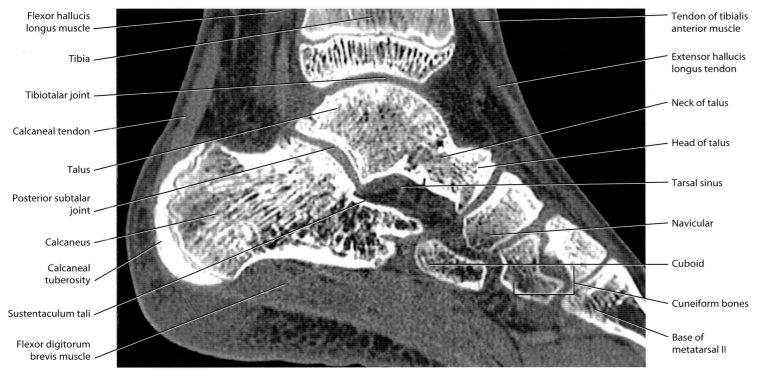

Flexor hallucis longus muscle

Tibia

Tibiotalar joint

Calcaneal tendon

Talus

Posterior subtalar joint

Calcaneus

Calcaneal tuberosity

Sustentaculum tali

Flexor digitorum brevis muscle

Tendon of tibialis anterior muscle

Extensor hallucis longus tendon

Neck of talus

Head of talus

Tarsal sinus

Navicular

Cuboid

Cuneiform bones

Base of metatarsal II

Figure 46.17 Ankle and foot joints – CT scan (sagittal view). The subtalar joints are well visualized. The talus bears the full weight of the body and transfers it anteriorly to the navicular bone and posteriorly to the calcaneus

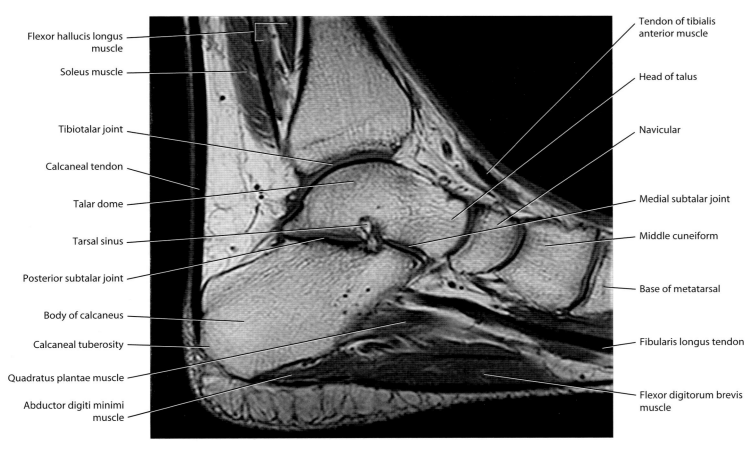

Flexor hallucis longus muscle

Soleus muscle

Tibiotalar joint

Calcaneal tendon

Talar dome

Tarsal sinus

Posterior subtalar joint

Body of calcaneus

Calcaneal tuberosity

Quadratus plantae muscle

Abductor digiti minimi muscle

Tendon of tibialis anterior muscle

Head of talus

Navicular

Medial subtalar joint

Middle cuneiform

Base of metatarsal

Fibularis longus tendon

Flexor digitorum brevis muscle

Figure 46.18 Ankle and foot joints – MRI scan (sagittal view). Note the excellent delineation of the joints in this scan. A fat pad (bright signal) is seen anterior to the calcaneal tendon (black signal void)

LOWER LIMB Ankle and foot joints

47 Foot

The foot is the arched part of the lower limb distal to the ankle joint. It consists of 26 bones bound together and strengthened by ligaments and muscles. The structure of the foot enables it to support the body's weight, act as a lever in forward locomotion, and serve as a shock absorber.

When standing, the body's weight is transferred from the tibia and fibula onto the seven tarsal bones of the foot: the talus, the calcaneus, the navicular, the three cuneiform bones (medial, intermediate, and lateral), and the cuboid.

The **talus** sits on the anterior two-thirds of the **calcaneus** and forms the weightbearing link between the bones of the leg and foot. The anterior aspects of the talus and calcaneus are flush and form the **transverse tarsal joint** by articulating with the **navicular** and **cuboid**, respectively. The three cuneiform bones are between the navicular and metatarsals I, II and III, whereas the cuboid articulates anteriorly with metatarsals IV and V. Weight is dissipated through the cuneiforms to the metatarsals. Distally, the metatarsals articulate with the phalanges (toe bones). The 14 phalanges are organized into five sets of bones (the digits) just like the fingers of the hand. Four digits have three phalanges (proximal, middle, and distal), but the great toe (toe I) has only two phalanges (proximal and distal). In addition, there is a variable number of sesamoid and accessory bones. The two most prominent sesamoid bones of the foot can be seen in the tendon of flexor hallucis brevis as it crosses the first metatarsophalangeal joint.

The intrinsic muscles of the foot are divided into dorsal and plantar groups. Each group has investing fascia as well as fascial bands (retinacula), which keep the muscles and tendons of the foot from protruding during muscle flexion.

DORSAL FOOT

The dorsal group of muscles includes the **extensor hallucis brevis** and **extensor digitorum brevis**, which originate from the dorsal surface of the calcaneus and extend the toes. The two muscles are closely connected with one another and the extensor hallucis brevis muscle is usually considered to be part of extensor digitorum brevis muscle.

The **deep fibular nerve** descends from the anterior compartment of the leg with the dorsalis pedis artery. On the dorsal surface of the foot it supplies extensor digitorum brevis and extensor hallucis brevis muscles. It terminates on the dorsum of the foot conveying sensation from a small patch of skin between toes I and II (first webspace) (Fig. 47.1). The rest of the dorsal skin of the foot is innervated mainly by the **superficial fibular nerve**, which originates in the leg. This nerve can be found within the superficial fascia of the leg as it descends inferiorly onto the dorsal surface of the foot just anterior to the lateral malleolus.

The blood supply to the dorsal foot comes from the **dorsalis pedis artery**, which is a continuation of the anterior tibial artery of the leg (Fig. 47.2). As the dorsalis pedis artery descends onto the foot next to the deep fibular nerve it gives off two branches – the **medial** and **lateral tarsal arteries** to the ankle joint. The dorsalis pedis artery then gives off some more unnamed branches to the proximal foot and continues anteriorly on the dorsum of the foot, where it terminates by giving off the **arcuate artery** to the lateral dorsum of the foot, and the **deep plantar artery**, which dives deep between

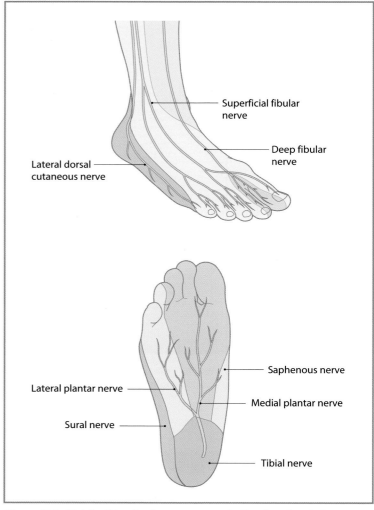

Figure 47.1 Distribution of cutaneous nerves to the dorsal and plantar surfaces of the foot

metatarsals I and II to anastomose with the **lateral plantar artery**, so forming the plantar arterial arch. Both the **deep plantar arch** and arcuate artery give off small metatarsal arteries, which divide into smaller digital arteries to supply each of the five digits (toes).

The venous and lymphatic drainage of the foot follows the route of the major arteries.

PLANTAR FOOT

The skin on the plantar surface of the foot is thickened, and beneath it are thick, fatty deposits that provide cushioning. Deep to the fat pad a plantar aponeurosis in the midline bridges the gap between the proximal and distal foot, providing support to the longitudinal arch of the foot. Two vertical septa arise from the deep surface of the aponeurosis and divide the plantar foot muscles into three compartments (medial, central, and lateral). This natural compartmentalization of the foot muscles is similar to the fascial separation in the hand, but for ease of understanding the structures of the plantar foot are discussed in four layers, from superficial to deep. There are two neurovascular planes – one between layers 1 and 2 and the second between layers 3 and 4 (Table 47.1):

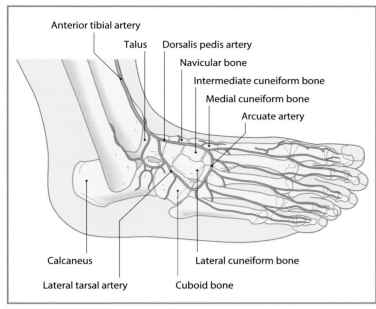

Figure 47.2 **Branches of the dorsal pedis artery**

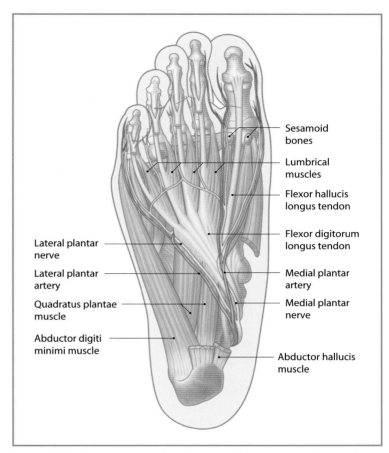

Figure 47.3 **Major nerves and blood vessels of the plantar surface of the foot**

- muscular layer 1 – abductor hallucis, flexor digitorum brevis, abductor digiti minimi;
- neurovascular plane 1 – medial and lateral plantar nerves, medial and lateral plantar arteries and veins;
- muscular layer 2 – quadratus plantae, lumbrical muscles I to IV, tendon of flexor hallucis longus (from the leg), tendon of flexor digitorum longus (from the leg);
- muscular layer 3 – flexor hallucis brevis, adductor hallucis (oblique and transverse heads), flexor digiti minimi brevis;
- muscular layer 4 – plantar interossei I to III, dorsal interossei I to IV, tendon of fibularis longus, tendon of tibialis posterior.

The plantar muscles are innervated by the terminal branches of the **tibial nerve**, which descends through the posterior compartment of the leg. Deep to the flexor retinaculum, the tibial nerve passes posterior to the medial malleolus and divides to become the medial and lateral plantar nerves (Fig. 47.3).

The **medial plantar nerve**, which is lateral to the medial plantar artery within the neurovascular plane, passes anteriorly to the distal foot, gives off branches that supply the abductor hallucis, flexor digitorum brevis, and flexor hallucis brevis muscles, and the most medial (first) lumbrical muscle. It terminates by conveying sensation from the skin over the medial three and a half toes.

The **lateral plantar nerve** is in the neurovascular plane, medial to the lateral plantar artery. It runs anteriorly in the foot and branches to the abductor digiti minimi, quadratus plantae, lumbrical muscles II to IV, adductor hallucis, and flexor digiti minimi, and all dorsal and plantar interosseous muscles. It terminates by giving off a superficial branch, which conveys sensation from the skin of the lateral one-and-a-half toes.

Cutaneous sensation from the plantar surface of the foot is conveyed by the sural nerve, calcaneal branches from the tibial nerve, and the saphenous nerve. The **sural nerve** enters the posterior aspect of the foot and conveys sensation from the lateral plantar foot and toe V, and the **calcaneal branches** of the tibial nerve supply the heel. The **saphenous nerve**, which is a continuation of the femoral nerve, enters the foot anterior to the medial malleolus to convey sensation from skin on the medial foot.

The plantar foot receives blood from the medial and lateral plantar arteries (Fig. 47.3), which are terminal branches of the posterior tibial artery (see Chapter 45):

- the smaller **medial plantar artery** begins in the posterior foot and passes between the abductor hallucis and flexor digitorum brevis muscles, and supplies the medial part of the foot and toe I.
- the larger **lateral plantar artery** runs obliquely on the plantar surface of the foot just lateral to the lateral plantar nerve, gives off several branches to the calcaneus and to the muscles and joints of the foot, and terminates by anastomosing with the **deep plantar branch** of the dorsalis pedis artery to form the plantar arterial arch.

Venous drainage of the deep foot is by vessels that follow the large arteries (dorsalis pedis, medial and lateral plantar); venous blood then drains to the deep veins of the leg. Superficial venous drainage originates in small unnamed vessels that drain to the **dorsal venous arch of foot** on the dorsum of the foot. The medial end of the dorsal venous arch of foot becomes the **great saphenous vein** and ascends up the medial foot, leg, and thigh to empty into the **femoral vein** in the groin. The lateral end of the dorsal venous arch becomes the **small saphenous vein**, which ascends up the leg and empties into the **popliteal vein** at the popliteal fossa.

Deep lymphatic drainage and superficial medial lymphatic drainage is to the **inguinal nodes**. Superficial lateral lymphatic

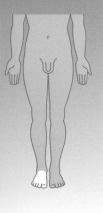

drainage follows the course of the small saphenous vein to the **popliteal nodes**.

■ CLINICAL CORRELATIONS

Bunion

Shoes that are too short or too tight can cause a deformity known as a bunion. Typical signs are an enlarged first metatarsophalangeal joint, which is painful to the touch and during movement, and an abnormal lateral deviation of the first phalanx (big toe). A bone spur forms, partly because of the prolonged wearing of tight-fitting shoes and partly because of the poor function of the abductor hallucis muscle. Definitive treatment is surgical, and is aimed at removing any bone spurs that have formed and realigning the first phalanx to its correct position.

Plantar fasciitis

Plantar fasciitis is caused by microinjuries to the proximal attachment of the plantar aponeurosis to the calcaneus as a result of repetitive motion and stress on the longitudinal plantar arch. It may be caused by extensive running. It usually results in pain over the proximal plantar surface of the foot, especially when stepping out of bed in the morning. Treatment is aimed at reducing the cause of the microinjuries and decreasing any local pain and swelling.

Deep fibular nerve paresthesia

One of the early clinical manifestations of injury after direct trauma to the distal anterolateral leg or with a compartment syndrome of the leg is paresthesia ('pins and needles') over the region innervated by the deep fibular nerve in the first web space – the lateral skin of toe I and the medial skin of toe II (Fig. 47.4). Surgical release of a high anterior compartment pressure can be attempted to prevent permanent nerve damage and muscle paralysis. If the trauma is minor, normal function of the cutaneous component of the nerve can usually be restored by allowing the injured area to rest. Severe injury leads to permanent nerve damage and muscle paralysis.

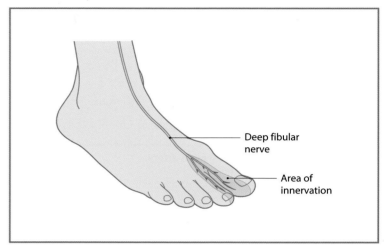

Figure 47.4 Cutaneous innervation by the deep fibular nerve

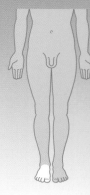

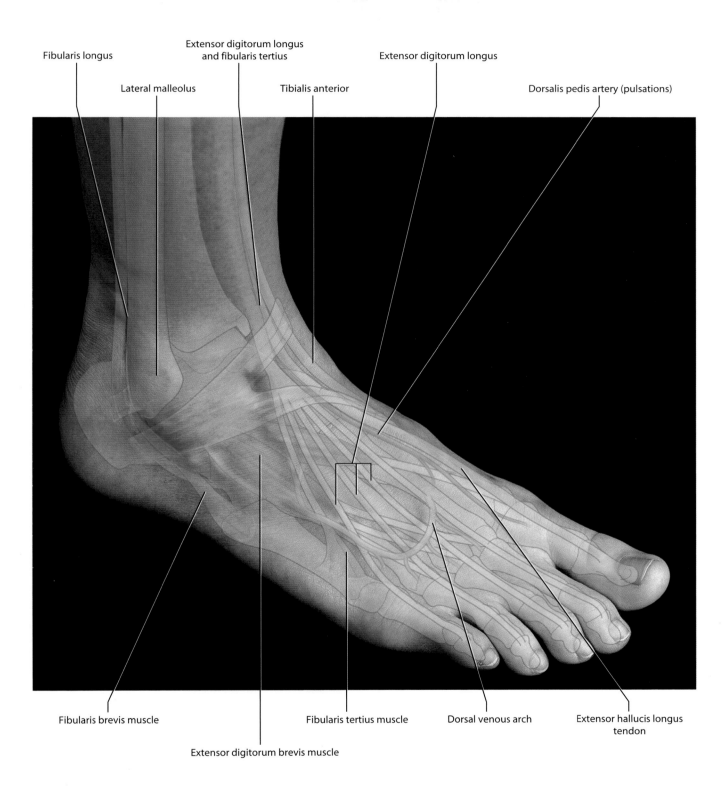

Fibularis longus

Extensor digitorum longus
and fibularis tertius

Extensor digitorum longus

Lateral malleolus

Tibialis anterior

Dorsalis pedis artery (pulsations)

Fibularis brevis muscle

Extensor digitorum brevis muscle

Fibularis tertius muscle

Dorsal venous arch

Extensor hallucis longus
tendon

Figure 47.5 Foot – surface anatomy 1. Superolateral view showing the dorsal venous network

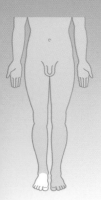

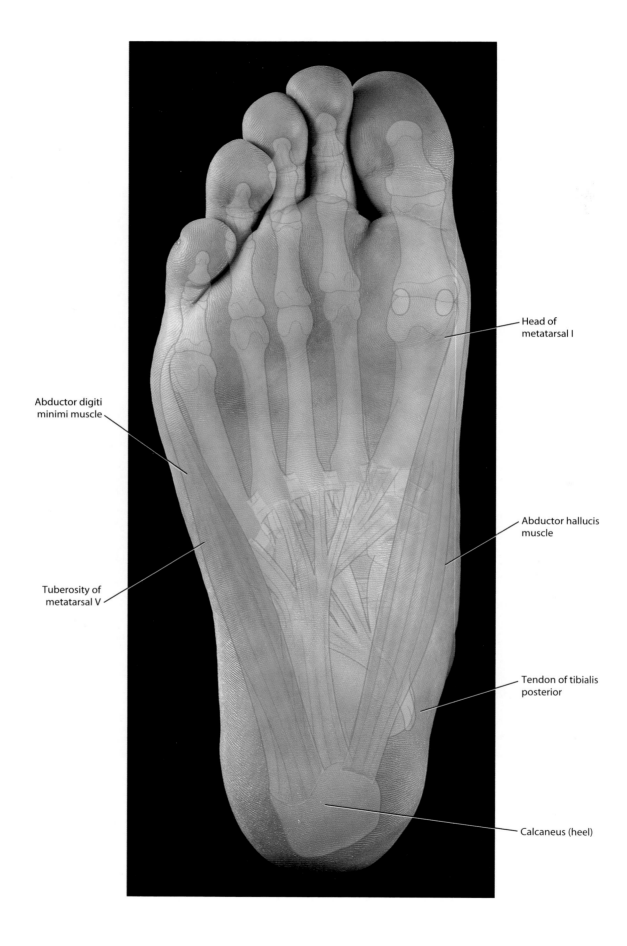

Head of
metatarsal I

Abductor digiti
minimi muscle

Abductor hallucis
muscle

Tuberosity of
metatarsal V

Tendon of tibialis
posterior

Calcaneus (heel)

Figure 47.6 Foot – surface anatomy 2. Plantar view of inferior right foot

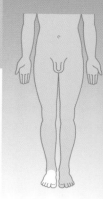

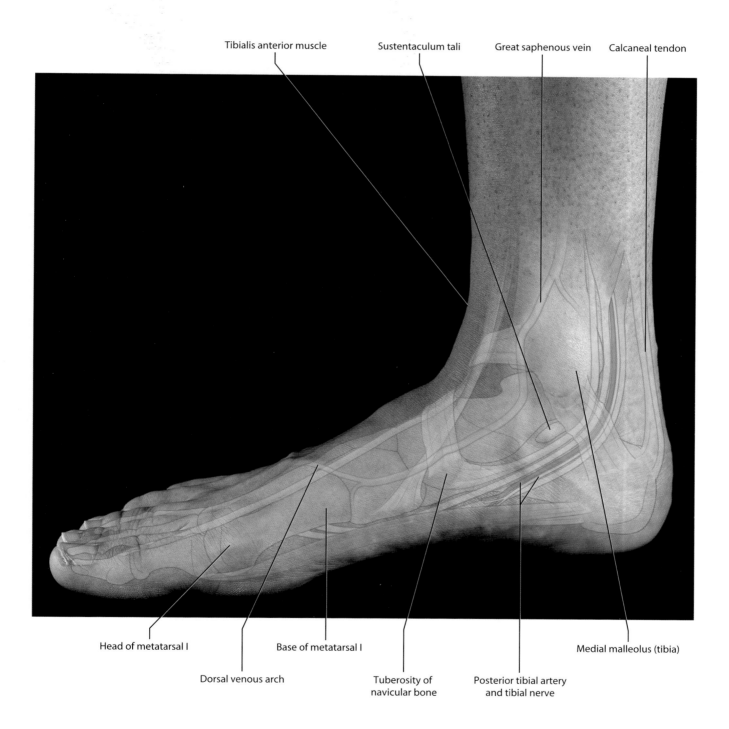

Tibialis anterior muscle   Sustentaculum tali   Great saphenous vein   Calcaneal tendon

Head of metatarsal I   Base of metatarsal I   Medial malleolus (tibia)

Dorsal venous arch   Tuberosity of navicular bone   Posterior tibial artery and tibial nerve

Figure 47.7 Foot – surface anatomy 3. Medial view showing the extent of the longitudinal arch

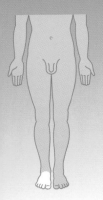

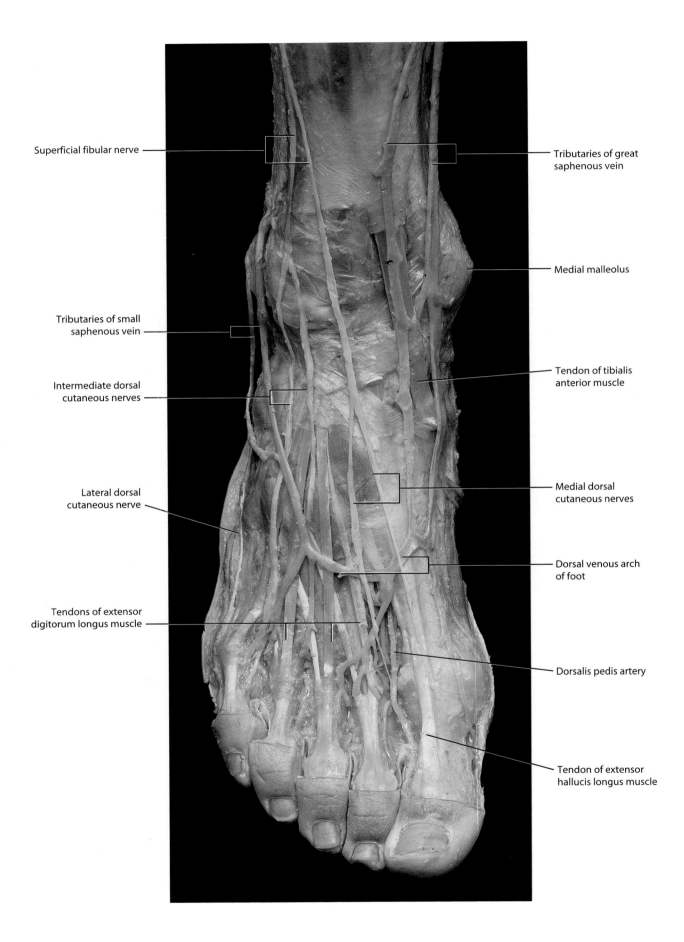

Superficial fibular nerve

Tributaries of great
saphenous vein

Medial malleolus

Tributaries of small
saphenous vein

Tendon of tibialis
anterior muscle

Intermediate dorsal
cutaneous nerves

Lateral dorsal
cutaneous nerve

Medial dorsal
cutaneous nerves

Dorsal venous arch
of foot

Tendons of extensor
digitorum longus muscle

Dorsalis pedis artery

Tendon of extensor
hallucis longus muscle

Figure 47.8 Foot – superficial dissection 1. Dorsum of the right foot, superficial layer, showing the dorsal venous network on top of the superficial tendons

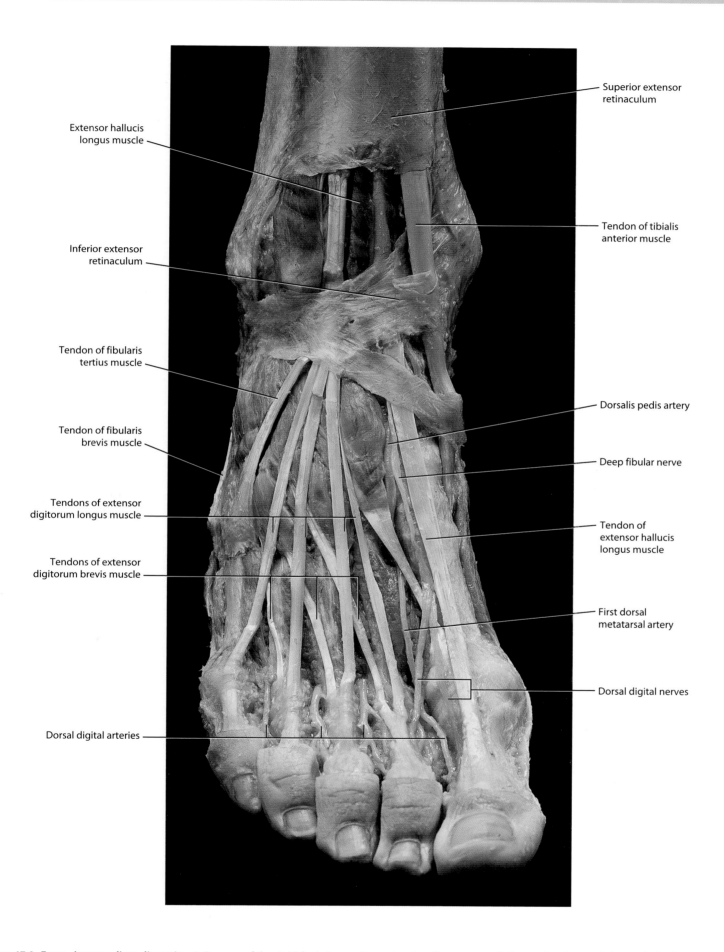

Extensor hallucis
longus muscle

Inferior extensor
retinaculum

Tendon of fibularis
tertius muscle

Tendon of fibularis
brevis muscle

Tendons of extensor
digitorum longus muscle

Tendons of extensor
digitorum brevis muscle

Dorsal digital arteries

Superior extensor
retinaculum

Tendon of tibialis
anterior muscle

Dorsalis pedis artery

Deep fibular nerve

Tendon of
extensor hallucis
longus muscle

First dorsal
metatarsal artery

Dorsal digital nerves

Figure 47.9 Foot – intermediate dissection 1. Dorsum of the right foot, deeper layer, showing the extensor digitorum brevis muscle beneath the long tendon of the anterior leg muscles

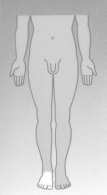

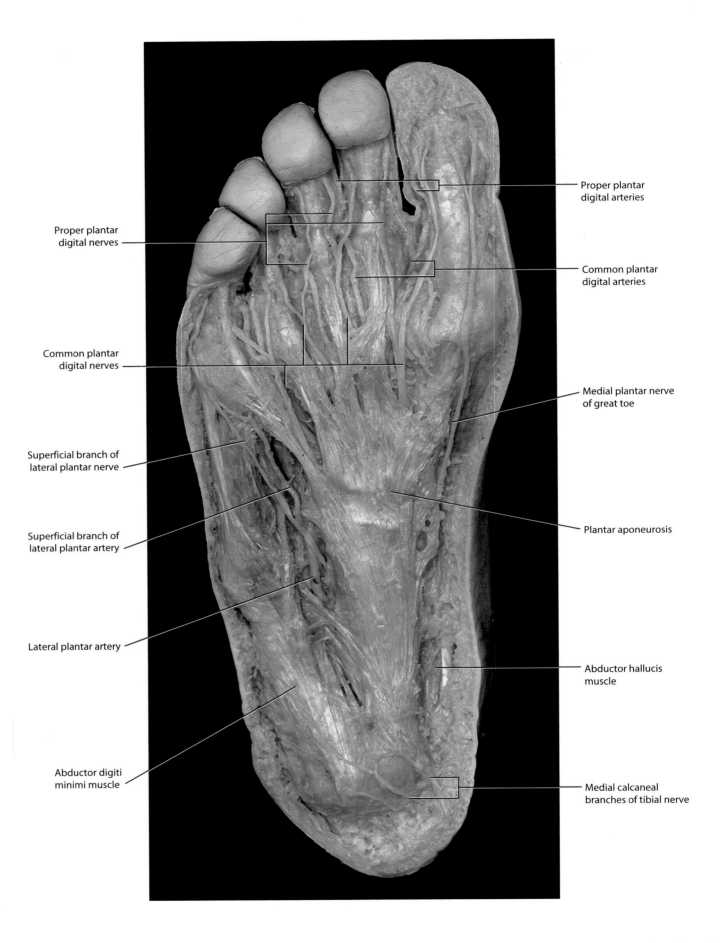

Proper plantar
digital arteries

Proper plantar
digital nerves

Common plantar
digital arteries

Common plantar
digital nerves

Medial plantar nerve
of great toe

Superficial branch of
lateral plantar nerve

Superficial branch of
lateral plantar artery

Plantar aponeurosis

Lateral plantar artery

Abductor hallucis
muscle

Abductor digiti
minimi muscle

Medial calcaneal
branches of tibial nerve

Figure 47.10 Foot – superficial dissection 2. Sole (plantar surface) of the right foot. The superficial layer shows the plantar aponeurosis overlying the intrinsic foot muscles

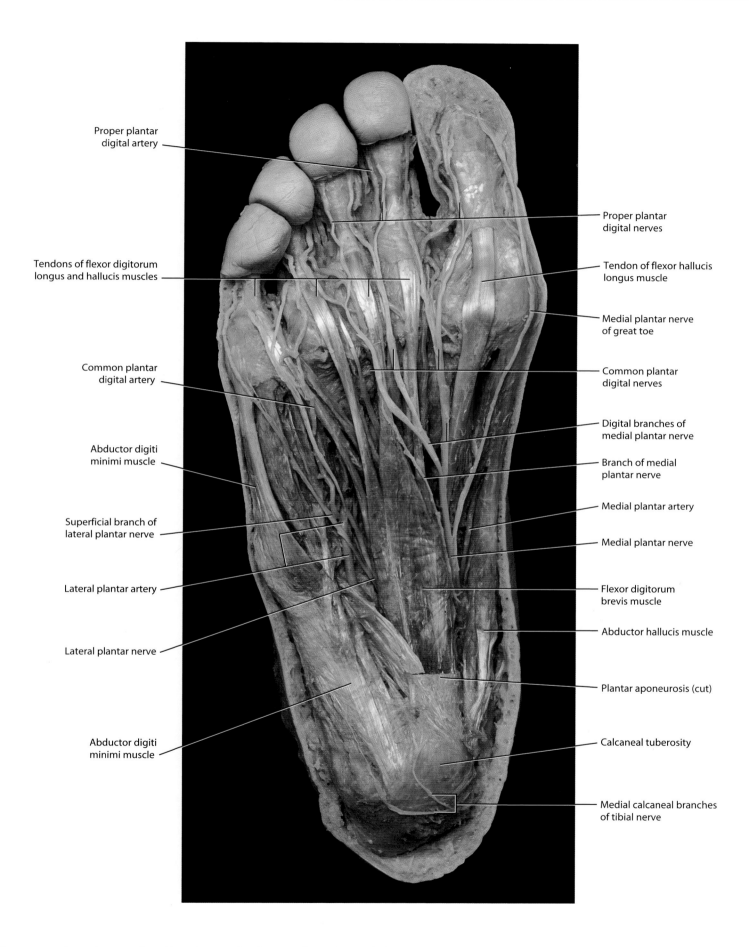

Proper plantar digital artery

Tendons of flexor digitorum longus and hallucis muscles

Common plantar digital artery

Abductor digiti minimi muscle

Superficial branch of lateral plantar nerve

Lateral plantar artery

Lateral plantar nerve

Abductor digiti minimi muscle

Proper plantar digital nerves

Tendon of flexor hallucis longus muscle

Medial plantar nerve of great toe

Common plantar digital nerves

Digital branches of medial plantar nerve

Branch of medial plantar nerve

Medial plantar artery

Medial plantar nerve

Flexor digitorum brevis muscle

Abductor hallucis muscle

Plantar aponeurosis (cut)

Calcaneal tuberosity

Medial calcaneal branches of tibial nerve

Figure 47.11 Foot – intermediate dissection 2. Sole (plantar surface) of the right foot, layer 1. The plantar aponeurosis has been removed to show the underlying flexor digitorum brevis muscle

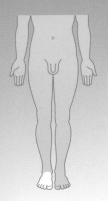

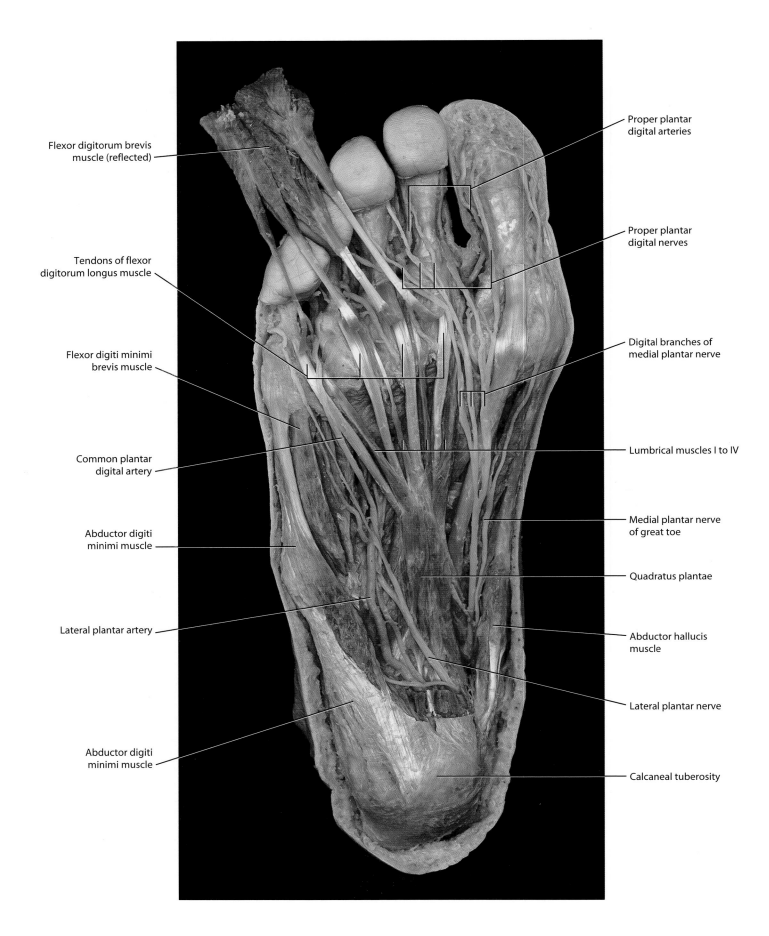

Flexor digitorum brevis
muscle (reflected)

Tendons of flexor
digitorum longus muscle

Flexor digiti minimi
brevis muscle

Common plantar
digital artery

Abductor digiti
minimi muscle

Lateral plantar artery

Abductor digiti
minimi muscle

Proper plantar
digital arteries

Proper plantar
digital nerves

Digital branches of
medial plantar nerve

Lumbrical muscles I to IV

Medial plantar nerve
of great toe

Quadratus plantae

Abductor hallucis
muscle

Lateral plantar nerve

Calcaneal tuberosity

Figure 47.12 Foot – intermediate dissection 3. Sole (plantar surface) of the right foot, layer 2. The flexor digitorum brevis muscle is reflected to show the quadratus plantae muscle and the four lumbricals alongside the tendons of flexor digitorum longus

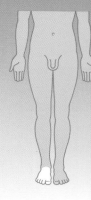

TABLE 47.1 MUSCLES IN SOLE OF FOOT					
Muscle	**Origin**	**Insertion**	**Innervation**	**Action**	**Blood supply**
Layer 1 Abductor hallucis	Medial process of calcaneal tuberosity, flexor retinaculum, plantar aponeurosis	Medial side of base of proximal phalanx of great toe	Medial plantar nerve (S2, S3)	Abducts and flexes great toe	Medial plantar artery
Flexor digitorum brevis	Medial process of calcaneal tuberosity, plantar aponeurosis	Middle phalanx of lateral four toes	Medial plantar nerve (S2, S3)	Flexes lateral four toes	Medial plantar artery
Abductor digiti minimi	Medial and lateral processes of calcaneal tuberosity, plantar aponeurosis	Lateral side of base of proximal phalanx of little toe	Lateral plantar nerve (S2, S3)	Abducts and flexes little toe	Lateral plantar artery
Layer 2 Quadratus plantae	Medial surface and lateral margin of plantar surface of calcaneus	Tendons of flexor digitorum longus	Lateral plantar nerve (S2, S3)	Assists flexor digitorum longus in flexing lateral four toes	Lateral plantar artery
Lumbricals	Tendon of flexor digitorum longus	Medial aspect of expansion over lateral four toes	*Medial one*: medial plantar nerve (S2, S3) *Lateral three*: lateral plantar nerve (S2, S3)	Flex proximal phalanges and extend middle and distal phalanges of lateral four toes	Plantar metatarsal artery
Layer 3 Flexor hallucis brevis	Plantar surfaces of cuboid and lateral cuneiforms	Medial and lateral side of proximal phalanx of great toe	Medial plantar nerve (S2, S3)	Flexes proximal phalanx of great toe	First plantar metatarsal artery
Adductor hallucis	Oblique head – bases of metatarsals II to IV Transverse head – plantar ligaments of metatarsophalangeal joints II to V	Tendons of both heads attach to lateral side of base of proximal phalanx of great toe	Deep branch of lateral plantar nerve (S2, S3)	Adducts great toe; assists in maintaining arch of foot	First plantar metatarsal artery
Flexor digiti minimi brevis	Base of metatarsal V	Lateral base of proximal phalanx of little toe	Superficial branch of lateral plantar nerve (S2, S3)	Flexes proximal phalanx of little toe	Lateral plantar artery
Layer 4 Plantar interossei (three muscles)	Bases and medial sides of metatarsals III to V	Medial sides of bases of proximal phalanges of toes III to V	Lateral plantar nerve (S2, S3)	Adducts toes II to IV and flexes metatarsophalangeal joints	Plantar metatarsal artery
Dorsal interossei (four muscles)	Adjacent sides of metatarsals I to V	*First*: medial side of proximal phalanx of second toe *Second to fourth*: lateral sides of toes II to IV	Lateral plantar nerve (S2, S3)	Abducts toes II to IV and flexes metatarsophalangeal joints	Dorsal metatarsal artery
Dorsum Extensor digitorum brevis	Superolateral surface of calcaneus	First tendon into dorsal base of proximal phalanx of great toe Tendons II to IV into lateral sides of tendons of extensor digitorum longus	Deep fibular nerve (L5 to S2)	Extends medial four toes	Dorsalis pedis artery, lateral tarsal artery

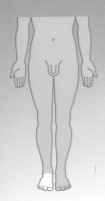

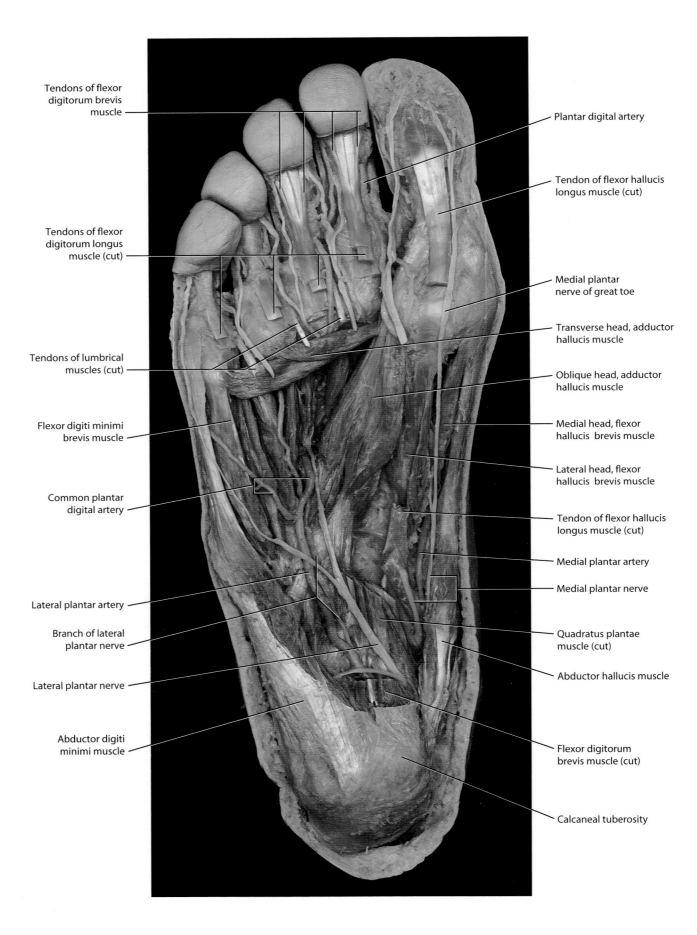

Tendons of flexor digitorum brevis muscle

Tendons of flexor digitorum longus muscle (cut)

Tendons of lumbrical muscles (cut)

Flexor digiti minimi brevis muscle

Common plantar digital artery

Lateral plantar artery

Branch of lateral plantar nerve

Lateral plantar nerve

Abductor digiti minimi muscle

Plantar digital artery

Tendon of flexor hallucis longus muscle (cut)

Medial plantar nerve of great toe

Transverse head, adductor hallucis muscle

Oblique head, adductor hallucis muscle

Medial head, flexor hallucis brevis muscle

Lateral head, flexor hallucis brevis muscle

Tendon of flexor hallucis longus muscle (cut)

Medial plantar artery

Medial plantar nerve

Quadratus plantae muscle (cut)

Abductor hallucis muscle

Flexor digitorum brevis muscle (cut)

Calcaneal tuberosity

Figure 47.13 Foot – deep dissection 1. Sole (plantar surface) of the right foot, layer 3. Note the adductor hallucis muscle and its two heads – transverse and oblique

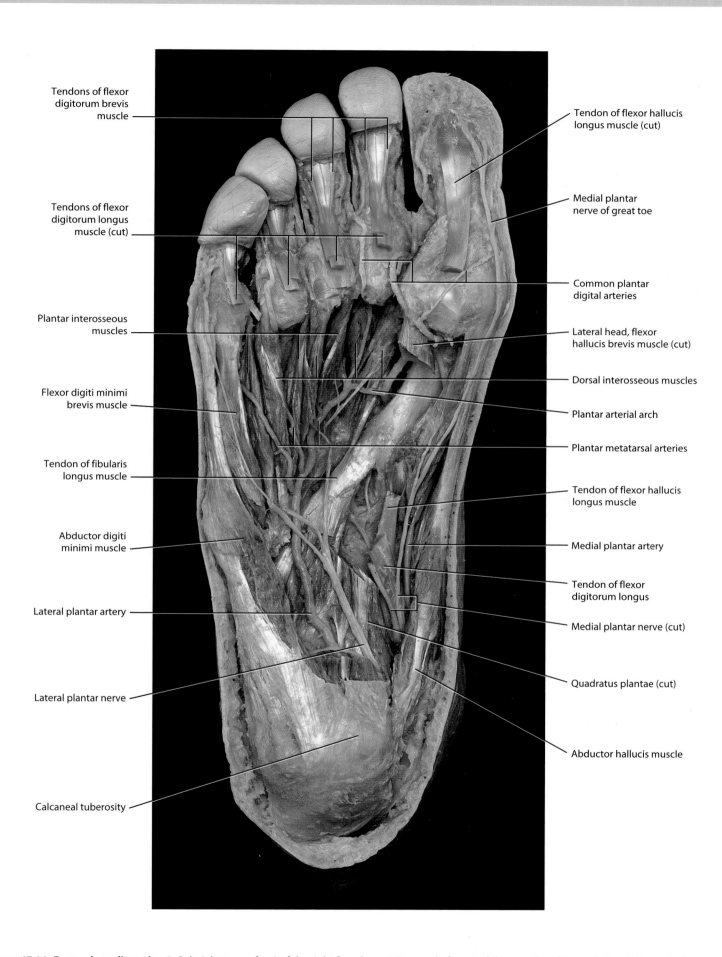

Tendons of flexor digitorum brevis muscle

Tendons of flexor digitorum longus muscle (cut)

Plantar interosseous muscles

Flexor digiti minimi brevis muscle

Tendon of fibularis longus muscle

Abductor digiti minimi muscle

Lateral plantar artery

Lateral plantar nerve

Calcaneal tuberosity

Tendon of flexor hallucis longus muscle (cut)

Medial plantar nerve of great toe

Common plantar digital arteries

Lateral head, flexor hallucis brevis muscle (cut)

Dorsal interosseous muscles

Plantar arterial arch

Plantar metatarsal arteries

Tendon of flexor hallucis longus muscle

Medial plantar artery

Tendon of flexor digitorum longus

Medial plantar nerve (cut)

Quadratus plantae (cut)

Abductor hallucis muscle

Figure 47.14 Foot – deep dissection 2. Sole (plantar surface) of the right foot, layer 4. Removal of most of the muscles of layers 1, 2, and 3 reveals the seven interossei – three plantar and four dorsal

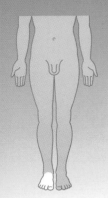

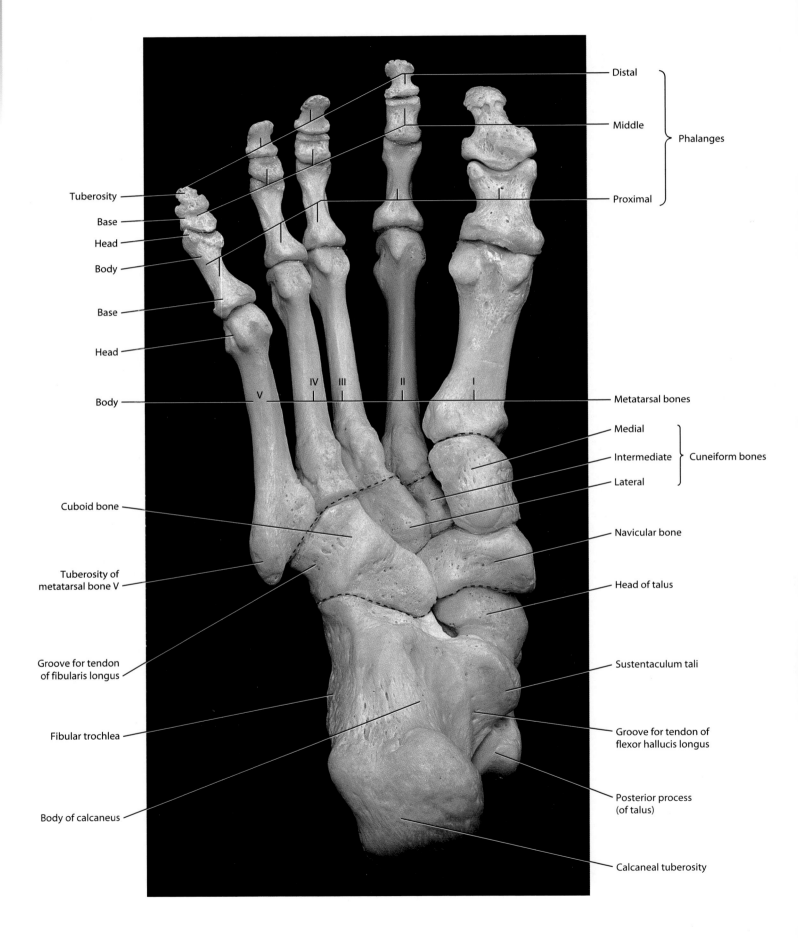

588   **Figure 47.15 Foot – osteology 1.** The plantar foot

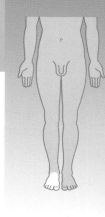

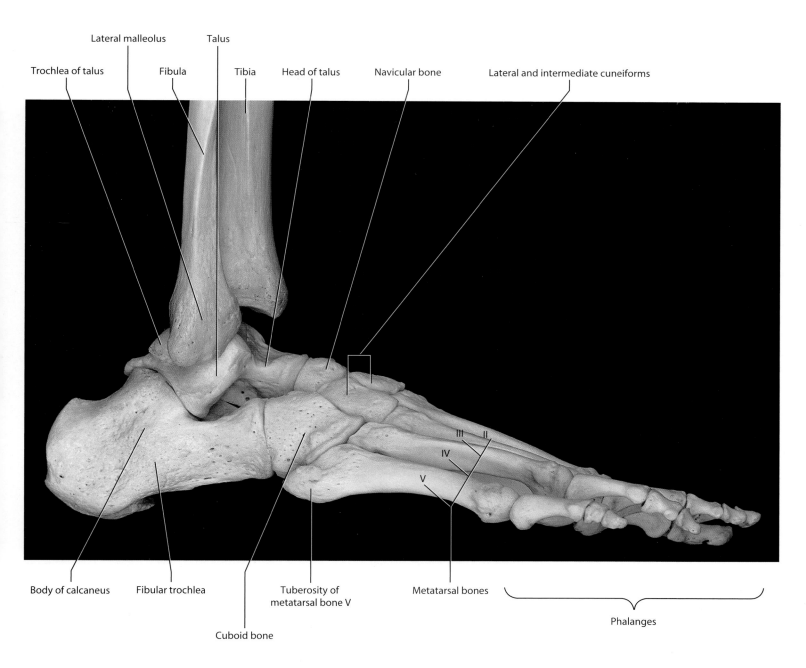

Lateral malleolus   Talus

Trochlea of talus   Fibula   Tibia   Head of talus   Navicular bone   Lateral and intermediate cuneiforms

III   II

IV

V

Body of calcaneus   Fibular trochlea   Tuberosity of   Metatarsal bones   Phalanges
metatarsal bone V

Cuboid bone

Figure 47.16 Foot – osteology 2. Lateral view of right foot

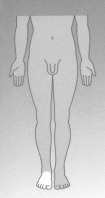

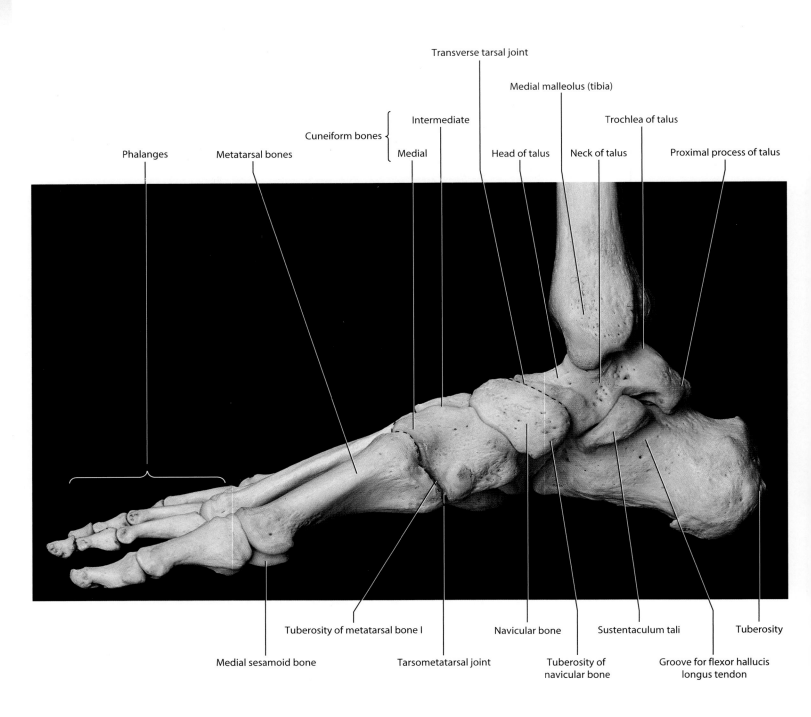

Transverse tarsal joint

Medial malleolus (tibia)

Cuneiform bones {

Intermediate

Trochlea of talus

Phalanges

Metatarsal bones

Medial

Head of talus

Neck of talus

Proximal process of talus

Tuberosity of metatarsal bone I

Navicular bone

Sustentaculum tali

Tuberosity

Medial sesamoid bone

Tarsometatarsal joint

Tuberosity of navicular bone

Groove for flexor hallucis longus tendon

Figure 47.17 Foot – osteology 3. Medial view of right foot

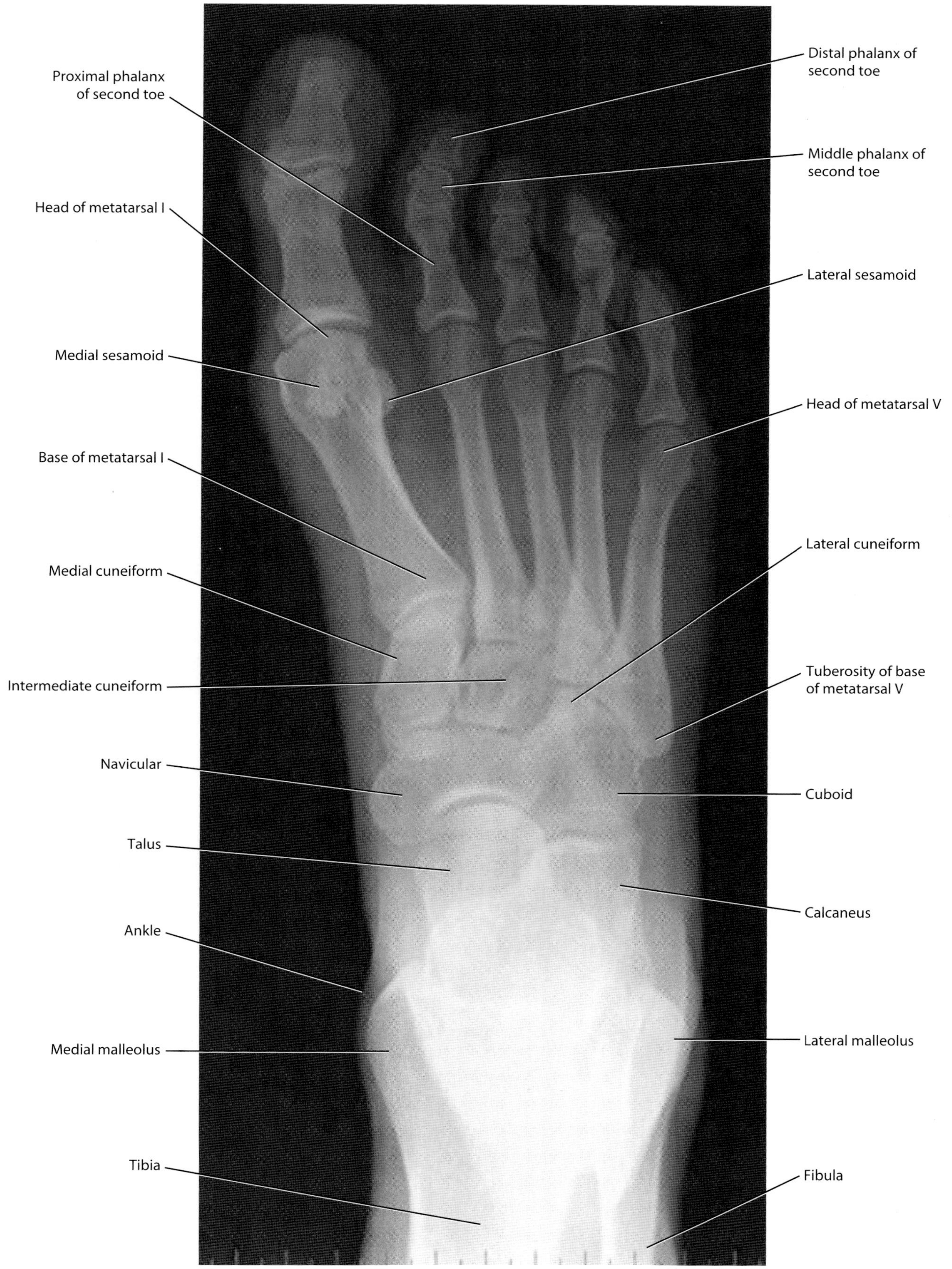

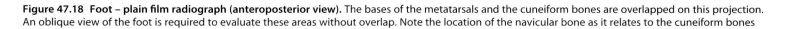

Proximal phalanx of second toe

Head of metatarsal I

Medial sesamoid

Base of metatarsal I

Medial cuneiform

Intermediate cuneiform

Navicular

Talus

Ankle

Medial malleolus

Tibia

Distal phalanx of second toe

Middle phalanx of second toe

Lateral sesamoid

Head of metatarsal V

Lateral cuneiform

Tuberosity of base of metatarsal V

Cuboid

Calcaneus

Lateral malleolus

Fibula

Figure 47.18 Foot – plain film radiograph (anteroposterior view). The bases of the metatarsals and the cuneiform bones are overlapped on this projection. An oblique view of the foot is required to evaluate these areas without overlap. Note the location of the navicular bone as it relates to the cuneiform bones

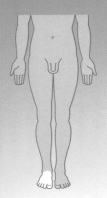

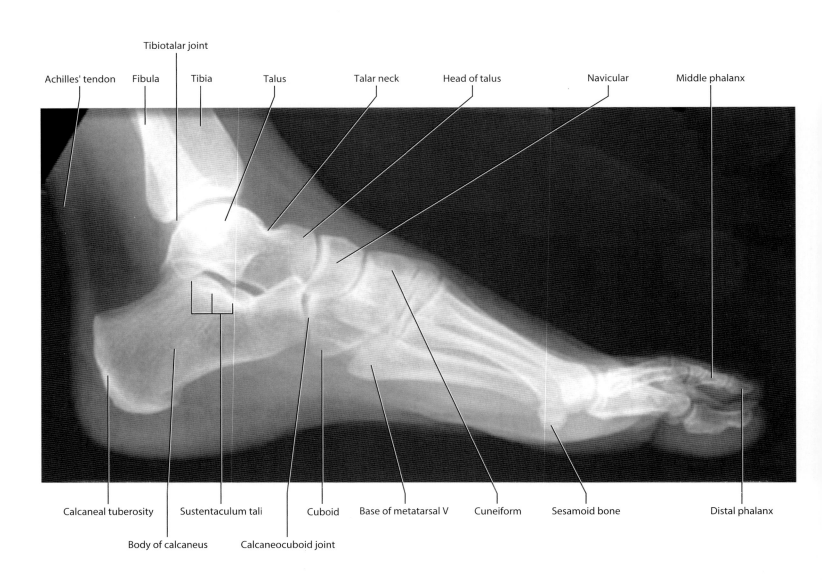

Tibiotalar joint

Achilles' tendon   Fibula   Tibia   Talus   Talar neck   Head of talus   Navicular   Middle phalanx

Calcaneal tuberosity   Sustentaculum tali   Cuboid   Base of metatarsal V   Cuneiform   Sesamoid bone   Distal phalanx

Body of calcaneus   Calcaneocuboid joint

Figure 47.19 Foot – plain film radiograph (lateral view). The tarsals, metatarsals and phalanges are all overlapped. Both anteroposterior and oblique views are required to evaluate these bones. Note the talus as it articulates with the calcaneus and navicular bones

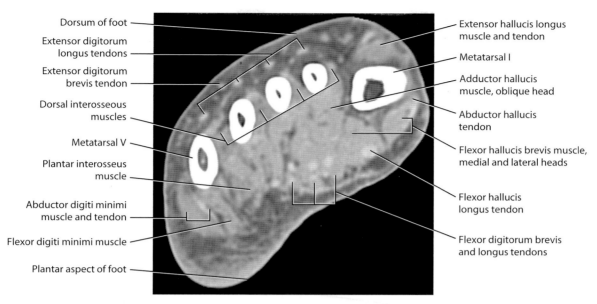

Dorsum of foot

Extensor digitorum longus tendons

Extensor digitorum brevis tendon

Dorsal interosseous muscles

Metatarsal V

Plantar interosseus muscle

Abductor digiti minimi muscle and tendon

Flexor digiti minimi muscle

Plantar aspect of foot

Extensor hallucis longus muscle and tendon

Metatarsal I

Adductor hallucis muscle, oblique head

Abductor hallucis tendon

Flexor hallucis brevis muscle, medial and lateral heads

Flexor hallucis longus tendon

Flexor digitorum brevis and longus tendons

Figure 47.20 Foot – CT scan (coronal view). In this scan at the level of the midtarsals, note how the tendons have a brighter signal than the muscles

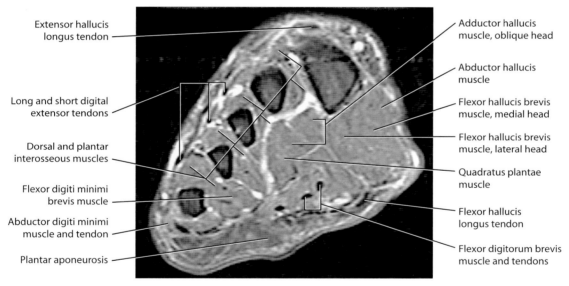

Extensor hallucis longus tendon

Long and short digital extensor tendons

Dorsal and plantar interosseous muscles

Flexor digiti minimi brevis muscle

Abductor digiti minimi muscle and tendon

Plantar aponeurosis

Adductor hallucis muscle, oblique head

Abductor hallucis muscle

Flexor hallucis brevis muscle, medial head

Flexor hallucis brevis muscle, lateral head

Quadratus plantae muscle

Flexor hallucis longus tendon

Flexor digitorum brevis muscle and tendons

Figure 47.21 Foot – MRI scan (coronal view). In this scan at the level of the metatarsals, the tendons have a black signal due to their fibrous nature

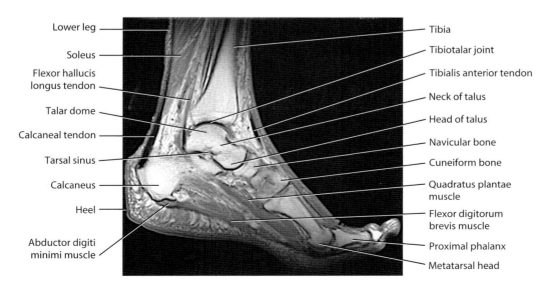

Lower leg

Soleus

Flexor hallucis longus tendon

Talar dome

Calcaneal tendon

Tarsal sinus

Calcaneus

Heel

Abductor digiti minimi muscle

Tibia

Tibiotalar joint

Tibialis anterior tendon

Neck of talus

Head of talus

Navicular bone

Cuneiform bone

Quadratus plantae muscle

Flexor digitorum brevis muscle

Proximal phalanx

Metatarsal head

Figure 47.22 Foot – MRI scan (sagittal view). Note the visualization of the plantar muscles in this projection

593

INDEX